Pancreatic Disease

Springer
London
Berlin
Heidelberg
New York
Barcelona
Budapest
Hong Kong
Milan
Paris
Santa Clara
Singapore
Tokyo

C.D. Johnson and C.W. Imrie (Eds)

Pancreatic Disease

Towards the Year 2000

Second Edition

With 87 Figures

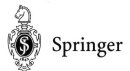

Springer

C.D. Johnson, MChir, FRCS
Senior Lecturer and Honorary Consultant Surgeon, Faculty of Medicine,
University Surgical Unit, Southampton General Hospital,
Tremona Road, Southampton SO1 6HU, UK

C.W. Imrie, ChB, FRCS
Consultant Surgeon, Surgical Unit, Royal Infirmary, Glasgow G4 OSF, UK

Cover illustration: Main photograph on front cover shows Chapter 32, Figure 1:
malignant peritoneal seedlings discovered during laparoscopy over the parietal
peritoneum of the left inguinal region.

ISBN 1–85233–037–6 2nd edition Springer-Verlag London Berlin Heidelberg

ISBN 3–540–19688–9 1st edition Springer-Verlag Berlin Heidelberg New York
ISBN 0–387–19688–9 1st edition Springer-Verlag New York Berlin Heidelberg

British Library Cataloguing in Publication Data
Pancreatic disease: towards the year 2000
   1. Pancreas – Diseases
   I. Johnson, C.D. (Colin David), 1952– II. Imrie, C.W.
   (Clement William)
   616.3'7
ISBN 1852330376

Library of Congress Cataloging-in-Publication Data
Pancreatic disease: towards the year 2000 / C.D. Johnson and C.W.
Imrie (eds.). – 2nd ed.
   p.   cm.
   Includes bibliographical references.
   ISBN 1–85233–037–6 (casebound : alk. paper)
   1. Pancreas–Diseases–Congresses.   I. Johnson, C.D. (Colin
David), 1952– . II. Imrie, C.W.
   [DNLM: 1. Pancreatic Diseases congresses. 2. Pancreatitis
congresses. 3. Pancreatic Neoplasms congresses. 4. Pancreas
Transplantation congresses. WI 800 P18932 1998]
RC857.P33   1998   98–17778
616.3'7–dc21   CIP
DNLM/DLC for Library of Congress

First published 1991
Second edition 1999

Typeset by EXPO Holdings, Malaysia
Printed and bound at the University Press, Cambridge
28/3830-543210 Printed on acid-free paper

Preface

Producing a book such as this is a delight for its editors. First we were able to welcome the contributors to an excellent meeting in Glasgow, where we spent two days discussing all aspects of pancreatic disease. Then we received chapters from each of the speakers, which, as the reader will discover, represent "state of the art" reviews in a wide variety of fields, with the most up-to-date information on the pancreas in the areas of basic sciences, inflammatory disease, endocrine problems and cancer. Finally we have the finished product, a book to read and re-read, and to keep on our shelves for handy reference.

We are very grateful to all the contributors for production of their excellent chapters, in a very short time. The publishers have done a marvellous job of putting together a high quality book in just a few months. This book is a true reflection of our current knowledge in pancreatic disease as we approach the new millennium.

C.D. Johnson and C.W. Imrie

Contents

Section 2: Transplantation

Section 3: Chronic Pancreatitis

Section 4: Endocrine–Exocrine Interactions

Section 5: Pancreatic Cancer

Laboratory Studies

Clinical Studies

List of Contributors

A. Agha
Klinik und Poliklinik für
  Chirurgie
Universität Regensburg
Franz-Josef-Strauß-Alle 11
D-93042 Regensburg
Germany

D. Alderson
Professor of Gastrointestinal
  Surgery
Department of Surgery
Bristol Royal Infirmary
Marlborough Street
BS2 8HW
UK

D. Al-Musawi
Senior Registrar
Department of Surgery
Imperial College School of
  Medicine
Hammersmith Hospital
Du Cane Road
London W12 0NN
UK

Å. Andrén-Sandberg
Department of Surgery
Hankeland Hospital
N-5021 Bergen
Norway

U. Arnelo
Department of Surgery
Karolinska Institutet at
  Huddinge University Hospital
S-14186 Huddinge
Sweden

J. Axelson
Hammersmith Hospital
Du Cane Road
London W12 0NN
UK

M. D. Barber
Research Fellow
University Department of
  Surgery
Royal Infirmary
Edinburgh EH3 9YW
UK

C. Bassi
Assistant Professor of
  Surgery
Surgical Department
Borgo Roma University
  Hospital
University of Verona
I-37134 Verona
Italy

H. G. Beger
Department of General
  Surgery
University of Ulm
Steinhövelstrasse 9
D-89075 Ulm
Germany

P. Berberat
Department of Visceral and
  Transplantation Surgery
University of Bern
Inselspital
Bern CH-3010
Switzerland

P. Bilchler
Department of Visceral and
  Transplantation Surgery
University of Bern
Inselspital
Bern 3010
Switzerland

C. Bloechle
Department of Surgery
Universitäts-Krankenhaus
  Eppendorf
Chirurgische Klinik und
  Poliklinik
Abteilung für
  Allgemeinchirurgie
Martinistraße 52
D-20246 Hamburg
Germany

H. A. Bruining
Professor of Surgery
Erasmus University Medical
  Center
Dr Molewaterplein 40
3015 GD Rotterdam
The Netherlands

M. M. Büchler
Professor of Surgery
Department of Visceral and
  Transplantation Surgery
University of Bern
Inselspital
Bern CH-3010
Switzerland

R. Carter
Department of Surgery
Royal Infirmary
16 Alexandra Parade
Glasgow G31 2ER
UK

R. Castoldi
Senior Registrar in Surgery
San Raffaele Hospital
Divisione Chirurgia II
Via Olgettina 62
Milan I-20132
Italy

A. G. Chalmers
Consultant Radiologist
CT/MR Unlt
The General Infirmary at Leeds
Clarendon Wing
Belmont Grove
Leeds LS2 9NS
UK

H. A. Clayton
Research Associate
Department of Surgery
University of Leicester
Robert Kilpatrick Building
Leicester Royal Infirmary
Leicester LE2 7LX
UK

M. Cremer
Department of Gastroenterology
ULB Hôpital Erasme
808 Route de Lennik
Brussels B-1070
Belgium

J. Cullingworth
Superintendent Radiographer
CT/MR Unlt
The General Infirmary at Leeds
Clarendon Wing
Belmont Grove
Leeds LS2 9NS
UK

J.-C. Dagorn
U.315 INSERM
46 Boulevard de la Gaye
F-13009 Marseille
France

J. Deviére
Director
Department of Gastroenterology
ULB Hôpital Erasme
808 Route de Lennik
Brussels B-1070
Belgium

V. Di Carlo
Professor of Surgery
San Raffaele Hospital

Divisione Chirurgia II
Via Olgettina 62
Milan I-20132
Italy

J. D. Evans
Research Fellow in Surgery
Department of Surgery
Royal Liverpool University
    Hospital
5th Floor UCD Building
Daulby Street
Liverpool L69 3GA
UK

M. Falconi
Surgical Department
Borgo Roma University Hospital
University of Verona
Verona I-37134
Italy

G. Farkas
Professor of Surgery
Department of Surgery
Albert Szent-Györgyi Medical
    University
PO Box 464
Szeged H-6701
Hungary

K. C. H. Fearon
Reader in Surgery
University Department of
    Surgery
Royal Infirmary
Edinburgh EH3 9YW
UK

M. D. Finch
Lecturer in Surgery
Department of Surgery
Royal Liverpool University
    Hospital
5th Floor UCD Building
Daulby Street
Liverpool L69 3GA
UK

D. Fitzsimmons
Research Fellow

University Surgical Unit
F Level, Centre Block
Southampton General
    Hospital
Tremona Road
Southampton SO16 6YD
UK

H. Friess
Department of Visceral and
    Transplantation Surgery
University of Bern
Inselspital
Bern CH-3010
Switzerland

F. Gansauge
Department of General
    Surgery
University of Ulm
Steinhövelstrasse 9
D-89075 Ulm
Germany

O. J. Garden
Professor of Hepatobiliary
    Surgery
University Department of
    Surgery
Royal Infirmary
Edinburgh EH3 9YW
UK

P. Ghaneh
Research Fellow in Surgery
Department of Surgery
Royal Liverpool University
    Hospital
5th Floor UCD Building
Daulby Street
Liverpool L69 3GA
UK

S. W. A. Gould
Specialist Registrar
Minimal Access Surgical Unit
4th Floor Stanford Wing
St Mary's Hospital
Praed Street
London W2 1NY
UK

G. Glazer
Consultant Surgeon
St Mary's Hospital
Praed Street
London W2 1NY
UK

C. N. Hacking
Consultant Radiologist
Department of Clinical
   Radiology
Southampton General Hospital
Tremona Road
Southampton SO16 6YD
UK

P. D. Hardt
Ill Medizinische Klinik und
   Poliklinik
Med Zentrum für innere Medizin
Justus-Liebig-Universität
Rodthohl Giessen
D-635385 Geissen
Germany

R. Heafield
Senior Registrar Radiology
Department of Clinical
   Radiology
Southampton General Hospital
Tremona Road
Southampton SO16 6YD
UK

E. Heinmöller
Institute of Pathology
Klinik und Poliklinik für
   Chirurgie
Universität Regensburg
Franz-Josef-Strauß-Alle 11
D-93042 Regensburg
Germany

C. W. Imrie
Consultant Surgeon
Department of Surgery
Royal Infirmary
16 Alexandra Parade
Glasgow G31 2ER
UK

M. J. R. Izbicki
Professor of Surgery
Universitäts-Krankenhaus
   Eppendorf
Chirurgische Klinik und
   Poliklinik
Abteilung für
   Allgemeinchirurgie
Martinistraße 52
D-20246 Hamburg
Germany

T. G. John
Consultant General Surgeon
North Hampshire Hospital
Aldermaston Road
Basingstoke RG24 9NA
UK

C. Johnson
Reader in Surgery
University Surgical Unit (816)
Southampton General Hospital
Tremona Road
Southampton SO16 6YD
UK

A. Kawesha
Research Fellow in Surgery
Department of Surgery
Royal Liverpool University
   Hospital
5th Floor UCD Building
Daulby Street
Liverpool L69 3GA
UK

J. Keller
Director of Department of
   Medicine
Department of Internal Medicine
Israelitisches Krankenhaus
Orchideenstieg 14
D-22297 Hamburg
Germany

A. N. Kingsnorth
Professor of Surgery
Postgraduate Medical School
Level 17

Derriford Hospital
Plymouth
Devon PL6 8DH
UK

J. Kleeff
Department of Visceral and
    Transplantation Surgery
University of Bern
Inselspital
Bern CH-3010
Switzerland

H. U. Klör
Ill Medizinische Klinik und
    Poliklinik
Med Zentrum für Innere
    Medizin
Justus-Liebig-Universität
Rodthohl Giessen
D-635385 Geissen
Germany

W. T. Knoefel
Department of Surgery
Universitäts-Krankenhaus
    Eppendorf
Chirurgische Klinik und
    Poliklinik
Abteilung für
    Allgemeinchirurgie
Martinistraße 52
D-20246 Hamburg
Germany

M. Korc
Professor of Medicine
Division of Endocrinology,
    Diabetes and Metabolism
Medical Sciences 1, C240
University of California
Irvine, CA 92697
USA

R. J. Laugier
Professor of Medicine-
    Gastroenterology
Gastroenterology Department
Hôpital de La Conception
147 Boulevard Baille

F-13385 Marseille Cedex 5
France

J. Larsson
Department of Surgery
Karolinska Institutet at
    Huddinge University
    Hospital
S-14186 Huddinge
Sweden

P. Layer
Director of Department of
    Medicine
Department of Internal Medicine
Israelitisches Krankenhaus
Orchideenstieg 14
D-22297 Hamburg
Germany

N. R. Lemoine
Professor of Molecular
    Pathology
ICRF Molecular Oncology
    Unit
Imperial College School of
    Medicine at Hammersmith
Hammersmith Hospital
Du Cane Road
London W12 0NN
UK

J. C. Limmer
Department of Surgery
Universitäts-Krankenhaus
    Eppendorf
Chirurgische Klinik und
    Poliklinik
Abteilung für
    Allgemeinchirurgie
Martinistraße 52
D-20246 Hamburg
Germany

K. H. Link
Department of General Surgery
University of Ulm
Steinhövelstrasse 9
D-89075 Ulm
Germany

N. J. M. London
Professor
Department of Surgery
University of Leicester
Robert Kilpatrick Building
Leicester Royal Infirmary
Leicester LE2 7LX
UK

E. J. T. Luiten
General Surgeon
Department of Surgery
St Anna Hospital
P.O. Box 90
5660 AB Geldrop
The Netherlands

S. Mann
Postdoctorate Assistant
Klinik und Poliklinik für
   Chirurgie
Universität Regensburg
Franz-Josef-Strauß-Alle 11
D-93042 Regensburg
Germany

U. Mann
Klinik und Poliklinik für
   Chirurgie
Universität Regensburg
Franz-Josef-Strauß-Alle 11
D-93042 Regensburg
Germany

I. J. Martin
Consultant General Surgeon
Princess Alexandra Hospital
Ipswich Road
Woolongabba
Queensland 4012
Australia

F. C. McCormick
Clinical Research Fellow
Department of Histopathology
Imperial College School of
   Medicine at Hammersmith
Hammersmith Hospital
Du Cane Road
London W12 0NN
UK

C. J. McKay
Lecturer in Surgery
University Department of
   Surgery
Western Infirmary
Glasgow G11 6NT
UK

J. P. Neoptolemos
Professor of Surgery
Department of Surgery
Royal Liverpool University
   Hospital
5th Floor UCD Building
Daulby Street
Liverpool L69 3GA
UK

S. A. Norton
Special Registrar in Surgery
Department of Surgery
Bristol Royal Infirmary
Marlborough Street
BS2 8HW
UK

C. Pasquali
Surgical Department
University of Padova
Padova I-35128
Italy

P. Pederzoli
Professor of Surgery
Surgical Department
Borgo Roma University Hospital
University of Verona
Verona I-37134
Italy

S. Pedrazzoli
Professor of Surgery
Surgical Department
University of Padova
Padova I-35128
Italy

J. Permert
Department of Surgery
Karolinska Institutet at
   Huddinge University Hospital

S14186 Huddinge
Sweden

O. H. Petersen
George Holt Professor of
    Physiology
The Physiological Laboratory
University of Liverpool
Crown St
Liverpool L69 3BX
UK

D. Ravichandran
Research Registrar
University Surgical Unit
F Level, Centre Block
Southampton General
    Hospital
Tremona Road
Southampton SO16 6YD
UK

C. Renou
Service Médicine Interne
Centre Hospitalier BP82
F-83407 Hyères Cedex
France

J. V. Reynolds
Consultant Surgeon
Department of Surgery
St James's Hospital
St James's Street
Dublin 8
Ireland

J. A. Ross
Non-Clinical Senior Lecturer
University Department of
    Surgery
Royal Infirmary
Edinburgh EH3 9YW
UK

J. Rüschoff
Klinik und Poliklinik für
    Chirurgie
Universität Regensburg
Franz-Josef-Strauß-Alle 11
D-93042 Regensburg
Germany

J. Schmidt
Klinik und Poliklinik für
    Chirurgie
Universität Regensburg
Franz-Josef-Strauß-Alle 11
D-93042 Regensburg
Germany

M. H. Schoenberg
Professor of Surgery
Department of Surgery
Rotkreuz Hospital
Nymphenburgerstrasse. 163
D-80634 Munich
Germany

R. Sutton
Senior Lecturer in Surgery
Department of Surgery
Royal Liverpool University
    Hospital
5th Floor UCD Building
Daulby Street
Liverpool L69 3GA
UK

S. M. Swift
Research Associate
Department of Surgery
University of Leicester
Robert Kilpatrick Building
Leicester Royal Infirmary
Leicester LE2 7LX
UK

S. Toh
University Surgical Unit (816)
Southampton General Hospital
Tremona Road
Southampton SO16 6YD
UK

W. Uhl
Department of Visceral and
    Transplantation Surgery
University of Bern
Inselspital
Bern CH-3010
Switzerland

S. K. Vyas
Consultant Gastroenterologist
Salisbury District Hospital
Salisbury SX2 8BJ
UK

J. B. Ward
Clinical Lecturer in Surgery
Department of Surgery
Royal Liverpool University
    Hospital
5th Floor UCD Building
Daulby Street
Liverpool L69 3GA
UK

R. C. N. Williamson
Professor of Surgery
Department of Surgery
Imperial College School of
    Medicine
Hammersmith Hospital
Du Cane Road
London W12 0NN
UK

H. Zirngibl
Professor of Surgery
University Witten/Herdecke
Chirurgischeklinik
Klinikum Wuppertal GmBH
Heusnerstrasse 40
D-42283 Wuppertal
Germany

Section 1

Acute Pancreatitis

1 Intracellular Calcium in the Pathogenesis of Acute Pancreatitis

J.B. Ward, O.H. Petersen and R. Sutton

Intracellular Calcium Signals in Normal Pancreatic Acinar Cells

The major function of the pancreatic acinar cell is the synthesis and secretion of digestive enzymes in an inactive form. Following discharge into the acinar lumen these pass via the pancreatic duct into the duodenum where trypsin is activated by the brush border enzyme enterokinase, to subsequently activate the other enzymes.

Within the pancreatic acinar cell the key messenger controlling enzyme secretion is cytosolic free ionised calcium. Pancreatic acinar cells isolated by enzymatic digestion have provided valuable models to study intracellular Ca^{2+} signals because they are both structurally and functionally polarised (37). Advances over the past 15 years have enabled the description of patterns of Ca^{2+} signals within acinar cells, largely using fluorescent dyes that are sensitive to changes in cytosolic calcium concentration ($[Ca^{2+}]_i$) (13), or indirectly by examining Ca^{2+}-dependent events, such as electrophysiological studies of Ca^{2+}-dependent Cl^- channels.

Normal "resting" $[Ca^{2+}]_i$ is in the order of 10^{-7} M, compared to levels of around 10^{-3} M outside the cell, a gradient that is maintained by a plasma membrane Mg^{2+}-dependent Ca^{2+}-ATPase and a Na^+-Ca^{2+} cotransporter (3,18). Calcium is also pumped into the endoplasmic reticulum (ER) by a specific Ca^{2+}-ATPase (2). Local increases in $[Ca^{2+}]_i$ in different regions of the cell can thus be utilised to control intracellular events. However, it is important that $[Ca^{2+}]_i$ is kept low because abnormal global elevations of $[Ca^{2+}]_i$ are known to be toxic to many cell types (25).

Pancreatic secretagogues, which include the neurotransmitter acetylcholine (ACh) and the gastrointestinal peptide cholecystokinin (CCK), bind to and activate G-protein-linked plasma membrane receptors on the basolateral aspect of the cell (29). The effects of secretagogue receptor binding are outlined in Figure 1. This leads to activation of G-proteins and generation of the intermediate cytosolic intracellular messengers inositol (1,4,5) trisphosphate (IP$_3$) from hydrolysis of phosphatidylinositol 4,5 bisphosphate (PIP$_2$), and cyclic adenosine diphosphate ribose (cADPr) from nicotinamide adenine diphosphate (NSAD$^+$) (4). These messengers act on IP$_3$ receptors (IP$_3$) and ryanodine receptors (cADPr) to induce release of Ca^{2+} from non-mitochondrial intracellular stores, resulting in

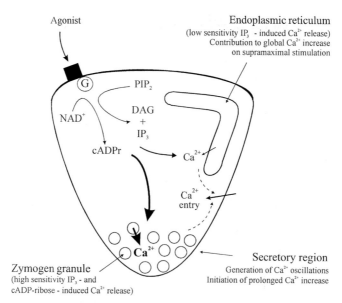

Figure 1. Calcium signalling in pancreatic acinar cells. Stimulation of G-protein linked receptors on the basolateral cell membrane leads to the formation of IP_3, from PIP_2 hydrolysis, and cADPr from NAD^+. These messengers induce the release of Ca^{2+} from intracellular stores, resulting in an increase in $[Ca^{2+}]_i$. The Ca^{2+} stores in the apical region of the cell are the most sensitive to these intermediate messengers. Depletion of intracellular stores initiates Ca^{2+} entry into the cytosol from outside the cell.

an increase in $[Ca^{2+}]_i$ (4). Depletion of intracellular Ca^{2+} stores stimulates Ca^{2+} entry from outside the cell into the cytosol to maintain the duration of the response (24).

Calcium stores in the apical region (secretory pole) of the acinar cell are highly sensitive to IP_3 and cADPr, and stimulation with low concentrations of ACh (25–100 nM) induces the generation of short-lasting repetitive increases (oscillations or spikes) in $[Ca^{2+}]_i$, at a frequency of several per minute, generally localised to the apical region. Physiological concentrations of CCK (5–20 pM (7)) induce short-lasting spikes of $[Ca^{2+}]_i$ at the secretory pole which are followed by longer repetitive transient increases in $[Ca^{2+}]_i$ occurring throughout the cell (37) (Figure 2a, b).

Calcium oscillations in the secretory pole are important in triggering bursts of exocytosis of zymogen granules from the apical membrane of the cell into the acinar lumen, signified by a change in membrane capacitance (22). The mechanism of oscillation production is still unknown, as is the means by which each rise in $[Ca^{2+}]_i$ triggers exocytosis, but such a system provides a powerful and variable signal enabling fine control of Ca^{2+}-dependent cellular processes, whilst avoiding large toxic increases in $[Ca^{2+}]_i$ throughout the cell. Localised $[Ca^{2+}]_i$ changes are important in maintaining the functional polarity of the acinar cell, controlling the discharge of zymogen granule contents from the apical cell membrane into the acinar lumen, and so into the pancreatic duct (15). In the pancreatic acinar cell, zymogen granules themselves have recently been shown to release Ca^{2+} in response to perifusion with the intermediate messengers IP_3 and cADPr, and they may be the organelles which initiate the physiological Ca^{2+} signal (8).

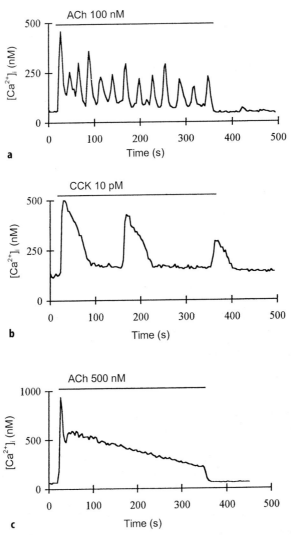

Figure 2. Patterns of calcium signals in normal acinar cells. **a** Stimulation with low does ACh (100 nM) initiates oscillations in $[Ca^{2+}]_i$ at a frequency of several per minute, generally localised to the apical region of the cell. **b** Physiological doses of CCK (10 pM) induce slower transients in $[Ca^{2+}]_i$ **c** Stimulation by high dose ACh (500 nM) produces a larger sustained increase in $[Ca^{2+}]_i$ which pervades throughout the cell after initiation in the secretory pole (see also Figure 3a). Adapted from Ward et al. (40) with permission.

Supramaximal stimulation by high doses of agonists induces a different type of Ca^{2+} signal. In this situation there is a larger, more sustained global rise in $[Ca^{2+}]_i$ throughout the cell (Figure 2c). This increase is still initiated in the secretory pole of the cell, but spreads basolaterally, with release of Ca^{2+} from the ER, which dominates the basolateral region of the cell (Figure 3a) (38). This type of global increase is known to be toxic in many cell types (25), and in the pancreas supramaximal stimulation *in vivo* leads to the production of cell injury and acute pancreatitis (19).

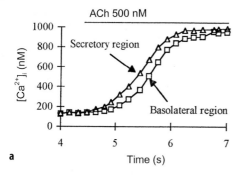

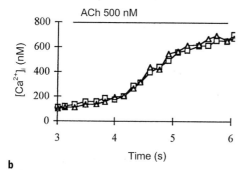

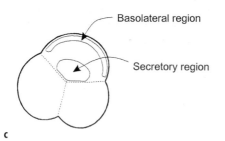

Figure 3. Subcellular patterns of calcium increase in normal and pancreatitic cells **a** Pattern of increase of $[Ca^{2+}]_i$ in normal cell in response to high dose of ACh. The initial $[Ca^{2+}]_i$ rise occurs in the secretory pole, before spreading to other regions of the cell. **b** $[Ca^{2+}]_i$ increase in cell from mouse having received five injections of caerulein. The normal initiation of $[Ca^{2+}]_i$ increase in the secretory pole is lost, with a diffuse increase in $[Ca^{2+}]_i$ across the cell being seen. **c** Cartoon of a pancreatic acinus demonstrating the areas of a cell studied using digital imaging micro fluorimetry with the fluorescent dye fura-2. From Ward et al. (40) with permission.

Early Cellular Events in Acute Pancreatitis

The conditions associated with the development of acute pancreatitis are well documented, but the mechanisms by which these conditions induce the disease are unclear. The inaccessibility of the pancreas in humans, together with delayed presentation and often uncertain diagnosis in patients with acute pancreatitis, has led to the development of several experimental models (34). The most widely used of these models induce pancreatitis either by supramaximal stimulation with secretagogues, or by ligation of, or injection of, various agents into the pancreatic duct, and by the administration of a choline-deficient ethionine supplemented diet to female mice. These models induce pancreatitis by very different mechanisms, but have several biological processes in common, suggesting a common disease pathway regardless of the nature of the initial insult.

Although the location of the earliest injury in acute pancreatitis has been the subject of considerable debate, it is now evident that the initial event involves acinar cell injury (35), with subsequent release of prematurely-activated pancreatic enzymes which damage pancreatic tissue and endothelium, resulting in a potentially lethal inflammatory cascade. Acinar cell uptake of amino acids and synthesis of proteins is unaltered during the early stages of all three experimental models described above (9,30,32). However, there does appear to be a disruption of the normal sorting of digestive enzyme precursors (zymogens) from lysosomal enzymes during the early stages of experimental pancreatitis, with subcellular fractionation experiments producing a pellet rich in both types of enzyme (17,31,32). The fact that lysosomal enzymes can activate trypsin (12) had led to the suggestion that the co-localisation of these enzymes in abnormal cytoplasmic vacuoles plays a role in the pathogenesis of the disease by allowing premature trypsin activation, but whether lysosomal enzyme redistribution is an important pathogenetic event or simply a response to cell injury is still unclear (11).

What is clear is that disruption of normal enzyme secretion by acinar cells is an early feature of all models of experimental pancreatitis. This was initially demonstrated in pulse chase experiments (9,30,32). More recent studies examining secretion both *in vitro* and *in vivo* have confirmed that disruption of secretion is a feature not only of caerulein-induced pancreatitis in both the rat and the mouse, but also of pancreatitis induced by the injection of taurocholate into the rat pancreatic duct, and of diet-induced pancreatitis (26). Detailed electron-micrographic studies have demonstrated that abnormal discharge of zymogen granules from the lateral cell membrane, rather than discharge confined to the apical pole, is a feature of human acute pancreatitis as well as of caerulein hyperstimulation of rat acini both *in vitro* and *in vivo* (1,16,33). Uncontrolled release of digestive enzymes into the interstitium of the gland could play an important role in producing the catastrophic tissue damage seen in acute pancreatitis.

Intracellular Calcium in Acute Experimental Pancreatitis

Because of the importance of Ca^{2+} signals in the control of normal enzyme secretion, we have examined pancreatic acinar cell Ca^{2+} signals during the early stages of pancreatitis induced *in vivo* by the administration of hourly intraperitoneal injections of caerulein to mice, at a dose of 50 μg/kg per hour, which in our laboratory induced mild oedematous disease (40). The pancreas was removed from each mouse after 1, 3, 5 or 7 injections of caerulein, and acini were isolated by collagenase digestion. Intracellular Ca^{2+} signals were then examined by loading cells with fura-2, a fluorescent dye sensitive to changes in $[Ca^{2+}]_i$, and studying the $[Ca^{2+}]_i$ response to stimulation by different doses of agonists and the tumour promoter thapsigargin.

In the presence of a physiological concentration of ACh (100 nM) the proportion of cells from control mice (administered saline injections) that demonstrated a normal oscillatory $[Ca^{2+}]_i$ signal upon physiological stimulation (Figure 2a) was maintained throughout the course of injections. However, the proportion of experimental cells maintaining this response progressively diminished with

Table 1. Oscillatory response of acinar cells to ACh during hyperstimulation *in vivo*

Injection	Control (saline) no. of cells (%)	Experimental (caerulein) no. of cells (%)
0	19 (79)	–
1	35 (81)	34 (74)
3	30 (81)	21 (78)
5	43 (90)	5 (20)
7	35 (97)	2 (6)

The number (%) of cells maintaining an oscillatory $[Ca^{2+}]_i$ response to 100 nM ACh during repeated injections of caerulein or saline. There was a significant difference between control and experimental cells after five and seven injections (x^2_Y, $P < 0.001$), and a significant linear trend in experimental results during the course of injections (x^2_{trend} = 46.72, $P < 0.001$). From Ward et al. (40) with permission.

Table 2. Oscillatory response to CCK during hyperstimulation

Injection	Control (saline) no. of cells (%)	Experimental (caerulein) no. of cells (%)
0	22 (92)	–
1	38 (83)	31 (57)
3	44 (79)	11 (44)
5	43 (96)	4 (13)
7	40 (98)	0 (0)

Number (%) of cells demonstrating an oscillatory $[Ca^{2+}]_i$ response to 10 pM following repeated injections of caerulein *in vivo*. There was a significant progressive loss of normal response in experimental cells, such that after seven injections no cells responded at all (x^2_{trend} = 35.75, $P < 0.001$).

repeated caerulein injections, such that only 20% of cells showed such a response after 5 injections (see Table 1), with more cells demonstrating a single abnormal response or no response at all. Similarly, the proportion of cells from experimental mice that demonstrated an oscillatory response to 10 pM CCK progressively diminished (see Table 2). In contrast, the sustained nature of the $[Ca^{2+}]_i$ response to a supramaximal dose of ACh (500 nM, Figure 2c) was maintained in the vast majority of cells until at least after the seventh injection of caerulein, when only 44% of cells showed this increase, and when the amplitude of the increase was significantly reduced. In spite of this, the subcellular pattern of the $[Ca^{2+}]_i$ response to this dose suggested that the signal was in fact abnormal at an earlier stage. In the normal acinar cell the initial $[Ca^{2+}]_i$ increase in response to maximal stimulation occurs at the secretory pole of the cell, despite the fact that secretagogue membrane receptors are situated on the basolateral aspect of the cell (15,29,38) (Figure 3a). In cells from experimental mice that had received caerulein injections the normal initiation of the Ca^{2+} signal in the secretory pole of the cell was progressively lost, as more cells demonstrated a diffuse increase in $[Ca^{2+}]_i$ across the cell (Figures 3b and 4) or an increase that was initiated in the basolateral region.

Thapsigargin is a tumour promoter that has been demonstrated to inhibit specifically the Ca^{2+}-ATPase which pumps Ca^{2+} into the ER (36). It is therefore a useful tool with which to assess the state of Ca^{2+} filling of the ER. We found that even in acinar cells from mice which had received seven injections of caerulein, the ability to replenish the ER following hyperstimulation was maintained, as

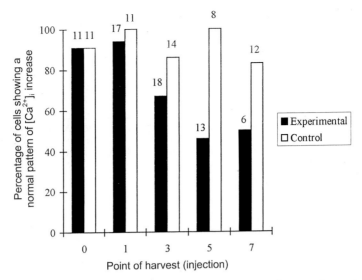

Figure 4. Percentage of cells showing normal pattern of $[Ca^{2+}]_i$ increase. Histogram demonstrating the percentage of cells from controls (received saline) and experimental mice (caerulein) which maintained the normal pattern of $[Ca^{2+}]_i$ increase in response to ACh, i.e. with initiation of increase in the secretory pole. Whereas a high percentage of control cells maintained a normal pattern of increase, this was progressively disrupted in experimental cells. From Ward et al. (40) with permission.

indicated by the increase in $[Ca^{2+}]_i$ due to leakage from the ER following inhibition of Ca^{2+}-ATPase by thapsigargin (Figure 5).

Examined together, these data indicate that early caerulein-induced pancreatitis is associated with the progressive disruption of acinar cell $[Ca^{2+}]_i$ signalling (40). This disruption is initially specific to the apical region of the cell, which is the site of generation of $[Ca^{2+}]_i$ oscillations in response to "physiological" stimulation and also the site of the initial increase in response to maximal stimulation, as indicated by the fact that both of these features were lost early in these experiments. In contrast, the ER, which dominates the basolateral region of the cell, was still replenished after seven caerulein injections, and contributed to the maintenance of the whole cell sustained increase in $[Ca^{2+}]_i$ in response to high dose ACh.

The loss of functional polarity of the acinar cell that we have demonstrated to occur in acute pancreatitis is accompanied by loss of structural polarity (1,21). *In vitro* studies have demonstrated disruption of the apical region of the acinar cell in response to caerulein hyperstimulation (27), and abnormal discharge of enzymes from the lateral plasma membrane has been described in both experimental and human disease (1,16). The mechanism of this disruption is not known, but could occur at any stage from binding of secretagogue to membrane receptor, through production of the intermediate intracellular messengers, to primary Ca^{2+} release from intracellular stores, or the reduction of $[Ca^{2+}]_i$ that occurs after each oscillation. Although heterologous receptor desensitisation leading to decreased production of IP_3 on subsequent stimulation could account for the abnormal signal, repeated stimulation of these membrane receptors is the principal means by which progressively severe pancreatitis is produced in this

Control

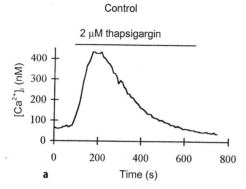

a

Experimental

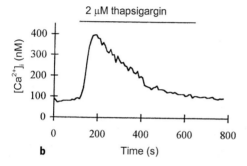

b

Figure 5. $[Ca^{2+}]_i$ response to thapsigargin in pancreatitis. Examples of $[Ca^{2+}]_i$ increase in response to the specific ER Ca^{2+}-ATPase inhibitor thapsigargin in both experimental and control cells, indicating that even cells from mice administered caerulein maintained the ability to replenish the ER with Ca^{2+}. From Ward et al. (40) with permission.

model, and so receptor desensitisation is not likely to be the means by which Ca^{2+} signals are disrupted. Decreased production of IP_3 is another possible explanation for the loss of the normal Ca^{2+} signal but during stimulation with physiological concentrations of agonist there is no measurable increase in IP_3 production, and it is possible that alteration of the sensitivity of IP_3 receptors on intracellular stores is the more important process (23,42).

It is now clear that Ca^{2+} stores in the secretory region of the acinar cell are very sensitive to the intermediate messengers IP_3 and cADPr (37). Recent evidence indicates that zymogen granules themselves release Ca^{2+} in response to stimulation with IP_3 and cADPr, and thus the granules themselves may be the Ca^{2+} store that initiates the physiological Ca^{2+} signal in the secretory region of the cell (8). It may be that during hyperstimulation *in vivo* both the zymogen granules and the ER become depleted of Ca^{2+}, but whereas the ER can be rapidly replenished (as indicated by the thapsigargin results, Figure 5) the zymogen granules are unable to refill their stores with Ca^{2+}, and thus are unable to initiate to $[Ca^{2+}]_i$ signals in the secretory region of the cell, thus leading to the abnormal secretion that is seen in acute pancreatitis, and to subsequent tissue damage.

Although the mechanism of disruption of normal physiological acinar cell Ca^{2+} signalling in the secretory region of the cell is as yet unknown, it is likely to account for the disruption of secretion in acute pancreatitis, and closer examination of these events may further elucidate the pathogenesis of the disease.

Possible Role of Intracellular Calcium in Initiation of Cell Damage

Despite characterisation of the early events, including the abnormal signals outlined above, the initial trigger of cell injury in acute pancreatitis is still unknown. As described earlier, one of the earliest intracellular events seen following abusive stimulation by supramaximal doses of secretagogues, which *in vivo* are associated with the production of acute pancreatitis, is a sustained elevation of $[Ca^{2+}]_i$ occurring throughout the cell, rather than being localised to the secretory region (37,38). Such abnormal elevations in $[Ca^{2+}]_i$ are known to be associated with damage in many cell types, by mechanisms including the excessive activation of cytosolic Ca^{2+}-dependent destructive enzymes, interference with normal cell signals, and disruption of the cytoskeleton, all of which are features of hyperstimulation (5,27,40). Other effects are mitochondrial dysfunction and nuclear changes such as the initiation of apoptosis (25).

Evidence is mounting that abnormal acinar cell Ca^{2+} homeostasis may play an important role in the pathogenesis of acute pancreatitis (39). Zhou and colleagues (44) found that hypercalcaemic rats developed acute pancreatitis when administered caerulein at a dose too low to cause cell injury in normocalcaemic animals. It may be that abnormally high Ca^{2+} levels in the interstitial fluid prevent efficient extrusion of Ca^{2+}, even after physiological stimulation, thereby preventing acinar cells from reducing $[Ca^{2+}]_i$ to low resting levels, leading to abnormal elevations and subsequent toxicity. In addition, hyperstimulation of isolated rat pancreatic acini induces the production of platelet activating factor (PAF), one of the key inflammatory mediators in acute pancreatitis, the production of which appears to be associated with a large increase in $[Ca^{2+}]_i$ (43). Moreover, the Ca^{2+} channel blocker verapamil has been reported to be of benefit in a human model of acute pancreatitis (20). Although verapamil is a voltage-gated Ca^{2+} channel blocker, recent evidence indicates that the transmembrane regions of ligand-gated Ca^{2+} channels, encoded by the *trp* gene, show some sequence homology to voltage-gated Ca^{2+} channels (28). If Ca^{2+} channel blockers do have some activity on the ligand-gated Ca^{2+} channels of pancreatic acinar cells, they may have reduced cell injury in these experiments by preventing excessive Ca^{2+} entry and subsequent abnormal $[Ca^{2+}]_i$ elevation.

What about the clinical situation? In humans, alcohol and gallstones account for 90% of cases of acute pancreatitis. Ethanol has been shown to interfere with cellular Ca^{2+} homeostasis in several cell types, including pancreatic acinar cells (6,41). In choledocholithiasis and other situations of pancreatic ductal hypertension, increased pressure in the acinar lumen may interfere with acinar cell extrusion of Ca^{2+}, thus preventing reduction of $[Ca^{2+}]_i$ to low resting levels following physiological stimulation (39). In fact CCK has been shown to exacerbate other models of acute pancreatitis (10), including biliary disease (14). Other causes of acute pancreatitis include hypoxia, infection, lipid abnormalities and certain drugs with anticholinesterase activity. Abnormalities of $[Ca^{2+}]_i$ homeostasis have been shown to be the mechanism by which these agents mediate damage in many other cell types (39).

The mechanisms of initiation of pancreatic acinar cell injury by such a diverse range of conditions, leading to a common disease pathway, are still very poorly understood. Cytosolic free ionised calcium plays an important role in the control of the normal functions of the acinar cell, and evidence suggests that abnormalities of Ca^{2+} homeostasis may play a key role in the pathogenesis of disease (39,40,44). Future studies examining the effects of such abnormalities on acinar cell structure and function, and the demonstration of these abnormalities in relevant experimental or clinical situations, may prove fruitful in further definition of the pathogenesis of this disease, in the endeavour to find new approaches to prophylaxis and therapy.

Acknowledgement

The author acknowledges kind permission from the publishers of *Gastroenterology* to reproduce Table 1 and Figures 2.5 (see reference 40).

References

1. Adler G, Rohr G, Kern HF (1982) Alteration of membrane fusion as a cause of acute pancreatitis in the rat. Dig Dis Sci 27:993–1002.
2. Bayerdorffer E, Streb H, Eckhardt L, Haase W, Schulz I (1984) Characterization of calcium uptake into rough endoplasmic reticulum of rat pancreas. J Membr Biol 81:69–82.
3. Bayerdorffer E, Haase W, Schulz I (1985) Na^+/Ca^{2+} countertransport in plasma membrane of rat pancreatic acinar cells. J Membr Biol 87:107–119.
4. Berridge MJ (1993) A tale of two messengers. Nature 365:388–389.
5. Bialek R, Willemer S, Arnold R, Adler G (1991) Evidence of intracellular activation of serine proteases in acute cerulein-induced pancreatitis in rats. Scand J Gastroenterol 26:190–196.
6. Davidson M, Wilce P, Shanley B (1990) Ethanol and synaptosomal calcium homeostasis. Biochem Pharmacol 39:1283–1288.
7. Dockray GJ (1982) The physiology of cholecystokinin in brain and gut. Br Med Bull 38:253–258.
8. Gerasimenko OV, Gerasimenko JV, Belan PV, Petersen OH (1996) Inositol trisphosphate and cyclic ADP-ribose-mediated release of Ca^{2+} from single isolated pancreatic zymogen granules. Cell 84:473–480.
9. Gilliland L, Steer ML (1980) Effects of ethionine on digestive enzyme synthesis and discharge by mouse pancreas. Am J Physiol 239:G418–426.
10. Gomez G, Townsend CM, Green DW et al. (1990) Protective action of luminal bile salts in necrotizing acute pancreatitis in mice. J Clin Invest 1990:323–331.
11. Gorelick FS, Matovcik LM (1995) Lysosomal enzymes and pancreatitis. Gastroenterology 109:620–625.
12. Greenbaum LM, Hirschkowitz A (1961) Endogenous cathepsin activation of trypsinogen in extracts of dog pancreas. Proc Soc Exp Biol Med 107:74–76.
13. Grynkiewicz G, Poenie M, Tsien RY (1985) A new generation of Ca^{2+} indicators with greatly improved fluorescence properties. J Biol Chem 260:3440–3450.
14. Jenkins SA, Ellenbogen S, Kynaston H et al. (1992) Effects of sandostatin on pancreatic bloodflow, structure and function during the development of experimentally induced pancreatitis. Br J Surg 79:S112.
15. Kasai H, Augustine GJ (1990) Cytosolic Ca^{2+} gradients triggering unidirectional fluid secretion from exocrine pancreas. Nature 348:735–738.
16. Kloppel G, Dreyer T, Willemer S, Kern HF, Adler G (1986) Human acute pancreatitis: its pathogenesis in the light of immunocytochemical and ultrastructural findings in acinar cells. Virchows Arch [A] 409:791–803.
17. Koike H, Steer ML, Meldolesi J (1982) Pancreatic effects of ethionine: blockade of exocytosis and appearance of crinophagy and autophagy precede cellular necrosis. Am J Physiol 242:G297–307.
18. Kribben A, Tyrakowski T, Schulz I (1983) Characterization of Mg-ATP-dependent Ca^{2+} transport in cat pancreatic microsomes. Am J Physiol 244:G480–490.
19. Lampel M, Kern HF (1977) Acute interstitial pancreatitis in the rat induced by excessive doses of a pancreatic secretagogue. Virchows Arch [A] 373:97–117.

20. Leahy A, Darzi A, Grace P, et al. (1992) Verapamil is beneficial in a model of acute pancreatitis after endoscopic retrograde cholangiopancreatography. Br J Surg 79:1241.

21. Lerch MM, Saluja AK, Dawra R, Ramarao P, Saluja M, Steer ML (1992) Acute necrotizing pancreatitis in the opossum: earliest morphological changes involve acinar cells. Gastroenterology 103:205–213.

22. Maruyama Y, Petersen OH (1994) Delay in granular fusion evoked by repetitive cytosolic Ca^{2+} spikes in mouse pancreatic acinar cells. Cell Calcium 16:419–430.

23. Matozaki T, Goke B, Tsunoda Y, Rodriguez M, Martinez J, Williams JA (1990) Two functionally distinct cholecystokinin receptors show different modes of action on Ca^{2+} mobilization and phospholipid hydrolysis in isolated rat pancreatic acini. Studies using a new cholecystokinin analog, JMV-180. J Biol Chem 265:6247–6254.

24. Muallem S (1989) Calcium transport pathways of pancreatic acinar cells. Ann Rev Physiol 51:83–105.

25. Nicotera P, Bellomo G, Orrenius S (1992) Calcium-mediated mechanisms in chemically induced cell death. Annu Rev Pharmacol Toxicol 32:449–470.

26. Niederau C, Niederau M, Luthen R, Strohmeyer G, Ferrell LD, Grendell JH (1990) Pancreatic exocrine secretion in acute experimental pancreatitis. Gastroenterology 99:1120–1127.

27. O'Konski MS, Pandol SJ (1990) Effects of caerulein on the apical cytoskeleton of the pancreatic acinar cell. J Clin Invest 86:1649–1657.

28. Petersen CCH (1996) Store operated calcium entry. SINS 8:293–300.

29. Rosenzweig SA, Miller LJ, Jamieson JD (1983) Identification and localization of cholecystokinin binding sites on rat pancreatic plasma membranes and acinar cells: a biochemical and autoradiographic study. J Cell Biol 96:1288–1297.

30. Saluja A, Saito I, Saluja M et al. (1985) In vivo rat pancreatic acinar function during supramaximal stimulation with caerulein. Am J Physiol 249:G702–710.

31. Saluja A, Hashimoto S, Saluja M, Powers RE, Meldolesi J, Steer ML (1987) Subcellular redistribution of lysosomal enzymes during caerulein-induced pancreatitis. Am J Physiol 253:G508–516.

32. Saluja A, Saluja M, Villa A et al. (1989) Pancreatic duct obstruction in rabbits causes digestive zymogen and lysosomal enzyme colocalization. J Clin Invest 84:1260–1266.

33. Scheele G, Adler G, Kern H (1987) Exocytosis occurs at the lateral plasma membrane of the pancreatic acinar cell during supramaximal secretagogue stimulation. Gastroenterology 92:345–353.

34. Steer ML (1988) Experimental models of acute pancreatitis. In: Glazer G, Ranson J (eds) Acute pancreatitis. Saunders, London, pp 207–226.

35. Steer ML, Saluja AK (1993) Experimental acute pancreatitis: studies of the early events that lead to cell injury. In: Go VLW, DiMagno EP, Gardner JD, Lebenthal E, Reber HA, Scheele GA (eds) The pancreas: biology, pathobiology and disease, 2nd edn. Raven Press, New York, pp 489–500.

36. Thastrup O, Cullen PJ, Drobak BK, Hanley MR, Dawson AP (1990) Thapsigargin, a tumour promoter, discharges intracellular Ca^{2+} stores by specific inhibition of the endoplasmic reticulum Ca^{2+}-ATPase. Proc Natl Acad Sci USA 87:2466–2470.

37. Thorn P, Lawrie AM, Smith PM, Gallacher DV, Petersen OH (1993) Local and global cytosolic Ca^{2+} oscillations in exocrine cells evoked by agonists and inositol trisphosphate. Cell 74:661–668.

38. Toescu EC, Lawrie AM, Petersen OH, Gallacher DV (1992) Spatial and temporal distribution of agonist-evoked cytoplasmic Ca^{2+} signals in exocrine acinar cells analysed by digital image microscopy. EMBO J 11-4:1623–1629.

39. Ward JB, Petersen OH, Jenkins SA, Sutton R (1995) Is an elevated concentration of acinar cytosolic free ionised calcium the trigger for acute pancreatitis? Lancet 346:1016–1019.

40. Ward JB, Sutton R, Jenkins SA, Petersen OH (1996) Progressive disruption of acinar cell calcium signalling is an early feature of cerulein-induced pancreatitis in mice. Gastroenterology 111:481–491.

41. Ward JB, Sutton R, Petersen OH (1996) Ethanol interacts with the CCK receptor and causes calcium release from intracellular pools in mouse pancreatic acinar cells. Br J Surg 83:1632.

42. Xu X, Zeng W, Muallem S (1996) Regulation of the IP_3 activated Ca^{2+} channel by activation of G proteins. J Biol Chem 271:11737–11744.

43. Zhou W, Levine BA, Olson MS (1993) Platelet-activating factor: a mediator of pancreatic inflammation during cerulein hyperstimulation. Am J Pathol 142:1504–1512.

44. Zhou W, Shen F, Miller JE, Han Q, Olson MS (1996) Evidence for altered cellular calcium in the pathogenetic mechanism of acute pancreatitis in rats. J Surg Res 60:147–155.

2 Monocytes and Mediators in Acute Pancreatitis

C. McKay

Many patients with severe pancreatitis have evidence of a systemic illness, characterised by varying degrees of respiratory and renal impairment. In the most severe cases, death results from multiple organ failure. Recent prospective clinical trials in the UK indicate that early mortality from organ failure continues to account for around 40% of all deaths in acute pancreatitis.

In 1988, Rinderknecht (1) first proposed the hypothesis that cytokines may play an important role in the pathophysiology of acute pancreatitis. He cast doubt on the conventional view that activated pancreatic proteases were responsible for the systemic manifestations of acute pancreatitis and suggested that excessive stimulation of neutrophils by phagocytosed cell debris may lead to production of harmful quantities of free oxygen radicals, leukotrienes and the newly described cachectin (tumour necrosis factor) in a situation analogous to septic shock. The role of cytokines and activated leucocytes has been widely studied since that time.

Pro-inflammatory Cytokines in Peripheral Blood

Tumour Necrosis Factor (TNFα)

TNFα is a pro-inflammatory cytokine produced predominately by cells of the monocyte/macrophage lineage although its production by NK-cells, antigen-stimulated T cells and mast cells has been documented (2). TNFα acts on endothelial cells to enhance procoagulant activity, increase permeability and induce the production of other inflammatory mediators including interleukin-1 and platelet activating factor (3). TNFα induces neutrophil margination and activation and is therefore an important stimulator of the non-specific immune response (4–7). TNFα also induces the maturation of myeloid cells to monocytes and macrophages and is capable of macrophage activation, thus stimulating its own production (8,9).

The first attempt to study the role of TNFα in acute pancreatitis was by Banks and colleagues (10) who measured serial plasma levels of TNFα in 27 patients with acute pancreatitis. They found raised levels of TNFα in some patients, including two who died of their illness, but found no statistically significant difference in TNFα levels between patients with mild and those with severe disease.

In those with raised levels, TNFα levels peaked within the first 3 days after admission but many patients had TNFα levels which were similar to those observed in healthy controls. The authors concluded that it was unlikely that TNFα played an important pathophysiological role in acute pancreatitis, although they did find evidence of neutrophil activation.

Subsequently, Exley and co-workers (11), in 38 patients with predicted severe acute pancreatitis taking part in a therapeutic trial of fresh frozen plasma, measured serum levels of TNFα during the first week of admission. They found detectable levels of TNFα on admission in 45% of non-survivors compared with 23% of survivors and, overall, the levels of TNFα were higher than those reported by Banks et al. In addition, endotoxin was detected on admission in 91% of non-survivors.

These studies demonstrate the problems associated with plasma TNFα measurement. TNFα is thought to act primarily at a paracrine level, and a cell-bound form has been described (12,13). Circulating levels therefore represent "spillover" into the circulation of excess TNFα and the absence of TNFα in the circulation does not imply that TNFα is not involved in a disease process. Circulating TNFα inhibitors rapidly bind TNFα (14,15) and can interfere with its detection in assays, which further complicates the interpretation of these studies (16). In addition, TNFα has a relatively short circulation half-life (17) so that transiently raised levels may be missed. It is therefore not surprising that these studies have inconclusive results.

Interleukin-6 (IL-6)

IL-6 is produced by mononuclear phagocytes, endothelial cells, fibroblasts and T-cells in response to cytokines including TNFα and IL-1β (18). IL-6 plays an important role in inducing the change of priority in hepatocyte protein synthesis in response to various injurious stimuli. This results in the increased synthesis of acute phase proteins such as C-reactive protein, fibrinogen and α-1-antitrypsin and the decreased synthesis of albumin (18,19). Several authors have documented raised IL-6 levels in patients with severe pancreatitis. Leser and colleagues (20) described elevated levels of IL-6, measured by bioassay, in patients with complicated acute pancreatitis, with normal or slightly elevated levels of IL-6 in patients with mild attacks. Similar findings were reported by Viedma et al. (21) who measured IL-6 by ELISA and by Heath and colleagues (22) who used a bioassay.

What is unclear from these papers is the time course of the rise in plasma IL-6 and the variation which occurs between individual patients. Leser (20) described the pattern of IL-6 activity in two individual patients with severe disease, showing peak levels on day 1, falling thereafter in one patient and on day 3 in the second patient. It is not clear how accurately this reflects the findings in the remaining patients or how this relates to the time from onset of symptoms. In the study by Viedma et al. (21), persistently raised levels of IL-6 were found but there was no obvious peak in IL-6 levels during the 7 days of study. Heath et al. (22) corrected their results for the time from onset of symptoms and found that IL-6 levels peaked between 24 and 48 hours after symptom onset. However, it is unclear what degree of variation there was between individual patients.

The relationship between C-reactive protein and IL-6 levels has been studied, because the rise in plasma IL-6 has been proposed as the main stimulus to hepatic acute phase protein production. Peak IL-6 levels correlated with peak CRP levels in the studies by Heath et al. (22) and Leser et al. (20) with the peak in IL-6 preceding the peak in CRP by 1 day. However, conflicting results have been reported by other authors (21).

Interleukin-8

IL-8 is secreted by activated monocytes and macrophages and induces neutrophil aggregation and activation. The activation of neutrophils induced by TNFα is, at least in part, a consequence of the effect of TNFα on IL-8 secretion (23). Early studies suggest that plasma IL-8 levels are increased in patients with complicated attacks of acute pancreatitis (24) but, compared with IL-6 and TNF, little is known of the role of this cytokine in acute pancreatitis.

Interleukin 1 (IL-1β)

The main source of IL-1β is the mononuclear phagocyte although production by endothelial cells, neutrophils and B-lymphocytes has been reported (25). As with TNFα, endotoxin is the main stimulus to its production although IL-1β production is also induced by other stimuli, including TNFα (3). There have been no reports of raised levels of circulating IL-1β in patients with acute pancreatitis.

Other Mediators in Acute Pancreatitis

Platelet Activating Factors (PAF)

PAF is a cytokine released from endothelial cells, activated leukocytes and platelets which has potent effects on neutrophil activation and which has been implicated in the pathophysiology of acute pancreatitis (26,27). PAF can induce acute pancreatitis when injected into the pancreaticoduodenal artery in an experimental model (28). In a rodent model of acute pancreatitis (29), increased pulmonary PAF levels were associated with the development of lung injury and PAF antagonists are protective against the local and systemic changes of experimental pancreatitis (29–31). Recent clinical trials have demonstrated a reduction in organ failure scores in patients with acute pancreatitis treated with the PAF antagonist, lexipafant (32,33). These findings have been confirmed in a multicentre study which also showed a reduction in mortality and complications after early treatment with lexipafant.

Nitric Oxide

Nitric oxide (NO) is produced by endothelial cells, macrophages, activated neutrophils and other cells and is an important mediator of the inflammatory response. Increased production of NO has been demonstrated in patients with sepsis (34,35) and burn injury (36) and NO has been shown to mediate the haemodynamic effects of TNFα (37).

In experimental acute pancreatitis, NO has been reported to be increased only after lipopolysaccharide (LPS) injection (38) suggesting that it may be an important mediator of the systemic effects of endotoxaemia in acute pancreatitis. However, inhibition of NO does not appear to influence the progression from oedematous to necrotising experimental AP (39) and in another study, NO inhibition was actually reported to increase the pulmonary effects of acute pancreatitis (40).

Endotoxin in Acute Pancreatitis

For activated leucocytes to be responsible for the systemic manifestations of acute pancreatitis, a factor capable of inducing leucocyte activation must be present in these patients. Bacterial endotoxin is a potent activator of mononuclear phagocytes and it induces the secretion of cytokines including TNF, IL-6, IL-1 and IL-8.

The presence of endotoxaemia in acute pancreatitis was first reported in 1974 in three patients (41), with disappearance of endotoxin from the circulation when the illness resolved. In 1982 Foulis et al. (42) reported 24 patients with acute pancreatitis in whom serial assays of serum endotoxin were carried out (42). Endotoxin was detected on two consecutive days in half of the attacks of acute pancreatitis and in six of the seven patients who developed systemic complications.

The limulus amoebocyte lysate assay for endotoxin has certain limitations. Therefore assays have been developed which measure the immunological response to endotoxin, and so measuring indirectly endotoxin exposure. Kivilaakso et al. (43) measured titres of antibodies to the enterobacterial common antigen in a series of patients with acute pancreatitis. The enterobacterial common antigen is spatially related to the lipopolysaccharride component of the bacterial cell wall and it was argued that plasma levels of antibodies to this antigen were a measure of exposure to enteric bacteria and thence to endotoxin. The authors reported decreased titres on admission in those patients with complicated or fatal pancreatitis, with a rise in levels during the course of the illness in survivors, suggesting endotoxin exposure. However, in five of six patients with fatal pancreatitis no rise in anti-enterobacterial titres was observed, despite proven Gram-negative septicaemia in two cases. This exemplifies the difficulty in interpretation of such indirect methods of endotoxin measurement.

More recently, an assay has been developed to detect titres of an antibody to the core glycolipid portion of the endotoxin molecule. Depletion of the IgM anti-endotoxin antibody has been demonstrated in patients with both mild and severe pancreatitis and falling IgG levels have been linked with a poor prognosis (44). This contradicts the argument that raised titres are an indicator of endotoxin exposure but it has been suggested that antibody depletion results in increased exposure to free endotoxin. At the present time the complex relationship between endotoxin, its circulating inhibitors and leucocyte activation has not been clearly defined.

Role of the Reticuloendothelial System (RES) in Acute Pancreatitis

In health, portal endotoxin is rapidly removed from the circulation by the hepatic Kupffer cells, thus preventing systemic endotoxaemia (45). The failure of hepatic reticuloendothelial function results in what has been termed "spillover" of endotoxin into the systemic circulation (45). In this way, suppression of reticuloendothelial function, increased endotoxin load or a combination of both may be associated with the development of systemic endotoxaemia and the subsequent activation of systemic mononuclear phagocytes.

In experimental sepsis, systemic endotoxaemia was associated with decreased hepatic RES phagocytic function (46). Similarly, depressed RES function associated with systemic endotoxaemia has been demonstrated in patients with obstructive jaundice (47). As discussed above, acute pancreatitis is also associated with systemic endotoxaemia. In experimental acute pancreatitis, the suppression of reticuloendothelial function with oleic acid was reported to increase mortality (48). In another study, stimulation of the RES with glucan reduced mortality (49).

There is indirect evidence from clinical studies that the RES is either overwhelmed or its function is suppressed as raised levels of complexed α-2-macroglobulin, normally removed by the RES, are present in the circulation in patients with severe attacks (50).

Monocytes in Acute Pancreatitis

Monocytes and macrophages are the main source of the pro-inflammatory cytokines and the up-regulation of cytokine synthesis is thought to be an important step in the development of organ failure in acute pancreatitis. Our group has examined the secretion of pro-inflammatory cytokines by peripheral blood monocytes isolated from patients with acute pancreatitis (51). In this study, blood was withdrawn on the first, third and fifth days after admission in 26 patients with predicted severe pancreatitis. In patients who developed systemic

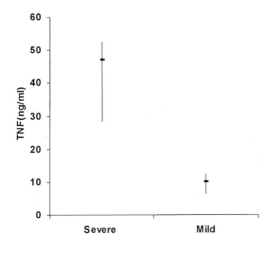

Figure 1. Peak tumour necrosis factor (TNFα) secretion by monocytes in acute pancreatitis. $P < 0.01$, Mann–Whitney U-test.

complications there was significantly greater production of TNFα, IL-8, IL-6 but not IL-1β when these cells were stimulated with endotoxin *in vitro* (TNFα data in Figure 1). This suggests that in patients with severe pancreatitis, monocytes are primed for an increased cytokine response. Workers in Edinburgh have reported similar results with regard to the secretion of IL-6 and IL-8 by peripheral blood mononuclear cells (52).

More recently we have measured monocyte free oxygen radical production as a further marker of monocyte priming. In 23 patients with predicted severe pancreatitis, we assessed intracellular H_2O_2 production by monocytes stimulated with phorbol myristate acetate (PMA). Significantly greater H_2O_2 production was observed in patients with acute pancreatitis when compared with healthy controls although there was no difference between patients with organ failure and those with uncomplicated attacks.

Neutrophil Function in Acute Pancreatitis

Many of the effects of TNFα, IL-8 and PAF on endothelial damage are mediated by activated neutrophils and each is associated with neutrophil priming *in vitro*. Widdison and Cunningham (53) reported increased neutrophil metabolic function in patients with acute pancreatitis compared with controls and suggested that this may be important in the development of organ failure.

We have recently reported the results of a study in which we measured neutrophil function in 23 patients with acute pancreatitis (54). Severe pancreatitis was associated with a significant increase in intracellular H_2O_2 production when compared with healthy controls. Similar levels of H_2O_2 production were seen in patients with sepsis. This increased respiratory burst was not a consequence of global neutrophil activation but was due to a subpopulation of primed neutrophils. As with monocyte respiratory burst, however, there was no association between the degree of neutrophil priming and the development of organ failure.

Conclusion

From the evidence presented here, there can be little doubt that the activation of monocytes, macrophages and neutrophils plays an important role in the development of the systemic complications of acute pancreatitis. However, it is still unclear what factors trigger the systemic activation of these cells resulting in the development of organ failure in some patients. It is also apparent that the presence of primed inflammatory cells in the peripheral blood is not in itself sufficient to induce organ failure.

It is likely that the monocyte and neutrophil priming which is seen in acute pancreatitis is a consequence of the normal inflammatory response to pancreatic damage in the early stages of acute pancreatitis and the extent of leucocyte priming may simply reflect the magnitude of the initial pancreatic insult. Patients with circulating primed cells may, however, be *at risk* of developing systemic complications if other factors contribute to the inflammatory response. In such patients, endotoxaemia as a result of splanchnic hypoperfusion and reticuloendothelial suppression, may induce further activation of circulating primed cells in systemic capillary beds. Ischaemia and subsequent reperfusion of the pancreas may cause the release of PAF into the systemic circulation which could cause the release of free oxygen radicals from primed neutrophils. It is also possible that spillover of pro-inflammatory cytokines such as TNFα and IL-8 could induce similar responses. In this hypothesis, organ failure in acute pancreatitis is not caused by any one factor but instead it may result from the presence of one of a number of possible systemic mediators acting on cells which are primed by exposure to small amounts of cytokines released in the early stages of pancreatic inflammation.

This hypothesis, if true, would suggest that prevention of organ failure in acute pancreatitis should be approached in several ways. Prevention of splanchnic hypoperfusion by adequate early resuscitation may help prevent systemic endotoxaemia. Antibiotics may also be indicated, particularly in the presence of gallstones where subclinical cholangitis is a possibility. Treatment with a PAF antagonist may help prevent further activation of primed neutrophils in the event of the release of PAF into the systemic circulation. Other approaches such as antiendotoxin and cytokine inhibitors and antioxidant supplements may also have a role as part of a multi-modality approach to treatment. It is hoped that further research will elucidate the nature of the relationship between cytokines, inflammatory cells and organ failure in acute pancreatitis and that this will lead to a therapeutic approach that reduces early mortality from this condition.

References

1. Rinderknecht H (1988) Fatal pancreatitis, a consequence of excessive leukocyte stimulation? Int J Pancreatol 3:105–112.
2. Aggarwal BB, Kohr WJ, Hasse PE et al. (1985) Human tumour necrosis factor production, purification and characterisation. J Biol Chem 260:2345–2354.
3. Tracey KL (1990) The role of cytokine mediators in septic shock. Adv Surg 23:21–56.
4. Shalaby MR, Aggarwal BB, Rinderknecht E et al. (1985) Activation of human polymorphonuclear functions by interferon gamma and tumour necrosis factor. J Immunol 135:2069–2073.
5. Moser L, Schleiffenbaum B, Groscurth P, Fehr J (1989) Interleukin-1 and tumour necrosis factor stimulate human vascular endothelial cells to promote transendothelial neutrophil passage. J Clin Invest 83:444–455.
6. Ulich TR, Castillo J, Keys M et al. (1987) Kinetics and mechanisms of recombinant human interleukin-1 and tumour necrosis factor α induced changes in circulating numbers of neutrophils and lymphocytes. J Immunol 139:3406–3415.
7. Gamble JR, Harlan JM, Kebanoff SJ et al. (1985) Stimulation of the adherence of neutrophils to umbilical vein endothelium by recombinant human tumour necrosis factor. Proc Natl Acad Sci USA 82:8667–8671.
8. Munker R, Gassoon J, Ogawa M et al. (1986) Recombinant human TNF induces production of granulocyte-macrophage colony stimulating factor. Nature 323:729–732.
9. Philip R, Epstein LB (1986) Tumour necrosis factor as immunomodulator and mediator of monocyte cytotoxicity induced by itself, gamma interferon and interleukin-1. Nature 323:86–89.
10. Banks RE, Evans SW, Alexander D, McMahon MJ, Whicher JT (1991) Is fatal pancreatitis a consequence of excessive leukocyte stimulation? The role of tumor necrosis factor alpha. Cytokine 3:12–16.
11. Exley AR, Leese T, Holliday MP, Swann RA, Cohen J (1992) Endotoxaemia and serum tumour necrosis factor as prognostic markers in severe acute pancreatitis. Gut 33:1126–1128.
12. Keogh C, Fong Y, Marano MA et al. (1990) Identification of a novel tumour necrosis factor from the livers of burned and infected rats. Arch Surg 125:79–85.
13. Peck R, Brockhaus M, Frey JR (1989) Cell-surface tumour necrosis factor (TNF) accounts for monocyte and lymphocyte mediated killing of TNF-resistant target cells. Cell Immunol 122:1–10.

14. Fernandez-Botran R (1991) Soluble cytokine receptors: their role in immunoregulation. FASEB J 5:2567–2574.
15. James KJ (1990) Interactions between cytokines and alpha-2-macroglobulin. Immunol Today 11:163–166.
16. McIntyre CA, Chapman K, Reeder S et al. (1992) Treatment of malignant melanoma and renal cell carcinoma with recombinant human interleukin-2: analysis of cytokine levels in sera and culture supernatants. Eur J Cancer 28:58–63.
17. Blick M, Sherwin S, Rosenbaum M et al (1987) Phase I study of recombinant tumour necrosis factor in cancer patients. Cancer Res 47:2986–2989.
18. Heinrich PC, Castell JV, Andus T (1990) Interleukin-6 and the acute phase response. Biochem J 265:621–636.
19. Nijsten MWN, DeGroot ER, TenDuis HJ (1987) Serum levels of interleukin-6 and acute phase responses. Lancet II:921.
20. Leser HG, Gross V, Scheibenbogen C et al. (1991) Elevation of serum interleukin-6 concentration precedes acute-phase response and reflects severity in acute pancreatitis. Gastroenterology 101:782–785.
21. Viedma JA, Perez-Mateo M, Dominguez JE, Carballo F (1992) Role of interleukin-6 in acute pancreatitis. Comparison with C-reactive protein and phospholipase A. Gut 33:1264–1267.
22. Heath DI, Cruickshank A, Gudgeon M, Jehanli A, Shenkin A, Imrie CW (1993) Role of interleukin-6 in mediating the acute phase protein response and potential as an early means of severity assessment in acute pancreatitis [see comments]. Gut 34:41–45.
23. DeForge LE, Kenney JS, Jones ML, Warren JS, Remick DG (1992) Biphasic production of IL-8 in lipopolysaccharide (LPS) stimulated human whole blood. J Immunol 148:2133–2141.
24. Gross V, Andreesen R, Leser HG et al. (1992) Interleukin-8 and neutrophil activation in acute pancreatitis. Eur J Clin Invest 22:200–203.
25. Dinarello CA (1984) Interleukin-1 and the pathogenesis of the acute phase response. N Engl J Med 311:1413–1418.
26. Ais G, Lopez Farre A, Gomez Garre DN et al. (1992) Role of platelet-activating factor in hemodynamic derangements in an acute rodent pancreatic model. Gastroenterology 102:181–187.
27. Bonavida B, Mencia-Huerta JM, Braquet P (1989) Effect of platelet activating factor (PAF) on monocyte activation and production of tumour necrosis factor (TNF). Allergy Appl Immunol 88:157–160.
28. Emanuelli G, Montrucchio G, Gaia E, Dughera L, Corvetti G, Gubetta L (1989) Experimental acute pancreatitis induced by platelet activating factor in rabbits. Am J Pathol 134:315–326.
29. Zhou W, McCollum MO, Levine BA, Olson MS (1992) Role of platelet-activating factor in pancreatitis-associated acute lung injury in the rat. Am J Pathol 140:971–979.
30. Tomaszewska R, Dembinski A, Warzecha Z, Banas M, Konturek SJ, Stachura J (1992) Platelet activating factor (PAF) inhibitor (TCV-309) reduces caerulein- and PAF-induced pancreatitis. A morphologic and functional study in the rat. J Physiol Pharmacol 43:345–352.
31. Formela LJ, Wood LM, Whittaker M, Kingsnorth AN (1994) Amelioration of experimental acute pancreatitis with a potent platelet-activating factor antagonist. Br J Surg 81:1783–1785.
32. Kingsnorth AN, Galloway SW, Formela LJ (1995) Randomised, double-blind phase II trial of lexipafant, a platelet-activating factor antagonist, in human acute pancreatitis. Br J Surg 82:1414–1420.
33. McKay C (1996) The use of lexipafant in the treatment of acute pancreatitis. In: Nigam S, Kunkel G, Prescott S (eds) Platelet activating factor and related lipid mediators in health and disease. Plenum Press, New York, pp 365–370.
34. Tanjoh K, Shima A, Aida M, Tomita R, Kurosu Y (1995) Nitric oxide and active oxygen species in severe sepsis and surgically stressed patients. Surg Today 25:774–777.
35. Endo S, Inada K, Nakae H et al. (1996) Nitrite/nitrate oxide (NOx) and cytokine levels in patients with septic shock. Res Comm Molec Pathol Pharmacol 91:347–356.
36. Preiser JC, Reper P, Vlasselaer D et al. (1996) Nitric oxide production is increased in patients after burn injury. J Trauma Injury, Infect Crit Care 40:368–371.
37. Baudry N, Vicaut E (1993) Role of nitric oxide in effects of tumor necrosis factor-alpha on microcirculation in rat. J Appl Physiol 75:2392–2399.
38. Kikuchi Y, Shimosegawa T, Satoh A et al. (1996) The role of nitric oxide in mouse ceruleininduced pancreatitis with and without lipopolysaccharide pretreatment. Pancreas 12:68–75.
39. Weidenbach H, Lerch MM, Gress TM, Pfaff D, Turi S, Adler G. (1995) Vasoactive mediators and the progression from oedematous to necrotising experimental acute pancreatitis. Gut 37:434–440.

40. O'Donovan DA, Kelly CJ, Abdih H et al. (1995) Role of nitric oxide in lung injury associated with experimental acute pancreatitis. Br J Surg 82:1122–1126.

41. Fossard DP, Kakkar VV, Elsey PA (1974) Assessment of limulus test for detecting endotoxaemia. Br Med J II:465–468.

42. Foulis AK, Murray WR, Galloway D et al. (1982) Endotoxaemia and complement activation in acute pancreatitis in man. Gut 23:656–661.

43. Kivilaakso E, Valtonen VV, Malkamaki M et al. (1984) Endotoxaemia and acute pancreatitis: correlation between the severity of disease and the anti-enterobacterial common antigen titre. Gut 25:1065–1070.

44. Windsor JA, Fearon KC, Ross JA et al. (1993) Role of serum endotoxin and antiendotoxin core antibody levels in predicting the development of multiple organ failure in acute pancreatitis. Br J Surg 80:1042–1046.

45. Bradfield J (1974) Control of spillover. The importance of Kupffer-cell function in clinical medicine. Lancet II:883–886.

46. Jones GE, Purves LR, de Chalain TMB et al. (1989) Reticuloendothelial function and plasma fibronectin in a murine model of intra-abdominal sepsis. J Hepatol 9:287–294.

47. Pain J (1987) Reticuloendothelial function in obstructive jaundice. Br J Surg 74:1091–1094.

48. Adham NF, Song MK, Haberfelde GC (1983) Relationship between the functional status of the reticuloendothelial system and the outcome of experimentally induced pancreatitis in young mice. Gastroenterology 84:461–469.

49. Browder IW, Sherwood E, Williams D, Jones E, McNamee R, diLuzio N (1987) Protective effect of glucan-enhanced macrophage function in experimental pancreatitis. Am J Surg 153:25–33.

50. Banks RE, Evans SW, Alexander D, van Leuvin F, Whicher JT, McMahon MJ (1991) Alpha-2-macroglobulin state in acute pancreatitis. Raised values of alpha-2-macroglobulin-protease complexes in severe and mild attacks. Gut 32:430–434.

51. McKay CJ, Gallagher G, Brooks B, Imrie CW, Baxter JN (1996) Increased monocyte cytokine production in association with systemic complications in acute pancreatitis. Br J Surg 83:919–923.

52. de Beaux AC, Ross JA, Maingay JP, Fearon KCH, Carter DC (1996). Proinflammatory cytokine release by peripheral blood mononuclear cells from patients with acute pancreatitis. Br J Surg 83:1071–1075.

53. Widdison AL, Cunningham S (1996) Immune function early in acute pancreatitis. Br J Surg 83:633–636.

54. Sinclair M, McKay C, Sharples C, McArthy A, Imrie C (1997) Patients with severe acute pancreatitis have increased priming of peripheral blood neutrophils. Br J Surg 84:4(abstract).

3 Therapeutic Plasma Exchange in Severe Acute Necrotising Pancreatitis

S. Mann, A. Agha, U. Mann, J. Schmidt and H. Zirngibl

Multiple organ failure (MOF) is the most frequent reason for a fatal outcome in severe acute necrotising pancreatitis (SAP). The pathophysiological pathways of SAP remain uncertain. In a retrospective study of 161 patients with necrotising pancreatitis admitted to the surgical department of the University in Erlangen, Germany, we demonstrated that there was no correlation between the extent of the extrapancreatic necroses and hospital mortality rate. However, there was a correlation between hospital mortality rate and the number of organ failures (1). In this group patients with no organ failure presented a mortality rate of 6%, patients with one or two organ failures had an overall mortality rate between 40% and 50%; 80% of patients with three organ failures died and the mortality rate was 100% in patients having four organs in severe distress.

The clinical course of SAP presents with two phases: in the first phase a systemic inflammatory response syndrome (SIRS) develops, finally ending in multiple organ failure. Inflammatory overfunction of the immunologically competent systems leads to their complete derangement. Specific antibodies and inhibitory proteases of cytokines are consumed rapidly. Macromolecular cytokine inhibitor complexes cannot be cleared by the reticuloendothelial system (RES) in the liver. High endogenous catecholamine output and dysfunction of the haemostatic system lead to a microcirculatory failure of the main abdominal organs and the brain.

In the second phase of SAP when necroses develop, mainly septic complications and immunological paralysis may be observed. As within this phase the microcirculation is maximally impaired, current therapeutic concepts are focused on the restoration of microcirculatory perfusion. Specific therapies like anti-proteases, anti-cytokines or even other immunologically competent agents have not shown positive effects on the course of SAP. Based on this knowledge, in the early 1980s therapeutic plasma exchange was introduced as a non-specific treatment to extract macromolecular paraproteins or proteins from the plasma of patients with SAP in order to clear the vasoactive mediators that stimulate inflammation. The substituted FFP (fresh frozen plasma) may give additional support to the inhibitor pool. After therapeutic plasma exchange (TPE) the disproportion of pro- and anti-inflammatory mediators should become restored to the normal range after a short time. This therapy may somehow partially reset the systemic inflammatory response so that the patient can find the opportunity to control the situation and to run down MOF. Good results of TPE in single cases of SAP or SIRS have been already reported by several authors (2–17).

Experimental Work

An animal experiment was started in 1985. The effects of therapeutic plasma exchange during SAP were studied in male mongrel dogs. The first group served as control in which plasma exchange was tested in the healthy dog. In the second group SAP induced by instillation of taurocholic acid into the pancreas was treated by therapeutic plasma exchange. The last group had SAP as in group 2 and did not receive plasma exchange. After 7 hours the animals were killed. In all groups extensive cardiovascular monitoring, laboratory tests of arterial and venous blood together with separated plasma and ascites were performed every 30 minutes. In the SAP group treated by therapeutic plasma exchange, heart frequency rate, cardiac output, mean arterial pressure, mean venous pressure, peripheral and pulmonary resistance were within normal ranges. On the histological examination within this group there were only marginal reactions within lung, kidneys, the heart and the liver. The difference from the SAP group without plasma exchange was highly significant. In summary we could demonstrate in the animal experiment that organ failure could be prevented by therapeutic plasma exchange (18–20).

Clinical Data

A pilot study started in 1989 which included 11 patients with SAP having an expected mortality of 80% at admission. Therapeutic plasma exchange was performed with a mean of 12 sessions per patient. Mean organ failure was 2.9. Ten of these 11 patients survived, one died.

Stimulated by these encouraging results a prospective two-centre-trial was started in 1992 in which patients with early SAP and multiple organ dysfunction syndrome (MODS) were randomised either to therapeutic plasma exchange or to standard intensive care. SAP was defined when necroses were present at more than 30% and at least one organ failure was noted. Surgical treatment was not performed in the early phase of SAP. When infection of necrosis was apparent,

Table 1. Clinical features of patients so far recruited to the study

	SAP with plasmapheresis (mean age 48 years)	SAP without plasmapheresis (mean age 65 years)
Biliary	3	4
Alcoholic	3	1
Idiopathic	1	1
Total	7	6
Necroses < 30%	2	2
Necroses 30–50%	2	3
Necroses > 50%	3	1

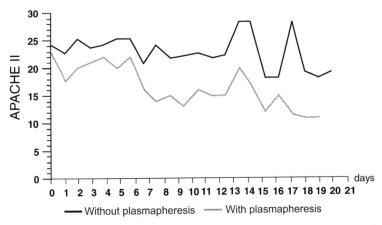

Figure 1. Mean APACHE II score in patients randomised to plasma exchange or control.

computed tomography (CT)-guided catheters were placed and in some cases even necrosectomy was performed radiologically. The study is not yet concluded. The first clinical results demonstrate that the expected mortality of SAP with multiple organ failure seems to be reduced dramatically by therapeutic plasma exchange. At present there are 13 patients included. The mean age in the group which received plasmapheresis was 40 years and in the group without plasmapheresis was 65 years (Table 1). There was a significant drop of APACHE II score in the plasmapheresis group from 23 to 10 within 3 weeks, whereas patients without plasmapheresis presented APACHE II scores of 20 after the same period of time. Figure 1 shows the evolution of the APACHE II score (mean) in both groups of patients with and without plasma exchange. There was a statistically significant difference between both groups ($P < 0.01$).

Within 3 weeks pulmonary failure had resolved in six of seven patients in the plasmapheresis group whereas in the other group this was only possible in one of five cases. Figure 2 shows the differences in duration of ventilation and intensive care in both groups. There was a significant difference noted ($P < 0.01$).

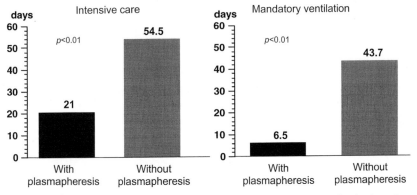

Figure 2. Duration of intensive care and artificial ventilation in patients randomised to plasma exchange or control.

Table 2. Operative interventions in patients entered into the study

Surgical therapy: plasmapheresis	After (days)	SAP with plasmapheresis	SAP without plasmapheresis
Necrosectomy	29	1	–
	13	1	–
	44	–	1
Programmed lavage	41	–	1
Necrosectomy + lavage	42	–	1

Although nearly every patient had interventionally placed drainages within the necroses it was not possible to reduce the septicaemia efficiently in five patients. In these cases surgical necrosectomy was performed. In the plasmapheresis group one patient (of seven) died and in the group without plasmapheresis four (of six) patients died. In the plasma monitoring we noted a reduced level of TNF receptor p55 and p75, in contrast to patients with therapeutic plasma exchange during SAP. High cytokine levels (IL-1 and IL-6) could be seen as signs of the severity of the disease and these correlated with the outcome of the patients. The same happens with TNF-α levels that may be observed throughout the disease and are noted to be strictly activated. This parameter also correlates directly with the patients' outcomes.

Summary and Conclusion

In SAP the inhibitor pool of cellular immunological response may not control the development of MOF. The extensive microcirculatory changes combined with decreased oxygen delivery to the organs causing reduced energy production finally leads to a total collapse. On the other hand the clearance of inhibitor complexes is maximally decreased, so that these vasoactive substances accumulate. Schranz and Bartels (14) published five cases of SAP and Larvin et al. (6) reported two cases where therapeutic plasma exchange showed favourable effects on the course of the disease. Bambauer (2) and Tobin and Fahy (16) confirmed these observations as well as several other authors in many case reports (3–17).

In the literature there are no prospective randomised trials available dealing with therapeutic plasma exchange in SAP. Gebhardt et al. (21) reported about 140 patients with severe acute necrotising pancreatitis where in 11 cases a continuous venovenous haemofiltration was applied when multiple organ failure was present. In this group one patient died. Similar results were presented by Miller et al. (22). In a subgroup where patients with SAP underwent haemofiltration ($n = 7$) five survived and two died. In the past 5 years several studies of plasmapheresis in SAP from Russia have also reported comparable good results (23–25).

We believe that therapeutic plasma exchange in the early course of SAP represents the most effective therapy to prevent the development of MOF. We finally conclude that plasmapheresis shows positive effects on the course of SAP as a first trend. As our patient groups are too small, statistical statements are not possible at this point. Primarily elevated cytokine levels reflect the severity of the disease and correlate directly with its clinical course. A randomised multicentre study is planned.

References

1. Zirngibl H, Mann S, Braun G (1993) Plasma separation and hemofiltration in acute necrotizing pancreatitis. In Beger, Büchler Malfertheiner (eds) Standards in pancreatic surgery. Springer, Berlin, pp 171–182.
2. Bambauer R (1988) Therapeutischer Plasmaaustausch und verwandte Plasmaseparationsverfahren. Schattauer Verlag, Stuttgart, pp 189–190.
3. Busund R, Rekvig OP, Lindsetmo R-O, Rokke O, Revhaug A (1990) Plasma exchange with albumin as replacement fluid in septicemia. An experimental study on survival and circulatory performance. Surg Res Comm 8:289–301.
4. Gardlund B, Sjolin J, Nilsson A, Roll M, Wickerts C-J, Wikstrom B, Wretlind B (1993) Plasmapheresis in the treatment of primary septic shock in humans. Scand J Infect Dis 25:757–761.
5. Janbon B, Vuillez JP, Carpentier F, Barnoud D, Andrepoyaud P, Barbe G, Guignier M (1992) Removal of circulating tumor necrosis factor: its role in septic shock treatment. Ann Med Interne 143:13–16.
6. Larwin M, Landsdown MRJ, Mcmahon MJ, Chalmers AG, Turner JH, Brownjohn AM (1988) Plasmapheresis: a rational treatment for fulminant acute pancreatitis? Br Med J: 288:297–593.
7. McClelland P, Williams PS, Yaqoob M, Mostafa SM, Bone JM (1990) Multiple organ failure: a role for plasma exchange? Intensive Care Med 16:100–103.
8. Nieter B, Sisova S, Klug C et al. (1991) Plasma exchange in septic-toxic diseases. Nieren- und Hochdruckkrankheiten 20:155–159.
9. Pollack M (1992) Blood exchange and plasmapheresis in sepsis and septic shock. Clin Infect Dis 15:432–433.
10. Rokke O, Rolf S, Revhaug A, Rekvig OP (1993) Plasma exchange, but not extracorporal recirculation nor removal of white blood cells, depresses plasma levels of IL-1 during severe Gram-negative septicemia. Transfusion Sci 14:173–182.
11. Rokke O, Rekvig OP, Giercksky K-E, Revhaug A (1990) Changes in the activity of polymorphonuclear granulocytes during septicemia and the influence of early plasma exchange. Surg Res Comm 8:63–72.
12. Rokke O, Rekvig OP, Lundgren TI, Revhaug A (1990) The treatment of severe Gram-negative septicemia with plasma exchange: Effects mediated by extracorporeal recirculation. Surg Res Comm 8:183–194.
13. Rokke O, Rasmussen L-T, Giercksky KE, Seljelid R, Rekvig OP, Revhaug A (1990) The influence of plasma exchange on shock mediators in septicemia. Surg Res Comm 8:173–182.
14. Schranz W, Bartels O (1986) Frühzeitiger Plasmaaustausch bei akuter Pankreatitis: Ein erfolgreiches Therapiekonzept bei extremer Hyperlipidämie. Fortschr Med 104:530–532.
15. Stegmayr BG, Jakobsen S, Rydvall A, Bjorsell-Ostling E (1995) Plasma exchange in patients with acute renal failure in the course of multiorgan failure. Int J Artif Org 18:45–52.
16. Tobin MV, Fahy LT (1988) Plasmapheresis and fulminant acute pancreatitis. Br Med J 288:297–979.
17. Zilow EP, Selle B, Zilow G (1994) Plasmapheresis in severe septic shock with disseminated intravascular coagulation. In: Sibrowski W, Stangel W, Wegener S (eds) Beiträge zur Infusionstherapie und Transfusionsmedizin. Band 32. Transfusionsmedizin S. Karger, Basel, pp 374–377.
18. Zirngibl H, Schild A, Werner B, Mann S, Köppendörfer H (1987) Phospholipase A in Serum and Aszites bei tierexperimenteller akuter Pankreatitis. Klinische Chemie (Clin Chem). Z Dtsch Ges. Klin. Chem 5:244–246.
19. Zirngibl H, Mann S, Schild A, Zech M (1989) Phospholipase A activities in ascites, serum, lymph, and urine in acute pancreatitis following pancreas stimulation with secretin: ceruletid. Klin Wochenschr 67:141–143.
20. Zirngibl H, Werner B, Braun G, Mann S (1987) Die Bedeutung der Plasmaseparation in der Behandlung der akuten nekrotisierenden Pankreatitis: eine tierexperimentelle Studie. Demeter Verlag, Gräfelfing Abstraktband der Deutschen Gesellschaft für Chirurgie (18).

21. Gebhardt C, Bödeker H, Blinzler L, Kraus D, Hergdt G (1994) Changes in the therapy of severe acute pancreatitis. Chirurgie 62:33–40; Discussion 40–41.

22. Miller BJ, Henderson A, Strong RW, Fielding GR, Dimacoar M, Oloughlin S (1994) Necrotising pancreatitis: operating for life. World J Surg 18:906–910.

23. Zaitsev VT, Krivoruchko IA, Klimova EM, Gusak IV, Khizhniak AA, Shaposhnikov GA (1993) Plasmapheresis and immunocorrective therapy in the combined treatment of patients with pancreatic necrosis. Klin Khir 11:3–5.

24. Neimark II, Ovchinnikov VA (1991) Experience with using extracorporal methods of detoxification in acute diseases of the organs of the abdominal cavity. Vestn Khir-Im-I-I-Grek 146:86–90.

25. Manucharov NK, Tavdidishvili IuD, AkhvledianiEN, Sychev MD, Tomaev KB, Kiladze MM (1991) The choice of an adequate method of detoxication and immunocorrection in destructive experimental pancreatitis. Biull Eksp Biol Med 112:517–519.

4 Prediction of Severity in Acute Pancreatitis

C.D. Johnson and S. Toh

Early assessment of the patient with acute pancreatitis leading to an accurate prediction of severe outcome is useful for two reasons. First, and better established, is the need to categorise groups of patients to allow comparison of published series, and to generate groups at risk of complications for clinical trials. Second, and only recently relevant, is the need to identify patients who are individually at risk of complications so that effective preventive management can be started before those complications develop.

A severe attack of pancreatitis is defined as one in which a complication has occurred (1). Complications may be systemic, that is failure of an organ or system distant from the pancreas, or local, which are probably all secondary to necrosis of pancreatic or peripancreatic tissues. Pancreatic necrosis is usually accompanied by at least one organ failure, often respiratory. Care must be taken to distinguish between features which diagnose severity, such as hypoxaemia or CT evidence of necrosis, and truly predictive markers of severity which precede objective evidence of complications.

The features which predict a severe outcome can be categorised as clinical, related to pancreatic enzyme activation, or inflammatory. In addition, there are disturbances of physiological and biochemical processes which can be demonstrated by simple clinical and laboratory measurement. These are often combined into multiple factor scoring systems.

Clinical Features

It is well established that subjective clinical assessment is inaccurate in predicting severity at the time of admission to hospital (2,3). This is because at that early stage in the disease, incipient organ failure is difficult to recognise clinically. Early clinical assessment is reasonably specific but has a very poor sensitivity. By 48 hours after admission, the sensitivity improves, and matches that achieved by multiple factor scoring systems. However, the accuracy of clinical assessment depends entirely on the experience and judgement of the clinical team, and it is difficult to standardise. A number of specific clinical features are associated with a severe outcome. Subcutaneous fat necrosis and body wall bruising are both individually associated with severe outcome. Subcutaneous fat necrosis is extremely rare and is thus of limited clinical usefulness. Body wall bruising is also uncommon, but is strongly predictive of poor outcome with a high risk of death in these patients (4). However, its appearance is often delayed by 2–4 days after onset of symptoms. This combined with its infrequent occurrence makes it of limited clinical usefulness.

Obesity

Several studies have demonstrated that obesity is strongly associated with the development of complications. Lankisch and Schirren (5) have demonstrated that patients with complications had a greater mean body mass index (BMI; kg/m²) than those who did not. Subsequently, others (6,7) showed that BMI > 30 was associated with an increased risk of complications, and death (7). We have confirmed these observations, and in a series of 186 patients we were able to demonstrate that even minor elevation of BMI (26–30) increases the risk of complications (Figure 1).

Radiological Markers

Appearances of the plain abdominal radiograph in acute pancreatitis are non-specific and do not help to predict outcome. The chest radiograph may show pulmonary infiltrates or basal pleural effusions, and both these signs have been associated with a severe outcome (8,9). The assessment of pulmonary infiltrates is potentially subjective, and pleural effusion is probably a more reliable marker. Left-sided or bilateral effusions on chest radiograph within 24 hours of admission were associated with a 76% and 88% risk of complications, and a 14% and a 42% risk of death, respectively (8).

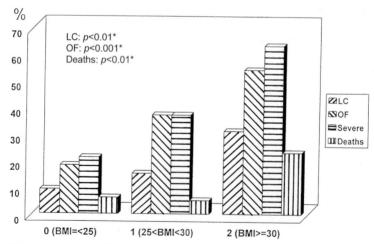

Figure 1. Relationship between BMI and outcome. Local complications (LC), organ failure (OF), all severe cases and deaths increased significantly with increasing BMI (*n* = 186).

Computed Tomography

Signs of pancreatitis on computed tomography (CT) are well known, and have been used to categorise severity (10,11). Strictly, when considering prediction of severity, it is necessary to separate early potentially reversible features such as fluid collections from features diagnostic of a complication such as failure of enhancement (i.e. necrosis). CT is extremely accurate for the diagnosis of local complications but its predictive value early in the course of the disease is limited, mainly due to the lack of specificity in the early stages (12,13).

Markers of Enzyme Activation and Release

It is well established that acute pancreatitis is diagnosed by detection of marked elevation of plasma levels of pancreatic enzymes. Amylase and lipase are the most frequently used for this. It is clear that the height of elevation of these enzymes is unreliable for prediction of severity or monitoring of progress. However, plasma levels of proteases may be more useful, although the assay systems needed are more demanding and are not commercially available for clinical application. Serum trypsinogen 2 has been reported to differentiate patients with complications with a sensitivity of 91% and a specificity of 71% (14). Pancreatic phospholipase has also been proposed as a marker of severity (15).

Activation Peptides

Pancreatic enzymes are synthesised as inactive proenzymes in which the active site is masked by a peptide chain of varying length. Cleavage of this peptide chain (activation peptide) exposes the active site of the enzyme. Activation peptides are generally short (the activation peptide of trypsin (TAP) contains only three amino acids), although that for carboxypeptidase B (CAPAP) is larger with a molecular weight of 10 kDa. These peptides are therefore more diffusible than the parent enzyme, and as they are released in a proportional amount to the number of molecules activated they have been proposed as markers of the extent of pancreatic injury (Figure 2).

TAP was the first of these activation peptides to be tested in clinical practice with promising results (16). Subsequent development of the assay has confirmed

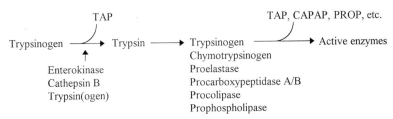

Figure 2. Production of activation peptides. Activation of trypsinogen releases TAP, and trypsin which activates all pancreatic proenzymes.

that high urinary levels of TAP are associated with a severe outcome (17) but this assay is still only available in a research-based format.

The activation peptide of prophospholipase (PROP) has also been proposed with promising preliminary results (18), but these require further validation.

The CAPAP is a promising marker of severity, partly because its greater molecular weight leads to a longer plasma half-life and less rapid fluctuation of plasma and urinary concentrations. An initial study (19) has shown a clear separation of urinary and serum CAPAP levels in patients with severe pancreatitis, using samples obtained within 3 days of onset of symptoms and within 48 hours of admission.

Further rapid progress appears likely in this field as various activation peptide assays are developed for clinical application.

Antiproteases

Release of activated proteases into the circulation is rapidly countered by binding of proteases to circulating antiproteases. These complexes are then cleared from the circulation, leading to depletion of the antiprotease. However, the complex interplay between the amount of activated protease released, initial circulating levels, and the rate of replenishment limits the value of antiprotease levels for prediction of severity. Estimation of $\alpha2$-macroglobulin can give some predictive information but it is less useful than other easily available markers (20).

Markers of the Immune Response

Current understanding of the mechanism of organ failure in acute pancreatitis invokes excessive stimulation of the immune response leading to the systemic immune response syndrome (SIRS). Factors thought likely to be involved in this chain of events include translocation of bacteria or absorption of endotoxin, stimulation of tumour necrosis factor alpha (TNFα) release from white cells, activation of neutrophils and production of various interleukins, particularly IL-8 and IL-6. This last then stimulates an acute phase protein response from the liver most easily identified by elevation of C-reactive protein concentration in plasma.

TNF Receptors

Demonstration of circulating endotoxin, and associated elevation of TNF levels in some patients with severe pancreatitis has been well documented. However, measurement of TNF is difficult and its release is intermittent, so many samples, even in patients with severe disease, have TNF levels below the limit of detection. When TNF binds to target cells the cells become unresponsive to further stimulation by shedding the TNF/TNF receptor complex. This soluble TNF receptor is more stable and has a longer half-life than TNF and can be demonstrated in high concentrations in patients with severe pancreatitis (21). Indeed there was good separation between the three groups of mild pancreatitis, those with organ failure, and patients with pancreatic necrosis.

Table 1. Diagnostic sensitivity and specificity of different pancreatic enzymes in the diagnosis of acute pancreatitis. Data are expressed as ranges reported in the literature. Further discussed in reference 29

	Sensitivity (%)	Specificity (%)
Total amylase	67–100	85–98
P-Lipase	67–100	83–98
Lipase	82–100	82–100
Trypsin	89–100	79–83
Elastase	97–100	79–96

Polymorphonuclear Neutrophil Elastase (PNME)

This marker of neutrophil activation is released early in the course of severe acute pancreatitis and had a positive predictive value for severe outcome of 75–80% (22,23). Although not all studies have been in agreement, because the predictive results depend on the assay system used, there is now substantial evidence that early estimation of PNME can provide a reliable prediction of severity (Table 1).

Interleukins (IL)

These inflammatory mediators are involved in the early events of the inflammatory response to injury, and are released in excess in the SIRS. A study of ERCP-induced acute pancreatitis has shown that IL-8 is released very early, and peaks within the first 12 hours after the causative stimulus (24). Although IL-8 has been suggested as a potential marker of severity, the rapid decline of IL-8 levels after 12 hours in this study suggests that its peak will be too early to be of clinical usefulness, given that most patients with acute pancreatitis present to hospital much later than 12 hours after of onset of symptoms.

IL-6 has been known for some time to be elevated in patients who will develop complications (25,26); however, estimation of this mediator is difficult and no clinically applicable assay system is available at present.

C-reactive Protein (CRP)

The acute phase protein response from the liver begins after the early peak of IL-6. The peak levels occur 48 to 96 hours after onset of symptoms, but because of the frequent delay in presentation to hospital elevated levels of CRP may be seen within the first 48 hours of admission in patients who subsequently develop complications (27,28,29). Current consensus is that a cut-off level of 120 mg/l within the first 48 hours of symptoms is extremely sensitive (90%) with an acceptable positive predictive value (29).

Multiple Factor Scoring Systems

A number of multiple factor scoring systems have been developed for assessing the severity of illness in patients suffering trauma, sepsis, or who need intensive therapy, in addition to the Ranson and Glasgow scoring systems which were devised specifically for acute pancreatitis. The general system which has emerged as most useful in the prediction of severe pancreatitis is the APACHE II score.

The Ranson and Glasgow Scores

Observation of multiple physiological and biochemical variables in patients with acute pancreatitis enabled the identification of a number of a factors which could be combined into a scoring system. These systems reflected the desire to quantify the subjective clinical assessment for detection or prediction of patients at risk of complications. Both the Ranson (30) and the Glasgow (31) systems categorise patients as predicted severe pancreatitis on the basis of three or more abnormal features observed within the first 48 hours of admission to hospital. Both systems were subsequently modified to improve sensitivity in patients with gallstones and the modified Glasgow system (32) has found widespread acceptance. These systems can identify patients who subsequently developed complications with sensitivity and overall accuracy in the region of 75–80%.

The multiple scoring systems are cumbersome to use and various attempts have been made to reduce their complexity. However, these have been generally unsuccessful, probably because the originators of the scoring systems required to incorporate many factors in order to achieve acceptable accuracy.

APACHE II

The main disadvantage of the Ranson and Glasgow scores is the need to collect data for 48 hours before a complete assessment can be made. Early assessment therefore lacks sensitivity although specificity will be high. The APACHE II system has found widespread acceptance in general intensive care, with scores on admission correlating well with outcome. It is now becoming clear that application of APACHE II within the first 24 hours of admission can give as good a prediction of severity as the Ranson and Glasgow scores (33,34) and performed well in clinical trials (35). Larvin and McMahon (33) showed that APACHE II was superior to other sepsis scores in this regard. Our own experience confirms these findings with a positive predictive value of 71% and an overall accuracy of 80% when a cut-off value > 9 is used.

Addition of further clinical features with specific independent predictive value in acute pancreatitis, such as obesity, can improve the predictive value of APACHE II. We categorised obesity on the basis of BMI score (26–30 = 1; > 30 = 2). The composite of this score added to APACHE II gave superior predictive values to APACHE II alone (Figure 3).

Categories and Probabilities

The multiple factor scoring systems have been specifically designed to assess the risk of complications in groups of patients with severe pancreatitis, and to categorise patients into groups at high risk. Their developers all point out that they

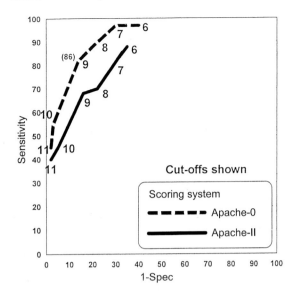

Figure 3. Receiver operating characteristic curve demonstrating the relative accuracies, APACHE-II and the sum of BMI score plus APACHE-II (APACHE-0) in 186 patients with acute pancreatis; numbers on the curves are the various cut-off values tested.

are not appropriate for directing management decisions in individual patients. Furthermore the categorisation of patients into a "predicted severe" group tends to mask the inherent inaccuracy (20–25%) of the prediction, and confusion may arise between predicted severity, and actual severity, which is based on outcome.

When no specific treatment existed which could prevent the onset of complications, these categorical predictive scores were sufficient to allow comparison between different groups of patients in published series, and to select high-risk groups of patients for clinical trials. We have now entered a new era in the treatment of severe acute pancreatitis, with several possible preventive strategies aimed at limiting the number of patients who develop complications. These are discussed elsewhere in this volume, and include endoscopic sphincterotomy, prophylactic antibiotics, enteral nutrition, and the platelet-activating factor antagonist lexipafant. Clearly there is now a need for a predictive system which will be suitable for assessing the risk of individual patients and assisting in individual management decisions.

We have begun to address this requirement by developing a logistic model using the three independent factors of age, obesity score, and the acute physiology score component of APACHE II. This calculation uses information which is readily available within the first 24 hours of admission, and can be easily performed with a hand-held scientific calculator. The outcome of the calculation is a probability value for the individual's risk of developing a complication. Initial assessment of this tool is encouraging, with a 20% incidence of complications in those with a predicted risk < 30%, and 67% incidence in those with a predicted risk > 60% (37).

Individual markers of severity such as measurement of CRP may be also be helpful for individual patients, but once again they categorise patients into high risk or low risk groups. It may be that a calculation of individual probability of complications will help to focus attention on the inherent inaccuracy of any predictive marker or system. Decisions about instituting therapy should be based on a clear assessment of risk for the individual patient.

Conclusion

Prediction of outcome in severe acute pancreatitis has moved into a new phase, with the availability of effective preventive strategies which can limit the number of patients developing complications. This has given urgency to the need to develop effective and accurate markers of severe outcome early in the course of the disease. To be of value, a prediction must be accurate within 48 hours of onset of symptoms, or within 24 hours of admission to hospital. Of the individual markers of severity, those which are clinically useful at present are obesity (BMI > 30), left-sided or bilateral pleural effusions, and C-reactive protein > 120 mg/l. The APACHE II system seems the best of the multiple factor scores because of its earlier availability, and because different cut-offs can be chosen for appropriate manipulation of sensitivity and positive predictive value. In future it may be that prediction will become more orientated towards individual risk assessment and we are moving away from categorisation into predicted severity groups.

References

1. Bradley E (1993) A clinically based classification system for acute pancreatitis: summary of the Atlanta International Symposium. Arch Surg 128:586–590.
2. McMahon MJ, Playforth MJ, Pickford IR (1980) A comparative study of methods for prediction of severity of attacks of acute pancreatitis. Br J Surg 67:22–25.
3. Corfield AP, Cooper MJ, Williamson RCN et al. (1985) Prediction of severity in acute pancreatitis: a prospective comparison of three prognostic indices. Lancet ii: 403–406.
4. Dickson AP, Imrie CW (1984) The incidence and prognosis of body wall echymosis in acute pancreatitis. Surg Gynecol Obstet 159:343–347.
5. Lankisch PG, Schirren CA (1990) Increased body weight as a prognostic parameter for complications in the course of acute pancreatitis. Pancreas 5:626–629.
6. Porter KA, Banks PA (1991) Obesity as a predictor of severity in acute pancreatitis. Int J Pancreatol 10:247–252.
7. Funnell IC, Hornman PC, Weakley SO, Terblanche J, Marks IN (1993) Obesity: an important prognostic factor in acute pancreatitis. Br J Surg 80:484–486.
8. Talamini G, Bassi C, Falconi M et al. (1996) Risk of death from acute pancreatitis. Int J Pancreatol 19:15–24
9. Pezzilli R et al. (1996) Chest X-ray in severity prediction in acute pancreatitis. Digestion 57:254
10. Balthazar EJ (1989) CT diagnosis and staging of acute pancreatitis. Radiol Clin North Am 27:19–37.
11. Balthazar EJ, Robinson DL, Megibow AJ, Ranson JH (1990) Acute pancreatitis: value of CT in establishing prognosis. Radiology 174:331–336.
12. Vesentini S, Bassi C, Talamini G Cavallini G, Campedelli A, Pederzoli P (1993) Prospective comparison of C-reactive protein level. Ranson score and contrast-enhanced computed tomography in the prediction of septic complications of acute pancreatitis. Br J Surg 80:755–757.
13. Kemppainen E, Sainio R, Haapiainen R, Kivisaari L, Kivilaakso E, Puolakkainen P (1996) Early localisation of necrosis by contrast-enhanced computed tomography can predict outcome in severe acute pancreatitis. Br J Surg 83:924–929.
14. Sainio V, Puolakkainen P, Kemppainen E et al. (1996) Serum trysinogen-2 in the prediction of outcome in acute necrotising pancreatitis. Scand J Gastroenterol 31:818–824
15. Bird NC, Goodman AG, Johnson AG (1989) Serum phospholipase A_2 activity in acute pancreatitis: an early guide to severity. Br J Surg 76:731–732.
16. Gudgeon M, Heath DI, Hurley P et al. (1990) Trypsinogen activation peptides assay in the early severity prediction of acute pancreatitis. Lancet 335:4–8.
17. Tenner S, Fernandez-del Castillo C, Warshaw A et al. (1997) Urinary trypsinogen activation peptide (TAP) predicts severity in patients with acute pancreatitis. Int J Pancreatol 21:105–110

18. Beechey-Newman N, Rae D, Sumar N, Hermon-Taylor (1995) Stratification of severity in acute pancreatitis by assay of trypsinogen and 1-prophospholipase A_2 activation peptides. Digestion 56:271.

19. Appelros S, Thim L, Borgstrom A (1998) Activation peptide of carboxypeptidase B in serum and urine in acute pancreatitis. Gut: 42:97–102.

20. McMahon MJ, Bowen M, Mayer AD, Cooper EH (1984) Relationship of α_2-macroglobulin and other anti-proteases to the clinical features of acute pancreatitis. Am J Surg 147:164–170.

21. de Beaux AC, Goldie AS, Ross JA, Carter DC, Fearon KCH (1996) Serum concentrations of inflammatory mediators related to organ failure in patients with acute pancreatitis. Br J Surg 83:349–353.

22. Dominguez-Munoz JE, Carballo F, Garcia MJ et al. (1991) Clinical usefulness of polymorphonuclear elastase in predicting the severity of acute pancreatitis: results of a multicentre study. Br J Surg 78:1230–1234.

23. Gross V, Scholmerich J, Leser H-G et al. (1990) Granulocyte elastase compared in assessment of severity in acute pancreatitis. Comparison with acute-phase proteins C reactive protein, alpha 1 antitrypsin, and protease inhibitor alpha-2 macroglobulin. Dig Dis Sci 35:97–105.

24. Messman H, Vogt W, Holstege A et al. (1997) Post ERCP pancreatitis as a model for cytokine induced acute phase response in acute pancreatitis. Gut 40:80–85.

25. Viedma JA, Perez-Mateo J, Agullo J, Dominguez J, Carballo F (1994) Inflammatory response in the early prediction of severity of acute pancreatitis. Gut 35:822–827

26. Heath DI, Cruikshank AC, Gudgeon M, Shenkin A, Imrie CW (1993) Role of interleukin-6 in mediating the acute phase response and potential as a means of severity assessment in acute pancreatitis. Gut 34:41–45.

27. Buchler M, Malfertheiner P, Beger HC (1986) Correlation of imaging procedures, biochemical parameters and clinical stage in acute pancreatitis. In: Malfertheiner P, Ditschuneit H (eds) Diagnostic procedures in pancreatic disease. Springer, Berlin Heidelberg New York, pp 123–129.

28. Wilson C, Heads A, Shenkin A, Imrie CW (1989) C-reactive protein, anti-proteases and complement factors as objective markers of severity in acute pancreatitis. Br J Surg 76:177–181.

29. Dervenis C, Bassi C, Bradley E et al. (1998) Diagnosis, objective assessment of severity and management of acute pancreatitis. (In press.)

30. Ranson JHC, Rifkind KM, Turner JW (1976) Prognostic signs and non-operative peritoneal lavage in acute pancreatitis. Surg Gynecol Obstet 143:209–219.

31. Imrie CW, Benjamin IS, McKay AJ, Mackenzie I, O'Neil J, Blumgart LH (1978) A single centre double blind trial of trasylol therapy in primary acute pancreatitis. Br J Surg 65:337–341.

32. Blamey SL, Imrie CW, O'Neil J, Gilmour WM, Carter DC (1984) Prognostic factors in acute pancreatitis. Gut 25:1340–1346.

33. Larvin M, McMahon MJ (1989) APACHE-II score for assessment and monitoring of acute pancreatitis. Lancet II:201–205.

34. Wilson C, Heath DI, Imrie CW (1990) Prediction of outcome in acute pancreatitis: a comparative study of APACHE-II, clinical assessment and multiple factor scoring systems. Br J Surg 77:1260–1264.

35. Johnson CD, Kingsnorth AN, Imrie CW et al. (1998) Prospective randomised trial of lexipafant in severe acute pancreatitis. (In press.)

36. Toh SKC, Walters J, Johnson CD (1996) APACHE-0: a new predictor of severity in acute pancreatitis. Gut 38 (Suppl 1): A35.

37. Johnson CD, Phillips S, Toh SCK, Campbell M (1998) An individual probability index for prediction of complications in acute pancreatitis. Gut 42 (Suppl 1): A10.

5 Prophylactic Antibiotics and Selective Digestive Decontamination in Severe Acute Pancreatitis

E.J.T. Luiten and H.A. Bruining

The use of antibiotics in acute pancreatitis has been continuously debated for more than half a century. In 1950 Lewis and Wangensteen (1) reported reduced mortality in dogs with acute haemorrhagic pancreatitis treated with penicillin. Persky et al. (2) demonstrated that aureomycin, given orally, resulted in 100% survival after bile-induced necrotising pancreatitis in mongrel dogs. Cultures of pancreatic necrosis from non-surviving dogs treated without antibiotics, showed an increase of secondary pancreatic infection, especially with Clostridia. Subsequently, they found a moderate reduction of mortality with polyvalent clostridial toxoid, neomycin and polymyxin B (3). However, Byrne and Joison (4), discussing the primary role of bacteria in the pathogenesis of necrotising pancreatitis, found that neomycin, tetracyclin, penicillin and sulfonamide instilled in a closed duodenal loop, prevented the onset of necrotising pancreatitis. Thal et al. (5) mentioned increased survival when *Escherichia coli*-induced necrotising pancreatitis was treated with aureomycin. Similar results were also reported when antibiotics were used in germ-free dogs with necrotising pancreatitis, casting some doubt on the essential role of bacteria in the pathogenesis (6).

While many investigators supported the clinical use of antibiotics in acute pancreatitis, Kodesch and DuPont in 1973 probably were the first to express scepticism about the protection against infectious complications (7–10). A few years later three controlled clinical trials with ampicillin in patients suffering from, mild, acute pancreatitis showed no benefit (11–13).

Since advances in critical care have greatly reduced the incidence of death caused by the early cardiopulmonary sequelae of acute necrotising pancreatitis, secondary pancreatic infections currently have emerged as the leading cause of mortality and morbidity (14–18).

After a decade of nihilism in the face of infected pancreatic necrosis, there is now optimism that infection may be preventable due to results of recent controlled clinical trials based on knowledge of penetration of different antibiotics into pancreatic tissue and on data regarding the microbial flora most frequently isolated from pancreatic necrosis (14,17–30).

Incidence of Infection

Secondary infections (i.e. infected necrosis, pancreatic abscess or infected pseudocyst) complicate 3–12% of cases of acute pancreatitis (17,21,29–34). It is estimated that acute necrotising pancreatitis develops in 10–20% of patients with acute pancreatitis and secondary infection of pancreatic necrosis occurs in 40–70% of these patients (14,22,26,29,30,33–42). Gram-negative aerobic microorganisms are isolated from 50–70% cultures of infected pancreatic necrosis suggesting an enteric origin (14,27–30,34,37,40). Development of Gram-negative infection of (peri-) pancreatic necrosis is, apart from the Glasgow score, the most important parameter determining outcome as compared with patients in whom infection does not (i.e. sterile necrosis) occur (43). Infection of necrosis with only Gram-positive microorganisms has the same prognosis as necrosis remaining sterile (43). Gram-negative infection of pancreatic necrosis has been found to be preceded by intestinal colonisation with identical Gram-negative microorganisms both experimentally and clinically (44–52).

Beger et al. (14) showed that infection of pancreatic necrosis increases with time during the course of the disease. However, only data of patients who were operated were analysed. We also found that the incidence of infected necrosis, when analysing the bacteriological status at the first laparotomy, increased with time, from 9% during the first week to 50% during the second and third weeks, as has also been reported by others (23,26,53). Mortality due to infection of pancreatic necrosis is significantly increased from 31% within 2 weeks to 77% thereafter (23).

Role of Antibiotics

Since infection of pancreatic necrosis is a secondary phenomenon, prophylactic antibiotics should be administered at an early stage of tissue injury before infection has developed, i.e. from the onset of the disease. Antibiotics should probably only be used in patients with severe acute pancreatitis (three or more positive Glasgow criteria), since mild acute pancreatitis is a self-limiting disease irrespective of the type of medical treatment (54–57). It is currently unknown whether antibiotics are more useful in acute pancreatitis due to gallstones or from alcohol abuse.

Three early controlled clinical trials using prophylactic ampicillin in patients with mild mostly alcohol-induced pancreatitis showed no benefit (11–13). However, ampicillin is a poor antibiotic choice for acute pancreatitis as it does not penetrate the pancreas and, perhaps more importantly, does not cover the Gram-negative microorganisms most frequently isolated from infected pancreatic necrosis, i.e. *Escherichia coli, Pseudomonas, Klebsiella* species and *Enterobacter* species (Table 1) (14,22–24,26,27). In addition, the patients recruited to those studies had mild disease not bearing the risk of pancreatic infection.

Based on pharmacokinetic data on several antibiotics from human pancreatic juice or pancreatic tissues from animals, several investigators have speculated about appropriate antibiotics to treat patients with acute pancreatitis (17,58–61). Büchler et al. (25) measured blood and pancreatic tissue concentrations of several antibiotics in patients undergoing elective pancreatic surgery. They calculated that, 120 minutes after intravenous infusion, imipenem, ofloxacin and ciprofloxacin have the highest pancreatic tissue levels and highest bactericidal activity against the microorganisms most often found in infected pancreatic necrosis. Aminoglycosides were not effective.

Table 1. Bacteriological analysis of infected necrosis in severe acute pancreatitis: presence of microorganisms[a]

Species	SD group ($n = 9$)	Control group ($n = 20$)
Gram-negative aerobic		
Acinetobacter spp.	–	3
Citrobacter spp.	–	3
Escherichia coli	1	12
Enterobacter spp.	–	5
Klebsiella spp.	1	5
Pseudomonas spp.	3	10
Proteus spp.	–	2
Morganella spp.	–	4
Serratia maresc.	1	–
Alicaligenes spp.	–	1
Gram-positive aerobic		
Staphylococci spp.	–	1
S. aureus	4	4
S. epidermidis	9	12
Streptococci	2	–
Enterococci	7	12
Yeasts		
Candida albicans	2	10

[a] Microorganisms may occur in combinations in each separate patient
From Luiten et al. (23)

Controlled Clinical Trials of Antibiotics

Based on these results, a controlled multicentre trial of imipenem prophylaxis in patients with necrotising pancreatitis was conducted by Pederzoli et al. in Italy (24). During a two-and-a-half-year period 74 patients were included, based on the presence of detectable pancreatic necrosis demonstrated by contrast-enhanced computed tomography (CE-CT) within 72 hours of onset of symptoms. Patients were randomised to receive standard medical treatment without ($n = 33$ patients) or with adjuvant imipenem (41 patients) for 2 weeks (500 mg every 8 hours intravenously). Ranson scores, which were not used as an inclusion criterion, ranged from 3 to 6 (mean 3.7). Almost 50% of the patients only had mild necrosis as found on CE-CT, bearing a lesser risk of infection. Nevertheless, a significant reduction of pancreatic sepsis (12% versus 30%) and non-pancreatic sepsis (15% versus 48.5%) was observed. However mortality (7% versus 12%) was not different, but overall mortality (9%) was rather low, probably reflecting the inclusion of patients with less severe disease. Results regarding a consecutive trial including only patients with moderate or severe necrosis (i.e. more than 30% necrosis) are expected shortly (Dr C. Bassi, personal communication).

A Finnish controlled study by Sainio et al. (62) reported reduced mortality in 60 patients, recruited during a 4-year period, with acute necrotising pancreatitis using cefuroxime (4.5 g/day). This was not associated with a reduction of pancreatic sepsis. Unfortunately the authors were forced to change from cefuroxime to alternative antibiotics in two-thirds of the patients after 9 days (2–28) and to initiate antibiotic therapy after 6 (2–16) days, on the basis of presumed or documented infection, in 23 of the 30 patients initially randomised to no therapy. The incidence of urinary sepsis and overall mortality were significantly decreased in the group of patients treated initially with cefuroxime.

A well-designed controlled German study of 26 patients, enrolled during a 4-year period, using ofloxacin and metronidazole reported no prevention of pancreatic infection (63). A controlled French study of 23 patients, recruited during a 5-year period, using ceftazidime, metronidazole and amikacin for only 10 days, reported reduction of pancreatic infection (64). Conclusions from these two studies should be interpreted with caution due to the very small number of patients included.

Selective Digestive Decontamination (SDD)

Following better knowledge about infected necrosis, its prevalent flora suggesting an origin in the gut, experimental evidence concerning the protective effect of reduction of intestinal flora and successful clinical reduction of Gram-negative intestinal flora from the digestive tract, a multicentre controlled randomised clinical trial using selective decontamination in 102 patients with acute necrotising pancreatitis, enrolled in a 3-year period, was conducted in the Netherlands (14,23,65–73). All patients had severe acute pancreatitis defined by Glasgow score $\geqslant 3$ and or Balthazar grade D or E (Table 2) (66,74). The selective decontamination regimen consisted of oral, and rectal (enema containing daily dose), administration of colistin sulphate (200 mg), amphotericin (500 mg) and norfloxacin (50 mg) every 6 hours. Also a sticky paste with the three drugs was smeared along the gums and tracheostomy, if present. Short-term systemic prophylaxis (mean 7 days) using low dose cefoxatime was given until the digestive tract was success-

Table 2. Prognostic systems used to select patients for inclusion in the trial

(1) Multiple laboratory criteria (Glasgow score)[a]	
Age	> 55 years
Serum uncorrected calcium	< 2.00 mmol/l
Serum urea	> 16 mmol/l
LDH	> 600 U/l
Blood glucose (no diabetes)	> 10 mmol/l
WBC	$> 15 \times 10^9$/l
Serum albumin	< 32 g/l
PaO$_2$	< 60 mmHg (7.5 kPa)

(2) Degree of disease severity according to Balthazar classification[b]

Grade A Normal pancreas
Grade B Focal or diffuse enlargement of the pancreas (including contour irregularities, non-homogeneous attenuation of the gland, dilatation of the pancreatic duct, and foci of small fluid collections within the gland, as long as there is no evidence of peripancreatic disease
Grade C Intrinsic pancreatic abnormalities associated with haziness and streaky densities representing inflammatory changes in the peripancreatic fat
Grade D As C plus single ill-defined fluid collection (phlegmon) in or adjacent to the pancreas
Grade E As C plus two or multiple, poorly defined fluid collections or the presence of gas in or adjacent to the pancreas

[a] The Glasgow score equals the number of separate criteria present (minimum: 0; maximum: 8)
[b] CT scan with use of oral (half an hour before) and intravenous contrast (rapid iv drip)
LDH, lactate dehydrogenase; WBC, white blood cell count; PaO$_2$, arterial oxygen concentration

fully selectively decontaminated. SDD was discontinued as soon as the risk of acquiring an infection had receded, i.e. the patient was extubated and without supplementary oxygen therapy or infusions, on regular diet and mobilised on the ward.

SDD significantly reduced overall mortality through its significant effect on Gram-negative pancreatic infection and late mortality (Figure 1, Table 3). The Glasgow score proved to be very valuable in identifying patients with increased risk of development of Gram-negative pancreatic infection and also at risk of dying (23,43). CT findings using Balthazar grades were less accurate as they tend to overestimate the severity of severe acute pancreatitis. SDD reduced mortality in treated patients with three or more positive Glasgow criteria from 55% to 31%

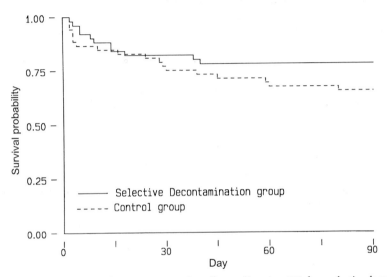

Figure 1. Overall survival according to treatment. Overall mortality rates at 90 days: selective decontamination group = 22%; control group = 35%. Adjusted for Glasgow score and Balthazar grade, $P = 0.048$. Difference in mortality rates equals 13% (95% confidence limits: −4%, +30%). (From Luiten et al. [23]).

Table 3. Multivariate analysis of mortality in relation to treatment, Glasgow score and Balthazar grade

Factor	Odds-ratio		P-value	
Treatment				
Control	1[a]	–	–	
SD	0.3	(0.3)	0.048	(0.049)
Glasgow score	3.7[b]	(3.9)	< 0.001	(< 0.001)
Balthazar grade				
C/D	1[a]	–	–	
E	1.8	(–)	0.354	(–)

[a] Reference category
[b] Relative to patients who have a Glasgow score of 1 point less
Data given are odds-ratios for mortality. (Odds-ratios > 1 indicate an increased mortality; < 1 indicate a decreased mortality.) Data in parentheses denote results when only treatment and Glasgow score are analysed regarding mortality
From Luiten et al. (23)

with a 95% confidence interval for the difference in mortality ranging from 0 to 48%. Failure of SDD to successfully maintain clearance of Gram-negative nosocomial flora from the digestive tract was seen in four patients, followed by development of a pancreatic infection. SDD-induced overgrowth of Gram-positive flora was not found (75–76).

There is general agreement that infected (peri-) pancreatic necrosis is an absolute indication for operation (14,26,37,39,77–79) which may need to be repeated. Even after operation, infected necrosis carries a threefold higher mortality rate (range 15–82%) in contrast to sterile necrosis (34,78,80). A significantly lower number of repeated laparotomies and lower surgery-related complication rate were achieved in patients treated with SDD through a significant reduction of Gram-negative pancreatic infections (23). More than 70% of these infections occurred within 1 week of first isolation from the digestive tract (52).

Persky and collegues (2) in 1951 were way ahead of their time when they found a much greater effectiveness of the oral as compared with intravenous aureomycin and postulated that the microorganisms responsible for secondary infection of the pancreas in dogs originated from the intestine. Favourable effects have been reported on the outcome of experimental necrotising pancreatitis in rats, reducing the intestinal flora by means of colectomy, caecostomy, intestinal lavage with the addition of oral kanamycin or colonic irrigation (72,81). Two recent experimental studies with selective decontamination reported reduction of pancreatic infection (47,82).

Since acute pancreatitis induces intestinal bacterial overgrowth and secondary pancreatic infections are gut-derived, the gut serves as the "motor" of pancreatic sepsis (50–52,83). Intravenous antibiotic prophylaxis, i.e. imipenem, does not affect the colonic pool of bacteria (47). In order to nip the danger of secondary pancreatic infection in the bud, early elimination of Gram-negative microorganisms from the digestive tract by means of SDD seems the most logical and effective step to reduce morbidity and mortality in acute necrotising pancreatitis.

Other Prophylactic Strategies

Initial enthusiasm for peritoneal lavage was dampened by a large controlled clinical trial showing no effect on the outcome of severe acute pancreatitis (84–88). However, inspiring results were reported by the late J.H.C. Ranson, comparing long (7 days) versus short (2 days) periods of peritoneal lavage (89). The operative technique advocated by Beger et al. (33) consists of necrosectomy and continuous closed postoperative lavage of the lesser sac. Currently an overall mortality rate of 15.4% is reported in cases of infected pancreatic necrosis (34). Initially a lower mortality rate of 8.4% (90) was reported, including results of patients operated for sterile necrosis. The very impressive results in cases of sterile necrosis may be partly due to the excessive lavage, initially with more than 24 litres per day, preventing secondary pancreatic infection.

Recommendations for Treatment

Only patients with acute necrotising pancreatitis (i.e. three or more positive Glasgow signs) will benefit from antibiotic therapy. As infection can occur during the first week after onset of the disease, prophylactic antibiotics should be given as soon as possible after admission and diagnosis.

Up to now selective decontamination of the digestive tract (SDD) (colistin, amphotericin and norfloxacin) combined with a short-term (average 7 days) systemic prophylaxis of cefotaxime, until SDD is established, is most effective in reducing morbidity as well as mortality. Antibiotic prophylaxis should be continued until the risk of pancreatic infection is absent.

The intravenous prophylactic antibiotics used should adequately penetrate (peri-) pancreatic tissues and should be effective against the prevalent flora found in infected necrosis. However imipenem, which meets these criteria, has only proven its efficacy with regard to reduction of pancreatic infection but not mortality.

Further controlled multicentre trials with adjuvant antibiotic prophylaxis, including large numbers of patients with severe acute pancreatitis after proper severity stratification, are warranted in order to answer the many outstanding questions, including the potential additional benefit of SDD over antibiotic therapy alone, the best combination of agents, and the most desirable length of treatment.

References

1. Lewis FJ, Wangensteen OH (1950) Antibiotics in the treatment of experimental acute hemorrhagic pancreatitis in dogs. Proc Soc Exp Biol Med 74:453–455.
2. Persky L, Schweinberg FB, Jacob S, Fine J (1951) Aureomycin in experimental acute pancreatitis of dogs. Surgery 30:652–656.
3. Schweinberg FB, Jacob S, Persky L, Fine J (1953) Further studies on the role of bacteria in death from acute pancreatitis in dogs. Surgery 33:367.
4. Byrne JJ, Joison J (1964) Bacterial regurgitation in experimental pancreatitis. Am J Surg 107:317–320.
5. Thal A, Tansathitaya P, Egner W (1956) An experimental study of bacterial pancreatitis. Surg Gynecol Obstet 103:459–468.
6. Tedesco VE III, Evans JT, Nance FC (1969) Antibiotic prevention of experimental hemorrhagic pancreatitis in germ-free and conventional dogs. Rev Surg 26:375.
7. Ponka JL, Landrum SE, Chaikof L (1961) Acute pancreatitis in the post-operative patient. Arch Surg 83:475–490.
8. Baker RJ (1972) Acute surgical diseases of the pancreas. Surg Clin North Am 52:239–256.
9. Rahman F, Geokas MC (1972) Pancreatitis: mortality, antibiotics. Ann Intern Med 76:1044–1045.
10. Kodesch R, DuPont HL (1973) Infectious complications of acute pancreatitis. Surg Gynecol Obstet 136:763–768.
11. Howes R, Zuidema GD, Cameron JL (1975) Evaluation of prophylactic antibiotics in acute pancreatitis. J Surg Res 18:197–200.
12. Craig RM, Dordal E, Myles L (1975) The use of ampicillin in acute pancreatitis. Ann Intern Med 83:831–832.
13. Finch WT, Sawyers JL, Schenker S (1976) A prospective study to determine the efficacy of antibiotics in acute pancreatitis. Ann Surg 183:667–671.
14. Beger HG, Bittner R, Block S, Buchler M (1986) Bacterial contamination of pancreatic necrosis. A prospective clinical study. Gastroenterology 91:433–438.
15. Wilson C, Imrie CW (1991) Systemic effects of acute pancreatitis. In: Johnson CD, Imrie CW (eds) Pancreatic disease. Springer, London, pp 287–97.
16. Renner IG, Savage WT III, Pantoja JL, Renner VJ (1985) Death due to acute pancreatitis. A retrospective analysis of 405 autopsy cases. Dig Dis Sci 30:1005–1018.
17. Bradley EL III. Antibiotics in acute pancreatitis. Am J Surg 158:472–478.
18. Lumsden A, Bradley EL III (1990) Secondary pancreatic infections. Surg Gynecol Obstet 170:459–467.
19. Buggy BP, Nostrant TT (1983) Lethal pancreatitis. Am J Gastroenterol 78:810–814.

20. Johnson CD (1996) Antibiotic prophylaxis in severe acute pancreatitis. Br J Surg 83:883–884.
21. Ranson JHC, Spencer FC (1977) Prevention, diagnosis and treatment of pancreatic abscesses. Surgery 82:99–106.
22. Isenmann R, Büchler MW (1994) Infection and acute pancreatitis. Br J Surg 81:1707–1708.
23. Luiten EJT, Hop WCJ, Lange JF, Bruining HA (1995) Controlled clinical trial of selective decontamination for the treatment of severe acute pancreatitis. Ann Surg 222:57–65.
24. Pederzoli P, Bassi C, Vesentini S, Campedelli A (1993) A randomized multicenter clinical trial of antibiotic prophylaxis of septic complications in acute necrotizing pancreatitis with imipenem. Surg Gynecol Obstet 176:480–483.
25. Büchler M, Malfertheiner P, Friess H et al. (1992) Human pancreatic tissue concentration of bactericidal antibiotics. Gastroenterology 103:1902–1908.
26. Gerzof SG, Banks PA, Robbins AH et al. (1987) Early diagnosis of pancreatic infection by computed tomography-guided aspiration. Gastroenterology 93:1315–1320.
27. Pederzoli P, Bassi C, Vesentini S et al. (1990) Retroperitoneal and peritoneal drainage and lavage in the treatment of severe necrotizing pancreatitis. Surg Gynecol Obstet 170:197–203.
28. Bradley EL III (1991) Operative management of acute pancreatitis: ventral open packing. Hepatogastroenterology 38:134–138.
29. Widdison AL, Karanjia ND (1993) Pancreatic infection complicating acute pancreatitis. Br J Surg 80:148–154.
30. Bittner R, Block S, Buchler M, Beger HG (1987) Pancreatic abscess and infected pancreatic necrosis. Different local septic complications in acute pancreatitis. Dig Dis Sci 32:1082–1087.
31. Becker JM, Pemberton JH (1984) Prognostic factors in pancreatic abscesses. Surgery 96:455–460.
32. Donahue PE, Nyhus LM, Baker RJ (1980) Pancreatic abscess after alcoholic pancreatitis. Arch Surg 115:905–909.
33. Beger HG, Buchler M, Bittner R, Block S, Nevalainen T, Roscher R (1988) Necrosectomy and postoperative local lavage in necrotizing pancreatitis. Br J Surg 75:207–212.
34. Beger HG, Rau B, Mayer J, Pralle U (1997) Natural course of acute pancreatitis. World J Surg 21:130–135.
35. Bradley EL III (1993) A clinically based classification system for acute pancreatitis. Arch Surg 128:586–590.
36. Allardyce DB (1987) Incidence of necrotizing pancreatitis and factors related to mortality. Am J Surg 154:295–299.
37. Bradley EL III, Allen K (1991) A prospective longitudinal study of observation versus surgical intervention in the management of necrotizing pancreatitis. Am J Surg 161:19–24.
38. Warshaw AL (1974) Inflammatory masses following acute pancreatitis. Phlegmon, pseudocyst, and abscess. Surg Clin North Am 54:621–636.
39. Beger HG (1991) Surgery in acute pancreatitis. Hepatogastroenterology 38:92–96.
40. Bassi C, Falconi M, Girelli R et al. (1989) Microbiological findings in severe acute pancreatitis. Surg Res Commun 5:1–4.
41. Smadja C, Bismuth H (1986) Pancreatic debridement in acute necrotizing pancreatitis: an obsolete procedure? Br J Surg 73:408–410.
42. Roscher R, Beger HG (1987) Bacterial infection of pancreatic necrosis. In: Beger HG, Buchler M (eds) Acute pancreatitis. Springer, New York, pp 314–320.
43. Luiten EJT, Hop WCJ, Lange JF, Bruining HA (1998) Differential prognosis of gram-negative versus gram-positive infected, and sterile pancreatic necrosis. Clin Inf Dis (in press).
44. Medich DS, Lee TK, Melhem MF, Rowe MI, Schraut WH, Lee KKW (1993) Pathogenesis of pancreatic sepsis. Am J Surg 165:46–52.
45. Tarpila E, Nystrom PO, Franzen L et al. (1993) Bacterial translocation during acute pancreatitis in rats. Eur J Surg 159:109–113.
46. Foitzik T, Mithöfer K, Ferraro MJ et al. (1994) Time course of bacterial infection of the pancreas and its relation to disease severity in a rodent model of acute necrotizing pancreatitis. Ann Surg 220:193–198.
47. Foitzik T, Fernández-del-Castillo C, Ferraro MJ et al. (1995) Pathogenesis and prevention of early pancreatic infection in experimental acute necrotizing pancreatitis. Ann Surg 222:179–185.
48. Gianotti L, Munda R, Alexander JW (1992) Pancreatitis-induced microbial translocation: a study of the mechanisms. Res Surg 4:87–91.
49. Gianotti L, Munda R, Alexander JW et al. (1993) Bacterial translocation: a potential source for infection in acute pancreatitis. Pancreas 8:551–558.
50. Runkel NS, Moody FG, Smith GS, Rodriguez LF, LaRocco MT, Miller TA (1991) The role of the gut in the development of sepsis in acute pancreatitis. J Surg Res 51:18–23.

51. Wang X, Andersson R, Soltesz V et al. (1996) Gut origin sepsis, macrophage function and oxygen extraction associated with acute pancreatitis in the rat. World J Surg 20:299–308.

52. Luiten EJT, Hop WCJ, Endtz HE, Bruining HA (1998) Prognostic importance of gram-negative intestinal colonization preceding pancreatic infection in severe acute pancreatitis. Intensive Care Med (Submitted).

53. Schwarz M, Büchler M, Meyer H et al. (1994) Effect of antibiotic treatment in patients with necrotizing pancreatitis and sterile necrosis. Pancreas 9:802.

54. Creutzfeldt W, Lankisch RG (1981) Intensive medical treatment of severe acute pancreatitis World J Surg 5:341–350.

55. Beger HG (1991) Acute pancreatitis: a challenge to gastroenterologists and surgeons. Hepatogastroenterology 38:90–91.

56. Ihse I, Lempinen M, Worning H (1994) A clinically based classification system for acute pancreatitis. Scand J Gastroenterol 29:95–96.

57. Banks PA (1994) Acute pancreatitis: medical and surgical management. Am J Gastroenterol 89:S78–S85.

58. Byrne JJ, Treadwell TL (1989) Treatment of pancreatitis. When do antibiotics have a role? Postgrad Med 85:333–339.

59. Trudel JL, Mutch DO, Brown PR, Richards GK, Brown RA (1982) Antibiotic therapy for pancreatic sepsis: differences in bioactive blood and tissue levels. Surg Forum 33:26–27.

60. Pederzoli P, Falconi M, Bassi C et al. (1987) Ciprofloxacin penetration in pancreatic juice. Chemotherapy 33:397–401.

61. Brattstrom C, Malmbory AS, Tyden G (1989) Penetration of imipenem in pancreatic juice following single intravenous dose administration. Chemotherapy 35:83–87.

62. Sainio V, Kemppainen E, Puolakkainen P et al. (1995) Early antibiotic treatment in acute necrotising pancreatitis. Lancet 346:663–667.

63. Schwarz M, Isenmann R, Meyer H, Beger HG (1997) Antibiotika bei nekrotisierender Pankreatitis. Dtsch Med Wochenschr 122:356–361.

64. Delcenserie R, Yzet T, Ducroix JP (1996) Prophylactic antibiotics in treatment of severe alcoholic pancreatitis. Pancreas 13:198–201.

65. Ranson JHC, Balthazar E, Caccavale R, Cooper M (1985) Computed tomography and the prediction of pancreatic abscess in acute pancreatitis. Ann Surg 201:656–665.

66. Balthazar EJ, Ranson JH, Naidich DP, Megibow AJ, Caccavale R, Cooper MM (1985) Acute pancreatitis: prognostic value of CT. Radiology 156:767–772.

67. Lange JF, Teng HT, Menu M, vd Ham AC (1988) The role of computed tomography in the management of acute pancreatitis. Acta Chir Scand 154:461–465.

68. Ranson JHC (1984) Acute pancreatitis: pathogenesis, outcome and treatment. Clin Gastroenterol 13:843–863.

69. Warshaw AL, Jin GL (1985) Improved survival in 45 patients with pancreatic abscess. Ann Surg 202:408–417.

70. Webster MW, Pasculle AW, Myerowitz RL, Rao KN, Lombardi B (1979) Postinduction bacteremia in experimental acute pancreatitis. Am J Surg 138:418–420.

71. Wells CL, Rotstein OD, Pruett TL, Simmons RL (1986) Intestinal bacteria translocate into experimental intra-abdominal abscesses. Arch Surg 121:102–107.

72. Lange JF, van Gool J, Tytgat GN (1987) The protective effect of a reduction in intestinal flora on mortality of acute haemorrhagic pancreatitis in the rat. Hepatogastroenterology 34:28–30.

73. Stoutenbeek CP, van Saene HK, Miranda DR, Zandstra DF (1984) The effect of selective decontamination of the digestive tract on colonisation and infection rate in multiple trauma patients. Intensive Care Med 10:185–192.

74. Blamey SL, Imrie CW, O'Neill J, Gilmour WH, Carter DC (1984) Prognostic factors in acute pancreatitis. Gut 25:1340–1346.

75. Jackson RJ, Smith SD, Rowe MI (1990) Selective bowel decontamination results in gram-positive translocation. J Surg Res 48:444–447.

76. Webb CH (1992) Antibiotic resistance associated with selective decontamination of the digestive tract. J Hosp Infect 22:1–5.

77. Bradley EL III (1987) Management of infected necrosis by open drainage. Ann Surg 206:542–550.

78. Rau B, Uhl W, Büchler MW, Beger HG (1997) Surgical treatment of infected necrosis. World J Surg 21:155–161.

79. Hiatt JR, Fink AS, King W, Pitt HA (1985) Percutaneous aspiration of peripancreatic fluid collections: a safe and effective diagnostic technique. Dig Dis Sci 30:974–977.

80. D'Egidio A, Schein M (1991) Surgical strategies in the treatment of pancreatic necrosis and infection. Br J Surg 78:133–137.

81. Sulkowski U, Boin C, Brockmann J, Bünte H (1993) The influence of caecostomy and colonic irrigation on the pathophysiology and prognosis in acute experimental pancreatitis. Eur J Surg 159:287–291.
82. Gianotti L, Munda R, Gennari R, Pyles T, Wesley Alexander J (1995) Effect of different regimens of gut decontamination in bacterial translocation and mortality in experimental acute pancreatitis. Eur J Surg 161:85–92.
83. Meakins JL, Marshall JC (1986) The gastro-intestinal tract: The "motor" of multiple organ failure. Arch Surg 121:197–201.
84. Ranson JHC, Spencer FC (1978) The role of peritoneal lavage in severe acute pancreatitis. Ann Surg 187:565–575.
85. Stone HH, Fabian TC (1980) Peritoneal dialysis in the treatment of acute alcoholic pancreatitis. Surg Gynecol Obstet 150:878–882.
86. Ihse I, Evander A, Holmberg JT, Gustafson I (1986) Influence of peritoneal lavage on objective prognostic signs in acute pancreatitis. Ann Surg 204:122–127.
87. Rosato EF, Chu WH, Mullen JL, Rosato FE (1972) Peritoneal lavage treatment of experimental pancreatitis. J Surg Res 12:138–140.
88. Mayer AD, McMahon MJ, Corfield AP et al. (1985) Controlled clinical trial of peritoneal lavage for the treatment of severe acute pancreatitis. N Engl J Med 312:399–404.
89. Ranson JHC, Berman RS (1990) Long peritoneal lavage decreases pancreatic sepsis in acute pancreatitis. Ann Surg 211:708–718.
90. Beger HG (1991) Operative management of necrotizing pancreatitis: necrosectomy and continuous closed postoperative lavage of the lesser sac. Hepatogastroenterology 38:129–133.

6 Platelet Activating Factor and Results of PAF Antagonist Therapy

A.N. Kingsnorth

Platelet activating factor (PAF) is a phospholipid released from cell membranes by the action of phospholipase A2 and it has been implicated in a variety of pathophysiological disorders including acute pancreatitis (1,2). The development of potent PAF receptor antagonists has lead to a greater understanding of the role of PAF in disease processes and the potential for development of these compounds as therapy for inflammatory diseases (3,4). PAF (1-0-alkyl-2-acetyl-sn-glycero-3-phosphocholine) was the term originally introduced for a soluble platelet aggregating substance released from IgE stimulated basophils. PAF is a component of structural membrane lipids and together with other classes of lipid mediators such as arachidonates and leukotrienes, it is involved in the trafficking of membrane phospholipids via transacetylation reactions. PAF is involved in both physiological (fertilisation, foetal development, pressor activity) and pathological processes such as asthma, ischaemia, the systemic inflammatory response syndrome, multiple organ failure and pancreatitis.

Biosynthesis of PAF occurs from one of two synthetic pathways: first, the remodelling pathway through the action of phospholipase A2 cleaves PAF from membrane lipids and it is from this source that PAF is generated during inflammation. Second, there is a *de novo* synthetic pathway to maintain intracellular levels of PAF during the resting state. The exact molecular mechanism of action of PAF is unknown although the receptor has now been identified and a cDNA synthesised. PAF acts via a receptor which is G protein-coupled. PAF does not work in isolation, its action is intertwined with many other cells signalling processes and mechanisms.

The principal mechanisms through which PAF exerts its biological effect is believed to be through enhancement of transmigration of activated polymorphonuclear white cells from post-capillary venules into the interstitium of organs such as lung, kidney, myocardium and liver. Once in the tissue spaces of these organs, activated polymorphs release tissue-damaging substances such as proteolytic enzymes, elastases, cathepsin B and superoxide ions. Amelioration of this process is likely to down-regulate the systemic inflammatory response with a beneficial effect on organ failure.

PAF in Experimental Pancreatitis

There are numerous models of acute pancreatitis which can be used to study the pathophysiology of the disease and the development of new therapeutic strategies

(5). Soling and Fest (6) were the first to show that guinea-pig pancreas was capable of synthesising PAF. Isolated pancreatic lobules were able to incorporate labelled acetate into PAF and exposure to cholecystokinin or caerulein led to a strong stimulation of this process. The newly synthesised PAF was partially released into the medium. Pulse chase experiments with radioactive lyso PAF indicated the stimulation of incorporation of radioactive lysoPAF into PAF represented increased net synthesis of PAF rather than increased PAF turnover. The authors suggested for the first time that PAF was a cellular hormone of a lipid nature. Studying effects *in vivo*, Emanuelli and colleagues (7) used a single injection of 50–500 nanograms of PAF into the superior pancreaticoduodenal artery of rabbits. This resulted in an increase in serum amylase and morphological changes of acute pancreatitis which at 72 hours by light microscopy showed oedema, polymorph infiltration, cell vacuolisation and acinar cell necrosis. Electron microscopy revealed an increase in zymogen granules in the apical region of acinar cells at 3 hours. The pancreatic lesions developed in the region supplied by the artery. It was recognised that the inflammatory response induced by PAF did not necessarily depend on a direct effect on acinar cells and it may be due to a release of secondary mediators by stimulated immune cells such as lymphocytes, macrophages or endothelial cells. Subsequent work from the same laboratory showed that endotoxin injected into the pancreatic arterial supply also dose-dependently induced acute pancreatitis; this was potentiated by PAF and could be completely blocked by a PAF antagonist (8). Similar results have been shown in a rat model in which exogenous PAF was injected intraperitoneally and induced biochemical and morphological changes in the pancreas similar to those induced by a 5-hour infusion of caerulein. A PAF antagonist given before the intraperitoneal injection of PAF gave a protective effect on tissue damage indicating a role for PAF in the pathogenesis of acute pancreatitis in this model. As a result of observations on blood flow measurements by Doppler flow-meter the authors suggested that the mechanism of action for PAF antagonist was by reducing blood flow and increases in vascular permeability (9).

These observations have been confirmed and expanded upon in other rat models of acute pancreatitis (10–15). In a rat model of acute pancreatitis induced by retrograde injection of sodium deoxycholate, systemic haemodynamic changes were assessed using radioactive microspheres. Very high levels of PAF were found in the peritoneal exudate from rats with pancreatitis together with high blood levels (10). Although a PAF receptor antagonist did not alter the haemodynamic changes, survival was improved. In a caerulein-induced model of acute pancreatitis, however, these alterations in blood flow were ameliorated by PAF antagonism as were alterations in pancreatic protein, PAF release and oedema (11). A further dimension was explored by Dabrowski and colleagues (12) who noted that PAF antagonism also reduced lipid peroxidation in pancreatic tissues in the caerulein-induced model of acute pancreatitis as well as reducing inflammatory cell infiltrate and pancreatic damage. Yotsumoto and colleagues (13) confirmed the effects of PAF when administered with caerulein by demonstrating ischaemia in the distribution of the gastroduodenal artery and microscopic changes in inflammatory cell infiltrate and scattered haemorrhages.

The lung injury associated with experimentally induced acute pancreatitis was initially investigated by Zhou et al. (14). Pulmonary tissue levels of PAF were increased gradually and reached levels six times that of control animals at 12 hours, at which time pancreatic PAF levels were undetectable and blood PAF levels remained unchanged. The local PAF accumulation occurred at approximately the same time as the progression of the lung injury. Acute pancreatitis had been induced by bile-salt infusion and pretreatment with PAF antagonists reduced PAF induction, polymorph infiltration and extravasation of Evans' blue as indicators of lung injury. The authors concluded that pancreatitis associated lung injury was the result of an endogenous inflammatory response in which PAF played the major role. Kald also demonstrated an increase in PAF content in lung and an increase in pancreatic and blood levels of PAF in bile-salt-induced acute pancreatitis (15). In the microembolic model of acute pancreatitis a microvascular injury to the lung is ameliorated by PAF antagonism started after induction of pancreatitis (16).

In summary there is abundant evidence which demonstrates that in experimental acute pancreatitis. PAF antagonism ameliorates the severity of the disease by reducing serum amylase, oxidative injury, morphological changes, polymorph infiltration, vascular permeability in pancreas and lung, pulmonary damage and levels of PAF blood and peritoneal exudate.

Clinical Studies of PAF Antagonists

On the background of this compelling evidence the PAF antagonist, lexipafant, has been tested in Phase II and Phase III trials in human acute pancreatitis. Lexipafant is one of the most potent PAF receptor antagonists binding to the receptor seven times more avidly than native PAF itself (17). Preclinical data with this compound had shown that unlike other PAF antagonists it was effective when administered after induction of the experimental acute pancreatitis and diminished pancreatic damage and pulmonary capillary permeability (16,18). In a Phase II study (19) the outcome measures were clinical and biochemical markers of severity. The main clinical measure was the effect on organ failure

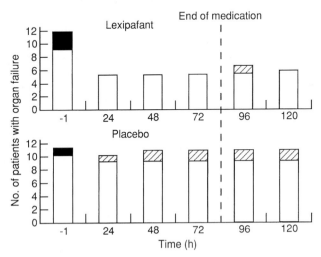

Figure 1. Number of patients with organ failure to day 5 in a study (19) which compared lexipafant 60 mg/day with placebo.

score as an indication of down-regulation of the systemic inflammatory response. Such down-regulation should ultimately be reflected in saving lives from multiple organ failure (20). Biochemical markers were used to measure the effect of lexipafant on the inflammatory response by the assessment of interleukin-8, interleukin-6, E-selectin and polymorphonuclear elastase, α1 antitrypsin and C reactive protein. Figure 1 shows the numbers of patients with organ failure plotted to day 5, the infusion of lexipafant having ceased at 72 hours. In the active treatment group 12 patients had at least one organ failure at entry to the study and in eight patients this had resolved by the end of the medication. In the placebo group 11 patients with organ failure were recorded at entry and at 72 hours there were still 11 patients with organ failure; in two patients with organ failure this had resolved and there were two in whom there was new organ failure. The mean organ failure scores are shown in Figure 2 and again demonstrate a significant treatment effect with lexipafant. The changes in the inflammatory mediators (Figure 3) were significant only for interleukin-8 although there were changes in E-selectin, interleukin-6 and polymorphonuclear elastase. Taken together the overall effect of reducing the concentration of inflammatory mediators in blood could result in a less activated endothelium, down-regulated

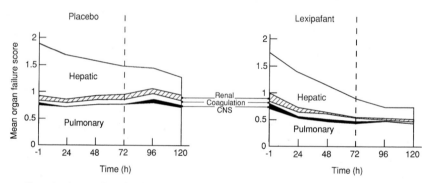

Figure 2. Changes from baseline mean organ failure scores in the same study as Figure 1.

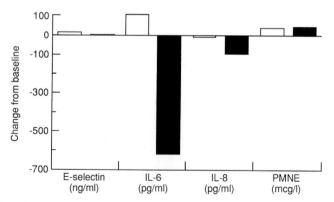

Figure 3. Mean changes from baseline on day 1 of inflammatory mediators in the same study as in Figure 1. PMNE, polymorphonuclear elastase.

polymorphs and less tissue damage; this would be consistent with the observed reduction in organ failure.

A similar study in Glasgow (21) looked at clinical outcome in 50 patients with predicted severe pancreatitis. Treated patients received infusion of lexipafant 100 mg per day for up to 7 days. There was a significant reduction in organ failure scores in the lexipafant group, and although the effect on mortality was not significant, three of the treated group died compared with six of the placebo group.

The encouraging results from these studies stimulated a multicentre double-blind placebo-controlled Phase III study with lexipafant (22). In this study 290 patients with predicted severe acute pancreatitis (APACHE II $\geqslant$ 6) received up to 7 days infusion with lexipafant.

Effects on organ failure were similar to those in the Phase II studies (Table 1). Moreover there was a significant reduction in local complications with fewer patients suffering pseudocysts (5.4% vs 13.8%; $P < 0.02$) and a non-significant reduction in necrosis (21% vs 15.5%) and abscess formation (4.3% vs 3.4%). Overall attributable mortality was reduced by lexipafant from 15.2% to 9.5% ($P = 0.13$). Analysis of 205 patients (70% of those entering the study) who received treatment within 48 hours of onset of symptoms revealed a significant reduction in mortality from 20.4% to 9.3% ($P < 0.04$). It was concluded from this study that lexipafant is associated with a more rapid resolution of systemic complications, fewer local complications and a reduction in mortality if treatment is started early.

Conclusion

The experimental evidence is convincing that PAF is a principal mediator of inflammation, both local and systemic, in acute pancreatitis. Two Phase II and one Phase III studies all show amelioration of systemic inflammation with PAF antagonist therapy. Early treatment (< 48 hours) appears to reduce mortality. We have entered a new era in the treatment of acute pancreatitis arising from improved understanding of the pathophysiology of the disease.

References

1. Formela LJ, Galloway SW, Kingsnorth AN (1995) Inflammatory mediators in acute pancreatitis. Br J Surg 82:6–13.
2. Kingsnorth AN (1997) Role of cytokines and their inhibitors in acute pancreatitis. Gut 40:1–4.
3. Venable ME, Zimmerman GA, McIntyre TM, Prescott SM (1993) Platelet activating factor: a phospholipid autacoid with diverse actions. J Lipid Res 34:691–702.
4. Koltai M, Guinot P, Hosford D, Braquet PG (1994) Platelet activating factor antagonists: scientific background and possible clinical applications. Adv Pharmacol 28:81–167.
5. Banerjee AK, Galloway SW, Kingsnorth AN (1994) Experimental models of acute pancreatitis. Br J Surg 81:1096–1103.
6. Soling H-D, Fest W (1986) Synthesis of 1-0-alkyl-2-acetyl-sn-glycero-3-phosphocholine (platelet-activating factor) in exocrine glands and its control by secretagogues. J Biol Chem 261:13916–13922.
7. Emanuelli G, Montrucchio G, Gaia E, Dughera L, Corvelli G, Gubetta L (1989) Experimental acute pancreatitis induced by platelet-activating factor in rabbits. Am J Pathol 134:315–326.

8. Emanuelli G, Montrucchio G, Dughera L et al. (1994) Role of platelet activating factor in acute pancreatitis induced by lipopolysaccharides in rabbits. Eur J Pharmacol 261:265–272.

9. Konturek SJ, Dembinski A, Konturek PJ et al. (1992) Role of platelet activating factor in pathogenesis of acute pancreatitis in rats. Gut 33:1268–1274.

10. Ais G, Lopez-Farre A, Gomez-Garre DN et al. (1992) Role of platelet activating factor in hemo-dynamic derangements in an acute rodent pancreatic model. Gastroenterology 102:181–187.

11. Tomaszewska R, Dembiniski A, Warzecha Z, Banas M, Konturek SJ, Stachura J (1992) Platelet activating factor (PAF) inhibitor (TCV-309) reduces caerulin and PAF-induced pancreatitis. A morphologic and functional study in the rat. J Physiol Pharmacol 4:345–352.

12. Dabrowski A, Gabrylelewicz A, Chyczewski L (1991) The effect of platelet activating factor antagonist (BN52021) on cerulein induced acute pancreatitis with reference to oxygen radicals. Int J Pancreatol 8:1–11.

13. Yotsumoto L, Manabe T, Kyogoku T et al. (1994) Platelet-activating factor involvement in the aggravation of acute pancreatitis in rabbits. Digestion 55:260–267.

14. Zhou W, McCollum MO, Levine BA, Olson MS (1992) Role of platelet-activating factor in pancreatitis associated acute lung injury in the rat. Am J Pathol 140:971–979.

15. Kald B, Kald A, Ihse I, Tagesson C (1993) Release of platelet-activating factor in acute experimental pancreatitis. Pancreas 8:440–442.

16. Galloway SW, Kingsnorth AN (1996) Lung injury in microembolic model of acute pancreatitis. Pancreas 13:140–146.

17. Whittaker M (1992) PAF receptor antagonists: recent advances. Curr Opin Ther Patents 2:583–623.

18. Formela LJ, Wood LM, Whittaker M, Kingsnorth AN (1994) Amelioration of acute pancreatitis in a rat model by a potent platelet activating factor antagonist. Br J Surg 81:1783–1785.

19. Kingsnorth AN, Galloway SW, Formela LJ (1995) Randomized, double-blind Phase II trial of lexipafant, a platelet activating factor antagonist, in human acute pancreatitis. Br J Surg 82:1414–1420.

20. Nathens AB, Marshall JC (1996) Sepsis, SIRS and MODS: what's in a name? World J Surg 20:386–391.

21. McKay C, Curran F, Sharples, Imine CW (1997) A placebo controlled randomised study of lexi-pafant in severe acute pancreatitis. Br J Surg 84 (in press).

22. Toh SKC and The British Acute Pancreatitis Study Group (1997) Lexipafant, a platelet activating factor antagonist, reduces mortality in a randomised placebo controlled study in patients with severe acute pancreatitis. Gut 40 (suppl 1):A12.

7 Incidence, Mortality Rate and Underdiagnosis of Acute Pancreatitis

C.W. Imrie and C.J. McKay

Despite advances in the knowledge of the pathophysiology of acute pancreatitis (AP), and advances in intensive care management for patients with severe AP, the mortality rate is still appreciable and improvements are slow. Mortality ranges overall from 2% to 10%, but in severe AP approaches 20% (1–13).

About 25% of patients will develop complications (9), but it can be difficult to predict from an individual patient assessment who will progress to severe disease and therefore require intensive care monitoring. Severe disease is characterised by organ failure and local complications such as abscess or pseudocysts. Complications can develop very quickly, particularly organ failure (especially respiratory and renal failure). Multiple organ failure is the most common cause of death within 7 days of disease onset (4–7,9).

The mortality rate is higher for elderly patients (11,12) probably due to a higher incidence of concomitant disease, but younger patients may also die early on in the course of the disease (10). Available data show that patients who survive a severe attack of AP have a good chance of returning to normal activity with good quality of life (14). Early and correct diagnosis is therefore vital if these patients are to receive appropriate care.

The reported incidence of AP and the accuracy of diagnosis in an individual patient depends on a number of factors such as: clinical awareness of the possibility of the diagnosis; availability of rapid and accurate enzyme measurements of amylase and lipase; availability of imaging equipment such as computed tomography (CT); and availability of autopsy information.

Other factors, such as the willingness to perform peritoneal aspiration (15) may also affect diagnosis of the disease. It is now many years since the publication of the verification of the safety and accuracy of peritoneal aspiration in the difficult differential diagnosis and, indeed, its usefulness in grading severity (16). This approach, which is very rapid and also safe when nasogastric tube and a urinary catheter are placed, is underutilised.

In the developed world, when genuine diagnostic doubt exists, CT can often identify pancreatic swelling and the accumulation of peripancreatic fluid in the difficult diagnostic situation. However, this approach is expensive and slower than peritoneal aspiration.

Disease Incidence and Clinical Awareness

In an 18-year study from 1950 to 1967 carried out in the Bristol area (UK), an increasing incidence of AP was documented during the first 6 years of the study and a further peak of incidence occurred from 1961 to 1964 (17). The initial increase was attributed to wider application of blood amylase measurements, and the later increase to locally heightened interest in the disease. Therefore, both surges of incidence were thought to be due to improvements in diagnosis rather than an absolute change in incidence (17). In a study extending from 1940 to 1969 in Rochester, Minnesota, USA, a similar experience was reported (18).

The original Bristol data were updated in a paper published in 1985 (19) and showed an increase in incidence of 26% over the previous two decades. However, the overall case mortality rate was little changed at approximately 20% throughout the 30-year period covered by both studies (17,19). The suggestion, therefore, was that improved understanding of fluid replacement and other supportive therapy for patients with AP had had little impact on mortality.

A study on the changing patterns of incidence and mortality from AP in Scotland from 1961 to 1985 (20) revealed a steady increase from 181 cases per year in 1961 to 1234 in 1085, an almost seven fold increase in diagnosis. Although there was a steady increase in diagnosis throughout the 1960s a sharp rise in diagnoses in both males and females occurred from 1971 onwards following the introduction and widespread acceptance of the Phadebas test (Pharmacia Diagnostics, Uppsala, Sweden), a simple reproducible assay for blood amylase. This test was probably a major factor in the surge of diagnosis of AP from 1971, when the total annual incidence in Scotland was less than 500 cases per year, reaching almost 1000 cases per year by 1975 (20). As already indicated, the incidence had increased to 1234 cases per year by 1985. However, the mortality rate showed a marked change, thus differing from the Bristol data. Indeed, in the Scottish study the case mortality had fallen from 17.8% in the period 1961 to 1965 to 5.6% in the period 1981 to 1985. It was concluded that the apparent increase in the incidence of AP was largely attributable to improved accuracy in diagnosis, with milder forms of AP being identified more often.

The data obtained from the Scottish study (20) were collated from the Scottish Hospital Inpatient Statistics, and were based on the discharge diagnosis recorded for each patient on a standard form (SMR1) required since 1961. Throughout that period from 1961 to 1985 the population of Scotland had remained remarkably stable at around 5.2 million, which is very similar to the national populations of Norway, Denmark and Finland.

A study of incidence and mortality of AP has been published from Finland (21) in which the incidence steadily rose from 1970 to 1989. These data identified *each pancreatitis discharge* (rather than individual patients) and showed an overall correlation with increased alcohol consumption ($r = 0.78$, $P = 0.0001$). The pancreatitis discharges correlated with liver cirrhosis for men ($r = 0.81$), with gallstone disease for women ($r = 0.77$). Overall episodes rose from 466 to 734 per million per year, mainly in men (from 591 to 1134), while in women the figure was constant at 350. Mortality rates decreased from 5.9% to 2.6% (21).

Our centre has performed a further study of incidence and mortality of AP in Scotland from 1985 to 1994, and this shows a steady increase in incidence, to a figure of over 380 patient episodes per million in 1994 (22).

A study from the Grampian region in Scotland through the years 1983 to 1985 examined the accuracy of hospital records against the record of amylase examinations carried out in a single regional laboratory (23). This study suggested that only 53% of the total number of patients with AP were accurately identified in the hospital's computer-linked diagnostic index. Extrapolating this result to all of the Health Boards in Scotland, then the data in the earlier Scottish study (3) may have underestimated the true incidence of AP by as much as 100%. Therefore, part of the explanation of increasing incidence in the past decade may be simply due to an improvement in the recording system. However, it is likely that there is a true increase in incidence when one considers the unchanged standard method of recording throughout that decade and the steady increase in figures year by year.

The real incidence of AP which was reported to be less than 60 cases per million of the population in the Bristol area of the UK by Trapnell and Duncan in 1975 (17) has more recently been shown to be in excess of 380 patient episodes per million of the population (22) in Scotland. Using similar diagnostic criteria, the Finnish national figures indicated an incidence of pancreatitis discharges at 734 per million per year in 1989, which was more than twice the Scottish incidence (21). However, it is very important to note that the Finnish figures related to pancreatitis discharges and with alcohol abuse being the most common aetiology for AP in that country, it would be essential to have the number of patients per year to obtain comparability of data. In the USA the National Inpatient Profile data indicate an increasing incidence of AP with just over 800 episodes per million of the population in 1991, and these data also relate to pancreatitis discharges from hospital. Therefore, as with Finland, a single patient with several episodes in one year may be counted many times, thus perhaps (with alcohol the main aetiology) explaining the seemingly higher incidence at 800 episodes per million per year. An additional factor to be taken into account is that in the USA twice the upper limit of normal serum amylase is acceptable as a diagnostic indicator, while in Europe an elevation to three times the upper limit of normal is usually considered the minimal criterion in a patient with an appropriate clinical presentation. Unfortunately, until national or regional data can be processed to analyse the exact number of patients with acute pancreatitis in any given year, we have to rely on the number of patient episodes. It has already been noted that the figures for Scotland, Finland and the USA are quite different at 382, 734 and 800 patient episodes (per million of the population per year), respectively. Furthermore, only the Scottish data have been analysed to identify exact numbers of acute pancreatitis patients in a year and the figure of 261 patients is very likely to be lower than the true figure because of missed diagnoses (22).

Availability of Amylase and Lipase Measurements

The experience of the surge in diagnostic incidence between 1971 and 1975 in Scotland has already been highlighted as coinciding with the ready acceptance of a standard cheap and efficient method of measurement of blood amylase. In developing areas of the world such standard availability of enzyme measurements does not exist, making biochemical verification of the likelihood of AP a rare event. However, when it is used, there are a considerable number of important facets of amylase measurement which are not always recognised.

1. Single blood amylase measurements are not particularly reliable because of the dynamics of change, especially in a patient who has good renal function. It is, therefore, possible that the diagnosis will be discounted or considered unlikely on an isolated blood sample, whereas the clinician who carries out a further blood sample a few hours later may obtain results in the diagnostic range (usually considered in excess of three times the upper level of normal).

2. Claims for the sensitivity of the amylase test are spurious, because of inbuilt bias due to the fact that hyperamylasaemia is a criterion for diagnosis of AP (24). Also the specificity is low, as there are several conditions that can result in hyperamylasaemia (25).

3. The importance of obtaining more than one blood sample where the initial result is only slightly elevated is further emphasised by the knowledge that 20% of AP patients have a rising blood amylase when admitted to hospital. This is particularly important for patients who are admitted within a few hours of onset of symptoms.

4. Urine amylase measurements can also be very helpful and are underused. When hyperlipidaemia is present, urine amylase measurements are more reliable than those in blood (26).

5. Blood lipase measurements are probably more accurate than amylase if only one enzyme can be measured. This was particularly highlighted by Gumaste and colleagues in 1993 (27) but there is a great reluctance to change, and the serum amylase test remains the most widely used diagnostic test for AP. The optimum, but obviously more expensive method, would be to check both enzymes in patients where the diagnosis was considered likely, particularly where the initial blood sample for either lipase or amylase was only moderately elevated.

Availability of Autopsy Information

The present autopsy rate of those who die in hospital varies from country to country. For example, Sweden had an almost 100% autopsy rate until 1991, when a change in the law lowered the figure to around 95%. On the other hand, in France very few patients have a hospital autopsy performed, and the rate in the UK varies between 12% and 35% (A.K. Foulis, personal communication). While this may initially seem of little consequence it is very important to note that between 1974 and 1984 in Glasgow Royal Infirmary, a period during which prospective studies of AP were being performed, 53 (42%) of the 126 patients recorded to have died from AP had the diagnosis first made in the post mortem room. At that time the hospital autopsy rate was 19%. A very similar study by Lankisch et al. (28) in Germany revealed that 13 (30.2%) of a total 43 patients dying from AP between 1980 and 1989 had the diagnosis first established at autopsy. Lower rates of autopsy diagnosis have been recorded in more recent publications from the London area where 7 (12.3%) of 57 deaths recorded in a 4.5-year period came into this category (7) and most recently 10 (15.4%) of 65 deaths over a 6-year period in the two city hospitals in Nottingham were first diagnosed by the pathologists (29). A more comprehensive scan of this problem going back to the early 1960s (30) is portrayed in Table 1, which includes 11 series of patients with a total of 839 fatal cases in which 299 (35.6%) were only diag-

Table 1. Incidence of diagnosis of acute pancreatitis (AP) at autopsy

Authors and reference		Total and fatal AP	Diagnosis at autopsy	
			Number	%
Wilson & Imrie	(3)	126	53	42.1
Mann et al.	(7)	52	7	12.3
Lankisch et al.	(28)	43	13	30.2
Banerjee et al.	(29)	65	10	15.4
Toffler & Spiro	(30)	25	9	36.0
Shader & Paxton	(31)	100	24	24.0
Read et al.	(32)	24	4	16.7
Hofler	(33)	270	145	53.7
Buggy & Nostrant	(34)	32	7	21.9
Banerjee et al.	(36)	65	10	15.4
Petersen & Brooks	(35)	40	17	42.5
Totals		839	299	35.6

nosed at autopsy. When one considers that the autopsy rate for patients dying within hospital rarely exceeds 20%, then the size of the problem begins to become much more clear. With a 100% autopsy rate it seems possible that more than half the patients who die with AP as a major factor contributing to death are not diagnosed with this disease during their lifetime by clinicians. Two of these studies came from university teaching hospitals engaged in prospective studies of patients with AP, namely the University of Gottingen Hospital (28) and Glasgow Royal Infirmary (3) where diagnostic awareness should have been high. However, these studies demonstrated autopsy diagnostic rates of 30.2% and 42.1%, respectively (3,28).

When analysing these studies it is pertinent to try to determine the reasons for the failure of diagnosis, and thus whether an early diagnosis may have altered the outcome. In our own study (3) the most common reason for failure of diagnosis was a *lack of consideration of the possibility of AP*, usually because of an *atypical presentation*. Therefore blood amylase had been measured in only 5 of 53 (9%) of the patients first diagnosed at autopsy. At that time the lipase assay was unreliable and not considered an option. Of those undiagnosed patients 36 (68%) had presented atypically as emergencies to the Medical Department of the hospital, rather than to the Surgical Department which would be the normal referral pattern. However, surgeons themselves were also unsuspecting of the possibility of AP in *patients who deteriorated postoperatively*, and 10 of these (19%) came into this category. Only seven (13%) of these patients had presented with abdominal pain (Table 2). Most of the patients had postoperative AP following upper abdominal surgery, and only three were cardiac surgery patients. In the similar

Table 2. Comparison of presentation in fatal AP

Clinical presentation	Autopsy diagnosis	In-life diagnosis
Abdominal pain ± vomiting	7 (13%)	54 (74%)
Postoperative AP	10 (19%)	1 (1%)
Atypical presentation	36 (68%)	18 (25%)
Totals	53	73

Data from Wilson and Imrie 1988 (3).

study by Lankisch et al. (28) blood amylase measurements were performed in 85% of the patients who died from AP, but in 70% of the remainder the amylase level was either normal, marginally elevated, or the result was obtained too late to be helpful. Indeed, in three or four patients who had blood amylase levels more than 3 times the upper limit of normal, death occurred within 3 days of admission. No patients in the Glasgow series and only two patients in the Gottingen series of patients had ultrasound examinations performed, and there is no record of CT scanning in any patient in either of the two studies.

Absence of Abdominal Pain

Patients with AP usually present with severe acute abdominal pain of sudden onset, which is often accompanied by nausea and vomiting. Occasionally patients do not experience such abdominal pain and this can lead to misdiagnosis. There was a reported absence of abdominal pain of significant note in 12 of the 13 deaths in the Lankisch study (28). While this may be partly due to lack of suspicion and accurate questioning of the patient, it seems evident that clamant pain was not a major presenting factor in these patients and that the AP was remarkable for this atypical presentation. As in the Glasgow study most of the "missed" patients presented as medical emergencies, but postoperative AP featured in 5 of the 13 deaths (46%). In our own study (3) we reported that only 13% of patients first diagnosed at autopsy had presented with severe abdominal pain, compared with 74% of those diagnosed in life (Table 2).

Would Early Diagnosis Have Altered Outcome?

This question is exceedingly difficult to answer from retrospective studies based on patients' case records. However, we did make an attempt to answer this question (3). We believe that for most of our patients the ultimate outcome would have been unaffected by early diagnosis of AP, but in 45% of patients the correct diagnosis should have favourably influenced therapy and thus survival. The intravenous fluid requirements of a patient suffering myocardial ischaemia or infarct differ greatly from those of someone with AP so that management in a proportion of patients would have been radically affected by early diagnosis.

Early Death in Course of AP

Finally, in most of the studies early death within the first week of admission is a feature of undiagnosed AP (28–36). This was greatly emphasised by the excellent review of 400 autopsy cases by Renner et al. in 1985 (37). They compared 405 deaths from AP (defined as the official primary cause of death) with a control autopsy population of over 38 000 patients. Sixty per cent of the AP patients died within 1 week of admission and lung pathology was predominant with both pulmonary oedema and congestion being significantly more prevalent within the AP group (37). Just under 50% of the Lankisch study patients (6 of 13) died within 8 days of admission (28) while the time to death in the Glasgow study (3) was less than a week in the majority of patients. In many studies on AP both sepsis associated with stones in the common bile duct and sepsis associated with infected necrosis of the pancreas were major features suggesting that early endoscopic retrograde cholangiopancreatography (ERCP), sphincterotomy and antibiotic therapy could potentially lower the mortality rate (38). Renner and his colleagues (37) particularly emphasise the predominance of infection in the 40% of patients who survived beyond the first week, only to die later. These authors also recommend a high degree of suspicion that patients with complicated diabetes may also have significant associated exocrine pancreatitis.

A Change in Approach?

In practical terms a greater degree of clinical suspicion of AP is necessary and there is a strong case that all patients reaching the emergency departments of hospitals with pain in the lower chest or upper abdomen should have appropriate biochemical screening tests. Of particular importance are the considerable number of patients who present with suspected myocardial infarction and have atypical ECG and/or atypical enzymes. This recommendation is particularly important for patients who fail to improve as expected after upper abdominal or cardiac surgery or ERCP procedures. Diagnostic doubt from an initial enzyme assay or amylase and/or lipase should prompt a repeat assay and arrangements should be made for either peritoneal aspiration or CT. Early diagnosis is essential for the appropriate energetic attention to intravenous fluid requirements, possible endoscopic intervention and appropriate intravenous antibiotic therapy. To this list may be added in the near future the use of the platelet-activating factor antagonist lexipafant, which has shown promise in double-blind randomised studies (4,6).

References

1. Bourke JB (1977) Incidence and mortality of acute pancreatitis. Br Med J II:1668–1669.
2. de Bolla AR, Obeid ML (1984) Mortality in acute pancreatitis. Ann R Coll Surg Engl 66: 184–186.
3. Wilson C, Imrie CW (1988) Deaths from acute pancreatitis: why do we miss the diagnosis so frequently? Int J Pancreatol 3:273–282.
4. Kingsnorth AN, Galloway SW, Formela LJ (1995) Randomised double-blind II trial of lexipafant, a platelet activating factor antagonist, in human acute pancreatitis. Br J Surg 82:1414–1420.
5. McKay C, Baxter J, Imrie CW (1997) A randomised controlled trial of octreotide in the management of patients with acute pancreatitis. Int J Pancreatol 21:13–19.
6. McKay C, Curran FJM, Sharples CE, Baxter JN, Imrie CW (1997) Prospective placebo-controlled randomised trial of lexipafant in predicted severe acute pancreatitis. Br J Surg 84:1239–1243.
7. Mann DV, Hershman MJ, Hittinger R, Glazer G (1994) Multicentre audit of death from acute pancreatitis. Br J Surg 81:890–893.
8. Heath D, Alexander D, Wilson C, Larvin M, Imrie CW, McMahon MJ (1995) Which complications of acute pancreatitis are most lethal? A prospective multi-centre study of 719 episodes. Gut 36:478.
9. Bradley EL (1994) The necessity for a clinical classification of acute pancreatitis: the Atlanta system. In: Bradley EL (ed) Acute pancreatitis: diagnosis and therapy. Raven Press, New York, pp 27–32.
10. Forsmark CE, Toskes PP (1995) Acute pancreatitis: medical management. Crit Care Clin 11:295–309.

11. Jacobs ML, Daggett WM, Civetta JM et al. (1977) Acute pancreatitis: analysis of factors inflencing survival. Ann Surg 185:43–51.
12. Fan ST, Choi TK, Lai CS, Wong J (1988) Influence of age on the mortality from acute pancreatitis. Br J Surg 75:463–466.
13. Leese T, Holliday M, Heath D, Hall AW, Bell PRF (1987) Multicentre trial of low volume fresh frozen plasma therapy in acute pancreatitis. Br J Surg 74:907–911.
14. Doepel M, Eriksson J, Halme L, Kumpulmainen T, Hockerstedt K (1993) Good long-term results in patients surviving severe acute pancreatitis. Br J Surg 80:1583–1586.
15. Pickard IR, Blackett RL, McMahon MJ (1977) Early assessment of severity of acute pancreatitis using peritoneal lavage. Br Med J II:1377–1379.
16. Corfield AP, Williamson RCN, McMohan MJ et al. (1985) Prediction of severity in acute pancreatitis: prospective comparison of three prognostic indices. Lancet I:404–407.
17. Trapnell JE, Duncan EHL (1975) Patterns of incidence in acute pancreatitis. Br Med J II:179–183.
18. O'Sullivan JN, Nobrega FT, Morlock CG, Brown AL, Bartholomew LG (1972) Acute and chronic pancreatitis in Rochester, Minnesota, 1940–1969. Gastroenterology 62:373–379.
19. Corfield AP, Cooper MJ, Williamson RCN (1985) Acute pancreatitis: a lethal disease of increasing incidence. Gut 26:724–729.
20. Wilson C, Imrie CW (1990) Changing patterns of incidence and mortality from acute pancreatitis in Scotland, 1961–1985. Br J Surg 77:731–734.
21. Jaakkola M, Nordback I (1993) Pancreatitis in Finland between 1970 and 1989. Gut 34:1255–1260.
22. McKay C, Sinclair M, Evans S, McCarthy A, Imrie CW Increasing incidence of acute pancreatitis in Scotland 1985–1994. (abstract).
23. Thomson SR, Hendry WS, McFarlane GA, Davidson AI (1987) Epidemiology and outcome of acute pancreatitis. Br J Surg 74:398–401.
24. Agarwal N, Pitchumoni CS, Sivaprasad AV (1990) Evaluation tests for acute pancreatitis. Am J Gastroenterol 85:356–366.
25. Pieper-Bigelow C, Strocchi A, Levitt MD (1990) Where does serum amylase come from and where does it go? Gastroenterol Clin North Am 19:793–810.
26. Dickson AP, O'Neill J, Imrie CW (1984) Hyperlipidaemia, alcohol abuse and acute pancreatitis. Br J Surg 71:685–699.
27. Gumaste VV, Roditis N, Mehta D, Dave PB (1993) Serum lipase levels in non-pancreatic abdominal pain versus acute pancreatitis. Am J Gastroenterol 88:2051–2055.
28. Lankisch PG, Schirren CA, Kunze E (1991) Undetected fatal acute pancreatitis: why is the disease so frequently overlooked? Am J Gastroenterol 86:322–326.
29. Banerjee AK, Kaul A, Bache E, Parberry AC, Doran J, Nicholson ML (1995) An audit of fatal acute pancreatitis. Postgrad Med J 71:472–475.
30. Toffler AH, Spiro HM (1962) Shock or coma as the predominant manifestation of painless acute pancreatitis. Ann Intern Med 57:655–659.
31. Shader AE, Paxton JR (1966) Fatal pancreatitis. Am J Surg 111:369–373.
32. Read G, Braganza JM, Howat HT (1976) Pancreatitis: retrospective study. Gut. 17:945–952.
33. Hofler H (1979) Todesursachen. Uberlebenszeit und whal des operationszeitpunktes. (English translation: Necrosis of the pancreas). Dsch Med Wochensch 104:315–317.
34. Buggy BP, Nostrant TT (1983) Lethal pancreatitis. Am J Gastroenterol 78:810–814.
35. Peterson LM, Brooks JR (1979) Lethal pancreatitis: a diagnostic dilemma. Am J Surg 137:491–496.
36. Bannerjee AK, Haggie SJ, Jones RB, Basran GS (1995) Respiratory failure in acute pancreatitis. Postgrad Med 72:327–330.
37. Renner IG, Savage WT, Pantoja JL, Renner VJ (1985) Death due to acute pancreatitis: a retrospective analysis of 405 autopsy cases. Dig Dis Sci 30:1005–1018.
38. Wilson C, Imrie CW, Carter DC (1988) Fatal acute pancreatitis. Gut 29:782–788.

8 The Role of Magnetic Resonance in Acute Pancreatitis

A.G. Chalmers and A.J. Cullingworth

At the time of writing, dynamic contrast enhanced computed tomography (CT) using conventional or more recently spiral/helical techniques, remains the accepted gold standard for imaging patients with severe acute pancreatitis. Any new imaging technique must provide significant advantages over established practice before being accepted as a satisfactory alternative or replacement. The respective roles of other techniques have been discussed elsewhere (1). In this chapter the relative advantages and disadvantages of magnetic resonance (MR) with respect to CT will be discussed and the strengths and weaknesses of each technique will be highlighted with respect to the particular requirements for imaging in acute pancreatitis.

The definitions agreed at Atlanta in 1992 (2) form a useful framework for this chapter and each will be discussed in turn with particular emphasis on the role of MR. The next section of this chapter will give a review of MR terminology, imaging sequences used with their advantages and disadvantages, and what MR means for the patient, because clinicians should be aware of what their patient will experience when such an examination is requested.

The Dutch physicist C.J. Gorter developed the concept of nuclear magnetic resonance in 1936 (NMR). NMR was demonstrated in bulk materials by the work of Bloch at Stanford and Purcell at Harvard in 1946. The key to adapting NMR to modern imaging techniques was Lauterbur's suggestion in 1973 to spatially localise a signal origin by using magnetic field gradients to encode the MR signal. Workers at the University of Nottingham were the first to produce images of human anatomy by a magnetic resonance technique in 1976 and 1977. Since then, engineering and computing advances along with developing scientific and clinical understanding have combined to produce the new diagnostic imaging tool we know as MR.

Terminology

Pulse Sequence Parameters

Magnetic resonance images are produced by pulse sequences which are made up of a series of radio frequency (RF) pulses, MR signal generation and intervening periods of relaxation.

Repetition time (TR). The time from the application of one RF excitation pulse to the application of the next RF excitation pulse is the repetition time (TR).

Echo time (TE). The time from the application of the RF excitation pulse to the peak signal induced in the receiver coil is the echo time (TE).

Image Contrast

T1 and T2 relaxation are the most important mechanisms to provide image contrast.

T1 relaxation. T1 relaxation is the process by which hydrogen nuclei lose energy to the surrounding environment and return to their equilibrium position.

T2 relaxation. T2 relaxation results from decay of the MR signal due to inter-actions between the magnetic fields of adjacent hydrogen nuclei.

T1 and T2 relaxation are independent processes but occur simultaneously, and as protons in different tissues relax at different rates, this gives us T1 and T2 contrast.

Image Weighting

To demonstrate either T1, proton density, or T2 contrast, specific values of TR and TE are selected for a given pulse sequence. It is possible to select values of TR and TE so that one contrast mechanism predominates in the resultant image. This is known as T1 or T2 weighting (T1W or T2W).

T1W images are of higher signal to noise ratio (SNR) when compared with T2W images and are useful to demonstrate abdominal anatomy including the fat planes between organs. Liver and pancreas have short T1 relaxation times and display a higher signal intensity on T1W images when compared with the spleen. Fat displays the highest signal intensity of all tissue on T1W images and will best demonstrate fatty infiltration of the pancreas.

T2W images best demonstrate pathology rather than anatomical detail as most pathological processes display a high water content which will show as an area of high signal intensity on these sequences. On T2W images the signal intensity of the pancreas is similar or slightly higher than the liver but is lower than the signal intensity of spleen.

Image Quality

Image quality is dependent on the signal to noise ratio (SNR), and spatial resolution. It is desirable to maximise SNR and spatial resolution while keeping scan times as short as possible. However, these factors are interrelated so that each factor must be optimised in relation to the others chosen.

Signal intensity. This is the amplitude of the MR signal induced in the receiver coil. A large signal will result in a bright area on the image, a low signal will result in a dark area on the image.

Signal to noise ratio (SNR). This is the ratio of the amplitude of the MR signal to the amplitude of background noise. As SNR increases, so image quality improves.

Spatial resolution. Spatial resolution is the ability to distinguish two adjacent structures as separate and distinct.

Temporal resolution. This is the time factor involved in acquiring scan data. Reducing the acquisition time of any sequence will improve temporal resolution.

Pulse Sequences

Spin echo sequences. For spin echo imaging, a 90° radiofrequency (RF) excitation pulse tips magnetisation into the transverse plane. This is followed by a 180° refocusing pulse which reforms the transverse magnetisation to produce an echo or MR signal. This process is repeated many times (typically 128–256) to produce a diagnostic MR image. Scan times for these sequences are around 5–8 minutes for T1W and 10–15 minutes for T2W spin echo sequences.

In dual echo SE sequences, the MR signal is sampled at two different echo times to produce a series of images that are T2W and also a series of images that are proton density weighted (PDW). PDW images reflect the number of protons in a particular tissue and there is no time penalty incurred for this additional information. PDW images are of higher SNR than the T2-weighted images and so provide better anatomical detail but are of lower contrast to noise ratio.

Fast spin echo sequences. Fast spin echo (FSE) or turbo spin echo (TSE) is now widely available. FSE uses multiple 180° refocusing pulses during each TR interval to generate a train of echoes following each excitation pulse. All the echoes contribute to the T2 FSE images and the number of echoes acquired is called the echo train length or turbo factor. The imaging time can be reduced in proportion to the echo train length so that high-quality T2W images can be obtained in typically 2–4 minutes. This represents a major time saving when compared with conventional spin echo images, and FSE sequences can be used to increase image quality or improve temporal resolution.

Proton density weighted images can be acquired using FSE sequences but there is a time penalty as some echoes are used to produce the proton density weighted images and some echoes are used to produce the T2-weighted images. The main limitation of FSE in the abdomen is some reduction in contrast differences between pathology and normal parenchyma compared with conventional spin echo sequences.

Gradient echo (GE) sequences. Gradient echo (GE) sequences use a single RF pulse and magnetic field gradients to form an echo or signal. This can be achieved in a much shorter time than for SE sequences. However, gradient echo sequences are of lower SNR and more prone to magnetic field inhomogeneity artefacts than SE sequences. Gradient echo sequences are used for dynamic contrast enhanced imaging.

Fat suppression sequences. T1W and T2W FSE fat suppressed sequences have improved the role of MRI in pancreatic disease. The resonant frequencies of fat and water are separated by about 3.5 ppm and it is possible to selectively saturate or suppress the signal from fat by using a frequency selective radio frequency pulse before imaging. Both the pancreas and adipose tissue are high-signal tissues on T1W images; fat suppression techniques can be used to improve visualisation of T1 contrast in the pancreas. T2W fat suppressed sequences demonstrate fluid collections.

2D and 3D imaging. It is possible to acquire information in the form of two-dimensional (2D) slices or as a three-dimensional (3D) volume. A 2D multislice sequence is one in which several slices are acquired during one scan period. In a 3D sequence, a volume of data rather than single slices are obtained. From this volume data set, single slices can be retrospectively constructed in any anatomical plane.

Motion-Related Artefacts

For both SE and FSE sequences, the scan times are in the order of minutes which allows image quality to be decreased by movement caused by respiratory motion, bowel peristalsis and blood flow. Motion causes ghost artefacts and image blurring. Respiratory motion, cardiac motion and blood flow cause discrete ghost artefacts which represent shadows of anatomical structures which have moved during the acquisition period and are repeated across the image often obscuring true anatomy. These artefacts may be reduced by the following strategies.

Multiple signal averaging. The number of signal averages is the number of times that data collection is repeated. Increasing the number of signal averages increases SNR and reduces the intensity of ghost artefacts but involves a penalty of a fourfold increase in scan time to achieve a 50% reduction in ghost artefacts. This is difficult to achieve for conventional T2W SE sequences because of the long acquisition times but high quality T1W SE images with relatively little motion-related artefact can be obtained with multiple signal averages.

Flow compensation which reduces respiratory artefact and artefact from flowing blood and cerebrospinal fluid (CSF).

Fat suppression techniques which reduce ghost artefacts arising from motion of subcutaneous fat in the chest or abdominal wall.

Respiratory compensation in which data collection is synchronised with the respiratory cycle.

Respiratory gating. The methods described above reduce ghost artefacts but not imaging blurring. Image blurring and ghost artefacts can be eliminated by ensuring that an object is in the same position during the acquisition of each view. This requires some means of controlling the effects of respiration and is accomplished by a technique called respiratory gating. With respiratory gating, the pulse sequence is triggered when the patient breaths out and continues until the patient breathes in again. This restriction in data collection is inefficient and as data are only acquired during part of the respiratory cycle, the scan time may be increased by 2–4 times. Although this is prohibitive for SE techniques, FSE with respiratory triggering is now available and is effective in eliminating respiratory ghosts and blurring.

Breath-hold sequences

The most effective way to reduce respiratory artefacts and blurring is to use breath-hold sequences. Using GE techniques, scan times can be reduced to seconds rather than the minutes required for SE imaging. Recent improvements in hardware and software permit very short echo times to generate multislice imaging in a breath-hold period of 15–20 seconds. These sequences have the disadvantage of low inherent contrast and SNR but fast imaging provides the temporal resolution necessary for dynamic studies. 3D gradient echo and multislice 2D GE sequences can be performed following a bolus injection of gadolinium DTPA. Both techniques provide 15–20 slices in a breath-hold period.

Field Strength, Types of Magnet and Magnet Environment

The magnets used in MR departments today involve field strengths ranging from under 0.03 Tesla(T) to 4 T. The SNR improves as magnetic field strength increases. There are two principal types of magnet:

Permanent Magnets

These are limited by their excessive weight (6–100 tons) and small field strengths (0.03 T to 0.3 T). Advantages of permanent magnets are that they require no power supply and have low operating costs. They have negligible fringe fields as the magnetic field runs vertically, which makes siting the magnet easier. This feature also enables an open magnet design to be used which is more "patient-friendly". However, at low field strengths, examination times are increased, limiting applications in the abdomen where patient motion is a problem and temporal resolution is needed for breath-hold imaging and dynamic contrast enhanced techniques.

Superconducting Electromagnets

These operate at temperatures near to absolute zero by using cryogens such as liquid helium and, in some older systems, liquid nitrogen as coolants. Superconducting magnets can produce field strengths ranging from 0.35 T to 4 T and are therefore considerably more powerful than permanent magnets. These systems have the advantage of high field homogeneity and stability when compared with permanent magnets.

The strength of the MR signal is directly proportional to the field strength of the system so that when using the same scan parameters, SNR at 1.5 T is approximately three times the SNR at 0.5 T. Conversely it is possible to produce comparable images in terms of SNR at 1.5 T in a third of the scan time required with 0.5 T. The reduction in scan time is most significant for breath-hold imaging which allows improved temporal resolution or an increase in the number of slices.

A disadvantage of a high field system is the increased prominence of artefacts such as respiratory motion artefact. T1 contrast is also reduced compared with images acquired on lower field strength systems. The requirements for siting and cooling high field superconducting magnets are complex and expensive. The direction of the main magnetic field in a superconducting magnet is along the bore of the magnet and the patient lies within the magnet bore throughout the examination. The magnet and its housing is 1.9–2.5 m long and 50–60 cm in diameter. A small but significant number of patients find this environment uncomfortably claustrophobic, which may lead them to refuse or prematurely terminate the examination.

Gradient coils perform spatial localisation of the MR signal by generating alternating magnetic fields within the main static magnetic field. Opposing magnetic fields generate vibration in the gradient coils which produces acoustic noise. For the patient, this means hearing a loud banging noise throughout the scan which can be distressing. Ear protection can help.

Safety

While MR avoids the use of ionising radiation there remain important safety issues related to the MR environment. Hazards related to the static magnetic field may cause pacemakers or other implanted devices and life support systems to malfunction. The detection and identification of foreign materials before the patient enters the MR suite is important because motion or displacement of these objects may cause injury to the patient or MR staff. It is therefore necessary for each patient to complete a screening questionnaire prior to examination. Patients in the following categories are excluded from MR examination:

Patients fitted with internal cardiac pacemakers, cochlear implants, retinal tacks, aneurysm clips

Patients known to have metal fragments lodged in the orbits

Consideration must also be given to certain electronic, electromechanical and metallic implants.

There is no convincing evidence to date that electromagnetic fields at the level used in clinical MR can cause any detrimental effect to the embryo or foetus but as a precautionary measure patients during the first trimester of pregnancy are excluded from MR examination unless there are overriding clinical grounds.

There is a potential missile effect when ferromagnetic materials are placed in the strong static magnetic field. The static magnetic field may cause loose ferromagnetic objects to become projectiles resulting in danger to persons close by or within the bore of the magnet as well as causing damage to the equipment. Ferromagnetic objects must be excluded from the examination room. These include standard hospital trolleys, wheelchairs and drip stands, gas cylinders, life support systems, tools, keys, scissors, pins, and jewellery which may be ferromagnetic. The static magnetic field may cause damage to electronic equipment such as infusion pumps and patient monitors. This raises practical problems for scanning acutely ill patients who require monitoring and ventilation as all such equipment must be MR compatible. Swapping from conventional to MR-compatible equipment in the scanning suite is time consuming. Before requesting an MR study for a patient on a life support system, careful liaison with the MR staff must take place so as to maintain an efficient and safe scanning service.

The Clinical Role of MR in Acute Pancreatitis

Interstitial Pancreatitis

The Atlanta Symposium (2) described mild acute pancreatitis as that condition associated with minimal organ dysfunction and an uneventful recovery. Mild attacks of acute pancreatitis can result in no significant change to the imaging appearances of the normal pancreas (3). With increasing disease severity the pancreas becomes swollen, displays reduced clarity at its margins, and may develop a mild heterogeneity of the parenchymal signal intensity. In approximately 20% of cases the pathological insult will be focal, most commonly involving the head.

Intravenous gadolinium is the MR contrast agent equivalent of iodinated contrast used for dynamic CT techniques. To date gadolinium has no reported significant adverse effects and can be safely used in patients with contrast allergy and renal dysfunction. Increasingly, high doses of intravenous gadolinium are being delivered during a variety of contrast-enhanced MR techniques with no adverse effects (11). The MR technique mirrors CT practice with a bolus delivery of gadolinium followed by a multislice acquisition through the pancreatic bed during the arterial phase of contrast enhancement.

Following intravenous gadolinium, the pancreatic parenchyma in mild acute pancreatitis enhances normally in analogous fashion to that found following contrast-enhanced CT (Figure 1a–c). Macroscopic areas of pancreatic necrosis are not found although minor degrees of peripancreatic necrosis may be present. The peripancreatic fat changes may be best seen on the non-contrast breath-hold gradient echo sequence performed prior to the post-gadolinium series (4).

Acute Fluid Collections

These occur early in the course of acute pancreatitis, are located in or around the pancreas, and always lack a capsule of fibrous or granulation tissue. The lack of a defined wall helps diagnostic differentiation from a pancreatic abscess. The majority of acute fluid collections spontaneously resolve without intervention although some progress to abscess formation or mature into pseudocysts (Figure 2).

MR has two significant advantages over CT in the display of acute fluid collections. First, the superior contrast sensitivity of MR enables the content of fluid collections to be characterised, and second, the multiplanar capabilities of MR provide optimum anatomical demonstration of the extent and location of any collection (5). CT is poor at differentiating between an inflammatory collection which is predominantly fluid and one which is predominantly solid. Both may appear of comparably low attenuation on CT. MR can accurately display the internal composition of fluid collections and by indicating the proportion of fluid and solid constituents, can more effectively predict which collections are drainable and which will not benefit from percutaneous intervention (Figure 3 and 4). Ultrasonography can provide similar information but has limitations in the demonstration of collections in the retroperitoneal compartments.

The ability to acquire directly information in a variety of anatomical planes enables MR to demonstrate elegantly the distribution of fluid collections as well

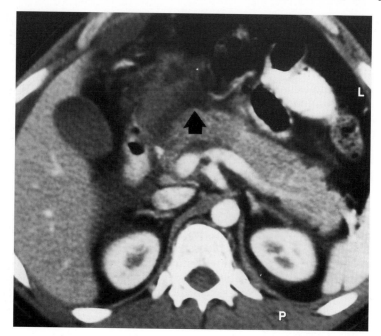

a

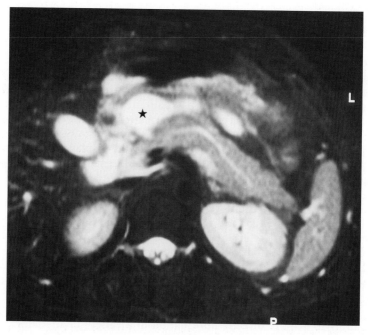

b

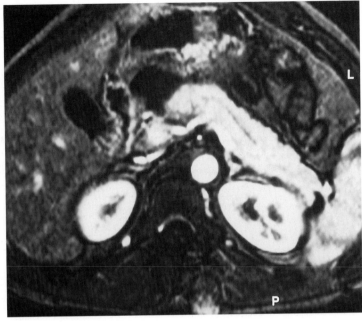

c

Figure 1. a Contrast-enhanced CT section through swollen pancreatic body and tail. Mild hetero-geneity of signal intensity within region of pancreatic neck/pancreatic body. Small acute fluid collections around pancreatic neck (*arrow*). **b** T2W TSE sequence with fat saturation performed several days after CT study. Anterior acute fluid collection shown as area of high signal intensity (*star*). **c** Breath-hold post-gadolinium 3D volume acquisition at comparable level to **a**. Pancreatic parenchyma displays normal enhancement with no evidence of necrosis.

as their composition. Coronal plane imaging in particular can be useful when collections extend remote from the pancreatic bed and can aid interventional or surgical planning (Figure 5).

Spiral CT using thin sections and an overlapping reconstruction index can provide images of similar anatomical display by using multiplanar reconstruction techniques. When the extent of a fluid collection involves a large anatomical area, CT coverage may be limited by tube cooling restrictions which may restrict the collimation chosen, leading to insufficient data acquisition to provide quality reformats. MR does not have this limitation.

Acute Pseudocysts

Defined at Atlanta (2) as a collection of pancreatic juice enclosed by a non-epithelialised wall which arises as a consequence of acute pancreatitis, pancreatic trauma or chronic pancreatitis and is of four or more weeks duration.

Pseudocysts are well demonstrated by MR with again two significant advantages over CT, namely superior contrast resolution for cyst content and a multiplanar anatomical display (Figure 6). Suspicion of haemorrhage into a

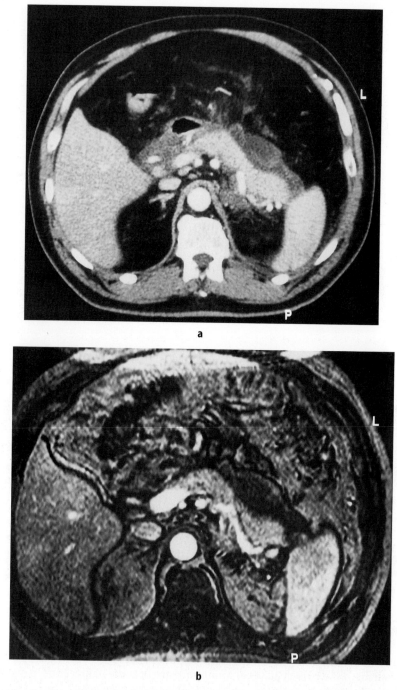

Figure 2. a Contrast-enhanced CT section through pancreatic body showing normal enhancement parenchyma of body and tail and well-defined adjacent acute fluid collection. **b** Analogous post-gadolinium breath-hold image showing comparable parenchymal enhancement to that shown on CT with anterior peripancreatic fluid collection.

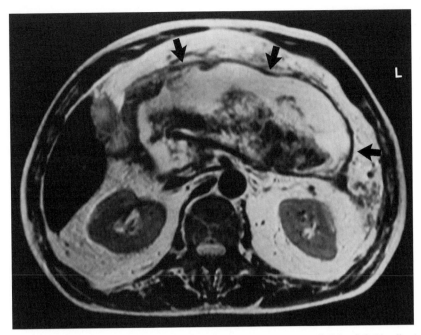

Figure 3. Axial T2W TSE image through pancreatic bed showing large well defined fluid collection (*arrows*) with excellent demonstration of internal residual pancreas/necrotic debris.

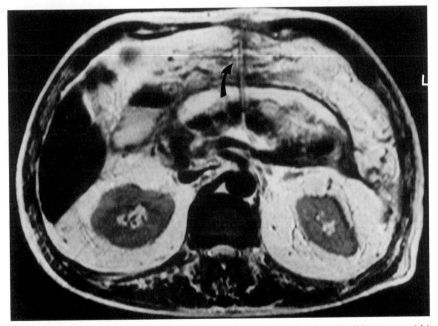

Figure 4. Axial T2W sequence through pancreatic bed showing extent of solid content within inflammatory collection. Note transgastric drainage catheter (*arrow*).

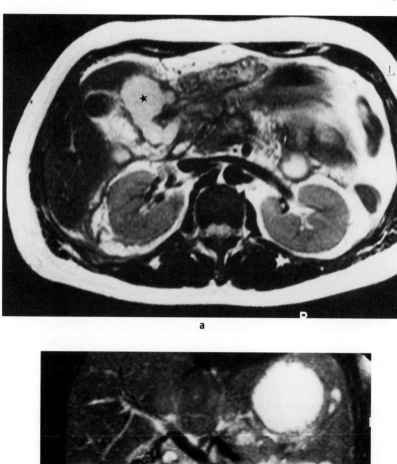

a

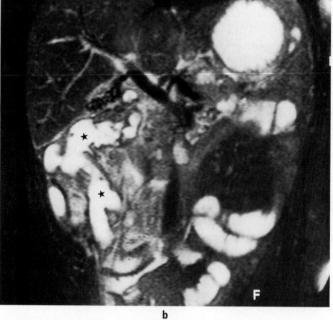

b

Figure 5. a Axial T2W TSE sections through pancreatic head showing fluid collection between pancreas and gallbladder fossa (*star*). **b** Coronal T2W TSE with fat saturation showing extent of fluid collection within right flank (*stars*).

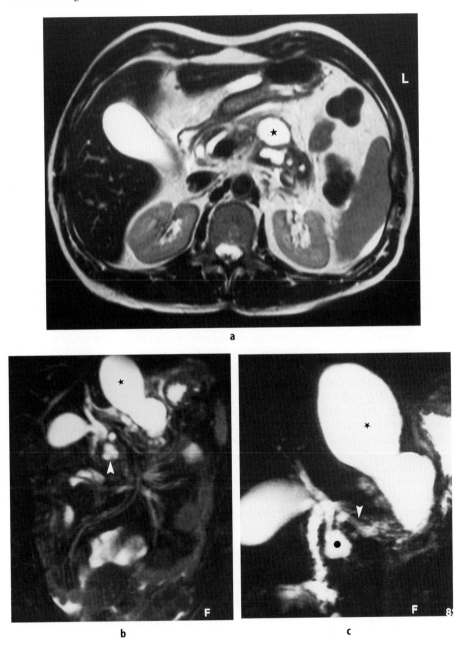

Figure 6. a Axial T2W TSE with fat saturation image through pancreatic body and tail showing patchily dilated pancreatic duct and inferior extent of mature pseudocyst (*star*). **b** Coronal T2W TSE with fat saturation showing lobulated pseudocyst (*star*) with further fluid-filled cavity within pancreatic head (*arrowhead*). **c** Breath-hold MRCP sequence showing pseudocyst (*star*) adjacent to dilated pancreatic duct (*arrowhead*). Pancreatic head cavity also demonstrated (*dot*).

pseudocyst can be confirmed by demonstrating high signal intensity on both T1W and T2W sequences. Dynamic post-gadolinium sequences with image acquisition during the arterial phase of contrast enhancement are used to detect any pseudoaneurysm formation.

Pancreatic Abscess

Defined at Atlanta (2) as a circumscribed intra-abdominal collection of pus, containing little or no pancreatic necrosis, which arises as a consequence of acute pancreatitis or pancreatic trauma. There is a need to differentiate pancreatic abscess from infected pancreatic necrosis as management will be different for the two conditions, and infected necrosis attracts twice to three times the mortality risk of abscess (6). In most cases sterile pancreatic necrosis can be managed conservatively whereas infected necrosis typically requires prompt surgical intervention.

Fine needle aspiration is required to confirm a diagnosis of abscess. Gas is present in only the minority of abscesses and infected necrosis, with figures of less than 30% being quoted in the CT literature. The MR diagnosis of small volume gas foci is difficult and the diagnosis is more easily and confidently made by CT, which gives it a significant advantage over MR when abscess or infected necrosis requires confirmation or exclusion. When conventional double echo T2W SE imaging is used, focal gas densities may be best demonstrated on the proton density sequence (5). Double echo T2W SE sequences are now performed less often on MR systems which have fast scanning capability and the ability to produce quality turbo spin echo images.

Although double echo TSE sequences can be performed, this increases the length of the examination and currently there are no publications assessing whether proton density TSE images offer any advantage over single echo TSE sequences in the detection of gas. Larger collections of gas are readily detected by MR (Figure 7). If MR is equivocal concerning the presence of gas, then a limited non-contrast CT study through the area of concern may be required.

Although MR-guided percutaneous aspiration is possible, the technique is time consuming and technically difficult compared with CT or ultrasound-guided procedures. For practical purposes percutaneous biopsy/aspiration under MR guidance is virtually never performed, the vast majority of interventions being carried out with either ultrasound or CT guidance. Recent developments with open magnet technology make interventions under MR guidance a more realistic proposition but open magnet systems in general cannot provide the level of image quality required for the diagnostic component of an acute pancreatitis study.

Pancreatic Necrosis

Pancreatic necrosis as defined at Atlanta (2) is a diffuse or focal area(s) of non-viable pancreatic parenchyma which is typically associated with peripancreatic fat necrosis. The difficulties of diagnosis using clinical findings and physiological scoring systems are well known, as are the limitations of direct surgical

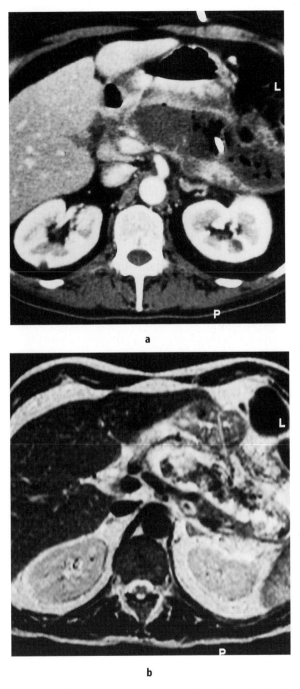

Figure 7. a Contrast-enhanced CT section through pancreatic bed showing fluid collection with transgastric drainage catheter. Multifocal gas densities within collection. **b** Analogous axial T2W TSE sequence showing collection contains much internal debris and focal gas densities.

assessment at the time of laparotomy (7). Publications throughout the 1980s and early 1990s evaluating the role of dynamic CT with contrast enhancement, led to the general acceptance that CT can diagnose pancreatic necrosis as well as indicating how much of the pancreatic parenchymal volume is involved. By combining an assessment of pancreatic and peripancreatic fluid collections with a quantitative assessment of pancreatic necrosis, a CT "severity index" was developed, which gave a prognostic indication of the likely disease outcome (8).

Establishing or excluding a diagnosis of pancreatic necrosis is one of the most important roles for diagnostic imaging as there is a strong correlation between the presence of necrosis and clinical outcome. The diagnosis of pancreatic necrosis is made by assessing the response of pancreatic parenchyma to intravenous iodinated contrast. The degree of parenchymal enhancement is either measured in Hounsfield units before and after intravenous contrast or the post-contrast appearances are compared with the degree of enhancement of the adjacent spleen. The Atlanta definition requires one third or more of the parenchyma to display compromised enhancement before a diagnosis of pancreatic necrosis can be established.

Typically some 100–150 ml of iodinated contrast is injected using a power injector. Some authors have shown little or no effect on subsequent renal function in patients with severe acute pancreatitis who have undergone contrast-enhanced CT (7). Others (9) have shown in animal models that the use of iodinated contrast can lead to an extension of the necrotic process although this view has not found widespread support (10). Nevertheless if large volumes of intravenous contrast can be avoided by using an alternative imaging technique, then there are at least theoretical benefits to the patient, which become more important when multiple examinations are required (10). Post-gadolinium dynamic studies provide an MR alternative to the information provided by contrast-enhanced CT (5) (Figures 8 & 9).

The need to avoid iodinated contrast in patients with multiorgan dysfunction, becomes more important when the often prolonged nature of an episode of severe acute pancreatitis is considered. This patient group typically requires a number of follow-up scans after the initial diagnostic study. The cumulative effects of radiation dose and repeated iodinated contrast delivery are important considerations especially in younger patients. Although contrast-enhancement studies are required in only the minority of follow-up studies, MR with or without gadolinium will avoid repeat iodinated contrast delivery and radiation exposure to the patient.

Recent Developments in MR Imaging of Abdomen and Pancreas

MR Cholangiopancreatography (MRCP)

MRCP aims to produce images comparable to those provided by endoscopic retrograde cholangiopancreatography (ERCP) in a non-invasive manner, avoiding endoscopic cannulation of the ampulla and avoiding the use of contrast media. For patients with gallstone pancreatitis, the demonstration of duct calculi early in the disease process means in some centres a requirement for ERCP

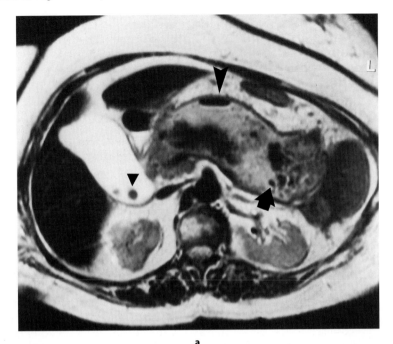

a

b

Figure 8. Series of images in an uncooperative patient who was unable to breath-hold. **a** Axial T2W TSE image through pancreatic bed showing inflammatory collection which contains much internal debris. Gas densities noted towards tail (*arrow*) and small air/fluid level anteriorly (*large arrowhead*). Note gallstones (*small arrowhead*). **b** Axial dynamic post-gadolinium sequence through comparable anatomy demonstrating minor areas of residual enhancement within posterior aspect of head and body (*arrows*). Extensive pancreatic necrosis.

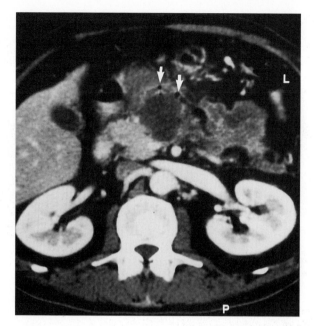

a

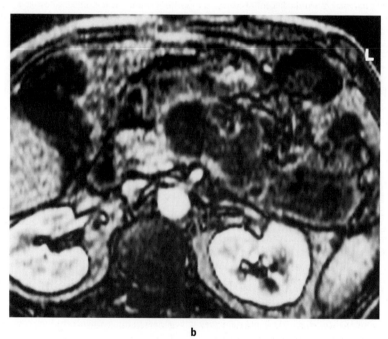

b

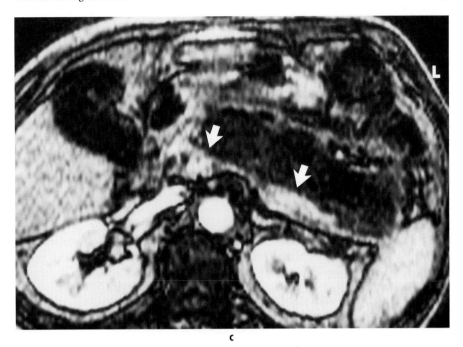

c

Figure 9. a Contrast-enhanced CT section through region of pancreatic neck and proximal body showing normally enhancing pancreatic head and adjacent necrosis in pancreatic body. Note gas foci anteriorly (*arrows*). **b** Analogous post-gadolinium breath-hold sequence showing corresponding enhancing parenchyma and adjacent necrosis. Gas densities cannot be identified. **c** Post-gadolinium breath-hold sequence through pancreatic body showing residual viable pancreatic parenchyma posteriorly within head and body (*arrows*). No evidence of the gas densities shown on analogous CT image.

and sphincterotomy. The role of sphincterotomy in patients with severe acute pancreatitis is controversial and has both its supporters and detractors (12,13).

Heavily T2-weighted sequences are used for MRCP. An extremely long TR (8000 msec) and TE (1200 msec) are used, which results in very little signal being contributed by solid tissue so that the image is largely produced by the high signal arising from static fluid in the biliary tree, pancreatic duct, stomach and duodenum and renal collecting systems.

Gradient echo and FSE methods can be used for MRCP. 2D FSE MRCP can be achieved in a single breath-hold using a single slice of 20–100 mm. A scan time of 2 seconds is possible at 1.5 T and several views in a variety of oblique planes can be obtained to best demonstrate biliary and pancreatic duct anatomy. As the acquisition times are short the image is less susceptible to motion artefact and a high-quality examination can be obtained in a very short time. Because of the short acquisition times, any images which fail to reach diagnostic quality can be repeated without significantly extending the duration of the study. By comparison, a 3D FSE volumetric acquisition has the advantage of higher SNR and spatial resolution than 2D techniques but suffers from much longer scan times. Typical acquisition times of 8 minutes at 1.5 T leads to problems with respiratory motion artefact. A recent technical development in MRI is the introduction of high power gradients, which enable shorter echo spacing, leading to reduction in scan times for breath-hold sequences or an increase in the number of slices possible. The shorter echo spacing also improves image sharpness.

Currently the most widely used technique for MRCP is a 3D volume heavily T2-weighted TSE sequence with maximum intensity projection (MIP). MIP is a mathematical manipulation of the scan data which takes only high signal information from the source images and displays this as a 3D projection. Both the MIP and source images are reviewed to fully evaluate the biliary and pancreatic ductal system allowing choledocholithiasis and pancreatic duct calculi to be identified. MRCP has lower spatial resolution but higher contrast resolution when compared with ERCP, which allows stones of only a few millimetres to be identified within the common bile duct (14). MRCP also demonstrates the pancreatic ductal system, a normal duct being identified in 69% of MIP images and 81% of single-slice images (15).

One limitation of MRCP is the non-dynamic nature of the study. With ERCP, injected contrast can be observed fluoroscopically to enter cavities, fistulate with bowel, etc., whereas MRCP simply displays static fluid with all other detail being effaced. MRCP does have the advantage of displaying ductal anatomy distal to a point of obstruction, a function ERCP cannot provide. Although the role of MRCP has not been fully evaluated in patients with acute pancreatitis, the addition of breath-hold sequences to the study does not prolong the MR examination unduly and the demonstration of choledocholithiasis may be an important diagnostic detail for management plans in these patients (Figure 10). Nevertheless,

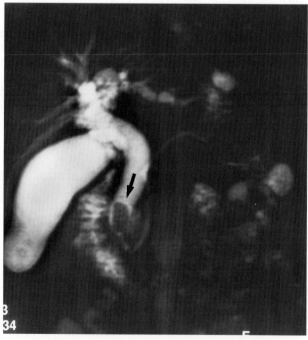

Figure 10. Breath-hold MRCP showing dilated extrahepatic biliary tree with calculus at the lower end of common bile duct (*arrow*). Stones within gallbladder and normal calibre pancreatic duct noted.

images of sufficient diagnostic detail may not be possible in very ill patients, who find the MR environment difficult to cope with.

The demonstration of gall stones by CT is poor. However, MR, using T2W sequences, is an excellent technique for showing gall stones (5) (Figure 8a).

MR Angiography

MR angiography has been available for some time. Most techniques have involved MR sequences such as phase contrast and time-of-flight which do not use intravenous contrast. Advances with fast scanning techniques have enabled MR vascular studies to give comparable anatomical display to that obtained with conventional angiography. These techniques involve the use of dynamic breath-hold 3D volume sequences with image acquisition following bolus delivery of intravenous gadolinium (16). Depending on the clinical problem being evaluated, images can be acquired in the arterial phase of contrast enhancement, the portal venous phase, or both (Figure 11). As well as using intravenous gadolinium to assess the presence and extent of parenchymal necrosis, magnetic resonance angiography techniques can be applied to demonstrate the vascular complications of acute pancreatitis, e.g. splenic vein thrombosis and pseudoaneurysm formation. The presence of a pseudoaneurysm is particularly important when interventional techniques are being considered.

Future Developments in MR

Developmental work in MR is largely aimed at producing ever faster scanning techniques. An example of this is echo planar imaging (EPI) in which the entire image is generated after a single RF excitation, accomplished by a series of gradient echoes generated by multiple gradient reversals. At present, the use of EPI in the abdomen has produced images with good T2 contrast characteristics but relatively low spatial resolution. Scan times of 100 msec or less are possible, which effectively eliminates motion artefact. EPI does require specialised hardware, which is not widely available. The development of such techniques will undoubtedly extend the application of MRI in the abdomen but, as yet, the clinical benefits of EPI in abdominal imaging have still to be established.

Summary

Magnetic resonance offers a realistic alternative to contrast-enhanced dynamic CT in the assessment of patients with acute pancreatitis. MR offers the advantage of excellent contrast sensitivity with a spatial resolution approaching that of CT but without the need for ionising radiation or large volumes of intravenous iodinated contrast agents. MR can confirm the diagnosis of acute pancreatitis when there is diagnostic doubt. It can diagnose pancreatic necrosis and can identify the various complications of acute pancreatitis.

There are, however, significant disadvantages to the use of MR in patients with acute pancreatitis. MR scanners provide an unfriendly environment with lower

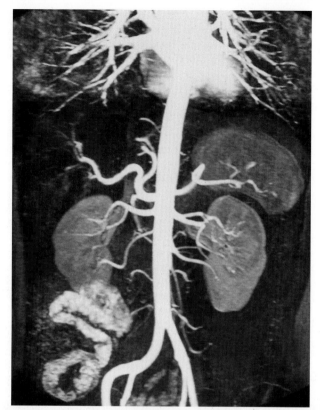

a

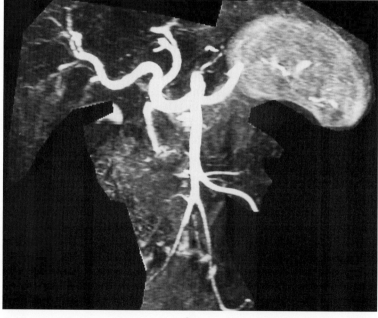

b

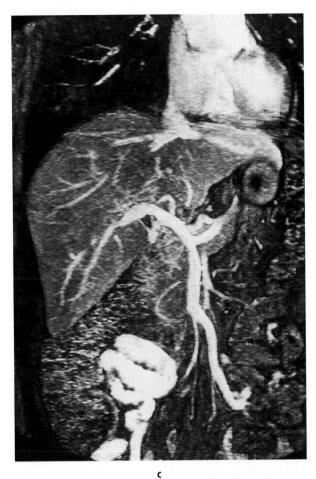

c

Figure 11. a Dynamic post-gadolinium breath-hold study abdominal aorta showing coeliac axis and renal arterial anatomy. **b** Similar breath-hold dynamic post-gadolinium image of coeliac axis. **c** Dynamic breath-hold post-gadolinium acquisition during portal venous phase of contrast enhancement displaying intra- and extrahepatic portal venous system. Patient has thrombosis of left portal vein. (By kind permission of Dr J.F.M. Meaney.)

patient acceptance when compared with CT. The practical difficulties of examining ventilated or high-dependency unit patients with their attendant life support systems may effectively preclude the use of MR and, currently, interventional procedures are not performed under MR guidance. In the UK, MR units remain a scarce and costly resource and are almost universally under significant pressure from multiple specialty groups requiring access for the more established indications for MR imaging.

For the present, contrast-enhanced CT remains the front-line imaging technique for the assessment of acute pancreatitis. However, MR offers a realistic alternative both for initial diagnostic and disease severity assessment, but especially for follow-up examinations and answering specific questions concerning extrapancreatic fluid collections and other complications.

Details of the scanning sequences currently used in our department are given in Appendix 1.

Appendix 1. Leeds General Infirmary MR protocol for acute pancreatitis

1. **Transverse T2 TSE with respiratory triggering, pancreatic bed**
   Scan time: 20 slices in 2 minutes.
   T2W TSE images give good anatomical display free from the ghost artefacts prevalent with T1W SE imaging, which are problematic in ill patients. Fluid collections can be demonstrated and characterised. Gallstones will be shown.

2. **Coronal T2W TSE with fat suppression**
   Scan time: 20 slices in 2 minutes.
   This fat suppression sequence emphasises the soft tissue/fluid differentiation but obliterates much of the anatomical display of the pancreas and peri-pancreatic tissues. Excellent sequence for fluid collections and their charac-terisation. Good for display of gallstones and occasionally common duct stones.

3. **Single-shot MRCP**
   Scan time: single slice in 2 seconds
   Using a short breath-hold heavily T2-weighted TSE sequence, excellent demonstration of the biliary tree and pancreatic duct can be obtained. Choledocholithiasis can be confirmed/excluded which may have significant management impact determining whether acute ERCP and sphincterotomy in gallstone pancreatitis is indicated. Even using relatively short breath-hold sequences, this technique can be technically unsuccessful in patients who are acutely unwell.

4. **Breath-hold T1W gradient echo pancreatic bed**
   Scan time: 20 slices in 16–23 seconds
   (a) Sequence obtained primarily to determine levels for post-contrast dynamic series. Also good for display of peripancreatic inflammatory changes.
   (b) Post-gadolinium dynamic 3D volume axial (± coronal) acquisition through pancreas
   The key sequence for diagnosis or exclusion of pancreatic necrosis. Can identify peripancreatic vascular complications, e.g. splenic vein thrombosis or pseudoaneurysm formation. Subsequent coronal dynamic sequence can be of value to show relationship of extrapancreatic inflammatory changes to enhanced pancreatic parenchyma.

Acknowledgements

The authors wish to thank Susan Lawrence and Janet Papuga for kindly typing the manuscript and Medical Illustration, Leeds General Infirmary. The majority of the cases were referred by Mr M.J. McMahon and Mr M. Larvin. We thank them for their kind permission to use these patients for illustration.

References

1. Chalmers AG (1997) The role of imaging in acute pancreatitis. Eur J Gastroenterol Hepatol 9:106–116.
2. Bradley EL III (1993) A clinically based classification system for acute pancreatitis. Arch Surg 128:586–590.
3. DiMagno EP (1994) Treatment of mild acute pancreatitis. In Bradley EL III (ed) Acute pancreatitis: diagnosis and therapy. Raven Press, New York.
4. Semelka RC, Ascher SM (1993) MR Imaging of the pancreas. Radiology, 188:593–602.
5. Ward J, Chalmers AG, Guthrie AJ, Larvin M, Robinson PJ (1997) T2 weighted and dynamic enhanced MRI in acute pancreatitis: comparison with contrast enhanced CT. Clin Radiol, 52:109–114.
6. Glazer G (1994) Epidemiology and pathology of pancreatic abscess. In: Bradley EL III (ed) Acute pancreatitis: diagnosis and therapy. Raven Press, New York.
7. Larvin M, Chalmers AG, McMahon MJ (1990) Dynamic contrast enhanced computed tomography: a precise technique for identifying and localising pancreatic necrosis. Br Med J 300:1425–1428.
8. Balthazar EJ, Robinson DL, Megibow AJ, Ranson JHC (1990) Acute pancreatitis: value of CT in establishing prognosis. Radiology, 174:331–336.
9. Foitzik T, Bassi DG, Schmidt J et al. (1994) Intravenous contrast medium accentuates the severity of acute necrotising pancreatitis in the rat. Gastroenterology, 106:207–214.
10. Balthazar EJ, Freeney P (1994) Intravenous contrast medium accelerates the severity of acute necrotising pancreatitis in the rat. Gastroenterology, 106:259–262 (editorial).
11. Prince MR, Arnoldus C, Frisoli JK (1996) Nephrotoxicity of high dose gadolinium compared with iodinated contrast. JMRI 6:162–166.
12. Neoptolemos JP, London NJ, James D (1988) Controlled trial of urgent endoscopic retrograde cholangiopancreatography and endoscopic sphincterotomy versus conservative treatment for acute pancreatitis due to gall stones. Lancet; II:979–983.
13. Fölsch U, Mitsche R, Lüdtke R, Hilgers RA Creutzfeldt W and The German Study group on acute biliary pancreatitis (1997) N Engl J Med 336:237–242.
14. Guibaud L, Bret PM, Reinhold C, Atri M, Barkun AN (1995) Bile duct obstruction and choledocholithiasis: Diagnosis with MR cholangiography. Radiology, 197:295–300.
15. Soto JA, Barisch MA, Yucel EK et al. (1995) Pancreatic duct: MR cholangiography with a three-dimensional fast spin echo technique. Radiology, 196:459–464.
16. Meaney JFM, Prince MR, Nostrant TT, Stanley James C (1997) Gadolinium-enhanced MR angiography of visceral arteries in patients with suspected chronic mesenteric ischaemia. JMRI7:171–176.

9 Surgical Treatment of Infected Pancreatic Necrosis

G. Farkas

Acute pancreatitis is an inflammatory process of variable severity, ranging from a mild, self-limited form with interstitial oedema of the pancreas to a severe form with extensive pancreatic necrosis and haemorrhage (1–3). Pancreatic necrosis combined with sepsis and organ failure is the leading cause of death in acute pancreatitis. Although aggressive organ system support has resulted in an improved survival rate in the early stage of the disease, patients continue to die at a later stage from septic complications, culminating in multiorgan failure (4). Overall infection rates in acute pancreatitis do not exceed 10%, but infected necrosis occurs in up to 70% of patients with necrotising pancreatitis (6,8,9). The reported mortality rate of these complications ranges from 15 to 80% (5,6). It is currently generally accepted that the initial treatment of acute pancreatitis should be conservative unless there is a specific indication for surgical intervention, but patients with infected necrosis should undergo urgent surgical debridement. It is thought that delay in the surgery of these patients results in higher mortality (5,12,13,58).

Definition of Pancreatic Infection

It has recently become apparent that there are three recognisable forms of pancreatic infection according to morphological, clinical and laboratory criteria: infected pancreatic necrosis, pancreatic abscess and an infected pseudocyst (8–15). *Infected pancreatic necrosis* is an infection of devitalised pancreatic and/or peripancreatic, retroperitoneal tissue with a positive smear or culture for bacteria or fungi. Usually, no major collection of pus is present; it occurs at an earlier stage of the disease and is associated with a worse prognosis. A *pancreatic abscess* consists of a walled-off collection of purulent material with little or no necrosis in the region of the pancreas. An *infected pancreatic pseudocyst* is a localised collection of infected fluid in the region of the pancreas and, like an abscess, is also walled off by a membrane of granulation tissue. The risk of death is not the same for the three clinical entities. The mortality rate for infected necrosis is double that for a pancreatic abscess, and more than triple that for an infected pseudocyst (8–10).

Incidence

The incidence of pancreatic infection, including infected necrosis, pancreatic abscesses and infected pseudocysts, ranges from 8% to 12% of all cases of acute pancreatitis (4,5,6). However, infected necrosis is reported to develop in 40% to 70% of all patients with necrotising pancreatitis (8,9,16) depending on the extent of the necrosis and the duration of the pancreatitis. The presence and extent of intra- and extrapancreatic necrosis is the main determinant for the development of infection (17). Although the time of presentation is variable, infection of necrosis is an increasing, time-dependent event up to the third week after the onset of symptoms. In prospective clinical studies, intraoperative bacteriology was positive in 24% during the first week, 36% during the second week, and reached a peak of 71% during the third week after the diagnosis of necrotising pancreatitis (21).

Pathophysiology

Clinical (21) and experimental (18) studies have confirmed a positive correlation between the risk of pancreatic infection in acute pancreatitis and the amount of tissue necrosis, which is believed to serve as a bacterial culture medium. Most cases of infected necrosis are caused by Gram-negative enteric bacteria, and generally one-third of the infections are polymicrobial (8,16,21). In our study, however, involving 123 patients with infected pancreatic necrosis, polymicrobial infections were found in 90% of patients, and a single organism in only 10% (19). *Enterobacter, Escherichia coli, Pseudomonas, Streptococcus* and *Klebsiella* were the most frequent bacteria, but in our patients *Candida* infection was also detected in 21%. The origin and the route of the bacteria resulting in pancreatic infection are still unclear. However, plausible ways appear to be direct transluminal penetration from the colon and/or spreading along the lymphatics from the gallbladder or the colon. Experimental work suggests this and indicates that the more important route of bacterial infection is by translocation from the small and large bowel. Other modes of infection are microperforation of the transverse colon and haematogenous infection. On the other hand, there is no doubt that the virulence of the microorganisms and the reduced defence capacity of the patient play a part (8). Under normal conditions, local and systemic factors clear the organism from the gland and prevent infection; depression of the phagocytic function and the immune system may play a role in the pathogenesis (20).

During the past few years, it has been recognised that pancreatic digestive enzymes may not play such a predominant role in the pathogenesis of complicated pancreatitis, which seems rather to result from the release of various inflammatory mediators from activated leucocytes. In fact, multiple organ failure and septic complications in acute pancreatitis are no different from the systemic complications of other diseases or injuries (sepsis, trauma and burn) which do not involve the release of digestive enzymes from the pancreas. The pathophysiological concept of severe acute pancreatitis is based on leucocyte activation as a key step leading from local to systemic inflammation (22). This concept is discussed in Chapter 2.

In our practice, we measured the serum TNF, IL-1β and IL-6 levels and the TNF-producing capacity of the leucocytes in patients with infected pancreatic necrosis following necrotising pancreatitis. ELISA revealed circulating TNF in 30% of patients with presumed sepsis following pancreatitis. There was no clear association between the TNF level and the development of shock or the fatal outcome of the disease, and TNF was detectable only at the onset of the clinical responses. The exact time that elapsed between the onset of symptoms and the collection of sera could not be assessed. The same tendency was observed in the kinetics of IL-1β production. The TNF-mediated cytotoxicity of the patients' leucocytes was significantly higher than that in the control group. The *in vitro* TNF-producing capacity was also higher in the study group. The decrease in inducibility before the fatal outcome of the disease might be due to the exhaustion of the leucocytes or a refractory condition of the leucocytes, which had been in a stimulated condition for a prolonged time *in vivo*. Paradoxically, therefore, the prolonged up-regulation of the TNF-producing cells was accompanied by a poor *in vitro* reactivity. This decrease in responsiveness might be of prognostic value. There was a close correlation between the IL-6 level and sepsis. However, a higher IL-6 level is a consequence of cytokine cascade activation rather than a cause of the pathogenesis of sepsis. Our results suggest that determination of the TNF-producing capacity of the leucocytes might be more informative than measurement of the serum TNF level for an evaluation of the severity or prognosis of septic complications following necrotising pancreatitis (24).

Clinical Features

Most patients with a pancreatic infection complain of a constant, severe upper abdominal pain which radiates to the back or flank. Fever, leucocytosis and a palpable abdominal mass should raise the index of suspicion of a pancreatic infection (8,9,17,19). However, these symptoms and signs are non-specific and, clinically, a pancreatic abscess, sterile or infected pancreatic necrosis, and an infected pancreatic pseudocyst cannot be distinguished with confidence. For an assessment of the severity of septic complications following necrotising pancreatitis, the APACHE II score is useful. It has been shown that the APACHE II score affords the most accurate prediction of the outcome in necrotising pancreatitis (29). Relative to the Ranson score (30), the APACHE II score is more complex and it may be useful for an accurate assessment of the prognosis of patients with a severe septic course, mainly in cases of infected pancreatic necrosis (31).

Diagnosis

The basis of appropriate treatment of infected pancreatic necrosis is an early, accurate diagnosis. Delayed diagnosis has been identified as a major factor resulting in poor outcome and death (12). Extensive clinical experience has shown that contrast-enhanced computed tomography (CT) is the gold standard for differentiating the morphological features of the pancreas (32–35). The introduction of helical CT scanners has allowed three-dimensional reconstruction of the intra-abdominal viscera, and volumetric assessment of the extent of intra- and extrapancreatic necrosis, and peripancreatic and retroperitoneal exudation. However, CT diagnosis of infection is rarely possible. A characteristic appearance, the "air bubble" phenomenon produced by gas-forming bacteria, is seen in only 20% to 55% of all patients with infected necrosis (9,35). The most appropriate diagnostic method for the early detection of infected pancreatic necrosis is guided percutaneous fine-needle aspiration (FNA) with Gram staining and culturing of the aspirate (34,36). Patients with suspected pancreatic necrosis should undergo CT or sonography-guided percutaneous FNA of the necrotic pancreas or peripancreatic fluid. Since bacterial colonisation in a necrotic pancreas and the peripancreatic region is likely to occur early in the course of acute necrotising pancreatitis, initial FNA is usually performed within the first 2 weeks of the illness (17,37). Infected necrosis can be documented by Gram staining and culturing of aspirate. FNA of the affected area is a safe, accurate method for the diagnosis of infected pancreatic necrosis, with a sensitivity of 96.2% and a specificity of 99.4% (38).

Non-surgical Supportive Treatment

Monitoring for respiratory, cardiovascular and renal insufficiency is one of the most important aspects in the treatment of patients with infected pancreatic necrosis. In addition, medical treatment includes total parenteral nutrition (TPN) and antibiotic therapy in accordance with the bacteriological findings in the abdomen, pancreas, blood and bronchial tree. Appropriate antibiotics must be active against Gram-negative organisms of intestinal origin commonly cultured in infected necrosis and they must be capable of penetrating the pancreatic juice and necrotic tissue (39). This supposition is provided by imipenem and cefuroxime. It is also noteworthy that the incidence of *Candida* infection in the infected necrotic pancreatic cases is close to 20%. *Candida* can be isolated in mixed cultures (fungal and bacterial infection) (19). Various authors have noted that bacterial sepsis and disseminated fungal infection are not mutually exclusive processes (40–42); medication is applied against both agents. In cases of disseminated fungal infection, fluconazole therapy is highly effective and well tolerated (43).

TPN is probably an important component of the management, because it allows nutritional intake to be maintained without stimulation of the synthesis of pancreatic enzyme although recent evidence suggests that enteral nutrition may help limit bacterial translocation. Glutamine is suggested as one of the more important components of TPN. Several observations support the concept that glutamine supplementation improves the organ function, and glutamine is a critical nutrient for the gut mucosa and immune cells (44). It has recently been clearly demonstrated that glutamine-enriched TPN exerts protein anabolic effects, improves the gut structure and immune cell number and function, and reduces morbidity (45).

To modify and decrease the cytokine production, supplementary administration of pentoxifylline (PTX; 400 mg/day) was applied in our practice (46,47). PTX is a well-known vasoactive drug, a phosphodiesterase inhibitor with proven clinical efficiency in various circulatory disorders. PTX raised new interest because it had been demonstrated to prevent or to attenuate the release of TNFα induced by lipopolysaccharide (48). PTX is a potent inhibitor of TNFα messenger RNA. PTX also exerts direct inhibitory effects on various neutrophil functions and it may influence other inflammatory cytokines (48). This drug may therefore improve the therapeutic strategy in the treatment of sepsis syndrome following necrotising pancreatitis.

Surgical Treatment

There is general agreement that infected pancreatic necrosis is an absolute indication for operation; non-operative or percutaneous management is usually associated with a fatal outcome. A variety of approaches have been advocated for the surgical management of infected pancreatic necrosis. They include different techniques, ranging from tissue-sparing methods to aggressive, extensive resection. During the 1980s, three main patterns of management could be identified in the surgical management of necrotic and infective complications of acute pancreatitis: (1) "conventional" treatment, including resection of the involved pancreatic tissue or necrosectomy, followed by simple drainage of the peripancreatic bed; (2) "lavage" treatment, in which necrosectomy is followed by continuous closed local irrigation or lavage of the involved pancreatic and retroperitoneal area; and (3) "open abdominal management" (laparostomy), involving necrosectomy followed by various combinations of planned and staged reoperations. Table 1 demonstrates the results of the three patterns, and indicates that the mortality rate was 42% (range 24–84%), 12.5% (range 6.3–23%) and 21% (range 11–55%) when "conventional" treatment, "lavage" treatment and "open abdominal management", respectively, were applied. However, these mortality figures also reflect case selection for operation, which are different in some of these series.

Table 1. Mortality in patients with infected pancreatic necrosis following different surgical procedures

Treatment/study	Patients (n)	Death (n)	Mortality (%)
Conventional			
Wilson et al. (50)	14	7	
Allardyce (49)	17	14	
Warshow and Jin (51)	45	11	
Total	76	32	42
Open			
Bradley (54)	71	10	
Wertheimer and Norris (55)	10	2	
Garcia-Sabrido et al. (56)	23	7	
Schlein et al. (57)	9	5	
Total	113	24	21
Lavage			
Larvin et al. (58)	14	3	
Bassi et al. (10)	55	13	
Rau et al. (37)	52	8	
Farkas	142	9	
Total	263	33	12.5

Conventional Treatment

When a conventional surgical approach (pancreatic resection or necrosectomy with simple drainage) is used for the treatment of infected necrosis, mortality rates are at a high level (24–84%) (49–51) with an overall mortality of 42% (Table 1). Reoperation, usually for persistent infection or abscess formation, is necessary in more than one-third of these patients. Nowadays, few centres still favour these methods, better results being attained through the application of aggressive debridement, wider drainage and insertion of multiple drains (52,53).

Open Abdominal Management

This surgical procedure entails an aggressive operative approach involving open packing and frequent, planned reoperation. After debridement the septic area is packed to protect intestinal surfaces and to prevent injury. Thereafter the abdomen is left open, and the packing is changed every 24 to 48 hours under sedation. The schedule of repeated intra-abdominal manipulation results in a significant number of postoperative local complications (bowel and pancreatic fistulas and haemorrhage) (54–57). The overall mortality was 21% in patients with infected necrosis treated according to this protocol (Table 1), but with this surgical treatment intensive care unit therapy is often mandatory for several weeks.

Lavage Treatment

Closed local lavage of the pancreatic bed and the affected area following necrosectomy has gained popularity in recent years because the combination of necrosectomy and postoperative local lavage allows the atraumatic and continuous removal of devitalized tissue, as well as the elimination of organisms and biologically active compounds (5,10,58,59). The overall mortality of closed management in infected necrosis in the reviewed series was 12.5% (Table 1).

Since 1986 we have adopted the "lavage" treatment in our practice, consisting of wide-ranging necrosectomy and other surgical interventions, combined with continuous widespread lavage (19). In all patients (142 patients), the operative management consisted of wide-ranging necrosectomy through the whole affected area, using bilateral subcostal laparotomy. The abdomen was explored for classification of the extent of pancreatic and extrapancreatic necrosis. Through division of the gastrocolic and the duodenocolic ligaments, the extent of necrosis in the head, body and tail of the gland could readily be assessed and measured. For accurate exploration of the retroperitoneum, Kocher's mobilisation of the duodenum and mobilisation of the right and left colon were performed. In our cases, the infected necrotising process was situated in the right and left retrocolic area in 67%, in the left subphrenic area in 21%, and in the retroduodenal and subhepatic area in 12%. Debridement or necrosectomy, either digitally or by the careful use of an instrument combined with continuous normal saline lavage, permitted the entire removal of all demarcated devitalized tissue, preserving vital pancreatic tissue (59) and removing the infected necrotic tissue from the whole

Table 2. Other surgical procedures performed in 142 patients undergoing pancreatic debridement

Distal pancreatectomy and splenectomy	25
Splenectomy	4
Subtotal pancreatectomy	4
Colon resection	3
Cholecystectomy	27
Cholecystectomy and bile duct drainage	5
Partial hepatectomy	1
Appendicectomy	2

affected retroperitoneal area. After surgical debridement, meticulous haemostasis and extensive intraoperative lavage with 8 to 10 litres of normal saline were applied, and for postoperative closed continuous local lavage 4 to 11 large (28–34fr) silicone rubber tubes were inserted into the whole affected area. They are inserted only into the pancreatic region and the retroperitoneal spaces, without any connection with the intraabdominal region. In 64 of the 142 cases (45%) some other surgical intervention was also performed (Table 2). Continuous washing and suction drainage was applied for an average of 41.5 days (range 21–90 days), with a median of 9.5 (range 5–20) litres of normal saline per 24 hours. In the first few postoperative days, the amount of lavage fluid was generally 15–20 litres, which was later reduced, depending on the clinical course and on the appearance and quality of the outflowing liquid. Reoperation was necessary in 24 (17%) patients. Of these patients 18 had developed a secondary abscess in the area of the original necrosis cavity and two had developed a colonic fistula, which was cured by large bowel resection, while massive diffuse local bleeding was responsible in four patients. Only one of the reoperated cases died following reoperation for local bleeding. Pancreatic fistulas were observed in 16 patients; in eight they closed spontaneously, but in the remaining eight they became long-standing, high-output ones with a high amylase concentration (mean 435 500 units/l). In all of these eight patients, octreotide therapy (3×0.1 mg/day) was combined with total parenteral nutrition, and all fistulas closed after a median of 13 days (range 7–19) (60). Systemic complications occurred mainly in connection with local complications and reoperation. In 12 patients respiratory failure required mechanical ventilation for over 24 hours. Renal and circulatory insufficiency developed in five and three patients, respectively.

Nine patients died following operation, and therefore the overall mortality rate was 6.3% (9 of 142 patients). The cause of death was bacterial sepsis in five patients, bacterial and fungal sepsis in one patient, fungal sepsis in one patient, myocardial infarction in one, and stroke in one. The hospital stay of surviving patients amounted to a median of 45 (range 24–95) days. The surgical management of our patients with infected pancreatic necrosis was directed towards removal of the devitalised intra- and extrapancreatic tissue in all affected areas. It seems very important to explore every possibly infected site because ineffective debridement can endanger the recovery of the patients and increase the likelihood of reoperation. In accord with several authors, it is not necessary to remove every small part of the devitalised tissue, because any necrotic or necrotising tissue is washed out by the lavage fluid later in the postoperative period (11,14,19,59). The success of postoperative closed continuous lavage depends on the number and the size of the drainage tubes (58,61). Generally, we applied 4–11 large silicone tubes inserted to all affected sites. As infected necrotic processes can extend into intra- and extrapancreatic areas, other surgical interventions can also be advised. This reason explains our surgical strategy, i.e. in 64 of 142 patients (45%) the necrosectomy and continuous lavage were combined with several surgical interventions (distal pancreatic resection, splenectomy, cholecystectomy, colon resection, etc.). We attribute the improved survival rate to adequate surgical debridement and additional surgical intervention combined with continuous widespread washing and suction drainage in all affected areas. A large volume of saline solution for continuous lavage through multiple drainage tube is safe and atraumatic and can eliminate the infected, necrotic tissue. Effective surgical treatment together with adequate supportive therapy can give good results in patients with infected pancreatic necrosis.

In conclusion, the improved result can be achieved by aggressive surgical treatment, continuous, long-standing washing and suction drainage, together with supportive therapy, including immunonutrition, modification of cytokine production, combined with adequate antibiotic and antifungal medication. This surgical strategy provides the possibility for recovery in cases of necrotising pancreatitis combined with septic complications.

References

1. Corfield AP, Cooper MJ, Williamson RCN (1985) Acute pancreatitis: a lethal disease of increasing incidence. Gut 26:724–729.
2. Gendell JH, Egan J (1987) Acute pancreatitis. West J Med 146:598–602.
3. Balthazar EJ (1989) CT diagnosis and staging of acute pancreatitis. Radiol Clin North Am 27:19–37.
4. Frey CF, Bradley EL III, Beger HG (1988) Progress in acute pancreatitis. Surg Gynecol Obstet 167:282–286.
5. Beger HG, Büchler M, Bittner R, Nevalainen T, Roschen R (1988) Necrosectomy and postoperative local lavage in necrotizing pancreatitis. Br J Surg 75:207–212.
6. Allardyce DB (1987) Incidence of necrotizing pancreatitis and factors related to mortality. Am J Surg 154:295–300.
7. Wilson C, McArdle CS, Carter DC, Imrie CW (1988) Surgical treatment of acute necrotizing pancreatitis. Br J Surg 75:1119–1123.
8. Bittner R, Block S, Büchler M, Beger HG (1987) Pancreatic abscess and infected pancreatic necrosis. Dig Dis Sci 32:1082–1087.
9. Schoenenberg MH, Rau B, Beger HG (1995) Diagnose und therapie des primaren pankreasabscesses. Chirurgie 66:588–596.
10. Bassi C, Vesentini S, Nifosi F, Girelli R, Falconi M, Elio A, Pederzoli P (1990) Pancreatic abscess and other pus-harboring collections related to pancreatitis: a review of 108 cases. World J Surg 14:505–512.
11. Imrie CW (1993) Indications for surgery: the surgeon's view. In: Beger HG, Büchler M, Malfertheiner P (eds) Standards in pancreatic surgery. Springer, Berlin Heidelberg New York, pp 148–156.
12. D'Egidio A, Schein M (1991) Surgical strategies in the treatment of pancreatic necrosis and infection. Br J Surg 78:133–137.
13. Bradley EL III (1993) A clinically based classification system for acute pancreatitis. Arch Surg 128:586–590.
14. Büchler M, Uhl W, Beger HG (1993) Surgical strategies in acute pancreatitis. Hepatogastroenterology 40:563–568.
15. Bradley EL III (1991) Operative management of acute pancreatitis: ventral open packing. Hepatogastroenterology 38:134–138.
16. Fedorak IJ, Ko TC, Djuricin G, McMahon M, Thomson K, Prinz A (1992) Secondary pancreatic infections: are they distinct clinical entities? Surgery 112:824–831.
17. Widdison AL, Karanjia ND (1993) Pancreatic infection complicating acute pancreatitis. Br J Surg 80:148–154.

18. Foitzik T, Mithöfer K, Ferraro MJ et al. (1994) Time course of bacterial infection of the pancreas and its relation to disease severity in a rodent model of acute pancreatitis. Ann Surg 220:193–198.

19. Farkas, G., Márton, J., Mándi, Y., Szederkényi, E (1996) Surgical strategy and management of infected pancreatic necrosis. Br J Surg 83:930–933.

20. Reber HA, Widdison AL (1994) Pathogenesis of infected pancreatic necrosis. In: Bradley EL III (ed) Acute pancreatitis: diagnosis and therapy. Raven Press, New York, pp 85–92.

21. Beger HG, Bittner R, Block S, Büchler M (1986) Bacterial contamination of pancreatic necrosis. Gastroenterology 91:433–438.

22. Gross V, Leser HG, Heinisch A, Schölmerich J (1993) Inflammatory mediators and cytokines, new aspects of the pathophysiology and assessment of severity of acute pancreatitis? Hepatogastroenterology 40:522–530.

23. McKay C, Brooks B, Gallagher G, Baxter JN, Imrie CW (1992) Monocyte activation in acute pancreatitis is related to the degree of systemic illness. Digestion 52:104–105.

24. Farkas, G., Mándi, Y., Márton, J (1995) Modification of cytokine production in septic condition following necrotizing pancreatitis. In: Papastamatiou L (ed) European IHPBA Congress "Athens '95". Monduzzi Editore, Bologna, pp 609–613.

25. McKay CJ, Gallagher G, Brooks B, Imrie CW, Baxter JN (1996) Increased monocyte cytokine production in association with systemic complications in acute pancreatitis. Br J Surg 83:919–923.

26. Grass V, Schölmerich J, Leser HG et al. (1990) Granulocyte elastase in assessment of severity of acute pancreatitis. Dig Dis Sci 35:97–105.

27. Uhl W, Büchler M, Malfertheiner P, Martini M, Beger HG (1991) PMN-elastase in comparison with CRP, antiproteases and LDH as indicators of necrosis in human acute pancreatitis. Pancreas 6:253–259.

28. Leser HG, Gross V, Scheibenbogen C et al. (1991) Elevation of interleukin-6 concentration recedes acute-phase response and reflects severity in acute pancreatitis. Gastroenterology 191:782–785.

29. Larvin M, McMahon MJ (1989) Apache-II score for assessment and monitoring of acute pancreatitis. Lancet I:201–204.

30. Ranson JHC, Rifkind KM, Roses DF (1974) Prognostic signs and the role of operative management in acute pancreatitis. Surg Gynecol Obstet 139:69–81.

31. Wilson C, Heath DI, Imrie CW (1990) Prediction of outcome in acute pancreatitis: a comparative study of Apache-II, clinical assessment and multiple, factor scoring systems. Br J Surg 77:1260–1264.

32. Freeny PC (1988) Radiology of acute pancreatitis: diagnosis, detection of complications, and interventional therapy. In: Glazer G, Ranson JHC (eds) Acute pancreatitis: experimental and clinical aspects of pathogenesis and management. Bailliere Tindall, London, pp 275–302.

33. Balthazar EJ, Robinson DL, Megibow AJ, Ranson JHL (1990) Acute pancreatitis: value of CT in establishing prognosis. Radiology 174:331–336.

34. Gerzof SG, Banks PA, Robbins AH et al. (1987) Early diagnosis of pancreatic infection by computed tomography-guided aspiration. Gastroenterology 93:1315–1320.

35. Freeny PC (1993) Incremental dynamic bolus computed tomography of acute pancreatitis. Int J Pancreatol 13:147–158.

36. Banks PA, Gerzof SG, Chong FK et al. (1990) Bacteriologic status of necrotic tissue in necrotizing pancreatitis. Pancreas 5:330–333.

37. Rau B, Uhl W, Buchler MW, Beger HG (1997) Surgical treatment of infected necrosis. World J Surg 21:155–161.

38. Banks PA, Gerzof SG, Langevin RE, Silverman SG, Sica GT, Hughes MD (1995) CT-guided aspiration of suspected pancreatic infection. Int J Pancreatol 18:265–270.

39. Büchler M, Malfertheimer P, Friess H, Beger HG (1989) The penetration of antibiotics into human pancreas. Infection 1:20–25.

40. Salomkin JS, Flohr A, Simmons RL (1982) *Candida* infections in surgical patients. Ann Surg 175:177–185.

41. Dyess DL, Garisson RN, Fry DE (1985) *Candida* sepsis. Arch Surg 120:345–348.

42. Stone HH, Kolb LD, Currie CA et al. (1974) *Candida* sepsis: pathogenesis and principles of treatment. Ann Surg 179:697–711.

43. Farkas G, Szendrényi V, Karácsonyi S, Mezey G (1993) *Candida* infection in pancreatic abscess. Dig Surg 10:254–256.

44. Heberer M, Babst R, Juretic A, Gross T, Horig H, Harder F (1996) Role of glutamine in the immune response in critical illness. Nutrition 12 (Suppl):71–72.

45. Van Der Hulst RRWJ, Von Meyenfeldt MF, Soeters PB. (1996) Glutamine: an essential amino acid for the gut. Nutrition 12 (Suppl):78–81.
46. Mándi Y, Farkas G, Ocsovszky I, Nagy Z (1995) Inhibition of tumor necrosis factor production and ICAM-1 expression by pentoxifylline: beneficial effects in sepsis syndrome. Res Exp Med 195:297–307.
47. Mándi Y, Farkas G, Ocsovszky I, Béládi, I, Balogh Å (1996) Effects of pentoxifylline and pentaglobin on cytokine production in septic patients. In: Faist E et al. (eds) The immune consequences of trauma, shock and sepsis-mechanisms and therapeutic approaches. Pabst Science Publishers, Berlin, pp 420–428.
48. Sullivan GW, Carper HT, Novick WJ Jr, Mandell GL (1988) Inhibition of the inflammatory action of interleukin-1 and tumor necrosis factor (alpha) on neutrophil function by pentoxifylline. Infect Immunology 56:1722–1729.
49. Allardyce DB (1987) Incidence of necrotizing pancreatitis and factors related to mortality. Am J Surg 154:295–299.
50. Wilson C, McArdle CS, Carter DC, Imrie CW (1988) Surgical treatment of acute necrotizing pancreatitis. Br J Surg 75:1119–1123.
51. Warshow AL, Jin G (1985) Improved survival in 45 patients with pancreatic abscess. Ann Surg 202:408–417.
52. Ranson JHC. discussion in Bradley EL III (1987) Management of infected pancreatic necrosis by open drainage. Ann Surg 206:542–550.
53. Stricker PD, Hunt DR (1986) Surgical aspects of pancreatic abscess. Br J Surg 73:644–646.
54. Bradley III EL (1994) Surgical indications and techniques in necrotizing pancreatitis. In: Bradley EL III (ed) Acute pancreatitis: diagnosis and therapy. Raven Press, New York, pp 105–117.
55. Wertheimer MD, Norris CS (1986) Surgical management of necrotizing pancreatitis. Arch Surg 121:484–487.
56. Garcia-Sabrido JL, Tallado J, Chistou NV, Polo JR, Valdecantos, E (1988) Treatment of severe intra-abdominal sepsis and/or necrotic foci by open-abdomen approach. Arch Surg 123:152–156.
57. Schein M, Hirschber A, Hashmonai M (1992) Current surgical management of severe intra-abdominal infection. Surgery 112:489–452.
58. Larvin M, Chalmers AG, Robinson PJ, McMahon MJ (1988) Debridement and closed cavity irrigation for the treatment of pancreatic necrosis. Br J Surg 76:465–471.
59. Büchler M, Uhl R, Isenmann R, Bittner R, Beger HG (1993) Necrotizing pancreatitis: necrosectomy and closed continuous lavage of the lesser sac. The Ulm experience. In: Beger HG, Büchler M, Malfertheiner P (eds) Standards in pancreatic surgery. Springer, Berlin Heidelberg New York, pp 191–202.
60. Farkas G, Leindler L, Szederkényi E (1993) Beneficial effect of Sandostatin, a long-acting somatostatin analog, in pancreatic surgery. Hepatogastroenterology 40 (Suppl.1):182–183.
61. Pederzoli P, Bassi C, Vesentini S et al. (1990) Retroperitoneal and peritoneal drainage and lavage in the treatment of severe necrotizing pancreatitis. Surg Gynecol Obstet 170:197–202.

10 Surgical Treatment of Infected Necrosis

H. Friess, P. Berberat, J. Kleeff, W. Uhl and M.W. Büchler

Acute pancreatitis is a diffuse and profound inflammation of the pancreas, caused in 80–90% of cases either by gallstones, which obstruct the biliary tract, or by drinking too much alcohol (1). The exact manner in which alcohol damages the exocrine pancreas is still not known. It has been suggested that gallstone-induced acute pancreatitis may be generated by reflux of bile into the pancreatic duct following blockage of the duodenal papilla by a gallstone (2), by reflux from the duodenal lumen through an incompetent sphincter in the pancreas, producing extensive damage by the already activated pancreatic proteases (3) or by the premature and intracellular activation of digestive enzymes. Severe acute pancreatitis is characterised by a strong infiltration with leucocytes, and by destruction and loss of the normal pancreatic cells and the intrapancreatic vessels, which can lead to haemorrhage, generation of pseudocysts and extended fat necrosis (4).

According to the morphological changes, acute pancreatitis can be classified histologically as interstitial-oedematous or necrotising pancreatitis. Approximately 80–85% of the patients with acute pancreatitis have an acute oedematous inflammation and will undergo a mild, self-limiting clinical course. But 15–20% of the patients develop severe, life-threatening disease (mortality rate up to 60%) with intra- and extrapancreatic necrosis (5,6). In the early phase – through the release of pancreatic enzymes and vasoactive substances – these patients suffer cardiovascular, pulmonary, and renal complications (7). If they survive this critical period, they are often faced in a second phase with severe septic complications due to pancreatic or peripancreatic infection of the necrosis (8–10).

With the impressive improvements in intensive care during past years, death has become increasingly rare in the first critical phase (11). In contrast, the local and systemic septic complications that follow bacterial contamination of the necrotic material continue to cause death in severe acute pancreatitis, and are an important challenge in clinical management. Although recent studies have undoubtedly proved that, in cases of infected necrotising acute pancreatitis, surgical therapy is superior to conservative treatment, there have been many uncertainties concerning the therapeutic schedule and prophylactic antibiotic therapy (12,13).

Taking into account recent findings from microbiological data and our own surgical experience, we have developed a new algorithm to be used in patients with acute pancreatitis. The goal is to reduce the mortality in patients with necrotising pancreatitis by using prophylactic antibiotic therapy (imipenem) and surgical intervention at the right time.

Infection of Pancreatic Necrosis

The development of pancreatic and peripancreatic necrosis is a critical point in the course of acute pancreatitis, and mainly determines the prognosis of the disease. The normal pancreas is generally sterile and resistant to infections because of extensive lymphatic drainage and the strong antibacterial activity of the pancreatic juice (14). But in acute pancreatitis, after the appearance of necrotic tissue, these protection mechanisms are no longer effective and the necrotic areas represent an ideal place for subsequent bacterial superinfection. Widdison et al. (15) demonstrated a positive correlation between the extent of necrosis and the rate of superinfection in necrotising pancreatitis. As already mentioned, pancreatic infection occurs in 40–70% of patients with necrotising pancreatitis and shows a time-dependent pattern of onset: it has been shown that the incidence of infected pancreatic necrosis is 24%, 36% and 71% in the first, second and third weeks following onset of acute pancreatitis, respectively (8). Animal studies have demonstrated that the most likely route of invasion by bacteria is the transmural route from the colon. This translocation is probably supported by an increased permeability of the colon wall and by the migration of bacteria-carrying macrophages. However, there may be other, less frequent, routes of infection as well: for example, haematogenous, via the circulation; by duodenobiliary reflux, via the main pancreatic duct; or from the portal vein and the liver, via the biliary duct system (16,17).

The most frequently isolated organisms in infected acute necrotizing pancreatitis arise from the intestinal flora, consisting primarily of Gram-negative bacteria, such as *Escherichia coli* and *Enterobacter*. However, in the three major studies which analysed bacterial contamination in infected pancreatic necrosis, either by performing intraoperative smears or by computed tomography (CT) guided fine needle aspiration microbiology, there was also frequently infection by Gram-positive bacteria, such as *Staphylococcus aureus*, *Streptococcus faecalis* and *Enterococcus* or anaerobes, and in some cases even fungi. It was found that 60–87% of the patients had infection with only one bacterium, whereas in 13–40% of the patients, more than one bacterium was present (8,18,19).

As it is well known that infectious complications such as sepsis and related systemic multiple organ failure are the causes of higher mortality rate, a longer hospital stay and a higher reoperation rate in patients with acute necrotising pancreatitis, which is triggered by the bacterial contamination of the necrotic tissue, it is of great importance to detect these cases as early as possible. First-phase acute necrotising pancreatitis can be differentiated from acute oedematous pancreatitis by contrast-enhanced CT and/or by the measurement of so-called necrosis markers in the serum. The accuracy rates of serum necrosis markers are 86% for C-reactive protein, 84% for polymorphonuclear granulocyte elastase, 82% for lactate dehydrogenase and 72% for $\alpha2$-macroglobulin (20,21). This differentiation is important, because the danger of subsequent bacterial contamination exists only in acute necrotising pancreatitis. Unfortunately, there are no reliable clinical or laboratory parameters that can accurately diagnose whether the necrosis is infected. The best approach to assess if an infection is present is CT or ultrasound-guided fine needle aspiration with Gram staining and culture of the aspirate. Gerzof et al. (19) demonstrated that with this method 80% of infected pancreatic necrosis could be detected by a single fine-needle aspiration. In the remaining 20% the diagnosis could be established after repeated fine-needle aspiration.

Antibiotics in Acute Pancreatitis

Whether antibiotic treatment can influence the infection rate of the pancreatic necroses and improve the patient's prognosis is still a subject of intense discussion (22,23). One problem is that many antibiotics do not attain therapeutic concentration in human pancreatic tissue. There is a blood–pancreas barrier which prevents antibiotics such as ampicillin from penetrating the human pancreas (24). Concentrations at the site of infection are regarded as the gold standard for evaluation of antibiotic treatment protocols. We have shown that imipenem, ciprofloxacin and ofloxacin are most efficacious and should be the preferred antibiotics for treatment of pancreatic infection (24). Recent clinical trials with various antibiotic regimens – such as cefuroxime or selective decontamination with norfloxacin, colistin and amphotericin – showed a significant reduction in morbidity and mortality (25,26). In another randomised, multicentre trial, imipenem (0.5 g twice a day) was used as a prophylactic antibiotic regimen in 74 patients suffering from necrotising pancreatitis. A significant reduction in the number of septic courses was observed in the imipenem-treated group (27). Although additional larger, controlled clinical studies with imipenem are needed, the results are promising (27,28).

Indication and Timing for Operation

Patients with proven necrotising pancreatitis (high levels of necrosis markers, CT evidence necrosis) should be treated in an intensive care unit for optimal management of the early complications, such as shock, lung and kidney failure, (see Chapters 3, 13). In this way, a certain percentage of patients with necrotising pancreatitis can be treated without surgery (29). In our institution, all patients with proven necrotising pancreatitis are treated with antibiotics (3 × 0.5 g imipenem) for 10 days prophylactically. However, surgical intervention will be indicated if signs of septic complications (fever, leucocytosis, organ failure) caused by bacterial infection of necroses occur, and the suspicion has been proven by fine-needle aspiration guided by imaging procedures. Also, if there has been persistent organ failure under maximum intensive care treatment, or nonresponse to conservative therapy, then an interdisciplinary discussion of the pros and cons of surgical therapy is called for (30–32).

The right time for the surgical intervention is still a matter of discussion: it can be done "early" if complications make operation absolutely necessary (2–5% of the patients with necrotising pancreatitis), but in general there is a tendency today to observe a minimum period of intensive-care therapy and to delay surgical intervention to the third week, when there are optimal surgical conditions for necrosectomy after demarcation of the necroses occurs (32).

Surgical Techniques

The goal of surgical therapy in the management of infected necrotising pancreatitis is to remove the necrotic extrapancreatic and pancreatic tissue and at the same time to preserve intact vital pancreatic tissue. Afterward, continuous evacuation of necroses and pancreatic fluids, which may contain further bacterial contamination, is performed.

The many surgical modalities proposed in the past for treatment of necrotising pancreatitis have met with variable success: (1) peritoneal dialysis alone failed to show any better patient outcome, since this procedure is restricted to the abdominal cavity and has no influence on the persistent necrotizing process in the retroperitoneal space (33). (2) The "triple tube drainage", consisting of implantation of several thick drainage tubes into the lesser sac, in combination with bile duct drainage, gastrostomy and jejunostomy, did not lead to a significant reduction in mortality or morbidity (34). Also, in this approach the removal of the necrotic tissue is missing. (3) Pancreatic resection, i.e. hemipancreatectomy, partial or total duodenopancreatectomy (35), showed to be – except for very rare cases of total pancreatic necrosis – an overtreatment, exposing the already severely ill patients, through removal of healthy organs (duodenum, part of the stomach, extrapancreatic ducts), to additional stress, with enhancement of the late morbidity and mortality due to endocrine and exocrine insufficiency. Furthermore, in a good number of cases the necroses are present only extrapancreatically or in the superficial part of the pancreas, and any classical resection of the gland would be the wrong method of therapy. (4) Many groups have tried to bring down the high morbidity and mortality rate by combining necrosectomy with additional intensive treatment protocols following surgical debridement, such as closed continuous local lavage of necrotic cavities (36), multiple sump drainage with lavage or planned frequent reoperations with or without zipper (37) and the application of open packing with multiple redressing (38). With the use of these three concepts in experienced hands, hospital mortality in severe acute pancreatitis has been reduced to less than 15%, and at present this approach represents the recommended standard technique of surgical management of necrotising pancreatitis. (5) More recently, a new, non-operative, percutanous technique of drainage has been introduced (39), but so far experience with this new procedure is limited. In addition, as with the older non-operative approaches, this method cannot guarantee complete removal of necrotic areas.

In our hospital we treat necrotising pancreatitis with necrosectomy supplemented by extensive intraoperative and postoperative closed continuous local lavage of the lesser sac and of the necrotic cavities involved in the retroperitoneum. After the abdominal cavity is opened, usually by an upper abdominal midline incision, the gastrocolic and duodenocolic ligaments are divided, and the pancreas is exposed. The extent of necrosis in the head, body, and tail of the gland can easily be assessed. Debridement or necrosectomy, either digital or with the careful use of instruments, permits the removal of all demarcated devitalized tissue, preserving the vital pancreatic parenchymal tissue. It is not necessary to remove every gram of devitalized tissue, because additional necrotic tissue is washed out by the lavage fluid later on. After surgical debridement, thorough homeostasis with transfixing stitches using monofilament suture material is mandatory (Novafil 3×0 or 4×0). After suturing of bleeding vessels, extensive intraoperative lavage is performed, using 20 or more litres of normal saline solution, to clear the surface of the pancreatic and peripancreatic tissues. For postoperative closed continuous local lavage, two to four double-lumen Salem sump tubes (20–32 charriere) and single-lumen silicone rubber tubes (28–32 charriere) are inserted, so that at least a regionally restricted lavage is effected. The gastrocolic and duodenocolic ligaments are sutured again to create a closed retroperitoneal lesser sac compartment for postoperative continuous lavage. In the first 7 postoperative days, the amount of lavage fluid is 24–48 litres/day, with rapid reduction over the following days, depending on the clinical course and appearance of the outflowing liquid (measurement of pancreatic enzymes and bacteriological examinations are repeated at regular intervals). For postoperative lavage, normal, slightly hyperosmotic, ambulatory peritoneal dialysis solution is usually used. The drainage tubes are generally removed 2–3 weeks post-operatively.

The Bern Experience with the Management of Patients with Acute Pancreatitis

From November 1993 to September 1995, a total of 64 patients with acute pancreatitis were admitted to the University Hospital of Bern. As predicted by indicators of necrosis (C-reactive protein > 120 mg/l), 32 patients suffered from acute necrotising pancreatitis, which was proven by contrast-enhanced CT. All patients with proven pancreatic necroses received imipenem therapy over at least 14 days at 0.5 g tid. In the case of clinical signs of sepsis, patients underwent fine-needle aspiration with Gram-staining and culture. All patients with acute necrotising pancreatitis were treated in the ICU with maximum conservative therapy measures. In 11 of 32 patients (34%), infected pancreatic necroses were found in this way (*E. coli*, *Enterococcus*, *S. aureus*, *Klebsiella* and *Candida*) a mean of 21 ± 3.3 days after the onset of the disease, leading to delayed surgical intervention. These 11 patients were treated with necrosectomy and closed continuous lavage of the lesser sac over a mean of 23 ± 7.8 days. One patient developed an abscess which was successfully managed by an interventional approach. No other reinterventions were necessary. The mean total length of hospital stay in sterile and infected acute necrotising pancreatitis was 25 ± 8.9 and 65 ± 13.5 days, respectively. Mortality rates were 18% (2/11) and 0% (0/21) in patients with infected and sterile pancreatic necrosis, respectively.

Conclusions

Most patients with acute pancreatitis have a mild, self-limiting disease and will improve with conservative medical therapy that includes fluid resuscitation and a close monitoring of the necrosis marker until the pain is gone. If the C-reactive protein is markedly elevated at onset or becomes elevated during the course of the disease, a contrast-enhanced CT will confirm if necrotising pancreatitis is present. In this case, the patient will receive antibiotic therapy for 10 to 14 days in addition to intensive-care measures. The former will reduce the number of septic courses and consequently reduce the need for surgical intervention, while the latter helps to effectively manage early cardiovascular, pulmonary and renal complications, significantly decreasing the first-week mortality. If signs of sepsis develop despite prophylactic antibiotic treatment, fine-needle aspiration will prove or disprove infection of the pancreatic necroses. At this point, surgical intervention, mostly delayed to the third week of the disease with optimal surgical conditions (demarcation of necrosis), is the therapy of choice. Although several surgical options for treating the problem of infected necrotising pancreatitis exist, our own experience shows that the best results concerning morbidity and mortality are obtained with necrosectomy and extended intraoperative and postoperative continuous lavage of the lesser sac. With necrosectomy the main source of the sepsis is removed, and then with the intense and continuous lavage, toxic substances and infected necrosis are constantly removed, so that we stop the ongoing necrotising process. This algorithm has been shown to significantly improve the outcome in the treatment of acute necrotising pancreatitis.

References

1. Kelly TR (1976) Gallstone pancreatitis: pathophysiology. Surgery 80:488–492.
2. Opie EL (1901) The etiology of acute hemorrhagic pancreatitis. Johns Hopkins Hosp Bull 12:182–188.
3. Lerch MM, Hernandez CA, Adler G (1994) Acute pancreatitis. N Engl J Med 331:948–949.
4. Bockman DE, Büchler M, Beger HG (1986) Ultrastructure of human acute pancreatitis. Int J Pancreatol 1:141–153.
5. Warshaw AL (1980) A guide to pancreatitis. Compr Ther 6:49–55.
6. Uhl W, Büchler M, Beger HG (1993) A clinicopathological classification of acute pancreatitis. In: Beger HG, Büchler MW, Malfertheiner P (eds) Standards in pancreatic surgery. Springer, Berlin Heidelberg New York, pp 34–43.
7. Beger HG, Bittner R, Büchler M, Hess M, Schmitz JE (1986) Hemodynamic data pattern in patients with acute pancreatitis. Gastroenterology 90:74–79.
8. Beger HG, Bittner R, Block S, Büchler M (1986) Bacterial contamination of pancreatic necrosis: a prospective clinical study. Gastroenterology 91:433–438.
9. Allardyce DB (1987) Incidence of necrotizing pancreatitis and factors related to mortality. Am J Surg 154:295–299.
10. Buggy BP, Nostrant TT (1983) Lethal pancreatitis. Am J Gastroenterol 78:810–814.
11. Sigurdsson GH (1994) Intensive care management of acute pancreatitis. Dig Surg 11:231–241.
12. Beger HG, Büchler M (1986) Decision-making in surgical treatment of acute pancreatitis: Operative or conservative management of necrotizing pancreatitis? Theor Surg 1:61–68.
13. Warshaw AL, Jin G (1985) Improved survival in 45 patients with pancreatic abscess. Ann Surg 202:408–417.
14. Bassi C, Fontana R, Vasentini S et al. Antibacterial and mezlocillin-enhancing activity of pure human pancreatic fluid. Int J Pancreatol 10:293–297.
15. Widdison AL, Karanjia ND, Alvarez C, Reber HA (1991) The association between pancreatic infection and the severity of acute pancreatitis. Gastroenterology 100:A304.
16. Widdison AL (1994) Microbiology and sources of pancreatic pathogens in acute pancreatitis. In: Pederzoli P, Cavallini G, Bassi C, Falconi M (eds) Facing the pancreatic dilemma. Springer, Berlin Heidelberg New York, pp 291–300.
17. Wells CL, Maddaus MA, Simmons RL (1988) Proposed mechanism for the translocation of intestinal bacteria. Rev Infect Dis 10:958–979.
18. Bassi C, Falconi M, Girelli R et al. (1989). Microbiological findings in severe pancreatitis. Surg Res Commun 5:1–4.
19. Gerzof SG, Banks PA, Robbins AH et al. (1987) Early diagnosis of pancreatic infection by computed tomography guided aspiration. Gastroenterology 93:1315–1320.
20. Büchler M, Malfertheiner P, Schoetensack C, Uhl W, Beger HG (1986) Sensitivity of antiproteases, complement factors and C-reactive protein in detecting pancreatic necrosis: results of a prospective clinical study. Int J Pancreatol 1:227–235.

21. Uhl W, Büchler M, Malfertheiner P, Martini M, Beger HG (1991) PMN-elastase in comparison with CRP, antiproteases, and LDH as indicators of necrosis in human acute pancreatitis. Pancreas 6:253–259.
22. Isenmann R, Büchler MW (1994) Infection and acute pancreatitis. Br J Surg 81:1707–1708.
23. Finch TA, Sawyers JL, Schenker S (1976) A prospective study to determine the efficacy of antibiotics in acute pancreatitis. Ann Surg 183:667–671.
24. Büchler MW, Malfertheiner P, Friess H et al. (1992) Human pancreatic tissue concentration of bactericidal antibiotics. Gastroenterology 103:1902–1908.
25. Sainio V, Kemppainen E, Puolakkainen P et al. (1995) Early antibiotic treatment in acute necrotising pancreatitis. Lancet 346:663–667.
26. Luiten EJ, Hop WC, Lange JF, Bruining HA (1995) Controlled clinical trial of selective decontamination for the treatment of severe acute pancreatitis. Ann Surg 222:57–65.
27. Isenmann R, Büchler MW, Friess H, Uhl W, Beger HG (1996) Antibiotics in acute pancreatitis. Dig Surg 13:365–369.
28. Friess H, Silva JC, Uhl W, Isenmann R, Büchler MW (1996) Acute pancreatitis: the role of infection. Dig Surg 13:357–361.
29. Büchler M, Malfertheiner P, Uhl W, Beger HG (1988) Conservative treatment of necrotizing pancreatitis in patients with minor pancreatic necrosis. Pancreas 3:592.
30. Kivilaakso E, Fräki O, Nikki P, Lempinem M (1981) Resection of the pancreas for acute fulminant pancreatitis. Surg Gynecol Obstet 152:493–498.
31. Poston GJ, Williamson RCN (1990) Surgical management of acute pancreatitis. Br J Surg 77:5–12.
32. Uhl W, Büchler MW (1996) The role of surgery in pancreatic sepsis. Dig Surg 13:374–380.
33. Mayer AD, McMahon MJ, Corfield AP, Cooper MJ, Williamson RRN (1985) Controlled clinical trial of peritoneal lavage for the treatment of severe acute pancreatitis. N Engl J Med 312:399–404.
34. McCarthy MC, Dickermann RM (1982) Surgical management of severe acute pancreatitis. Arch Surg 117:476–480.
35. Alexandre JH, Guerreri MT (1981) Role of total pancreatectomy in the treatment of necrotizing pancreatitis. World J Surg 5:369–377.
36. Beger HG, Krautzberger W, Bittner R, Block S, Büchler M (1984) Results of surgical treatment of necrotizing pancreatitis. World J Surg 9:972–979.
37. Sarr MH, Nagorney DM, Much P, Farnell MB, Johnson CD (1991) Acute necrotizing pancreatitis: management by planned, staged pancreatic necrosectomy/debridement and delayed primary wound closure over drains. Br J Surg 78:576–581.
38. Bradley EL III (1987) Management of infected pancreatic necrosis by open drainage. Ann Surg 206:542–550.
39. Gerzof SG, Robbins AJ, Johnson WC, Birkett DH, Nabseth DC (1981) Percutaneous catheter drainage of abdominal abscess: a five-year experience. N Engl J Med 305:653–657.

11 The Management Costs of the Most Severe Acute Pancreatitis

C.W. Imrie

In the present time of great interest in the audit of hospital expenses incurred in the management of common conditions, the management costs of the most severe cases of acute pancreatitis are especially important. In terms of clinical endeavour few conditions are so demanding. Access to expensive investigations and therapy are part and parcel of the management of this type of patient with contrast-enhanced computed tomography (CT) and early endoscopic retrograde cholangiopancreatography (ERCP) with sphincterotomy and duct clearance being necessary adjuncts to the management in addition to the costs of surgery and intensive care or high-dependency care.

The only paper in the literature to examine this question in detail was based on an analysis of 10 consecutive patients admitted between August 1990 and August 1991 to Glasgow Royal Infirmary. All had pancreatic necrosis confirmed at operation and in six of these patients the necrotic tissue was infected (1).

Patients and Methods

There were eight men and two women with a median age of 63 (range 29–73). Seven had a gallstone aetiology and three suffered from alcohol abuse. One patient died during initial hospitalisation and this patient had infected pancreatic necrosis. Gram-negative septicaemia was documented and multiorgan failure (MOF) was the cause of death.

The patients had a mean Glasgow prognostic score (2) of 3.8 and a median Glasgow score of 4. The time spent in intensive care ranged from 2 to 29 days with a median of 7 days. The median total hospital stay was 74 days and the range 40–150 days.

Surgical Procedures

All patients had at least one operation and the average was two operations per patient with a total of 22 procedures being carried out in the 10 patients. Only 2 of the 10 were successfully treated with one operation.

Management Costs

The median cost of management at the time of the study (1990–1991) was £18 441. The range of costs was from just over £9000 to almost £34 000 (£9296–£33 796). Hospitalisation accounted for 65% of the costs while the surgical procedures and endoscopic procedures accounted for 20% and laboratory costs the remaining 15%.

Flaws in the Costings

In the paper by Fenton-Lee and myself (1) there was no adequate provision made for high-dependency care. The patients spent a total of 74 days in hospital with a median of 7 days in intensive care, and most of the remaining 67 days were effectively in a high-dependency set-up. The Greater Glasgow Health Board Financial Department had no provision for costing this so that patients were costed at the average cost for those in a standard Nightingale ward. It is my belief that there was an estimated deficit of at least £125 per day for hospital costs over a minimum period of 50 days for an average patient so that the total deficit over the study period was £6250 per patient. This would correct the total cost per patient to be an average £24 650. Updating this figure to 1997 costs would be £28 200.

Nutrition Costs

In the original calculations there was an allowance for intravenous nutrition which is an expensive add-on to the cost. At the present time, enteral nutrition is being given early and utilised regularly by our team and this would be likely to reduce hospital costs because it is both safer and cheaper (3,4). It may also reduce hospital stay so that future impact of routine enteral nutrition may be considerable in lowering hospitals' costs. The study by McClave et al. (4) reckoned enteral nutrition to be less than 25% of the cost of total parenteral nutrition.

Quality of Life Measurements

In order to assess the quality of life benefits from the procedure, the measurement of quality of life adjusted life years (QALY) is utilised. This standard unit can be used when quality of life is related to life expectancy and in the study it is assumed that a normal life expectancy was 75 years. One QALY represented a year of quality life expectancy gained after treatment. The cost of treatment to individual patients is then related to the number of QALYs to give a cost for an individual QALY. In the study of severe acute pancreatitis management of 10 consecutive patients, the mean benefit was 8.5 QALYs obtained at a cost of £2157 each.

In comparison with other common diseases, the corresponding figure in the UK for coronary artery bypass surgery in 1991 was £1500 per QALY. The similar figure for renal transplantation was just over £6000. The cost of treatment in very severe acute pancreatitis is therefore considerably cheaper than renal transplantation and only a little more expensive than coronary artery bypass surgery, thus putting the management costs into perspective.

Comparison of Costs of Sterile and Infected Necrosis

In the Glasgow study where four patients had sterile necrosis and six had infected necrosis it was more expensive to manage the patients with infected necrosis largely due to the extended hospital stay and the greater severity of illness. The differences were not statistically significant although there was a cost difference of 16.5%. In a larger study it is likely that the difference for infected patients would be statistically significant. The average cost of the uninfected quartet of patients was £16 770 while the infected group cost £19 582 per patient. A similar adjustment to that used above would bring the management costs of infected necrotising AP management to a little more than £26 000 per patient at the present time.

Therapeutic Interventional Scoring System (TISS, Table 1)

This is a system of costing which has been specifically designed for intensive care units (ICU) by Cullen and his colleagues (5). There are 57 individual items in the Therapeutic Interventional Scoring System (TISS) and each has a grading on the scale of 1–4 according to the intensity of the procedure involved. Points are therefore acquired per patient per 24 hours and each TISS unit has a specific cost. This cost is reviewed on an annual basis in the USA for intensive care and an intermediate system for TISS is currently being calculated, which will be applicable to high-dependency care for patients.

The Therapeutic Interventional Scoring System Costs each intervention appropriately giving weighted scores for different items such as urinary catheterisation of the insertion and maintenance of a central venous pressure line. Some items have only one cost while others have a cost associated with the original procedure and thereafter the monitoring which is necessarily associated. In 1991 a TISS unit for intensive care in the USA was priced at $379. The cost of management of severe acute pancreatitis in the USA tends to be much higher than the figures which have been quoted from the UK. The most critically ill patients average 43 TISS points/day.

TISS Pricing Approach

The comparable pricing for the TISS system would be much greater per patient with infected necrotic peripancreatic/pancreatic tissue. This pricing is achieved by calculating the number of days in ICU care and then high-dependency unit (HDU) care. Costing for ICU at an average 7 days per patient would be $7 \times 43 \times 400 = \$120\,400/£75\,250$. Even halving this cost indicates a large disparity between the Fenton-Lee and Imrie calculation (1) and those used by the TISS pricing approach, before adding in the costs of the remaining 67 days in hospital. At a

Table 1. Therapeutic Intervention Scoring System

1 Point

a. ECG monitoring
b. Hourly vital signs or neuro vital signs
c. "Keep open" iv route
d. Chronic anticoagulation
e. Standard intake and output
f. Frequent STAT chems
g. Intermittent iv medications
h. Multiple dressing changes
i. Complicated orthopaedic traction
j. Iv antimetabolite therapy
k. Decubitus ulcer treatment
l. Urinary catheter
m. Supplemental oxygen (nasal or mask)
n. Antibiotics iv
o. Chest physiotherapy, IPPB
p. Extensive irrigations, packings or debridement of wound, fistula or colostomy
q. Gastrointestinal decompression

2 Points

a. CVP (central venous pressure)
b. 2 iv lines
c. Haemodialysis for chronic renal failure
d. Fresh tracheostomy (less than 48 hours)
e. Spontaneous respiration via endotracheal tube or tracheostomy
f. Tracheostomy care
g. Replacement of excess fluid loss
h. Chemotherapy pump

3 Points

a. Hyperalimentation or renal failure fluid
b. Pacemaker on standby
c. Chest tubes
d. Assisted respiration
e. Spontaneous PEEP
f. Concentrated K drip (>60 mEq/l)
g. Nasotracheal or orotracheal intubation
h. Endotracheal suctioning (non-intubated patient)
i. Complex metabolic balance (frequent intake and output, Brookline scale)
j. Multiple ABG, bleeding and STAT studies
k. Frequent infusions of blood products
l. Bolus iv medication
m. Multiple (>3) parenteral lines
n. Vasoactive drug infusion
o. Continues antiarrhythmia infusions
p. Cardioversion
q. Hypothermia blanket
r. Peripheral arterial line
s. Acute digitalisation
t. Active diuresis for fluid overload or cerebral oedema
u. Active Rx for metabolic alkalosis or acidosis
v. Emergency thora-, para- and pericardiocenteses
w. Acute anticoagulation
x. Phlebotomy (include with active diuresis)
y. Coverage with more than 2 iv antibiotics
z. Rx of seizures or metabolic encephalopathy (within 48 hours of onset)

4 Points

a. Cardiac arrest and/or countershock within 48 hours
b. Controlled ventilation with or without PEEP
c. Controlled ventilation with intermittent or continuous muscle relaxants
d. Balloon tamponade of varices
e. Continuous arterial infusion
f. Pulmonary artery line
g. Arterial or ventricular pacing
h. Haemodialysis in unstable patient
i. Peritoneal dialysis
j. Induced hypothermia
k. Pressure-activated blood infusion
l. G-suit
m. Measurement of cardiac output
n. Platelet transfusions
o. IABA (intra-aortic balloon assist)
p. Membrane oxygenation
q. Emergency operative procedures (within 24 hours)
r. Lavage of acute GI bleeding
s. Emergency endoscopy or bronchoscopy

conservative estimate it would be likely that the TISS scoring approach to pricing our patients would treble the cost, e.g. 5 TISS points average/day for 67 days at 50% of ICU cost/TISS unit would be $5 \times 67 \times 200$ or $67\ 000$/patient. The total hospital bill would be \$187 400 dollars (£117 125). This may well actually represent the difference in health care costs between UK and USA for the therapy of this most complicated group of patients. By the same token the UK costs may exceed that in other countries.

One of the really important facets of successful treatment of severe acute pancreatitis is the minimal further costs to the health care system incurred by these patients, especially if free from diabetes. Most patients recover and return to normal activities, which is a strong argument in support of the huge investment of time and resources needed to achieve this (6,7).

References

1. Fenton-Lee D, Imrie CW (1993) Pancreatic necrosis: assessment of outcome related to quality of life and cost of management. Br J Surg 80:1579–1582.
2. Osborne DH, Imrie CW, Carter DC (1981) Biliary surgery in the same admission for gallstone-associated acute pancreatitis. Br J Surg 68:758–761.
3. De Beaux AC, Plester C, Fearon KCH (1996) Flexible approach to nutritional support in severe acute pancreatitis. Nutrition 10:246–249.
4. McClave SA, Greene LA, Snider ML et al. (1997) Comparison of safety of early enteral vs parenteral nutrition in mild acute pancreatitis. J Parenteral Enteral Nutr 21:14–20.
5. Cullen DJ (1997) Results and costs of intensive care. Anaesthesiology 47:203–216.
6. Doepel VI, Eriksson J, Halme L, Kumpulainen T, Höckerstedt K (1993) Good long-term results in patients surviving severe acute pancreatitis. Br J Surg 80:1583–1586.
7. Carter DC (1993) Acute pancreatitis: the value of life. Br J Surg 80:1499–1500.

12 Enteral Nutrition in Acute Pancreatitis

J.V. Reynolds

Acute pancreatitis is a model of local and systemic immunoinflammation with a clinical spectrum incorporating the systemic inflammatory response syndrome (SIRS), sepsis, multiple organ failure (MOF), and death (1,2). A failure of the gut barrier to exclude endogenous bacteria, toxins and antigens from the portal and systemic circulation is incriminated in the modern paradigm of SIRS, sepsis and MOF (3). The gut has enhanced nutritional, metabolic and oxygen requirements in an established immunoinflammatory state (4). The rationale for feeding the gut using enteral nutrition is to support these needs and thus enhance local immune and barrier functions. Early enteral feeding has shown clinical benefit in other models of systemic immunoinflammation, including burns (5) and trauma (6), but its value as a therapeutic modality in acute pancreatitis has received scant experimental or clinical attention.

The major barrier to studying this is that acute pancreatitis has traditionally been considered to represent a relative, if not absolute, contraindication to enteral nutrition. This dogma is underpinned primarily by two assumptions. The first is that feeding the gut will stimulate pancreatic exocrine secretions and that this will aggravate the clinical condition. Second, since pancreatitis may be associated with gastric and intestinal atony, we are programmed since medical school to consider that enteral nutrition, however desirable it may be, would not be tolerated and may exacerbate symptoms.

The conventional approach to acute pancreatitis is thus at variance with our current understanding of the role of the gut and its nutritional requirement and ignores the modern paradigm of SIRS and sepsis. The purpose of this review is to question the evidence-base for this traditional dogma and to highlight the rationale for and data supporting the use of enteral nutrition in acute pancreatitis.

Effects of Feeding in Acute Pancreatitis

Does Enteral Nutrition Exacerbate Pancreatitis?

Theoretically this should be the case. Ingested and luminal nutrients may stimulate exocrine pancreatic secretion by three potential mechanisms: activation of enteropancreatic reflexes, release of enteral hormones and direct effects on the pancreas after absorption (7). Total parenteral nutrition (TPN), in contrast, bypasses the first two mechanisms. Direct experimental and clinical data, however, are sparse and conflicting. Animal studies have shown that intraduodenal administration of elemental diets results in less pancreatic stimulation than whole food but greater stimulation than TPN (7,8). Jejunal infusions do not appear to produce an increase in pancreatic secretion. Ragins et al. (9) created a pancreatic fistula in mongrel dogs, infused elemental diets successively into stomach, duodenum and jejunum and studied their effects on pancreatic secretion. Infusion into the stomach increased the volume, protein and bicarbonate content. Infusion into the duodenum produced minimal stimulation, whereas infusion into the jejunum at neutral pH produced no stimulation. Other studies have confirmed that delivery of nutrients as far distally as possible in the upper gastrointestinal tract can minimise pancreatic secretion (10). This concept may be supported by studies in man. Keith (11) showed that a low-fat elemental diet did not increase pancreatic ductal secretions which were directly measured by silastic tubes inserted into the pancreatic duct during surgery for chronic pancreatitis.

There are three small non-randomised clinical reports on enteral nutrition in acute pancreatitis (12–14). Two of these studies (12,13) simply showed that a small number of patients with complications of pancreatitis tolerated oral or nasogastric feeding with no exacerbation of their disease. Kudsk et al. (14) studied 11 patients following surgery for severe pancreatitis or complications. All patients were fed postoperatively via a jejunostomy catheter. Two patients did not tolerate enteral feeding. The remainder tolerated enteral nutrition with no increase in amylase and made a complete clinical recovery.

A randomised clinical trial has recently been reported which attests to the safety of enteral nutrition in acute pancreatitis. McClave et al. (15) randomised 32 admissions with predominantly mild acute pancreatitis (mean Ranson criteria: 1.3) to enteral or parenteral nutrition commenced within 48 hours of admission. Enteral nutrition was administered via a nasojejunal tube. This was well tolerated in all patients. Overall clinical outcome was the same in both groups. There was a significant improvement in Ranson criteria in the enteral group 6 days after admission compared with the TPN group. Stress-induced hyperglycaemia was worse in the TPN group, and the mean cost of nutrition per patient was over four times greater in the TPN group compared with the enteral group.

In summary, despite theory and anecdotal concerns to the contrary (16), there is no evidence from clinical or experimental studies that enteral nutrition, in particular jejunal administration of nutrients, stimulates pancreatic secretion or exacerbates pancreatitis.

Does Gut Rest and Total Parenteral Nutrition Improve Outcome?

A number of experimental studies have shown that TPN does not increase pancreatic exocrine secretion (7). In the clinical situation a direct therapeutic benefit of TPN was suggested after an uncontrolled, retrospective review of 200 patients demonstrated a reduction in mortality rate in patients with severe pancreatitis from 22% in conventionally managed patients to 14% in patients receiving TPN (17). Two prospective non-randomised studies have suggested a direct therapeutic benefit in patients with moderate and severe acute pancreatitis. Sitzman et al. (18), in a study of 73 patients, reported that 81% of patients had significant improvement in nutritional indices. Patients who remained in negative nitrogen balance had a significantly increased mortality rate (from 2 to 21%). Kalfarentzos et al. (19) in a trial of 67 patients showed a reduction in complications and mortality if TPN was started within 72 hours of admission to the ICU. Other retrospective studies have not, however, reported clinical benefit with TPN (7).

There is just one randomised controlled trial comparing TPN with no feeding (20). In 54 patients randomised to receive either conventional therapy (intravenous fluids, analgesics, antacids and nasogastric suction) or conventional therapy with early (within 24 hours of admission) TPN, the group receiving early TPN had significantly longer hospitalisation (16 vs 10 days, $P < 0.04$), and a higher rate of catheter sepsis (10.5% vs 1.5%, $P = 0.003$). This study is open to criticism since the patients had predominantly mild pancreatitis.

In summary, TPN does not appear to modulate the natural history of acute pancreatitis. There is no compelling evidence that TPN modulates pancreatic inflammation or improves outcome compared with no nutritional support in most patients with acute pancreatitis, and there is clearly no indication for TPN in mild acute pancreatitis. TPN has, however, a proven valuable supportive role in patients with severe pancreatitis or complications of the disease.

The Rationale for Enteral Feeding

Role of the Gastrointestinal Tract

Acute necrotising pancreatitis develops in 10–20% of patients with acute pancreatitis of whom about 30% develop pancreatic necrosis (21). Approximately 3–6% of patients with acute pancreatitis develop infected pancreatic necrosis, and pancreatic abscesses develop in a further 3–4% of patients. Enteric Gram-negative bacteria, in particular *Escherichia coli*, are the most common pathogens isolated from both infected pancreatic necrosis and other systemic organs and tissues in patients with pancreatitis. There is emerging consensus that pancreatic infection in severe acute pancreatitis arises as a result of bacterial translocation from the gut which permits colonisation of necrotic tissue (22). This is akin to the concept of the gut as the "undrained abscess" in septic patients who die of Gram-negative sepsis although no specific focus can be identified at autopsy (3).

The second line of evidence linking the gut and pancreatitis is linked to the recent conceptual advances in understanding SIRS and sepsis. Traditional dogma equated sepsis with infection, and progression to MOF was considered a sign of uncontrolled or occult infection. Infection is identified, however, in only approximately 50% of patients with clinical sepsis. Severe pancreatitis, major trauma, burns and shock may all result in this picture, now called SIRS, and this may progress to MOF in the absence of microbiological evidence of infection. An infectious focus is not identified in severe pancreatitis in about 25% of patients with MOF (23). In this situation, gut barrier failure with subclinical infection, endotoxaemia, and perhaps increased systemic antigen or splanchnic cytokine generation is purported to be the motor or fuel of MOF (24).

Irrespective of the initiating stimulus, SIRS and sepsis are the result of disordered activation of the host's immune system. Uncontrolled infection, necrotic tissue or gut barrier failure may alone or in combination prime and activate mononuclear phagocytes, neutrophils and endothelial cells (see Chapters 2 and 6).

There is no direct evidence for bacterial translocation in acute pancreatitis. However, Ryan et al. (25) in an experimental rat model showed that gut macromolecular permeability was increased, and that this increase was associated with the severity of disease and histological changes. We have also shown in preliminary unpublished studies that intestinal permeability to sugar probes is increased in pancreatitis in man.

The relevance of the gut to pancreatitis is also emphasised by the demonstration that selective gut decontamination improves outcome in severe acute pancreatitis (26, see Chapter 5). Intravenous cefuroxime alone has also been shown by workers in Finland (27) to decrease infectious complications and mortality in patients with severe alcoholic pancreatitis. These studies at least suggest that decreasing translocation or eliminating translocating bacteria may prevent colonization of necrotic tissue and modulate outcome.

Gastrointestinal microbes, endotoxins and splanchnic cytokines are thus linked to the complications of acute pancreatitis. Enteral nutrition is purported to support the nutritional, metabolic and immune requirements of the gastrointestinal tract and thus improve barrier function compared with bowel rest and TPN. This thesis is well proven in the animal model. In humans, the effect of TPN on gut barrier function is unknown. TPN, however, is associated with an exaggerated acute phase and metabolic response following injury which is attenuated by enteral nutrition (28).

A Randomised Study Comparing Enteral versus Bowel Rest ±TPN in Acute Pancreatitis

The above rationale was the basis for a randomised controlled trial comparing enteral and parenteral nutrition (29). The objective was to see if enteral nutrition affected outcome in patients with acute pancreatitis with respect to parameters that may relate to modulation of gut barrier function (Figure 1). Clinically, these included the incidence of SIRS and intra-abdominal sepsis, defined by Bone's criteria (30), the incidence of MOF, defined by Tran et al. (31), the need for operative intervention, intensive care unit stay and 30-day mortality. C-reactive protein was monitored as a marker of immunoinflammation and the acute phase response. Acute endotoxin exposure was monitored using IgM anti-core endotoxin antibodies. Total antioxidant capacity (TAC), which is decreased when the balance of free oxygen radical production exceeds consumption, was also measured.

Patients with a serum amylase of greater than 1000 IU and clinical evidence of acute pancreatitis were enrolled. Patients were then stratified according to their admission Glasgow score. Three or more Glasgow points predict severe disease and less than three mild/moderate disease. All patients underwent dynamic CT within 48 hours (32). Patients were randomised within 48 hours to receive either 7 days of enteral or parenteral nutrition. CRP, TAC and endotoxin measurements

Acute Pancreatitis

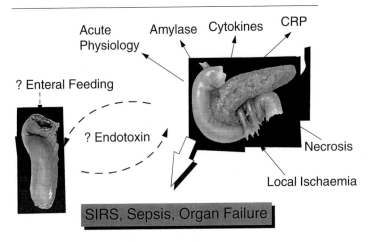

Figure 1. The study hypothesis. This study was set up to determine whether enteral nutrition modulated bacterial and endotoxin translocation (measured indirectly by IgM endotoxin antibodies and total antioxidant capacity), the hepatic acute phase response (CRP: C-reactive protein) and clinical outcome (SIRS, sepsis and organ failure).

were repeated following this period of nutritional support. Clinical parameters were monitored until discharge.

In patients with severe pancreatitis, the enteral feed (Osmolite, Ross Products, Kent, UK) was administered via a nasojejunal tube. In mild pancreatitis, the patients had access to modular nutritional supplements such as Entera (Fresenius, Cheshire, UK). Up to five cartons of supplement were taken each day, but no attempt was made to enforce an isocaloric, isonitrogenous intake in the enterally fed compared with the parenterally fed groups.

Thirty-four consecutive patients with pancreatitis fulfilled the enrolment criteria; 16 were randomised to enteral feeding and 18 to parenteral feeding. Both groups were matched for age, sex and severity stratification, including APACHE II score, Glasgow score, CT score and CRP. Eight patients in each group had predicted severe pancreatitis. No patient randomised to the enteral feeding group required conversion to parenteral nutrition.

Clinical outcome measures all improved in the enterally fed patients when compared with the parenterally fed patients. In the enterally fed group, SIRS was present in 11 patients prior to nutritional support but in only two patients after nutritional support ($P < 0.05$). There was no significant change (12 versus 10) in the incidence of SIRS following 7 days of parenteral feeding. Three patients in the parenterally fed group developed microbiologically proven intra-abdominal sepsis, two with pancreatic infection and one with a liver abscess. The two patients with pancreatic infection required necrosectomy and drainage of the infected material. Five parenterally fed patients also developed organ failure: three with single organ failure (pulmonary) and two with three organs failed (pulmonary, renal, cardiovascular). Two of these patients died, one at 7 days without documented sepsis and one at 14 days with evidence of pancreatic necrosis and infection following surgical intervention.

In addition to the clinical benefits of enteral nutrition, enteral feeding also attenuated the acute phase response and improved physiological scores. Following the nutritional support period there was a significant reduction in CRP (156 [117–222] to 84 [50–141] $P < 0.005$) and APACHE II scores (8 [6–10] to 6 [4–8] $P < 0.0001$) in the enterally fed group. No significant change in CRP (125 [49–168] to 124 [73–169]) or APACHE II scores (9.5 [8–13] to 8 [6–12]) was seen in the parenterally fed patients. The changes in CRP suggest that enteral feeding modulates the acute phase response while reprioritising hepatic visceral protein synthesis.

Acute endotoxin exposure and oxidative tissue injury appeared also to be favourably modulated by enteral nutrition. Serum IgM EndoCAb antibodies increased by a mean of 74% (± 19%) following 7 days of nutritional support in the parenterally fed group but remained unchanged in those enterally fed, suggesting that lack of luminal nutrition leads to significant systemic exposure to endotoxin. This may also explain the decrease in total antioxidant capacity, which fell by a mean of 30% (± 9%) in the parenterally fed group while this increased by a mean of 20% (± 14%) in the enterally fed patients.

Perspectives and Future Research

The cost implications of these observations as a whole are enormous. As a crude estimate parenteral feeding costs an estimated £75 per day not including disposables. Enteral feeding costs an estimated £5 not including disposables. If one takes into account the need for intensive therapy unit stay and potential com-

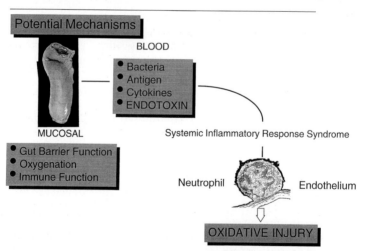

Figure 2. Possible mechanisms. The study showed decreased SIRS is associated with decreased exposure to endotoxin and oxidative stresses in the enterally fed group. Other potential contributory mechanisms at gut (splanchnic), systemic, pancreatic and end-organ sites are schematically indicated and merit experimental and clinical evaluation.

plications in the parenterally fed patients the net cost of parenterally feeding the patients with acute pancreatitis in this study would be considerably more than enteral feeding.

The early findings from this study suggest that contrary to conventional wisdom, enteral feeding is both feasible and desirable in the management of acute pancreatitis. Furthermore, despite the heterogeneity within the patient groups, the study provides evidence that enteral feeding appears to improve disease severity and clinical outcome by modifying the acute phase response, decreasing endotoxin exposure and modulating oxidative injury (Figure 2). The mechanism of action is unclear, and it is likely to be complex and multifactorial. Further research should address whether enteral feeding modulates gut barrier function, gut immune and cytokine parameters, and splanchnic blood flow. In the clinical setting it seems that the role of enteral nutrition merits further prospective evaluation, particularly in a large homogeneous group of patients with severe acute pancreatitis who are at high risk of SIRS, sepsis and MOF.

References

1. Formela LJ, Galloway SW, Kingsnorth AN (1995) Inflammatory mediators in acute pancreatitis. Br J Surg 82:6–13.
2. Steinberg W, Tenner S (1994) Acute pancreatitis. N Engl J Med 330:1198–1210.
3. Deitch EA (1992) Multiple organ failure. Pathophysiology and potential future therapy. Ann Surg 216:117–132.
4. Wilmore DW, Smith RJ, O'Dwyer ST, Jacobs DO, Ziegler TR, Wang XD (1988) The gut: a central organ after surgical stress. Surgery 104:917–923.
5. Alexander JW, MacMillan BG, Stinnett JD et al. (1980) Beneficial effects of aggressive protein feeding in severely burned children. Ann Surg 192:505–517.
6. Moore FA, Feliciano DV, Andrassy RJ et al. (1992) Early enteral nutrition, compared with parenteral, reduces postoperative septic complications. The results of a meta-analysis. Ann Surg 216:172–183.
7. Pisters PWT, Ranson JHC (1992) Nutritional support for acute pancreatitis. Surg Gynecol Obstet 175:275–284.
8. Marulendra S, Kirby DF (1995) Nutrition support in pancreatitis. Nutr Clin Pract 10:45–53.
9. Ragins H, Levenson SM, Singer R et al. (1973) Intrajejunal administration of an elemental diet at neutral pH avoids pancreatic stimulation. Am J Surg 126:606–614.
10. Kelly GA, Nahrwold AL. (1976) Pancreatic secretion in response to an elemental diet and intravenous hyperalimentation. Surg Gynecol Obstet 143:87–91.
11. Keith RG (1980) Effect of a low fat elemental diet on pancreatic secretion during pancreatitis. Surg Gynecol Obstet 151:337–343.
12. Voitk A, Brown RA, Echave V et al. (1973) Use of an elemental diet in the treatment of complicated pancreatitis. Am J Surg 125:223–227.
13. Parekh D, Lawson HH, Sigal I (1993) The role of total enteral nutrition in pancreatic disease. S Afr J Surg 31:57–61.
14. Kudsk KA, Campbell SM, O'Brien T, Fuller R (1990) Postoperative enteral feeding following complicated pancreatitis. Nutr Clin Pract 5:14–17.
15. McClave S, Greene LM, Snider H et al. (1997) Comparison of the safety of early enteral vs parenteral nutrition in mild acute pancreatitis. JPEN 21:14–20.
16. Ranson JHC, Spencer FC (1977) Prevention, diagnosis and treatment of pancreatic abscess. Surgery 82:99–106.
17. Feller JH, Brown RA, MacLaren-Toussant GP et al. (1974) Changing methods in the treatment of severe pancreatitis. Am J Surg 127:196–201.
18. Sitzmann JV, Steinborn PA, Zinner MJ et al. (1989) Total parenteral nutrition and alternate energy substrates in treatment of severe acute pancreatitis. Surg Gynecol Obstet 168:311–317.
19. Kalfarentzos FE, Karafios DD, Karatzas TM et al. (1991) Total parenteral nutrition in severe acute pancreatitis. J Am Coll Nutr 10:156–162.

20. Sax HC, Warner BW, Talamini MA et al. (1987) Early total parenteral nutrition in acute pancreatitis: lack of beneficial effects. Am J Surg 153:117–124.

21. Isenmann R, Buchler MW (1994) Infection and acute pancreatitis. Br J Surg 81:1707–1708.

22. Johnson CD (1996) Antibiotic prophylaxis in severe acute pancreatitis. Br J Surg 83:883–884.

23. Tran DD, Cuesta MA, Scneider JA, Wesdorp RIC (1993) Multiple organ failure in patients with acute pancreatitis. J Crit Care 8:145–153

24. Reynolds JV (1996) Gut barrier function in the surgical patient. Br J Surg 83:1668–1669.

25. Ryan CM, Schmidt J, Lewandrowski K et al. (1993) Gut macromolecular permeability in pancreatitis correlates with severity of disease in rats. Gastroenterology 104:890–895.

26. Luiten EJT, Hop WCJ, Lange JF, Bruining HA (1995) Controlled clinical trial of selective decontamination for the treatment of severe acute pancreatitis. Ann Surg 222:57–65.

27. Sainio V, Kemppainen E, Pouillakkainen P et al. (1995) Early antibiotic treatment in acute necrotising pancreatitis. Lancet 346:663–667.

28. Peterson VN, Moore EE, Jones TN et al. (1988) Total enteral nutrition versus total parenteral nutrition after major torso injury: attenuation of hepatic protein reprioritization. Surgery 104:199–207.

29. Windsor ACJ, Li A, Gurthrie A et al. (1996) Feeding the gut in pancreatitis: a randomised clinical trial of enteral versus parenteral nutrition. Br J Surg 83:689 (abstract).

30. Bone RC, Sibbald WJ, Sprung CL (1992) The ACCP-SCCM consensus conference on sepsis and organ failure. Chest 101:1481–1483.

31. Tran DD, Groeneveld AB, van der Muelen J et al. (1990) Age, chronic disease, sepsis, organ system failure and mortality in a medical intensive care unit. Crit Care Med 18:474–479.

32. Balthazar EJ, Robinson DL, Megibow AJ, Ranson JHC (1990) Acute pancreatitis; value of CT in establishing the prognosis. Radiology 1990;174:331–336.

13 The Burden of Acute Pancreatitis

S.W.T. Gould and G. Glazer

Acute pancreatitis is a disease with a significant mortality and has been reported as the principal diagnosis in 2% of all admissions with abdominal pain to hospitals in the UK (1). The management of acute pancreatitis involves a multidisciplinary approach, and requires a considerable investment of time and expertise. It can at times test the skill and patience of medical and paramedical staff, as well as consuming considerable hospital resources.

The reported incidence of acute pancreatitis varies greatly depending on such variables as geography and aetiological factors, but it has been accepted for some time that the incidence is in the range of 200–300 cases per million population per year (2). There is some evidence that this figure is increasing and is an underestimate. The incidence in Scotland appears to have risen from 200 to over 350 cases per million population in recent years (see Chapter 7). The rise in incidence may be partly due to an increase in alcohol consumption in the general population (3), although the incidence of gallstones, the other major aetiological factor in Western countries, is also probably rising (4). There is considerable variation in incidence between countries, the reported figure for Finland being 734 per million population per year, and the figure for the United States is even higher (over 800 per million population per year). This may reflect not only the varying aetiological factors at work, but also other issues such as national variations in autopsy rates and the availability and interpretation of diagnostic tests (see below).

The true incidence of acute pancreatitis is very difficult to assess accurately as the diagnosis depends upon clinical awareness of its varying and diverse patterns of presentation (including asymptomatic presentations), the availability and timing of the use of serum amylase and other diagnostic tests, and the availability of appropriate imaging facilities, particularly computed tomography (CT). The reported incidence of acute pancreatitis will also depend on the level at which a diagnostic test is said to be positive for the condition. Elevation of serum amylase to a level twice above normal is taken as diagnostic in North America, whereas a level of three times normal or greater than 1000 IU/ml is generally taken as the cut-off point in the UK. It is because of these factors, and also because of poor clinical acumen both in hospital and primary care practice that a significant number of cases probably go unreported. Further evidence for this comes from autopsy studies from a number of countries. These demonstrate that in up to 40% of cases the diagnosis of acute pancreatitis was made by the pathologist after death, and had not been suspected during the course of the patient's admission

(5). Since the autopsy rate in different countries varies (greater than 70% of hospital deaths in Sweden, approximately 15% in the UK) it is likely that some of the most severe cases of acute pancreatitis are not being reported at all. Despite the fact that acute pancreatitis found in some cases at autopsy may not have been the main cause of death, i.e. in hypothermia, the overall burden of acute pancreatitis is likely to be greater than is currently reported.

There have been a number of improvements in the management of acute pancreatitis in the past decade. These include a clearer understanding of the methods available to stratify patients early in an attack into either a predicted mild or severe category (see below) and an increased provision and use of intensive therapy unit (ITU) facilities to manage severe cases with multisystem organ failure (MOF). There is now widespread recognition of the many and varied complications of this disease which has been assisted by CT and other radiological techniques. The armamentarium of therapeutic techniques now available to the interventional radiologist, endoscopist and surgeon has resulted in improved and possibly more rational management strategies.

Current Practice and Outcome

Despite these "improvements" the mortality rate for acute pancreatitis has remained stubbornly constant for over 20 years (6) and is usually reported at around 10–12% in controlled clinical trials. This may not reflect the true death rate since some cases remain undiagnosed and comparison between different studies is hampered because the calculation of the true overall mortality rate should include patients in whom the diagnosis was established at autopsy. In addition many cases are misdiagnosed in life. It is also unclear in what proportion of cases the disease is the major contributing factor to death and, as severe co-morbid and lethal conditions will vary in different populations, this further contributes to the variability in the overall mortality rates. Furthermore the disease course is unpredictable and, since no specific cure is available, treatment has of necessity been supportive and reactive. Because of these variable factors, meaningful audits of the management process and patient outcome have been difficult to obtain.

Although the overall mortality has not changed over the past two decades, there may be changes in the pattern of mortality. Approximately 30% of deaths now occur in the early stages of an attack from MOF (6), a reduction compared with previous decades (7). Deaths after the first week are related to infectious complications, particularly infected pancreatic necrosis (8). Sterile pancreatic necrosis is associated with a mortality of 0–11% (9), infected necrosis 40–70% or greater (10). Outcome depends on a number of factors such as age, premorbid conditions, degree of pancreatic necrosis, onset of infection and form of surgical debridement (11).

Severity Prediction

There has been considerable interest and work in the early stratification of acute pancreatitis into mild and severe forms. This has considerable implications for management, provision of appropriate health care resources and prognostication. Failure to stratify patients accurately in this way can be identified as a cause of management deficiencies and may result in potentially avoidable mortality (6).

Clinical assessment of the severity of an attack will misclassify around 50% of patients and is therefore unreliable (12), unless failure of one or more organ systems is present to indicate a severe attack (13). A number of multifactorial biochemical scoring systems have been devised by multivariate analysis. The most frequently used examples are the Ranson (14) and Glasgow criteria (15). The latter has been validated on the UK population and these give a prognostic accuracy of 70–80%.

The serum C-reactive protein (CRP), measured in the first week of the attack, has been shown to have independent predictive value, with a prognostic accuracy again of approximately 80% (16). Other inflammatory markers have been used but their value has not been proven. Clinical severity scoring methods such as APACHE II have also been shown to be accurate in assessing the initial severity of the disease, and can be used on a daily basis for ongoing assessment (17). However its accuracy is also no greater than 80%.

Specific Treatments

The treatment of acute pancreatitis has been largely supportive with no specific remedies having been shown to be effective in properly controlled trials. Aprotinin (Trasylol), glucagon, fresh frozen plasma and peritoneal lavage have all failed to show any benefit. The place of emergency endoscopic retrograde cholangiography (ERCP) and sphincterotomy in early severe gallstone pancreatitis has its proponents (18) but there is some evidence that in non-jaundiced patients there is no benefit (19). There are other contentious issues in management such as the place of antibiotics, the value of selective decontamination of the gut and whether or not early enteral feeding improves outcome.

Imaging

Contrast-enhanced dynamic CT scanning need only be performed in those patients who have an attack predicted as severe. This scan has also been assessed as a prognostic aid as it allows the degree of pancreatic necrosis (measured by the areas of non-enhancement) and the number of peripancreatic fluid collections to be estimated. From this a quantitative score can be produced (the CT severity index, CTSI) which correlates well with the severity of the attack with a prognostic accuracy of approximately 85% (20). Any patient with a high prediction of developing infected necrosis (i.e. with 50% or more necrosis of the gland or with 30% necrosis and three or more fluid collections) should be treated in a specialist unit with multidisciplinary expertise and all the necessary facilities.

Costs

The financial costs of this complex disease are also high. Assuming on a conservative basis that the annual incidence of acute pancreatitis in the UK is

200 cases/million population/year (with the provisos noted above) and knowing the disease outcome probabilities, it is possible to predict approximately 8000 mild cases a year, with a mean hospital stay of 6–7 days. There would be 1000 severe cases a year without local pancreatic complications (mean stay 14 days) and 1000 severe cases with local complications (mean stay 60 days). These lengths of stay are based on our own practice and may be different elsewhere. The actual cost of this morbidity is extremely hard to calculate accurately, but if one estimates 1 day in a general ward with associated treatment and consumables to cost £350, with added costs for cholecystectomy, the overall cost of mild gallstone pancreatitis can be estimated to be approximately £6400 per case assuming that the patient has the surgery on the first admission and within 2 weeks of onset.

Of the 2000 patients per year with severe pancreatitis, even those patients with no complications associated with the disease would cost approximately £9000 per case. This may rise to as much as £100 000 per case if complications develop and the patient requires intensive and prolonged treatment, associated with the need for complex and expensive investigations and interventional procedures. Added to these figures is the cost to the economy of the prolonged convalescence that these patients often require, many of whom are of working age.

Guidelines and Audit Goals

With the complexity of this unpredictable disease, the limitations and deficiencies of current practice and the financial cost of managing it, a UK Acute Pancreatitis Consensus Group was formed to develop guidelines using the best current evidence. An ideal management protocol for patients with acute pancreatitis has been proposed and some broad audit goals have been set so that clinicians can measure their effectiveness against a standard. These key objectives are to keep the overall mortality to 10% or less and below 30% in severe cases; to achieve a correct diagnosis of acute pancreatitis in all patients within 24 hours, to stratify severity in all cases within 48 hours using a combination of the methods described above and to obtain a diagnosis of the aetiology in at least 75% of cases. Patients with mild gallstone pancreatitis should have their cholecystectomy performed within 2–4 weeks of the onset of the attack (Table 1).

Other criteria state that all severe cases should be observed and treated in a high-dependency unit (HDU) or intensive care unit (ICU), depending on severity and comorbid factors. The degree of pancreatic necrosis and site and number of acute fluid collections in these patients should be assessed by dynamic contrast-enhanced CT within 3–10 days, and the CT severity score calculated as an aid to stratification and as a baseline for comparison with scans performed later in the

Table 1. Outcome measures

UK consensus group: audit objectives

- Mortality: overall < 10%, severe < 30%
- Correct diagnosis within 24 hours: 100%
- Severity stratification within 48 hours: 100%
- Assessment of aetiology: idiopathic < 25%

Table 2. Process measures

UK consensus: audit objectives

- Mild gallstone pancreatitis. Definitive management of lithiasis within 2–4 weeks: 100%
- Severe acute pancreatitis. HDU/ITU monitoring and treatment: 100%
- Severe acute pancreatitis. Dynamic CT within 3–10 days: 100%
- ERCP available for selected cases of severe gallstone pancreatitis and/or cholangitis
- Early referral of complex cases to specialist unit with surgical control and multidisciplinary expertise

patient's management. Facilities for ERCP should be available for selected cases of gallstone pancreatitis and/or cholangitis early in the attack (Table 2).

Bearing in mind the factors described above, the ideal management protocol for patients with acute pancreatitis should begin with an accurate diagnosis within 24 hours, followed over the next 24–48 hours by severity stratification into predicted mild or severe cases. Mild cases should be managed in a ward area in a routine manner, with assessment and treatment of precipitating factors. Management of severe cases involves dynamic contrast-enhanced CT, possibly an urgent ERCP, and more intensive treatment and monitoring in an HDU or ICU. The main priority in these patients is to anticipate, diagnose and treat the possible local and systemic complications associated with the disease (Figure 1).

Patients with severe acute pancreatitis, or those with local complications, should be treated in specialist units with all the necessary expertise available. These units should be directed by a surgeon experienced in all aspects of management of patients with pancreatitis, supported by a multidisciplinary team. There is also a requirement for expertise in the full range of interventional radiological and ERCP procedures needed in the management of these patients. Patients with MOF, or those with established or (ideally) predicted local complications such as infected necrosis (based on early CT grading), should be transferred to these facilities.

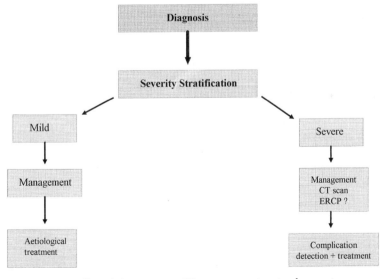

Figure 1. Acute pancreatitis: management protocol.

The development of specialist units, and the concentration of the most severe cases in the most expert hands available may be a step towards reducing the static mortality rate from this disease. Although these units will be expensive to develop and will have high running costs, if they succeed in reducing the magnitude of morbidity and mortality from the disease they will be an important step in the battle to ease the burden of acute pancreatitis.

Note added in proof

The UK guidelines for the management of acute pancreatitis have now been published as a supplement to *Gut* (June 1998).

References

1. De Dombal F (1991) Diagnosis of acute abdominal pain, 2nd edn. Churchill Livingstone, Edinburgh.
2. Graham D (1977) Incidence and mortality of acute pancreatitis. Br Med J II:1603.
3. Corfield A, Cooper M, Williamson, R (1985) Acute pancreatitis: a lethal disease of increasing incidence. Gut 26:724–729.
4. De Bolla A, Obeid M (1984) Mortality in acute pancreatitis. Ann R Coll Surg Eng 66:184–186.
5. Lankisch P, Schirren C, Kunze E (1991) Undetected fatal acute pancreatitis: why is the disease so frequently overlooked? Am J Gastroenterol 86:322–326.
6. Mann D, Hershmann M, Hittinger R, Glazer G (1994) Multicentre audit of death from acute pancreatitis. Br J Surg 81:890–893.
7. Storck G, Pettersson G, Edlund Y (1976) A study of autopsies upon 116 patients with acute pancreatitis. Surg Gynecol Obstet 143:241–245.
8. Renner I, Savage W, Pantoja J, Renner V (1985) Death due to acute pancreatitis: a retrospective analysis of 405 autopsy cases. Dig Dis Sci 30:1005–1018.
9. Bradley E, Allen K (1991) A prospective longitudinal study of observation versus surgical intervention in the management of necrotizing pancreatitis. Am J Surg 161:19–25.
10. Widdison A, Karanjia N (1993) Pancreatic infection complicating acute pancreatitis. Br J Surg 80:148–154.
11. Lumsden A, Bradley E (1990) Secondary pancreatic infections. Surg Gynecol Obstet 170:459–467.
12. Corfield A, Williamson R, McMahon M et al. (1985) Prediction of severity in acute pancreatitis: prospective comparison of three prognostic indices. Lancet II:403–407.
13. Bradley E III (1993) A clinically based classification system for acute pancreatitis. Arch Surg 128:586–590.
14. Ranson J, Rifkind K, Roses D (1974) Prognostic signs and the role of operative management in acute pancreatitis. Surg Gynecol Obstet 139:69–81.
15. Blamey S, Imrie C, O'Neill J, Gilmour W, Carter D (1984) Prognostic factors in acute pancreatitis. Gut 25:1340–1346.
16. Wilson C, Heads A, Shenkin A, Imrie C (1989) C-reactive protein, antiproteases and complement factors as objective markers of severity in acute pancreatitis. Br J Surg 6:177–181.
17. Wilson C, Heath D, Imrie C (1990) Prediction of outcome in acute pancreatitis: a comparative study of APACHE II, clinical assessment and multiple factor scoring systems. Br J Surg 77:1260–1264.
18. Neoptolemos J, Carr-Locke D, London N (1988) Controlled trial of urgent endoscopic retrograde cholangiopancreatography and endoscopic sphincterotomy versus conservative treatment for acute pancreatitis due to gallstones. Lancet II:979–983.
19. Folsch UR, Nitsche R et al. (1997) Early ERCP and papillotomy compared with conservative treatment for acute biliary pancreatitis. New Engl J Med 336:237–242.
20. Balthazar E, Robinson D, Megibow A (1990) Acute pancreatitis: value of CT in establishing prognosis. Radiology 174:331–336.

Section 2

Transplantation

14 Pancreas Transplantation

V. Di Carlo and R. Castoldi

Diabetes mellitus (DM) is a major health problem as it is widely spread in both Europe and USA. In North American epidemiological researches it seems that about 6% of the population suffer from DM, with approximately 30 000 new cases a year (1). Due to its classical complications, notably renal failure, neuropathy, retinopathy and cardiovascular disease, the life expectancy of the diabetic patient is about one-third less than that of the general population.

Evidence from the literature shows that such microvascular complications of DM are linked to long-term hyperglycaemia and that they could be reduced by intensive control of blood glucose level (2). Although exogenous insulin therapy is effective in preventing acute metabolic decompensation and is life saving, an intensive insulin replacement regimen cannot achieve the perfect glucose balance.

Pancreas transplantation is currently the only known therapy that establishes a long-term insulin-independent euglycaemic state with complete normalisation of glycosylated haemoglobin levels. Since 1966, more than 7000 pancreas transplants have been performed all over the world and in the majority of cases (87% in the USA), were associated with simultaneous kidney graft (SPK) in insulin-dependent diabetes mellitus (IDDM) patients with end or pre-end stage renal failure. The remaining pancreas transplants have been performed as a sequential pancreas after kidney transplant (PAK, 7%), as a pancreas transplant alone (PTA, 5%), or in conjunction with other organs than the kidney (1%).

In the past few years results have improved markedly. In the International Pancreas Transplant Registry (IPTR), the overall 1-year patient survival after pancreas transplant reaches 91%, with a 1-year pancreas graft survival of 75% (3). Results according to the different ways of managing the pancreatic duct after pancreas transplantation in the USA and Europe are shown in Table 1. According to these results pancreas transplantation, and particularly SPK

Table 1. Pancreas graft survival by duct management

	1-year		5-year	
	USA	Europe	USA	Europe
Bladder drainage	76%	78%	60%	73%
Enteric drainage	57%	63%	48%	49%
Duct injection	–	61%	–	59%

transplant, has become an accepted treatment for appropiately selected diabetic patients (4). The penalties for this are the surgical risk of the procedure and those linked to chronic immunosuppression.

Therefore indications for pancreas transplantation are a critical problem, and the criteria for selection of patients continue to evolve due to the availability of new immunosuppressive drugs with minimal toxicity and to improved surgical techniques.

Indications: Present and Future

Currently SPK must be considered in IDDM patients with end-stage renal failure, pre-end stage renal failure (creatinine clearance less than 30 ml/min), or failure of a previous kidney transplant, along with the usual option of kidney transplant alone. Contraindications are usually considered to include age greater than 60 years, left ventricular ejection fraction less than 40%, presence of active infection or malignancy, active smoking, severe obesity, recent history of substance abuse or non-compliance with treatment (5). In those patients in whom immuno-suppression is already mandatory for the presence of the kidney graft, the additional surgical risk of the pancreas procedure is justified by the excellent results and the evidence that diabetic complications can be prevented or stabilised by the euglycaemic state.

Of course patients with limited secondary complications of diabetes are considered optimal candidates for SPK. So it is now increasingly evident that pancreas transplantation should be performed early in the course of diabetes, and some pioneering centres have opened the discussion about pre-emptive SPK transplantation and single pancreatic graft in order to prevent secondary complications. The rationale for pre-emptive SPK transplantation, before the start of dialysis, would be the improved surgical results, reduced costs and morbidity and potential stabilisation of diabetic complications. A creatinine clearance greater than 70 ml/min is required for candidates for PTA, as current immuno-suppression can cause an accelerated deterioration of renal failure. For patients with a creatinine clearance between 40 and 70 ml/min, oral cyclosporine or an FK 506 challenge test is advised (6).

Another problem concerning PTA is that experience is at present more limited and results are currently less favourable than SPK (3). In fact, being almost constantly concomitant, rejection is easier to detect in the presence of the kidney graft and the kidney may have a protective immunological role versus the pancreas (7). For these reasons, although very fashionable from the perspective of preventing secondary complications, the indications for PTA are not yet well defined, apart from the rare entity of hyperlabile diabetes, and the procedure is currently adopted only in a few centres and within strict protocols. Finally, living-related pancreas donation is beginning to be performed in selected highly sensitised patients (8).

Advances in Surgical Techniques

Further progress in candidate selection protocols depends also on diminishing surgical morbidity. Pancreas transplantation techniques currently used are whole organ pancreaticoduodenal graft with bladder (BD) or enteric drainage (ED) of exocrine secretions and systemic venous drainage of insulin, segmental pancreas transplant with duct injection (DI) and segmental pancreas transplant with enteric or bladder drainage. Advantages of whole versus segmental pancreas graft include a greater islet cell mass, lower risk of thrombosis due to better blood flow and a reduced incidence of pancreatitis and fistula because of integrity of the pancreatic parenchyma.

Currently whole pancreas transplantation with duodenocystostomy is the procedure of choice in most US and European centres (94% of pancreas transplants in the USA) and IPTR data continue to show better results for BD in terms of pancreas graft survival compared with other techniques (3). Nevertheless current discussion of the BD technique concerns two problems. First is the non-physiological systemic drainage of insulin. Recent studies have investigated surgical and metabolic results in pancreas transplantation with enteric exocrine drainage and portal venous anastomosis (9). The second problem is the urological and metabolic complications due to the presence and activation of pancreatic enzymes in the urinary tract and the chronic loss of bicarbonate (10). Severe and refractory complications may necessitate conversion to enteric diversion. The most frequent urological complications are chemical cystitis, urethritis, balanitis, urethral disruption and stricture, haematuria and recurrent urinary tract infections. The incidence of the problem is about 40% in the different series (10,11). Usually these complications may be managed with urethral catheter drainage, alkalinisation of the urine, antibiotics, and very rarely may require surgery.

Metabolic acidosis and dehydration usually are self-limiting and can be treated by supplementation with fluids and bicarbonate; enteric conversion is performed for this complication in 5–7% of cases (12). Duodenal leak or perforation may be linked to vascular, immunological or infective problems (ischaemia, rejection, cytomegalovirus infection), and usually necessitate a surgical repair.

Reflux pancreatitis, fistulas and peripancreatic collection may be generally treated by urethral catheter drainage, somatostatin therapy and percutaneous drainage, but, if a peripancreatic infection develops, a laparotomy is required and the risk of graft loss rises to 30–50%. So, to avoid these problems, different authors have recently suggested the possibility of readopting a modified enteric drainage technique. The procedure consists in a duodenopancreatic graft with a duodeno-jejuno-anastomosis with or without a Roux-loop. Recent experiences report a low rate of complications (13). Nevertheless, if a complication such as leakage or pancreatitis appears, the consequences may be lethal. Thus caution should be used before changing a winning technique. Also, considering that the overall reported enteric conversion rate in different series ranges from 10% to 20%, the procedure is simple, safe, with surgical complications in about 10–20% of cases; graft loss and death after enteric conversion are exceptional (12,14,15).

Progress in Immunosuppression Strategies

There is currently great interest in new immunosuppressive agents in pancreas transplantation: the goal is to improve prevention and treatment of rejection while minimising risks to the patient. Currently most centres utilise a quadruple regime with antilymphocyte induction (ALG, ATG or OKT3), cyclosporine, prednisone and azathioprine. Pancreas graft loss is one of the major causes of graft loss (in different series about 40%) (3). In our experience 7.8% of patients with BD lost the pancreas due to rejection. Recently a new microemulsion formulation of cyclosporine (Neoral) has been introduced: it appears to have a better oral absorption and bioavailability which is particularly useful in the case of recipients with autonomic neuropathy.

FK 506 (Prograf) therapy has been utilised in a few protocols in place of cyclosporine for induction and rescue treatment after pancreas transplantation and results are promising (16). Mycophenolate mofetil (MMF-Cellcept) has begun to be used in substitution of azathioprine in kidney transplantation (17): experience in SPK is in progress. Great efforts are being made to diminish pancreas graft immunogenicity by means of monoclonal antibody technology, or to promote donor-specific tolerance of the host.

Metabolic Results and Effects of Pancreas Transplantation on Secondary Complications of DM

The effects of a functioning pancreas graft on glucose and lipid metabolism are well studied (18,19,20). In fact pancreas transplantation is able to achieve and mantain a long-term euglycaemic insulin-independent state with normal glycosylated haemoglobin levels, that is superior to any other form of therapy today. Also lipid metabolism is improved, in these cardiovascular high risk patients for cardiovascular disease. Nevertheless, hyperinsulinaemia is frequently demonstrated and may be linked to systemic venous drainage. No major complication of hyperinsulinaemia, however, has been described.

These satisfactory metabolic results justify the effects on secondary diabetic complications. The literature shows that SPK transplantation prevents the recurrence of diabetic nephropathy in the transplanted kidney (21), even if there is no demonstration of reversal of pre-existing nephropathy after long-term insulin independence.

Sensory and motor neuropathy, especially when mild, can be ameliorated and even reversed by a long-term euglycaemic state (22), and recent data about autonomic neuropathy are promising (23).

Retinopathy seems to be stabilized after a long-term successful pancreas transplantation but amelioration of the complication is not yet definitely proved (24). In conclusion the demonstrated improvement of quality of life after successful SPK (5), and the possibility of returning to normal activity are factors of great influence on the balance of benefit to risk. Thus pancreas transplantation and especially SPK, today offers very satisfactory results in terms of patient, pan-creas and kidney survival, and beneficial effects on most secondary diabetic complications.

Islet transplantation cannot at present be considered an alternative therapy to the used a vascularised graft, as long-term insulin independence has been achieved up to now in only a few cases. Nevertheless the advantages of the low-risk surgical procedure and the potential possibility of islet immunoalteration and eventual transplantation without immunosuppression render islet cell and foetal pancreas transplantation a fascinating research field (26).

The promising data about secondary diabetic complications and the new immunosuppressive strategies, with better prevention and treatment of rejection and less long-term risk of overimmunosuppression, will result in the future in more extensive and precise indications for pancreas transplantation.

Personal Experience

Our experience began in July 1985, with 29 segmental neoprene duct injected transplantations (DI); since October 1989, 69 duodenopancreatic transplants with bladder drainage (BD) have been performed.

Segmental pancreas was duct-injected with Neoprene according to DuBernard's technique (27) and grafted to the iliac vessels. Duodenopancreatic transplants (28), according to Sollinger's bladder drainage technique, were grafted in all cases to the external iliac artery. In most cases an extended iliac artery graft and an extended iliac or caval vein graft was anastomosed on to the portal vein.

The characteristics of the two groups (demographic data, organ procurement, surgical procedure, antithrombotic and antibiotic prophylaxis and immuno-suppressive therapy) are reported in Table 2. Immunosuppressive protocol included azathioprine (2.5 mg/kg per day, maintenance 1 mg/kg per day), prednisone (10 mg/kg per day, progressively reduced to 10 mg/d), and anti-lymphocyte globulines (ALG) (8 mg/kg per day for 10 days). ALG was then with-drawn and 6–8 mg/kg per day of cyclosporin was administered. Acute rejection episodes were treated by methylprednisolone boluses (500 mg). From October 1989 the immunosuppressive protocol was modified in the following way: prednisone (0.25 mg/kg per day) was used, and unresponsive acute rejection episodes were treated with OKT3.

Perioperative mortality was 6.9% in the DI group: one patient died of a myocardial infarction with both organs functioning and one patient of septic

Table 2. Characteristics of patients in duct injection (DI) and bladder drainage (BD)

	DI (n=29)	BD (n=69)
Sex (male/female)	0.8:1	1.06:1
Age (mean years ± SD)	39 ± 7	36 ± 3
Duration of IDDM (mean months ± SD)	25 ± 5	24 ± 2
Duration of dialysis (mean months ± SD)	23 ± 15	22 ± 5
Degenerative complications	all cases	all cases
Multiorgan donation	46% of cases	97% of cases
Preservation solution	Collins (75% of cases)	UW (all cases)
Cold ischaemia (mean min ± SD)	291 ± 70	612 ± 181
Warm ischaemia (mean min ± SD)	43 ± 12	43 ± 10
Duration of surgery (mean min ± SD)	466 ± 74	435 ± 49
Hospital stay (mean days ± SD)	548 ± 16	32 ± 17
Prevention of graft thrombosis	Anticoagulation	Antiaggregation
Antibiotic prophylaxis	Cefotaxime (all cases)	
Immunosuppression	Quadruple sequential per prednisone 1 mg/kg per day	Quadruple sequential pred [0.25 mg/kg/per day] OKT3 in steroid Refractory rejections

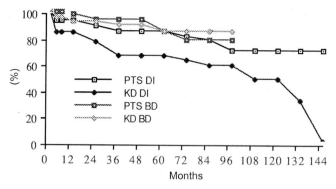

Figure 1. Patients (PTS) and kidney (KD) actuarial survival in duct injection (DI) and bladder drainage (BD) series.

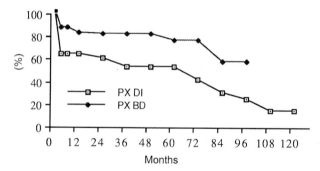

Figure 2. Pancreas graft (PX) actuarial survival in DI and BD series.

bleeding after the retrieval of both the organs. In the BD series one patient died of systemic sepsis due to mycobacterium tubercolosis secondary to lymphoma (1.4%). One-year patient survival in DI and BD series were 92% and 97%, and kidney 1-year survival 82% and 90%, respectively. Overall pancreas 1-year survivals were 61% in DI and 81% in BD series. One-year pancreas graft survival in technically successful cases was 96% in both series (Figures 1 and 2).

Technical failures in both groups were respectively 8/29 (28%) and 7/51(10%). Causes of graft failures are reported in Table 3. Fifteen patients (55%) in the DI group and 24 (40%) in the BD series had a postoperative surgical complication (Table 4). In eight patients (28%) in the DI series, the surgical complication led to graft failure, in one case (3.5%) to death and in eight patients relaparotomies were needed (28%). In seven patients (10%) in the BD series, complications determined pancreas failure, no patient died of surgical complications and in 14 patients relaparotomies were needed (20%). Arterial or venous thromboses were the leading complications (24% in DI group versus 7% in BD). Graft pancreatitis was infrequent in the BD series (10% versus 1%) but, in the DI group, five patients (17%) developed a pancreatic fistula. which healed in less than 2 weeks. One further patient developed a pancreatic fistula which was complicated by peritonitis requiring relaparotomy.

Table 3. Causes of graft failure

Pancreas failures	DI		BD	
Thrombosis	7	(24%)	5	(7%)
Rejection	6	(21%)	4	(6%)
Death with functioning graft	4	(14%)	2	(3%)
Neoplasm	–		1	(1%)
Septic bleeding	1	(3%)	2	(3%)
Primary non-function	1	(3%)	3	(4%)
Exhaustion of function	8	(28%)	2	(3%)
Overall	27	(93%)	19	(27%)
Technical	8	(28%)	7	(10%)

Table 4. Pancreas surgical complications at San Raffaele Hospital

Complication	DI ($n = 29$)		BD ($n = 69$)	
Thrombosis	5	(24%)	5	(7%)
Pancreatitis	3	(10%)	1	(1%)
Peripancreatic abscesses	–	–	2	(3%)
Pancreatic fistula	5	(17%)	–	–
Septic bleeding	2	(7%)	2	(3%)
Hemoperitoneum	2	(7%)	3	(4%)
Duodenum dehiscence	–	–	5	(7%)
Ileus	–	–	1	(1%)
Peritonitis	1	(4%)	1	(1%)
Wound infection	5	(19%)	10	(14%)
Wound dehiscence	3	(11%)	1	(1%)

In the DI series the heavy anticoagulant protocol during the earlier experience led to haemoperitoneum in two of eight patients. One of them required relaparotomy. No advantage has been reported in thrombosis prevention with the randomised trial antithrombin III + heparin (one venous thrombosis) versus Dextran (one arterial and one venous thrombosis and two chronic rejection).

Two patients in the DI series developed a septic haemorrhagic complication. In one with a thrombosed pancreas, vasculitis of the anastomosis secondary to peripancreatic abscess led to septic bleeding: the pancreas graft was removed and the patient died on the sixth day after the relaparotomy. In the second patient, localised stump pancreatitis, complicated by infection, led to septic bleeding. In the BD series one case of septic bleeding also occurred and required pancreas retrieval. Overall pancreas-related surgical complications were 11 (24%) in DI versus 12 (17%) in BD.

Conclusion

Pancreas transplantation using the whole organ with bladder drainage continues to give good results, especially when combined with kidney transplantation. Newer approaches to insulin substitution, such as islet cell transplantation, must be judged against this standard.

References

1. Libman I, Songer T, Laporte R (1993) How many people in the U.S. have IDDM? Diabetes Care 16:841–842.
2. Strowig SM, Raskan P (1995) Glycemic control and the complications of diabetes. Diabetes Rev 3:23–357.
3. Sutherland DER, Gruessner A, Gruessner RWG (1995) International Pancreas Transplant Registry: pancreas transplant results in the USA comparison to non-USA data in the International Registry. IPTR Annual Report.
4. Pirsh JD, Andrews C, Hricik DE (1996) Pancreas transplantation for diabetes mellitus. Am J Kidney Dis 27:444–450.
5. Stratta RJ, Taylor RJ, Wahl T (1993) Recipient selection and evaluation for vascularized pancreas transplantation. Transplantation 55:1090–1096.
6. Brennan DC, Stratta RJ, Lowell JA (1994) Cyclosporine challenge in the decision of combined kidney-pancreas versus solitary pancreas transplantation. Transplantation 57:1606–1011.
7. Gruessner RWG, Nakhleh R, Tzardis P (1994) Differences in rejection grading after simultaneous pancreas and kidney transplantation in pigs. Transplantation 57:1021–1028.
8. Sutherland DER, Gruessner R, Dunn D (1994) Pancreas transplants from living-related donors. Transplant Proc 26:443–445.
9. Gaber AO, Shokouh-Amiri MH, Hathaway DK (1995) Results of pancreas transplantation with portal venous and enteric drainage. Ann Surg 221:613–624.
10. Sollinger HW, Messing EM, Eckhoff DE (1993) Urological complications in 210 consecutive simultaneous pancreas-kidney transplants with bladder drainage. Ann Surg 218:561–570.
11. Taylor RJ, Bynon JS, Stratta RJ (1994) Kidney-pancreas transplantation: a review of the current status. Urol Clin North Am 21:343–354.
12. Sollinger HW, Sasaki TM, D'Alessandro AM (1992) Indications for enteric conversion after pancreas transplantation with bladder drainage. Surgery 112:842–846.
13. Tibell A, Brattstroem C, Wadstroem J, Tyden G, Groth CG (1994) Improved results using whole organ pancreatico-duodenal transplants with enteric exocrine drainage. Transplant Proc 26:412–413.
14. Stephanina E, Gruessner RWG, Brayman K (1992) Conversion of exocrine secretions from bladder to enteric drainage in recipients of whole pancreaticoduodenal transplants. Ann Surg 216:663–672.
15. Ploeg RJ, Eckhoff DE, D'Alessandro AM (1994) Urological complications and enteric conversion after pancreas transplantation with bladder drainage. Transplant Proc 26:458–459.
16. Gruessner RWG, Burke GW, Stratta RJ (1996) Multicenter analysis of the first experience with FK506 for induction and rescue therapy after pancreas transplantation. Transplantation 61:261–273.
17. Sollinger HW, for the US Renal Transplant Mycophenolate Mofetil Study Group (1995) Mycophenolate mofetil for the prevention of acute rejection in primary cadaveric renal allograft recipients. Transplantation 60:225–232.
18. Morel P, Goetz FC, Moudry-Munns KC, Freier E, Sutherland DER (1991) Longterm metabolic control in patients with pancreatic transplants. Ann Intern Med 115:694–699.
19. Diem P, Abid M, Redmon JB, Sutherland DER, Robertson RP (1990) Systemic venous drainage of pancreas allograft as independent cause of hyperinsulinemia in Type I diabetic recipients. Diabetes 39:534–540.
20. Luzi L, Groop LC, Perseghin G et al. (1996) Effect of pancreas transplantation on free fatty acid metabolism in uremic IDDM patients. Diabetes 45:354–360.
21. Wilczek HE, Jaremko G, Tyden G, Groth CG (1995) Evolution of diabetic nephropathy in kidney grafts: evidence that a simultaneous transplanted pancreas exerts a protective effect. Transplantation 59:51–57.
22. Secchi A, Martinenghi S, Galardi G (1991) Effects of pancreatic transplantation on peripheral and autonomic neuropathy. Transplant Proc 23:1658–1659.
23. Hathaway DK, Abell T, Cardoso S (1994) Improvement in autonomic and gastric function following pancreas-kidney versus kidney-alone transplantation and the correlation with quality of life. Transplantation 57:816–822.
24. Wang Q, Klein R, Moss SE (1994) The influence of combined kidney-pancreas transplantation on the progression of diabetic retinopathy: a case series. Ophthalmology 101:1071–1076.
25. Hathaway DK, Hartwig MS, Milstead J (1994) A prospective study of changes in quality of life reported by diabetic recipients of kidney-only and pancreas-kidney allografts. J Transplant Coord 4:1217.

26. Goss JA, Flye MW, Lacy PE (1996) Induction of allogenic islet survival by intrahepatic islet preimmunization and transient immunosuppression. Diabetes 45:144–147.

27. DuBernard JM, Traeger J, Neyra P, Touraine JL, Tranchant D, Blanc-Brunat N. (1978) New method of preparation of a segmental pancreatic graft for transplantation: trials in dogs and in man. Surgery 84:634–639.

28. Sollinger HW, Stratta RJ, D'Alessandro AM, Kalayoglu M, Pirsch JD, Belzer FO (1988) Experience with simultaneous pancreas-kidney transplantation. Ann Surg 208:475–482.

15 Islet Transplantation

H.A. Clayton, S.M. Swift and N.J.M. London

The transplantation of insulin-secreting tissue provides a potential treatment for insulin-dependent diabetes mellitus (IDDM), and can be achieved by using either the vascularised pancreas, or isolated islets. Success removes the need for exogenous insulin therapy, providing physiological control of blood glucose and thereby reducing the risk of developing the complications commonly associated with IDDM (retinopathy, neuropathy, nephropathy and microvascular damage). Purified beta cell transplantation has also been used in rodent models, but has never been demonstrated to be successful in larger animals. One of the major problems with this form of therapy is that it is considered to be life enhancing rather than life saving, as for heart and liver transplantation. Therefore, the risks related to the procedure of transplantation and the subsequent immuno-suppressive therapy have to be weighed against those of the complications which may develop with long-term IDDM. In practice, this means that pancreas or islet transplantation into diabetic patients is currently undertaken mainly in individuals who have already received a kidney, receive a simultaneous kidney transplant, or who are on the renal transplant waiting list, and therefore are already taking (or imminently will be prescribed) immunosuppressive drugs to prevent rejection of the kidney.

Vascularised pancreas transplantation was first undertaken in 1966 (19), and the results have continued to improve. Data collated by the International Pancreas Transplant Registry demonstrate 1-year patient and graft survival rates of up to 100% and 88%, respectively (45). However, there are two main problems with vascularised pancreas transplantation: first, it is a major operation with resulting morbidity and mortality rates, second, long-term immunosuppression is required. These factors preclude the application of this treatment to children with recent-onset IDDM, who may never develop complications associated with the disease, as the risks outweigh the potential benefits provided by the transplant.

Isolated islet transplantation offers several advantages over vascularised pancreas transplantation. First, only the tissue required is transplanted, as islet tissue constitutes approximately 2% of the tissue mass of the pancreas (14,41). In vascularised pancreas transplantation, one of the problems is that of drainage of the unwanted exocrine secretions. Second, it is a relatively minor procedure to transplant islet tissue. This can be achieved under local anaesthetic in under an hour, thus removing the risks of a major invasive operation and reducing all the associated health care costs relative to the vascularised transplant. Third, because the islets are a cellular transplant, there is potential for manipulation prior to transplantation, allowing the possibility of immunomodulation of the tissue. The latter point is of major importance, as the ability to transplant tissue without the requirement of immunosuppression, whether by pretreatment of the islets or by induction of tolerance in the recipient, would allow the potential for islet transplantation in young children without the associated risks of the drug therapy.

Islet Isolation

Detailed morphometric studies on a range of pancreata have determined that the islet tissue normally constitutes between 1% and 2% of the total pancreatic volume (14,41). The challenge for islet isolation, therefore, is to release these islets from the surrounding acinar tissue, ensuring maximum yield and purity. The original methodology for islet isolation was developed in animal models (1), and later applied to the human organ (11). However, a variety of factors can affect the success of the process in the human pancreas, problems which would not normally be associated with standardised animal models. For example, donor age and length of cold ischaemia time can play a significant role in islet isolation (25).

Method of Isolation

The methodology for preparing purified islets from the pancreas involves two stages: digestion of the pancreas, followed by purification of the digest to separate the islets from the acinar tissue.

Briefly, the pancreatic duct is cannulated and the organ distended with a solution of collagenase. The pancreas is placed into a digestion chamber (37), which is constantly shaken throughout the digestion procedure, and which forms part of a circuit through which warmed medium circulates. Dithizone, a dye which binds to the zinc present in beta cell granules, staining islets red, allows frequent monitoring of the resulting digest. Once cleaved islets are present, the flow of medium round the system is switched from a "closed" recirculation to an "open" flow from a reservoir to collecting bottles. Collection of the digest into new-born calf serum and storage of the pooled digest in UW (University of Wisconsin cold storage solution) on ice help to inhibit any further enzyme activity. Constant monitoring of the state of the digest and resulting alterations to the temperature and flow rate of the medium allow the conditions to be stabilised such that the enzyme breaks down the pancreatic tissue to liberate the islets, but does not cause fragmentation of the islets into single cells.

Once all the digested tissue has been pooled, density gradient centrifugation is undertaken to purify the islets from the acinar tissue, with Ficoll-based gradient media the most commonly used. Islets are less dense than exocrine tissue, so appear higher in the gradient than the acinar tissue. Adaptation of the COBE cell separator (23) has allowed large scale purification of the pancreatic digest on continuous density gradients (39). In practice, although a variable proportion of the islets will be free of any contamination, there is usually an overlap where islets and acinar tissue are of a similar buoyant density. A decision then has to made between collecting a small number of very pure islets, or accepting a degree of acinar contamination and retrieving a greater number of islets. As stated above, the successful outcome of an islet transplant appears to be partially dependent on the number of islets transplanted. Consequently, as the liver appears to be able to tolerate the presence of some acinar tissue, less pure islets would be retrieved from the gradient for transplantation to increase the numbers. However, the total volume of tissue transplanted into the liver is also a factor to be considered.

Collagenase

Although the methodology for islet isolation has been well documented, there are several factors involved which still remain variable and can have a significant effect on the final yield of islets. One of the most significant of these is collagenase. This enzyme, produced by the bacterium *Clostridium histolyticum*, breaks down collagen which forms part of the extracellular matrix of the pancreas. This product is crude and undefined, leading to variable activity between different batches (Figure 1). For example, some batches may have no effect on the

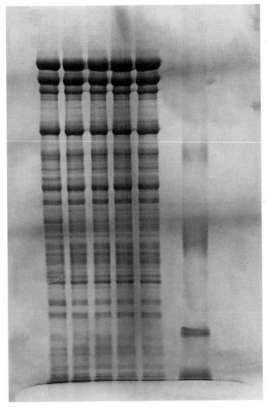

Figure 1. Polyacrylamide gel of a sample of collagenase. The large number of bands demonstrates the complexity of the crude preparations of the enzyme.

organ, leaving it apparently untouched, while others are too active and cause the islets to become fragmented into a single cell suspension. The ideal situation is to have an enzyme which cleaves between the acinar and islet tissue, without causing any fragmentation. In practice, however, most collagenases produce a range of cleaved and uncleaved islets, plus fragments of islet tissue. Much effort has been invested in trying to determine which components of collagenase are essential for successful pancreatic digestion, and some progress has been made with enzyme preparations specifically developed for islet isolation becoming commercially available. However, the production of a reproducible enzyme able to isolate large numbers of high-quality islets remains an elusive goal.

Culture

Once islets have been purified, it is possible to maintain them in a viable state in liquid culture medium, placed in humidified incubators, with 5% CO_2. Some studies have demonstrated that maintaining the islets at 37 °C reduces the amount of tissue more rapidly than if a lower temperature of 22 °C is used (24). Experimentally, islets can be maintained for prolonged periods (32), and this has allowed many studies on various aspects of islet biology to be undertaken. However, the risks of infection while replacing the medium, and significant losses of tissue, even after a brief period of culture, make this inadvisable prior to transplantation. The ability to culture islets, however, allows the purified islets to be maintained while the recipient is prepared, and the necessary clinical arrangements organised.

Cryopreservation

As stated above, considerable loss of tissue during culture makes that system unsuitable for long-term storage. Cryopreservation of islets is a technique which has been developed to allow islets to be stored for prolonged periods of time, and involves the use of dimethylsulphoxide (DMSO) as the cryoprotectant. The islets are slowly equilibrated with the DMSO, are cooled at a rate of 0.25 °C per minute to a temperature of –40 °C, then are plunged into liquid nitrogen in which they can be stored indefinitely. Thawing of islets is achieved at a rate of 200 °C per minute, and the islets can then be placed back into culture medium for a period of recovery prior to transplantation (35). Studies on the recovery and function of islets has demonstrated losses of approximately 40% (36). However, these islets provide a pool of potentially transplantable tissue, and the ability to store islets in this way allows preparations which cannot be used for immediate transplantation to be kept until a suitable recipient is available. In practice, cryopreserved islets are usually used for transplantation in conjunction with freshly prepared islets.

Human Islet Transplantation

The Islet Transplant Registry has recommended that islet transplantation should be performed by embolisation into the liver. The islets lodge in the portal triads and become vascularised by in-growth of capillaries. This may take up to 6 weeks to complete, and reinnervation may take much longer, resulting in a delay of up to 6 months for the islets to attain their full functional potential (48). One of the main advantages conferred by the intrahepatic site is that of portal delivery of the insulin. Successful transplantation has been undertaken in animal models using various other sites including the renal subcapsular space and the spleen; however, these have proved less successful in human transplantation.

If islets are transplanted at the same time as a kidney, the islets are embolised into the liver via a mesenteric vein, leading to infusion of the tissue throughout the whole organ. If the islets are grafted after a kidney transplant, percutaneous transhepatic cannulation allows the procedure to be undertaken under local anaesthesia, with islets being localised into the left lobe of the liver (28). Normal pulsatile insulin release has been demonstrated from islets transplanted into this site in patients undergoing islet autotransplantation following pancreatectomy for chronic pancreatitis (34).

Results of Human Islet Allotransplantation

Data from the International Islet Transplant Registry (16) show that since 1974, a total of 270 adult islet allografts have been undertaken in IDDM patients, 74% of which were single donor transplants. Of these 1:1 transplants, 7% have become insulin independent for more than 7 days, with 43% of these being free of exogenous insulin therapy for at least a year. The longest follow-up of a patient with insulin independence has been 4 years. Overall patient survival 1 year after transplant is 95% with a graft function rate, defined as basal C-peptide of $\geqslant 1$ ng.ml^{-1}, of 27% (normal basal C-peptide is approximately 1.5 ng.ml^{-1}).

Analysis of the data collated by the International Registry has demonstrated four main criteria which contribute to the successful function of islet grafts. First, a cold ischaemia time for the pancreas of under 8 hours before digestion; second, transplantation of at least 6000 IEQ per kg body weight (IEQ, or islet equivalents are a standardised measure of islet volume (38); third, intraportal transplantation into the liver; and last, the use of T cell antibodies for induction of immunosuppression. In patients receiving transplants who met all four criteria, 70% had functioning grafts (C-peptide $\geqslant 1$ ng/ml), 83% had glycosylated haemoglobin levels below 7% (a long-term indication of blood glucose control), and 20% were insulin independent for at least a year.

A recent study of a group of 15 islet transplant recipients has provided a more detailed insight into the metabolic function of the implanted tissue (29). Patients with functioning grafts ($n = 8$) had similar basal hepatic glucose production rates to normal controls, whilst levels were elevated in the group with non-functioning grafts; tissue glucose disposal was lowered in both groups when compared with controls, but was significantly higher in those with a functioning graft compared with non-functioning grafts. Also, the first phase insulin peak was blunted in those with graft function, although the second phase secretion was similar to normal. Therefore, although a functioning islet graft did not completely restore glucose metabolism in this group of patients, it clearly improved the parameters measured in the study when compared with patients without any graft function.

Function of Non-beta Cells Following Islet Transplantation

Inevitably, the success of islet grafts has focused largely on C-peptide secretion as an indicator of insulin release and hence β cell function. However, it is important to remember that islets are mini-organs composed of different cell types involved in the overall regulation of glucose homeostasis. Therefore, the normal function of the α, δ and PP cells is relevant following islet transplantation. Recent studies have indicated abnormalities of glucagon secretion following intraportal islet transplantation in dogs (12,20). Pancreatic polypeptide secretion has also been demonstrated to be either absent or abnormal (3,12).

Rejection and Recurrence of Autoimmune Disease

As with whole organ allotransplantation, islets are prone to rejection, making immunosuppression essential. As already stated above, this precludes the routine transplantation of young diabetic patients, as the risks associated with long-term immunosuppressive therapy are considered too great. In addition, many of the commonly used immunosuppressive drugs have been demonstrated to be diabetogenic. The problem of rejection is further complicated by the potential for the recurrence of the autoimmune disease process which originally causes the onset of IDDM. This problem was identified when a segmental pancreas transplant was undertaken between non-diabetic donor and diabetic recipient monozygotic twins (44). Due to the identical major histocompatibility complex (MHC), no immunosuppression was administered, and diabetes was initially successfully reversed. However, onset of hyperglycaemia within a few weeks was demonstrated to be a result of specific β cell destruction, indicating a return of the autoimmune disease process. This has since been demonstrated to be MHC restricted (31) and as it is only in the case of identical twins that the donor tissue will be of the same MHC type, this is unlikely to be a significant problem in routine transplantation.

Results of Human Islet Autotransplantation

Islet transplantation has also been applied to patients undergoing elective pancreas resection for the treatment of chronic pancreatitis. This procedure has the advantage of not requiring immunosuppression as the patient receives their own tissue, and as more data are collected, these cases should provide a valuable source of information on islet function without the complicating issues of rejection and immunosuppression. Data reported to the International Islet Transplant Registry (16) demonstrated that in well-documented cases, up to 77% of patients achieve insulin independence, with 67% remaining free of insulin therapy for at least a year. The longest follow-up of an autotransplanted patient with insulin independence is 13 years.

The autotransplantation data compare very favourably with the data for patients with pancreatectomy-induced insulin-dependent diabetes who receive allotransplanted islets: of a total of 15 reported to the International Registry, only seven received islets from a single donor. Overall insulin independence was 60%, with independence for at least a year in 40%. For the single donor transplants, these figures were 43% (three of seven) and 14% (one of seven), respectively. (It should be noted that two of the three patients with graft function died within a year of the transplant.) The longest follow-up of insulin independence is 5 years. It has been suggested that the lower success rates of the allotransplants into pancreatectomised patients is in part a reflection of the limited efficacy and the diabetogenic effects of the available immunosuppressive regimes (16).

Future Prospects

Immunomodulation and Tolerance

The small size of islets relative to a whole vascularised organ, and the ability to maintain them in culture have allowed the opportunity to modify the tissue, rendering the islets less susceptible to rejection. This is achieved by depletion of the dendritic or antigen-presenting cells (APCs) which are present within islets and which are involved in initiation of the rejection response (22). In theory, if such treatment were successful, it would allow long-term survival of the islet graft with only a short course of immunosuppression at the time of transplant.

Experimental work undertaken in rodent models of diabetes has demonstrated techniques such as gamma irradiation (17) ultra-violet irradiation (2,18) low temperature culture (21) and culture in 95% oxygen (7) to have some success. Also pretreatment of the islet grafts with monoclonal antibodies directed against specific molecules involved in rejection (e.g. anti-CD4, anti-MHC class II and anti-ICAM-1) have demonstrated prolongation of islet graft survival (30,51,52).

More recent interest in islet immunomodulation has concentrated on genetic manipulation to block the rejection response. For example, co-transplantation of muscle cells transfected with cDNA for CTLA4Ig (a fusion protein that prevents T cell activation by blocking the interaction of CD28 with CTLA4) together with monoclonal antibody treatment to block LFA-1 (a ligand involved in APC–T cell interaction) demonstrated prolonged graft function. In addition, CTLA4Ig was detectable in the recipients for up to 60 days after transplantation, suggesting that this type of genetic engineering has potential for production of the protein to allow islet graft survival (5).

The induction of a state of unresponsiveness or "tolerance" to an islet graft has also been developed in conjunction with islet immunomodulation. In these cases, pretreatment of the graft, usually by a period of culture, together with a short course of immunosuppressive therapy has demonstrated long-term graft function (10,50). The site of islet transplantation has been demonstrated to be important in these cases, with the intrahepatic site being more successful than renal subcapsular transplantation. Other methods demonstrated to achieve tolerance to islet grafts include simultaneous donor bone marrow transplantation (27) and intrathymic islet transplantation (4).

Unfortunately, however, despite the encouraging results of many of these studies, the majority have been undertaken in rodent models of diabetes, and it remains for their success to be transferred to larger animal models, or directly to human islet transplantation.

Xenotransplantation

As with all areas of transplantation, one of the major problems facing islet transplantation is that of the poor supply of islets relative to the numbers of potential recipients. This has led to the possibility of using animal organs for transplantation to meet this demand, with porcine tissue being considered the most suitable source. The major obstacle to be overcome with xenotransplantation is that of hyperacute rejection (HAR) in which naturally occurring antibodies react with the vasculature of the donor organ causing immediate graft failure. As islets are not transplanted as a vascularised graft, it had been thought that HAR may not be a problem. However, in practice xenogeneic islets are rapidly rejected with complement, cytotoxic IgG and IgM antibodies and neutrophils all implicated in the process (13,42,46).

It has been demonstrated that pretreatment of recipients to deplete them of complement and T cells, and culture of islets to deplete the APCs can overcome primary non-function in rats receiving canine islet xenografts. However, prolonged graft survival was not achieved, indicating the difficulties involved, even with graft and recipient modulation (8).

One line of approach to the problem of HAR has been the application of transgenic technology, in which appropriate gene expression is induced in the donor cells to prevent rejection. The majority of the work in this area has been directed at incorporation of human decay accelerating factor (hDAF) into the endothelial and vascular smooth muscle cells of pigs. The action of hDAF is to prevent the assembly of C3 and C5 convertases and to accelerate the decay of C3 convertase, thus blocking the complement cascade and thereby preventing HAR. Expression of the gene has been successfully achieved, although its distribution and intensity within different animals is variable (40). Attempts have also been made to induce the expression in pigs of membrane cofactor protein (49) and CD59 (9), both complement regulatory proteins involved in blocking or down-regulating the complement system. However, it is clear that more developmental work will be required if this approach is to become routinely applicable in humans.

In addition to the problems of HAR, xenotransplantation raises many issues related to the ethics and safety of using animal tissue for transplantation into man. These were addressed by the Nuffield Council on Bioethics (33). The conclusions and recommendations were that xenotransplantation could supplement the supply of human organs, thereby saving and improving quality of life. To this end, breeding pigs specifically for this purpose was considered ethically justified. However, assessment of the potential risks to public health by any infectious organisms, establishment of precautionary measures prior to clinical human trials and protection of the interests of recipients of xenotransplants were recommended to be investigated by the Advisory Committee on Xenotransplantation, and that the resulting safeguards should be in place before xenotransplantation could be offered to suitable recipients.

Encapsulation

Encapsulation is a process in which the islets are encased inside individual capsules (microencapsulation), or in a hollow fibre or diffusion chamber (macroencapsulation), thus physically separating them from the recipient's immune

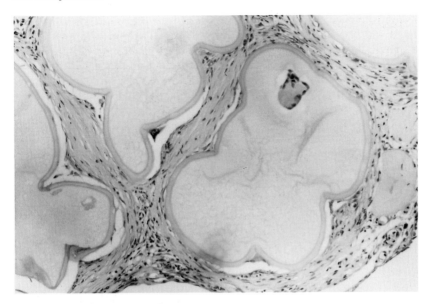

Figure 2. Encapsulated islet graft removed following intraperitoneal transplantation in the rat. The intense fibrotic reaction to the capsule wall, the resulting damage to the shape of the capsules, and remnants of a necrotic islet, can be clearly seen. (Stained with H & E, capsules approximately 500 μm in diameter.)

system and preventing rejection without the need for immunosuppression. A semi-permeable membrane forms an integral part of the device or capsule which has pores small enough to prevent the passage of immunoglobulins and cells of the immune system, but large enough to allow the passage of insulin, glucose and other nutrients. Two of the major attractions of this system are that it would allow the transplantation of xenogeneic tissue, without the associated problems of hyperacute rejection, and that removing the need for immunosuppression would allow the potential for transplanting young patients before any of the complications associated with IDDM had a chance to develop.

Although recent reports have demonstrated some success with this technique (26,43), there are still many problems relating to capsule biocompatibility (Figure 2) and the size of the graft (6), the kinetics of insulin absorption (47) and antigen shedding from the islets which can trigger a response against the tissue following passage of the antigens through the capsules (15). In conclusion, although much work and interest continues in the field of islet encapsulation, it is clear that these issues are currently preventing the successful routine application of the technique to diabetic patients, and much more work will be required before this process can fulfil its considerable potential.

Summary

Islet transplantation provides a potential treatment for diabetic patients, relieving them of the need for exogenous insulin therapy and providing physiological glycaemic control which should prevent the onset of the complications commonly associated with the condition. Recent results from allo- and autotransplanted patients have allowed the criteria for successful graft function to be determined, and have demonstrated that islet transplantation can lead to prolonged normoglycaemia with a near-normal metabolic profile. The potential for circumventing the rejection response, by immunomodulation and tolerance, and the scope for increasing the supply of transplantable tissue from xenogeneic sources, make the goal of transplanting young diabetic patients early in the course of their disease, without the need for long-term immunosuppression, a realistic possibility. However, widespread application of islet transplantation is unlikely until further development of these techniques and improved supply of islet tissue has been successfully achieved.

References

1. Ballinger WF, Lacy PE (1972) Transplantation of intact pancreatic islets in rats. Surgery 72:175–186.
2. Benhamou PY, Kenmochi T, Miyamoto M et al. (1995) Fetal pancreas transplantation in miniature swine. V. The functional and immunomodulatory effects of ultraviolet light on fetal pig islets. Transplantation 59:1660–1665.
3. van der Burg MPM, Guicherit OR, Jansen JBMJ et al. (1996) Function and survival of intrasplenic islet autografts in dogs. Diabetologia 39:37–44.
4. Campos L, Posselt AM, Deli BC et al. (1994) The failure of intrathymic transplantation of non-immunogenic islet allografts to promote induction of donor-specific unresponsiveness. Transplantation 57:950–953.
5. Chahine AA, Yu M, McKernan MM et al. (1995) Immunomodulation of pancreatic islet allografts in mice with CTLA4Ig secreting muscle cells. Transplantation 59:1313–1318.
6. Clayton HA, James RFL, London NJM (1993) Islet microencapsulation: a review. Acta Diabetol 30:181–189.
7. Coulombe M, Gill RG (1994) Tolerance induction to cultured islet allografts. I. Characterisation of the tolerant state. Transplantation 57:1195–1200.
8. Deng S, Ketchum RJ, Levy MM et al. (1996) Long-term culture or complement inhibition improves early islet function in dog to rat islet xenotransplantation. Transplantation Proc 28:805–806.
9. Diamond LE, McCurry KR, Martin MJ et al. (1996) Characterisation of transgenic pigs expressing functionally active human CD59 on cardiac endothelium. Transplantation 61:1241–1249.
10. Goss JA, Nakafusa Y, Finke EH et al. (1994) Induction of tolerance to islet xenografts in a concordant rat-to-mouse model. Diabetes 43:16–23.
11. Gray DWR, McShane P, Grant A, Morris PJ (1984) A method for isolation of islets of Langerhans from the human pancreas. Diabetes 33:1055–1061.
12. Gupta V, Wahoff DC, Rooney DP et al. (1997) The defective glucagon response from transplanted intrahepatic pancreatic islets during hypoglycaemia is transplantation site determined. Diabetes 46:28–33.
13. Hamelmann W, Gray DWR, Cairns TDJ et al. (1994) Immediate destruction of xenogeneic islets in a primate model. Transplantation 58:1109–1114.
14. Hellman, B. (1959) The frequency distribution of the number and volume of the islets of Langerhans in man. Acta Soc Med Upsal 64:432–60.
15. Horcher A, Zekorn T, Siebers U et al. (1994) Transplantation of microencapsulated islets in rats: evidence for induction of fibrotic overgrowth by islet alloantigens released from microcapsules. Transplantation Proc 26:784–786.
16. International Islet Transplant Registry (1996) Newsletter No 7.
17. James RFL, Lake SP, Chamberlain J et al. (1989) Gamma irradiation of isolated rat islets pretransplantation produces indefinite allograft survival in cyclosporine-treated recipients. Transplantation 47:929–933.
18. Kanai T, Porter J, Gotoh, M, Monaco AP, Maki T (1989) Effect of γ-irradiation on mouse pancreatic islet allograft survival. Diabetes 38:154–156.

19. Kelly WD, Lillehei RC, Merkel FK, Idezuki Y, Goetz FC (1967) Allotransplantation of the pancreas and duodenum along with the kidney in diabetic nephropathy. Surgery 61:827–837.
20. Kendall DM, Teuscher AU, Robertson RP (1997) Defective glucagon secretion during sustained hypoglycaemia following successful islet allo- and autotransplatation in humans. Diabetes 46:23–27.
21. Lacy PE, Davie JM, Finke EN (1979) Prolongation of islet allograft survival following *in vitro* culture (24 °C) and a single injection of ALS. Science 204:312–313.
22. Lafferty KJ, Prowse SJ, Simeonovic CJ (1983) Immunobiology of tissue transplantation: A return to the passenger leucocyte concept. Annu Rev Immunol 1:143–173.
23. Lake SP, Bassett PD, Larkins A et al. (1989) Large-scale purification of human islets utilising discontinuous albumin gradient on IBM 2991 cell separator. Diabetes 38 (Suppl 1):143–145.
24. Lakey JRT, Warnock GL, Kneteman NM et al. (1994) Effects of pre-cryopreservation culture on human islet recovery and *in vitro* function. Transplantation Proc 26:820.
25. Lakey JRT, Warnock GL, Rajotte RV et al. (1996) Variables in organ donors that affect the recovery of human islets of Langerhans. Transplantation 61:1047–1053.
26. Lanza RP, Kuhtreiber WM, Ecker D et al. (1995) Xenotransplantation of porcine and bovine islets without immunosuppression using uncoated alginate microspheres. Transplantation 59:1377–1384.
27. Li H, Ricordi C, Demetris AJ et al. (1994) Mixed xenogeneic chimerism (mouse + rat > mouse) to induce donor-specific tolerance to sequential or simultaneous islet xenografts. Transplantation 57:592–598.
28. London NJM, James RFL, Robertson GM et al. (1992) Human islet transplantation: the Leicester experience. In Ricordi C (ed) Pancreatic islet transplantation. RG Landes, Austin, pp. 454–462.
29. Luzi L, Hering BJ, Socci C et al. (1996) Metabolic effects of successful intraportal islet transplantation in insulin-dependent diabetes mellitus. J Clin Invest 97:2611–2618.
30. Marchetti P, Scharp DW, Finke E et al. (1994) Anti-CD4 antibody treatment in xenografts of differently immunomodulated porcine islets. Transplantation Proc 26:1132.
31. Markmann JF, Posselt AM, Bassiri H et al. (1991) Major histocompatibility complex restricted and nonrestricted autoimmune effector mechanisms in BB rats. Transplantation 52:662–667.
32. Nielsen JH (1981) Human pancreatic islets in tissue culture. In Federlin K, Bretzel RG (eds) Islet isolation, culture and cryopreservation: Giessen Workshop 1980. G. Thieme Verlag, Stuttgart, pp. 69–83.
33. Nuffield Council on Bioethics (1996) Animal-to-human transplants. The ethics of xenotransplantation. Nuffield Council, London.
34. Pyzdrowski KL, Kendall DM, Halter JB, Nakhleh RE, Sutherland DER, Robertson RP (1992) Preserved insulin secretion and insulin independence in recipients of islet autografts. N Eng J Med 327:220–226.
35. Rajotte RV, Warnock GL, Coulombe MG (1988) Islet cryopreservation: methods and experimental results in rodents, large mammals and humans. In van Schilfgaarde R, Hardy MA (eds) Transplantation of the endocrine pancreas in diabetes. Elsevier, Amsterdam, pp. 125–135.
36. Rich SJ, Swift S, Thirdborough SM et al. (1994) Islet cryopreservation: a detailed study of total functional losses. Transplantation Proc 26:823–824.
37. Ricordi C, Lacy PE, Finke EH, Olack BJ, Scharp DW (1988) Automated method for isolation of human pancreatic islets. Diabetes 37:413–20.
38. Ricordi C, Gray DWR, Hering BJ et al. (1990) Islet isolation assessment in man and large animals. Acta Diabetol Lat 27:185–195.
39. Robertson GSM, Chadwick DR, Contractor H et al. (1993) The optimisation of large scale density gradient human islet isolation. Acta Diabetol 30:93–98.
40. Rosengard AM, Cary NRB, Langford GA et al. (1995) Tissue expression of human complement inhibitor, decay accelerating factor, in transgenic pigs: a potential approach for preventing xenograft rejection. Transplantation 59:1325–1333.
41. Saito K. Iwama N, Takahashi T (1978) Morphometric analysis on topographical difference in size distribution, number and volume of islets in the human pancreas. Tohoku J Exp Med 124:177–186.
42. Schaapherder AFM, Wolvekamp MCJ, Te Bulte MTJW et al. (1996) Porcine islet cells of Langerhans are destroyed by human complement and not by antibody-dependent cell-mediated mechanisms. Transplantation 62:29–33.
43. Sun Y, Ma X, Zhou D et al. (1996) Normalization of diabetes in spontaneously diabetic cynomologus monkeys by xenografts of microencapsulated porcine islets without immunosuppression. J Clin Invest 98:1417–1422.

44. Sutherland DER, Goetz FG, Sibley RK (1989) Recurrence of disease in pancreas transplants. Diabetes 38 (Suppl 1):85–87.

45. Sutherland D, Gruessner A, Moudry-Munns K (1994) International Pancreas Transplant Registry Report. Transplantation Proc 26:407–411.

46. Tze WJ, Tai J, Cheung SSC et al. (1993) A diabetic rabbit model for pig islet xenotransplantation. Transplantation 56:1348–1352.

47. de Vos P, Vegter D, De Haan BJ et al. (1996) Kinetics of intraperitoneally infused insulin in rats. Functional implications for the bioartificial pancreas. Diabetes 45:1102–1107.

48. Warnock GL, Kneteman NM, Ryan EA, Rabinovitch A, Rajotte RV (1992) Long-term follow-up after transplantation of insulin-producing pancreatic islets into patients with Type 1 (insulin-dependent) diabetes mellitus. Diabetologica 35:89–95.

49. Yannoutsos N, Langford GA, Cozzi E et al. (1995) Production of pigs transgenic for human regulators of complement activation. Transplantation Proc 27:324–325.

50. Yasunami Y, Ryu S, Ueki M et al. (1994) Donor-specific unresponsiveness induced by intraportal grafting and FK506 in rat islet allografts: importance of low temperature culture and transplant site on induction and maintenence. Cell Transplantation 3:75–82.

51. Zeng Y, Gage A, Montag A et al. (1994) Inhibition of transplant rejection by pretreatment of xenogeneic pancreatic islet cells with anti-ICAM-1 antibodies. Transplantation 58:681–689.

52. Zeng Y, Peterson L, Levisetti M et al. (1995) Immunomodulation of human islets results in prolonged in vivo islet graft survival. Transplantation Proc 27:611–612.

Section 3

Chronic Pancreatitis

16 Growth Factors and Cytokines in Chronic Pancreatitis

S.K. Vyas

Introduction

The pathological appearances of chronic pancreatitis are characterised by parenchymal fibrosis, ductal stones and strictures, acinar cell atrophy and inflammatory infiltration by macrophages, neutrophils and lymphocytes. One of the key features of pancreatic fibrosis is an abundant presence of fibroblasts and an accumulation of a dense extracellular matrix which is rich in fibril-forming collagens type I and III. Deposition of extracellular matrix in a diseased pancreas must therefore be regarded as a wound-healing response, much as in fibrosis due to chronic injury in the lung, liver, kidney or joints.

In response to chronic injury, cytokines, growth factors and metabolites produced by resident and recruited cells in the pancreas may contribute to the disturbance of the physiological state. Such injury may produce changes in the amount and type of cells and in the qualitative and quantitative nature of the matrix components produced by these cells. Additionally, in response to chronic pancreatic injury, an increased number of endogenous non-parenchymal cells is seen histologically. This is in part due to the local proliferation of stromal fibroblasts but also due to the recruitment of new cells – leucocytes, macrophages/monocytes and lymphocytes – from the circulation, in response to chemotactic substances, growth factors and cytokines, with diverse effects on cell growth, differentiation, matrix synthesis and degradation. The relative importance of these inflammatory cells may vary between histological types of chronic pancreatitis. For example, increased abundance of lymphocytes is seen with immunohistochemical evidence for the class II major histocompatibility antigen HLA-DR, expressed in chronic obstructive and chronic calcifying but not in the diffuse fibrosing form of chronic pancreatitis (1).

This chapter will review the current literature on growth factors and cytokines which may be important in the pathogenesis of chronic pancreatitis. The bulk of our knowledge of the various important mediators of the wound-healing response is derived from studies of non-pancreatic tissues and inferences drawn from such studies need to be tested in pancreas-specific models; recent advances in maintaining different pancreatic cell types in primary culture and increasing evidence from transgenic studies have begun to facilitate this.

Mechanism of Action of Growth Factors

Growth factors and cytokines are small extracellular polypeptide molecules that bind to a target cell-surface receptor and trigger a response usually mediated via a signal transduction pathway. The cellular response may be altered differentiation or cell proliferation effected through the activation of specific gene expression. For a soluble protein to mediate an effect on a cell, it must first be in close proximity to that cell in a biologically active state while the target cell must be capable of responding to it (i.e. expressing specific receptors). A considerable complexity of cooperation between different mediators exists with discoordinate effects of individual cytokines on different tissues (see below).

A major emerging concept in pancreatic fibrogenesis is the modulation of cellular matrix synthesis and fibroblast proliferation. Some key growth factors have already been identified in pancreatic fibrosis and the evidence for their relevance in pancreatic fibrosis will be discussed. However, further studies of the cellular origin, effects on matrix turnover and regulation are required to understand their role in the pathogenesis of chronic pancreatitis.

Growth Factors in Chronic Pancreatitis

Transforming Growth Factor-beta

Transforming growth factor-beta (TGFβ) is a multifunctional protein capable of influencing cell proliferation, differentiation and a variety of cellular functions. This family of ubiquitous homodimeric 25-kDa cytokines (TGFβ 1–3) is secreted in latent, inactive forms that are not recognised by cellular receptors (2). When the molecule is latent, the precursor region remains dimerised; loss of this dimerisation leads to generation of the active species (3). Activity may be regulated by the isoform expressed, its rate of secretion and activation, its rate of release from the extracellular matrix or by the extent of receptor binding of active TGFβ.

In general, TGFβ stimulates growth of cells of mesenchymal origin, but inhibits growth of hepatocytes, epithelial cells, T and B lymphocytes. TGFβ has been shown to enhance the synthesis of extracellular matrix proteins including collagens, fibronectin and proteoglycans in many systems including the pancreas. In addition to stimulation of matrix synthesis, it also enhances fibrogenesis by inhibiting matrix degradation. TGFβ has been shown to decrease the synthesis of proteases (2,4) but the synthesis of protease inhibitors such as plasminogen activator inhibitor (5) and tissue inhibitors of metalloproteinases (TIMPs; see below) is down-regulated by TGFβ. TGFβ is expressed primarily in acinar and stromal cells of the intact pancreas (6). However, in pancreatic injury local expression and release of TGFβ is increased, predominantly in pancreatic ductal cells, islet cells and in vascular smooth muscle and endothelium (7). Overexpression of TGFβ-1 in murine pancreas induces massive fibrosis and diabetes (8) while repeated administration of recombinant TGFβ induces pancreatic fibrosis after repeated courses of acute pancreatitis (9). Transgenic TGFβ overexpression in the pancreas also leads to fibroblast proliferation, enhanced matrix deposition including fibronectin and laminin and induction of plasminogen activator inhibitor (10). In contrast to stimulating fibroblast growth, TGFβ inhibits pro-liferation of murine acinar cells *in vivo* (10) and rat ductal cells *in vitro* (11,12).

In human tissue, TGFβ-1 mRNA detected by reverse transciptase polymerase chain reaction, was not expressed or only faintly present in normal pancreatic tissue, whereas intense signals were found in chronic pancreatitis (13). Latent TGFβ-1 binding protein was present predominantly in mononuclear cells and in the extracellular matrix around them, suggesting an important role of inflammatory cells in chronic pancreatitis although transgenic TGFα overexpression may lead to pancreatic fibrosis in the absence of chronic inflammation (14).

TGFβ may induce indirect effects on mesenchymal cell fibrogenesis by stimulating chemotaxis (15) or modulating the proliferative activity of other cytokines. At low concentrations, TGFβ stimulates smooth muscle cell proliferation by inducing expression of platelet-derived growth factor (PDGF) A chain (16), whereas at high concentrations it inhibits proliferation by down-regulating expression of PDGF receptors (17). Transmodulation of one cytokine by another is increasingly being recognised as an important mode of cell growth regulation. Such findings are consistent with the evidence for the importance of TGFβ in non-pancreatic fibrosis. It is highly likely that similar mechanisms of TGF-induced fibrogenesis will be in operation since generation of transgenic mice overexpressing TGFβ_1 in murine pancreas resulted in massive fibrosis of the pancreas, with most of the acini in adult mice replaced by fibrotic and adipose tissues (8).

Epidermal Growth Factor and Related Proteins

Epidermal growth factor (EGF) is a 6-kDa polypeptide which is structurally similar to TGFα and is mitogenic for a wide variety of epidermal and epithelial cells including fibroblasts, glial cells, mammary epithelial cells, vascular and corneal endothelial cells (18). Both TGFα and EGF bind the EGF receptor which is a single pass transmembrane protein that stimulates intracellular secondary messages via phospholipase (PLC) C gamma 1 activation (19). Cripto, a further member of the EGF family, is a 188 amino acid protein containing a central domain that shares amino acid sequence homology with EGF and TGFα. Normal pancreas contains moderate levels of immunoreactive cripto in ductal cells and is rarely seen in acinar cells; however, a fourfold increase in cripto mRNA, and much higher levels of immunoreactive protein have been detected in ductal and acinar cells of pancreatic tissues from patients with chronic pancreatitis by Northern blot analysis and immunohistochemistry respectively (20).

A series of interesting transgenic studies has recently highlighted the important role of TGFα and EGF receptor in the pathogenesis of experimental lesions in mice which resemble the pathology of human chronic pancreatitis. Transgenic mice overexpressing TGFα have been proposed as a model for studying the initiation of fibrosis and redifferentiation in human pancreas since these mice develop an enlarged firm pancreas, with increased connective tissue (mainly collagen type I), fibroblast proliferation and redifferentiation of acinar cells, which develop into tubular complexes and demonstrate metaplasia into a duct cell-like appearance (14). Further studies have demonstrated high levels of TGFα, EGF receptor and PLC gamma 1 proteins in pancreatic ductal and acinar cells from patients with chronic pancreatitis by immunohistochemistry as well as increased

TGFα and EGF receptor mRNA by Northern blot analysis of chronic pancreatitis tissues compared with normal controls (21). TGFα has been shown to be expressed in normal pancreatic duct epithelial cells (22) and its expression is increased in ductal adenocarcinomas and chronic pancreatitis compared with normal pancreas (20,21,23). This suggests that TGFα may act via autocrine and paracrine mechanisms to activate EGF receptors overexpressed in acinar and ductal cells in chronic pancreatitis via a PLC gamma 1-dependent secondary messenger pathway. Stimulation of EGF receptors mediated through EGF and TGFα up-regulation has been shown to be associated with acinar redifferentiation into proliferating duct-like structures in γ-interferon transgenic mice (24).

Interleukins

The interleukins are a family of at least 15 related but distinct gene products which were originally described in lymphocytes, monocytes, leukaemic cells and epithelial cells. They are one of the body's key effector molecules in infection, tissue injury and inflammation (25). Only those interleukins which have been studied in the pancreas will be discussed (IL-1, IL-2 and IL-6) as a full review of this family of growth factors is beyond the scope of this chapter.

Interleukin-1 (IL-1), known previously as lymphocyte activating factor (LAF) and expressed primarily by monocytes/macrophages but also by other cells (26), activates T cell lymphocytes which then proliferate and secrete IL-2 (27). IL-1 is thought to play a key role in inflammatory and immune reponses (28) and has two closely related forms, IL-1α and IL-1β of M_r 17 kDa. They share 62% amino acid homology and elicit nearly identical biological responses. IL-1α and IL-1β have been studied with respect to pancreatic cancer tumour invasiveness and associated diabetes, with high levels of IL-1α associated with pancreatic cancer spread (29). Serum IL-1β detected by radioimmunoassay and ELISA has been implicated as a marker for chronic pancreatitis (30). The biological effects of IL-1 and TNFα are synergistic (25) leading to chemotaxic recruitment of neutrophils, monocytes, lymphocytes and enhanced collagen production (31) although the effects of IL-1 in the pancreas are uncertain.

Interleukin-2 (IL-2), also known as T cell growth factor, is an immunomodulatory factor produced by certain subsets of T lymphocytes (32) which promotes long-term growth of activated T cells, activation and proliferation of natural killer (NK) cells, and induction of secretion of γ-interferon and B cell growth factor (33–36). IL-2 has been little studied in chronic pancreatitis but an increase in serum levels of soluble IL-2 receptor has been observed in patients with either chronic pancreatitis or pancreatic cancer (37,38).

Interleukin 6 (IL-6) is a multifunctional protein originally discovered in the media of cells stimulated with double-stranded RNA (39) which may be involved in cooperation with IL-1 and tumour necrosis factor α (TNFα) in the acute phase response to infection and injury (40,41). It acts upon a variety of cells including fibroblasts, myeloid progenitor cells, T cells, B cells and hepatocytes, inducing multiple effects as indicated by its numerous synonyms, including plasmacytoma growth factor (PCT-GF), interferon-β_2, monocyte derived human B cell growth factor. Its principal effect is to stimulate growth of responsive target cells which are primarily of immunological origin. It is not surprising, therefore, that IL-6 has been associated with islet inflammation and hyperplasia in IL-6-overexpressing transgenic mice, but an interesting histological observation of this study was the finding of pancreatic fibrosis and a scant mononuclear cell infiltration with recruitment of B lymphocytes, macrophages and CD4- and CD8-positive T lymphocytes, suggesting a role for this cytokine in pancreatic inflammatory processes (42).

Fibroblast Growth Factors

Fibroblast growth factors (FGF) are a growing family of at least nine related molecules involved in a diverse array of physiological, developmental and pathological processes which share a high degree of cross-reactivity to the four known FGF tyrosine kinase receptors (43). The best characterised are two closely related polypeptides, acidic and basic fibroblast growth factors (aFGF and bFGF respectively) which exert similar mitogenic actions on a variety of mesoderm-derived cells, including BALB/3T3 fibroblasts, capillary endothelial cells, myoblasts, vascular smooth muscle cells, mesothelial cells, glial and astroglial cells and adrenal cortex cells (44). Both aFGF and bFGF share common cellular receptors but differ in their specific activities depending on the particular cell type studied (45).

Basic FGF may be sequestered in the extracellular matrix in an inactive state through binding to heparan sulphate proteoglycans (46). It may become available in the microenvironment of target cells after liberation from its protein binding in a biologically active state by the action of proteases released during tissue injury. These two mitogenic polypeptides have been identified in pancreatic acinar and ductal cells at the mRNA and protein levels by *in situ* hybridisation and immunohistochemistry (47). Increased mRNA and protein levels for both aFGF and bFGF were demonstrated by Northern and Western blotting respectively, in whole pancreas homogenates from patients with chronic pancreatitis compared with normal controls (47). These results demonstrate that aFGF and bFGF may either be involved in the pathogenesis of chronic pancreatitis or that their up-regulation is a consequence of other perturbations that occur in this disorder.

Platelet Activating Factor

Platelet activating factor (PAF) is a potent phosphoacylglycerol which acts through specific target cell receptors to mediate a wide variety of physiological and pathophysiological effects in various tissues (48). Evidence of its importance as a mediator in pancreatic inflammation has been demonstrated in the rat pancreatic duct ligation model of obstructive pancreatitis (49). In this model, a substantial (12-fold) increase in PAF bioactivity was shown in association with the chronic phase of obstructive pancreatitis after ligation when parenchymal atrophy, fibrosis and pancreatic insufficiency evolve. In another study, inhibition of PAF through specific receptor antagonism attenuated pancreatic damage and inflammation. Chronic PAF antagonism resulted in a decreased level of pancreatic acinar cell regeneration *in vitro* (50).

Growth Factors and the Extracellular Matrix

The extracellular matrix (ECM) is a complex network of secreted proteins and carbohydrates that occupies the spaces between cells. Current evidence suggests that such a network of proteins serves many purposes including binding cells together and providing tensile strength as well as signalling cellular differentiation and growth. The composition of the ECM varies between tissues, each specialised for a particular function such as strength (in a tendon), filtration (in the renal glomerulus), cell differentiation (in the liver) or adhesion. The ECM may act as a reservoir of various growth factors or cytokines and thus may affect their biological activity. In contrast, different growth factors have diverse effects on the nature of the ECM secreted during organ development, inflammation and repair.

Immunolocalisation studies have confirmed the presence of collagen types I, III and V (51), laminin and fibronectin (52) in normal human pancreas whereas the ECM in chronic pancreatitis is abundant in fibrillar type I collagen (53). The predominant cellular source of the increased deposition of ECM in pancreatic fibrosis is undetermined.

Modulation of the biological activity of cytokines by different components of the ECM may vary according to the particular mediator. For example, laminin contains a series of 25 EGF-like repeats which, when cleaved, may explain the mitogenic effect that this matrix protein has on cells expressing EGF receptors (54). Similar properties have been described for two other matrix proteins, tenascin and thrombospondin (55). Yet more growth factors may bind to matrix proteins rather than form integral domains, and, in so doing may either be activated or made biologically inert. These include basic fibroblast growth factor (bFGF) which is inactive whilst bound to the highly negatively charged side chains of heparan sulphate proteoglycans (56), which acquires biological activity when released from this binding by proteolysis of its matrix carrier. In contrast, $TGF\beta_1$ binds to type IV collagen, thus enhancing its biological activity either through protection or presentation of this molecule (56). Interestingly decorin, another matrix proteoglycan, is a natural inhibitor of $TGF\beta_1$ when it is bound to this growth factor (57). The array of cytokines bound by the extracellular matrix is wide and includes interferon-γ (IFNγ), platelet derived growth factor (PDGF), acidic fibroblast growth factor (aFGF) and granulocyte-macrophage colony stimulating factor (GM-CSF) (56). Furthermore, soluble proteins such as insulin-like growth factor (IGF) binding protein may bind certain cytokines (IGF) and maintain their inactivity until cleaved to release the active cytokine (58).

Regulation of Matrix Turnover

It has been postulated that fibrosis may result not only from alterations in matrix synthesis, but also through inhibition of matrix degradation (59). This underlines the potential importance of a family of zinc-dependent proteases known as the matrix metalloproteinases and their specific inhibitors known as tissue inhibitors of metalloproteinases (TIMPs) (60).

The matrix metalloproteinases comprise a family of related enzymes with common biochemical properties which are capable of degrading a variety of extracellular matrix proteins. They may loosely be classified according to their substrate profile: collagenases with degradative activity against fibrillar (interstitial) collagens; type IV (61,62) collagenases/gelatinases which degrade basement-membrane type IV collagen and gelatin; and stromelysins which have the broadest substrate profile including proteoglycans, laminin, fibronectin, type IV collagen and gelatin. Recently a fourth, and so far unique, membrane type metalloproteinase (MT-MMP) has been discovered on the surface of invasive tumour cells (63) with a potential integral transmembranous domain at the C-terminus heralding a new class of metalloproteinases. Although the complete substrate specificity of this new metalloproteinase is unknown, an important feature of its biological activity is that it is able to activate progelatinase A (64).

The regulation of metalloproteinase activity is tightly controlled and operates on at least three levels: gene transcription, activation of the proenzyme and specific inhibition of either the active enzyme or prevention of proenzyme activation by TIMPs. Many of these regulatory mechanisms are common to all the metalloproteinases, but some are disparate and more specific to individual members of this family. Matrix metalloproteinase gene expression is largely controlled through the action of growth factors, hormones and cytokines. Most of our current understanding of these regulatory mechanisms is based on studies of interstitial collagenase and stromelysin in cultured skin or synovial fibroblasts, with some data from other cell types in relation to other metalloproteinases (61,62,65–67).

Expression of most metalloproteinases is generally upregulated by inflammatory cytokines such as TNFα, PDGF, bFGF, EGF, IFNα and IL-1α (62). The effects some of these cytokines may be mediated through expression of the proto-oncogenes c-*jun* and c-*fos* (61).

The effects of TGFβ_1 on metalloproteinase gene expression are particularly interesting as this growth factor has discoordinate effects on different metalloproteinase genes; interstitial collagenase and stromelysin are inhibited (68,69) whereas gelatinase A (72 kDa type IV collagenase/gelatinase) expression is stimulated (68). Current evidence indicates that its effect on stromelysin expression is probably mediated through a TGFβ inhibitory element (TIE) in the promoter region of this gene and may also involve c-*fos* (70). Regulation of metalloproteinase synthesis in macrophages is mediated through different mechanisms. Endotoxin (71,72) and a mixture of lymphokines (73) are potent stimulators whilst interferon-γ inhibits macrophage metalloproteinase synthesis (74). Stimulation of macrophage metalloproteinase synthesis is mediated through synthesis of prostaglandin E2 and increase in intracellular cyclic AMP (75–77), and can be inhibited by corticosteroids (78,79) or prostaglandin synthetase inhibitors (75,77).

Metalloproteinase activation from the proenzyme is dependent on the plasminogen activating cascade reviewed by Murphy et al. (80,81). Plasmin is formed by the activation of circulating plasminogen and this process is inhibited by plasminogen activator inhibitors (PAI). Therefore cells expressing plasminogen activators (PA) and PAI have the potential to regulate metalloproteinase activation. Common transcription factors are present upstream of the genes encoding interstitial collagenase, stromelysin, PAI and urokinase-type plasminogen activator (uPA), providing a framework for coordinating expression of the activation cascade. Prostromelysin is at the top of this activation cascade which, when activated by plasmin to stromelysin can complete the partial activation of procollagenase by plasmin. A further degree of control is added by the effects of TGFβ which up-regulates PAI and down-regulates tissue plasminogen activator (tPA), thereby reducing matrix degradation by decreasing metalloproteinase activation. Moreover, TGFβ is activated by plasmin from pro-TGFβ thus providing a negative feedback loop on plasmin activation.

Matrix degradation in the extracellular space is further regulated by metallo-proteinase inhibitors. There are at least four members of this group of specific TIMPs of which two are well characterised, TIMP-1 and TIMP-2. In addition, other more general protease scavengers may inhibit metalloproteinases (e.g. α-2 macroglobulin). TIMP-1 gene expression may be co-regulated with metallo-proteinases (e.g. by EGF and bFGF) (82) or inversely co-regulated, e.g. by TGFβ which down-regulates expression of interstitial collagenase and stromelysin but up-regulates expression of TIMP-1 (82). TIMP-2 expression is regulated independently of TIMP-1; TIMP-2 expression is down-regulated by TGFβ (83).

In summary the regulation of matrix turnover is complex; mediating factors include cytokines, growth factors, matrix degradation products, retinoids, endo-toxin and autocrine signals. The intracellular messenger pathways and our understanding of the promoter regions and transactivating factors for the metalloproteinase genes and TIMPs are being elucidated. These data indicate that metalloproteinase gene expression is involved in a variety of important biological processes, including regenerative and neoplastic cell proliferation, tissue injury and inflammation.

Conclusions

During the past two decades it has become increasingly apparent that pancreatic fibrosis results from a complex interaction of multiple factors. While this chapter has dwelt on those growth factors which may be instrumental in pancreatic fibrosis, other factors will also be shown to be important in this process. A large body of information exists on the cellular origins, regulation, physiological and pathological importance of these factors in various tissues. Future studies using primary cultures of pancreatic fibroblasts, ductal and acinar cells, as well as transgenic and gene knockout biological models promise to improve our under-standing of the principal cellular and molecular mechanisms of pancreatic fibrosis.

References

1. Bedossa P, Bacci J, Lemaigre G, Martin E (1990) Lymphocyte subsets and HLA-DR expression in normal and chronic pancreatitis. Pancreas 5:415–420.
2. Sporn MB, Roberts AB, Wakefield LM, de Crombrugghe B (1987) Some recent advances in the chemistry and biology of transforming growth factor-beta. J Cell Biol 105:1039–1045.
3. Brunner AM et al. (1989) Site-directed mutagenesis of cysteine residues in the pro-region of the transforming growth factor beta-1 precursor. J Biol Chem 264:13660–13664.
4. Matrisian LM, Leroy P, Ruhlman C, Gesnel M-C, Breathnach R (1986) Isolation of the oncogene and epidermal growth factor-induced transin gene: complex control in rat fibroblasts. Mol Cell Biol 6:1679–1686.
5. Keski-Oja J, Raghow R, Sandey M (1988) Regulation of mRNAs for type I plasminogen activator inhibitor, fibronectin and type I procollagen by transforming growth factor-β. J Biol Chem 263:3111–3115.
6. Gress T, Müller-Pillasch F, Elsässer HP et al. (1994) Enhancement of transforming growth factor-β1 expression in the rat pancreas during regeneration from caerulin-induced pancreatitis. Eur J Clin Invest 24:679–685.
7. Slater SD, Williamson RC, Foster CS (1995) Expression of transforming growth factor-beta 1 in chronic pancreatitis. Digestion 56:237–241.

8. Sanvito F, Nichols A, Herrera PL et al. (1995) TGF-β1 overexpression in murine pancreas induces chronic pancreatitis and, together with TNF-alpha, triggers insulin-dependent diabetes. Biochem Biophys Res Comm 217:1279–1286.

9. Van Laethaem JL, Robberecht P, Resibois A, Deviere J (1996) Transforming growth factor-beta promotes development of fibrosis after repeated courses of acute pancreatitis in mice. Gastroenterology 110:576–582.

10. Lee MS, Gu D, Feng L et al. (1995) Accumulation of extracellular matrix and developmental dysregulation in the pancreas by transgenic production of transforming growth factor-beta 1. Am J Pathol 147:42–52.

11. Smith FE, Reitz P, Schuppin GT, Bonner-Weir S (1993) Transforming growth factor-β is involved in regulation of rat pancreatic regeneration following 90% pancreatectomy. Pancreas 8:773 (abstract).

12. Bisgaard HC, Thorgeirsson SS (1991) Evidence for a common cell of origin for primitive epithelial cells isolated from rat liver and pancreas. J Cell Physiol 147:333–343.

13. Van Laethem JL, Deviere J, Resibois A et al. (1995) Localization of transforming growth factor-beta 1 and its latent binding protein in human chronic pancreatitis. Gastroenterology 108:1873–1881.

14. Bockman DE, Merlino G (1992) Cytological changes in the pancreas of transgenic mice overexpressing transforming growth factor-α. Gastroenterology 103:1883–1892.

15. Lucas PA, Caplan AI (1988) Chemotactic response of embryonic limb bud mesenchymal cells and muscle derived fibroblasts to transforming growth factor-beta. Connect Tissue Res 18:1–7.

16. Makela TP et al. (1987) Regulation of platelet-derived growth factor gene expression by transforming growth factor-beta and phorbol ester in human leukaemia cell lines. Mol Cell Biol 7:3656–3662.

17. Battegay EJ et al. (1990) TGF-beta induces bimodal proliferation of connective tissue cells via complex control of an autocrine PDGF loop. Cell 63:515–524.

18. Carpenter G, Cohen S (1979) Epidermal growth factor. Annu Rev Biochem 48:193.

19. Todaro G, Fryling C, De Larco JE (1980) Transforming growth factors produced by certain human tumour cells: polypeptides that interact with epidermal growth factor receptors. Proc Natl Acad Sci USA 77:5258–5262.

20. Friess H, Yamanaka Y, Buchler M, Kobrin MS, Tahara E, Korc M (1994) Cripto, a member of the epidermal growth factor family is over-expressed in human pancreatic cancer and chronic pancreatitis. Int J Cancer 56:668–674.

21. Korc M, Friess H, Yamanaka Y, Kobrin MS, Buchler M, Beger HG (1994) Chronic pancreatitis is associated with increased concentrations of epidermal growth factor receptor, transforming growth factor-alpha and phospholipase C gamma. Gut 35:1468–1473.

22. Barton CM, Hall PA, Hughes CM, Gulli WJ, Lemoine NR (1991) Transforming growth factor-alpha and epidermal growth factor in human pancreatic cancer. J Pathol 163:111–116.

23. Tomioka T, Toshkov I, Kazakoff K et al. (1995) Cellular and subcellular localisation of transforming growth factor alpha and epidermal growth factor-receptor in normal and diseased human and hamster pancreas. Terat Carcinog Mutagen 15:231–250.

24. Arnush M, Gu D, Baugh C et al. (1996) Growth factors in the regenerating pancreas of c-interferon transgenic mice. Lab Invest 74:985–990.

25. Dinarello CA (1988) Interleukin-1. Dig Dis Sci 33:25S–35S.

26. Oppenheim JJ, Kovacs EJ, Matsushima K, Durum SK (1986) There is more than one interleukin-1. Immunol Today 7:45–56.

27. Gery I, Gershon RK, Waksman BH (1972) Potentiation of the T lymphocyte reponse to mitogens I. The responding cell. J Exp Med 136:128–142.

28. Durum SK, Schimdt JA, Oppenheim JJ (1985) Interluekin-1: an immunological perspective. Annu Rev Immunol 3:263–287.

29. Basso D, Plebeni M, Fogar P et al. (1995) Insulin-like growth factor, interleukin-1 alpha and beta in pancreatic cancer: role in tumour invasiveness and associated diabetes. Int J Clin Lab Res 25:40–43.

30. Bamba T, Yoshioka U, Inoue H, Iwasaki Y, Hosoda S (1994) Serum levels of interleukin-1 beta and interleukin-6 in patients with chronic pancreatitis. J Gastroenterol 29:314–319.

31. Cavalis E (1986) Interleukin-1 has independent effects on DNA and collagen synthesis in cultures of rat calvariae. Endocrinology 118:74–81.

32. Smith KA (1988) Interleukin-2: inception, impact and implications. Science 240:1169.

33. Morgan DA, Ruscetti FW, Gallo R (1976) Selective in vitro growth of T lymphocytes from normal human bone marrows. Science 193:1007–1008.

34. Ortaldo JR, Mason A, Gerard JP et al. (1984) Effects of natural and recombinant interleukin-2 on regulation of interferon-c production and natural killer cell activity: lack of involvement of the Tac antigen from these immunoregulatory effects. J Immunol 133:779–783.

35. Farrar JJ, Benjamin WR, Hifiker ML, Howard M, Farrar WL, Fuller-Farrar J (1982) The biochemistry, biology and role of IL-2 in the induction of cytotoxic T cell and antigen-forming B cell responses. Immunol Rev 63:129–166.

36. Inaba Kl, Grannelli-Piperno A, Steinman RM (1983) Dendritic cells induce T lymphocytes to release B cell stimulating factors by an IL-2 dependent mechanism. J Exp Med 158:2040–2057.

37. Pezzilli R, Billi P, Beltrandi E et al. (1994) Serum soluble interleukin-2 receptor in pancreatic cancer and chronic pancreatitis. Ital J Gastroenterol 26:137–140.

38. Rabbitti PG, Pacelli L, Uomo G et al. (1994) Soluble interleukin-2 receptor; a new marker in pancreatic adenocarcinoma? Minerva Gastroenterol Dietol 40:101–103.

39. Billau A (1987) Interferon β_2 as a promoter of growth and differentiation of B cells. Immunol Today 8:84–87.

40. Gauldie J, Richards C, Harnish D, Lansdrop P, Baumann H (1987) Interferon beta-2/B cell stimulating factor type 2 shares identity with monocyte derived hepatocyte-stimulating factor and regulates the major acute phase protein response in liver cells. Proc Natl Acad Sci USA 84:7521–7525.

41. Van Snick J (1990) IL-6: an overview. Annu Rev Immunol 8:253–278.

42. Campbell IL, Hobbs MV, Dockter J, Oldstone MB, Allison J (1994) Islet inflammation and hyperplasia induced by the pancreatic islet-specific overexpression of interleukin-6 in transgenic mice. Am J Pathol 145:157–166.

43. Sandor S, Zsuzsa S (1996) Basic fibroblast growth factor and PDGF in GI diseases. In: Goodland RA, Wright NA (eds) Bailliere's clinical gastroenterology, 10:7. Saunders, London, pp 97–112.

44. Gospodarowicz D, Ferrara N, Schweigerer L, Neufeld G (1987) Structural characterisation and biological functions of fibroblast growth factor. Endocrine Rev 8:95–114.

45. Neufeld G, Gospodarowicz D (1986) Basic and acidic fibroblast growth factors interact with the same cell surface receptors. J Biol Chem 261:5631–5637.

46. Folkmann J, Klagsbrunn M, Sasse J, Wadzinski M, Ingber D, Vlodavsky I (1988) A heparin-binding angiogenic protein – fibroblast growth factor – is stored within basement membrane. Am J Pathol 130:393–400.

47. Friess H, Yamanaka Y, Buchler M, Beger HG, Do DA, Kobrin MS, Korc M (1994) Increased expression of acidic and basic fibroblast growth factors in chronic pancreatitis. Am J Pathol 144:117–128.

48. Izumi T, Shimizu T (1995) Platelet-activating factor receptor: gene expression and signal transduction. Biochim Biophys Acta 1259:317–333.

49. Zhou W, Levine BA, Olson MS (1994) Lipid mediator production in acute and chronic pancreatitis in the rat. J Surg Res 56:37–44.

50. Zhou WG, Chao W, Levine BA, Olson MS (1990) Evidence for platelet activating factor as a late-phase mediator of chronic pancreatitis in the rat. Am J Pathol 137:1501–1508.

51. Van Deijnen JHM, Van Suylichem PTR, Wolters GHJ, Van Schilfgaarde R (1994) Distribution of collagens type I, type II and type V in the pancreas of rat, dog, pig and man. Cell Tissue Res 277:115–121.

52. Uscanga L, Kennedy RH, Choux R, Deuget M, Grimaud J-A, Sarles H (1984) Immunolocalization of collagen types, laminin and fibronectin in normal human pancreas. Digestion 30:158–164.

53. Kennedy RH, Bockman DE, Uscanga L, Grimaud J-A, Sarles H (1987) Pancreatic extracellular matrix alterations in chronic pancreatitis. Pancreas 2:61–17.

54. Panayotou G, End P, Aumailley M et al. (1989) Domains of laminin with growth factor activity. Cell 48:989–996.

55. Schuppan D, Somasundaram R, Just M (1992) The extracellular matrix: a major signal transduction network. In: Clement B Guillouzo A (eds) Cellular and molecular aspects of cirrhosis. Colloque INSERM/John Libbey Eurotext, London, pp 115–134.

56. Bissell DM (1992) Effects of extracellular matrix on hepatocyte behaviour. In: Clement B Guillouzo A (eds) Cellular and molecular aspects of cirrhosis. Colloque INSERM/John Libbey Eurotext, London, pp 187–197.

57. Border WA, Noble NA, Yamamoto T et al. (1992) Natural inhibitor of transforming growth factor-beta protects against scarring in experimental kidney disease. Nature 360:361–364.

58. Fowlkes JL, Suzuki K, Nagase H, Thrailkill KM (1994) Proteolysis of insulin-like growth factor binding protein-3 during rat pregnancy: a role for matrix metalloproteinases. Endocrinology 135:2810–2813.

59. Arthur MJP, Iredale JP (1994) Hepatic lipocytes, TIMP-1 and liver fibrosis. J R Coll Phys Lond 28:200–208.
60. Nagase H, Barrett AJ, Woessner JF Jr (1992) Nomenclature and glossary of the matrix metalloproteinases. Matrix (Suppl 1):421–424.
61. Matrisian LM (1990) Metalloproteinases and their inhibitors in matrix remodelling. Trends Genet 6:121–125.
62. Murphy G, Hembry RM, Hughes CE, Fosang AJ, Hardingham TE (1990) Role and regulation of metalloproteinases in connective tissue turnover. Biochem Soc Trans 18:812–815.
63. Sato H, Takino T, Okada Y et al. (1994) A matrix metalloproteinase expressed on the surface of invasive tumour cells. Nature 370:61–65.
64. Cao J, Sato H, Takino T, Seiki M (1995) The C-terminal region of membrane type matrix metalloproteinase is a functional transmembrane domain required for pro-gelatinase C activation. J Biol Chem 270:801–805.
65. Murphy G, Hembry RM (1992) Proteinases in rheumatoid arthritis. J Rheumatol 19:61–64.
66. Murphy G, Docherty AJP, Hembry RM, Reynolds JJ (1991) Metalloproteinases and tissue damage. Br J Rheumatol 30(Suppl 1):25–31.
67. Marbaix E, Donnez J, Courtoy PJ, Eeckhout Y (1992) Progesterone regulates the activity of collagenase and related gelatinase-A and gelatinase-B in human endometrial explants. Proc Natl Acad Sci USA 89:11789–11793.
68. Overall CM, Wrana JL, Sudek J (1989) Independent regulation of collagenase, 72kDa progelatinase, and metalloendoproteinase inhibitor expression in human fibroblasts by transforming growth factor-beta. J Biol Chem 264:1860–1869.
69. Edwards DR, Murphy G, Reynolds JJ et al. (1987) Transforming growth factor-beta modulates the expression of collagenase and metalloproteinase inhibitor. EMBO J 6:1899–1904.
70. Lafyatis R, Kim S-J, Angel P et al. (1990) Interleukin-1 stimulates and all-trans-retinoic acid inhibits collagenase gene expression through its 5′ activator protein-1-binding site. Mol Endocrinol 4:973–980.
71. Wahl LM, Wahl SM, Mergenhagen SE, Martin GR (1974) Collagenase production by endotoxin-activated macrophages. Proc Natl Acad Sci USA 71:3598–3601.
72. Cury JD, Campbell EJ, Lazarus CJ, Albin RJ, Welgus HG (1988) Selective up-regulation of human alveolar macrophage collagenase production by lipopolysaccharide and comparison to collagenase production by fibroblasts. J Immunol 141:4306–4312.
73. Wahl LM, Wahl SM, Mergenhagen SE, Martin GR (1975) Collagenase production by lymphokine-activated macrophages. Science 187:261–263.
74. Shapiro SD, Campbell EJ, Kobayashi DK (1990) Immune modulation of metalloproteinase production in human macrophages. J Clin Invest 86:1204–1210.
75. Bhatnagar R, Schade U, Rietschel ET, Decker K (1982) Involvement of prostaglandin E and adenosine 3′5′-monophosphate in lipopolysaccharide-stimulated collagenase release by rat Kupffer cells. Eur J Biochem 124:125–130.
76. McCarthy JB, Wahl SM, Rees JC, Olsen CE, Sandberg AL, Wahl LM (1980) Mediation of macrophage collagenase production by 3′-5′ cyclic adenosine monophosphate. J Immunol 124:2405.
77. Wahl LM, Olsen CE, Sandberg AL, Mergenhagen SE (1977) Prostaglandin regulation of macrophage collagenase production. Proc Natl Acad Sci USA 74:4955–4958.
78. Wahl LM, Winter CC (1984) Regulation of guinea pig macrophage collagenase production by dexamethasone and colchicine. Arch Biochem Biophys 230:661–667.
79. Werb Z, Foley R, Munck A (1978) Glucocorticoid receptors and glucocorticoid-sensitive secretion of neutral proteinases in a macrophage line. J Immunol 121:115–121.
80. Murphy G, Docherty AJP (1992) The matrix metalloproteinases and their inhibitors. Am J Respir Cell Mol Biol 7:120–125.
81. Murphy G, Atkinson S, Ward R, Gavrilovic JJ, Reynolds JJ (1992) The role of plasminogen activators in the regulation of connective tissue metalloproteinases. Ann NY Acad Sci 667:1–12.
82. Edwards DR, Murphy G Reynolds JJ et al. (1987) Transforming growth factor-beta modulates the expression of collagenase and metalloproteinase inhibitor. EMBO J 6:1899–1904.
83. Stetler-Stevenson WG, Brown PD, Onisto M et al. (1990) Tissue inhibitor of metalloproteinases-2 (TIMP-2) mRNA expression in tumour cells and human tumour tissues. J Biol Chem 265:13933–13938.

17 Endoscopic Therapy of Chronic Pancreatitis

J. Devière and M. Cremer

Chronic pancreatitis (CP) is a rare disease in Western countries (incidence 2–10/100 000 per year). It ultimately leads to irreversible damage of the pancreas with exocrine and endocrine insufficiency. Pain is the major clinical symptom and is present early in the course of the disease in most cases (1–3).

With the exception of the very rare hereditary CP which is associated with a mutation in the cationic tripsinogen gene on chromosome 7 (4,5), the aetiology of CP has not already been demonstrated. Chronic alcoholism is a precipitating factor and it dramatically increases the probability of development of CP, but the disease can develop in non-alcoholic subjects and is then described as "idiopathic" CP.

The pathophysiology of CP is still controversial. The theories of pathogenesis include the "stone theory" in which the primary abnormality is the formation of protein plugs due to a congenital lack of lithostatine (6), and the "necrosis fibrosis" theory in which fibrosis and ductal stricture are the consequence of focal inflammation and necrosis (7–9). Pain is most often associated with interstitial hypertension and further ischaemia resulting in both ductal hypertension and a lack of compliance of the diseased pancreas (10). It is also probable that, when CP is established, these repeated episodes of ischaemia participate in the irreversible process of fibrosis and further worsening of the disease ultimately leading to destruction of the gland.

Until recently, endoscopic retrograde cholangiopancreatography (ERCP) has been the gold standard for the morphological diagnosis of CP. The main features of ductal abnormalities observed have been described in different classifications using ERCP as a criterion of severity (11–13). These classifications are useful for the differential diagnosis of CP but also as a guide to choose the most appropriate management.

Magnetic resonance cholangiopancreatography (MRCP) is a major advance in depicting ductal anatomy of the pancreas (Figure 1). This technique gives satisfactory pancreatograms in most cases of CP, without the need for any ductal or intravenous contrast medium injection and without irradiation (14). Furthermore, the development of the dynamic secretin MRP (DSMRP) has improved the quality of the morphological information (Figure 2) especially for patients without abnormalities on computed tomography (CT) or ultrasonograph (15). It also detects anatomical variations and the presence of a dominant dorsal duct which indicates the necessary approach to the minor papilla if a stricture is shown and endotherapy is required. DSMRP allows the clinician to decide if

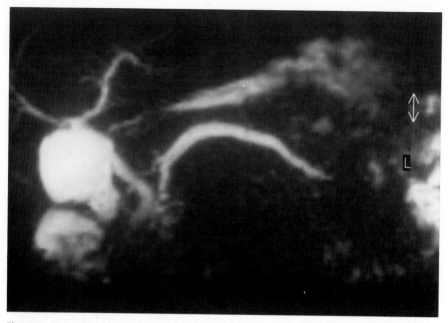

Figure 1. Magnetic resonance cholangiopancreatography (MRCP) in a patient with chronic pancreatitis (CP). (Image courtesy of C. Matos, MD.)

endotherapy is needed and to choose the appropriate treatment without any morbidity related to the diagnostic procedure. This information could become an important tool to detect, before ERCP, those patients with painful pancreatitis who could benefit from drainage procedures. With the development of these techniques, it is highly probable that within the next few years, it will become contraindicated to perform an ERCP just for imaging the pancreas.

Despite these sophisticated improvements in imaging techniques, the plain film of the pancreatic area remains mandatory to detect small or large calcified calculi responsible for obstruction of the main pancreatic duct (MPD). For diagnostic purposes, the detection and location of tiny calcifications is only possible using CT without contrast injection. In patients presenting with a normal pancreatography, the presence of tiny calcifications on the "CT plain film" is the best criterion for the differential diagnosis between acute pancreatitis and chronic pancreatitis at the early stage.

This chapter discusses endoscopic treatment of chronic pancreatitis. It is important to note that these drainage procedures are indicated for patients with pain and marked morphological changes of CP (12,13) (Figure 3) and do not concern patients with anatomical variants or mild pancreatitis in whom no stone or stricture is shown in the MPD. In patients with morphological evidence of MPD obstruction, improving MPD drainage has the best chance of improving the pain syndrome. In other cases, only a papillary dysfunction with a normal MPD is likely to benefit. Then, not only the risk associated with manipulation of normal ducts is higher but the results of these manipulations are largely inconsistent (16) and the implantation of material in the normal MPD could precipitate the development of morphological lesions of CP (17). Therefore, in the absence of demon-

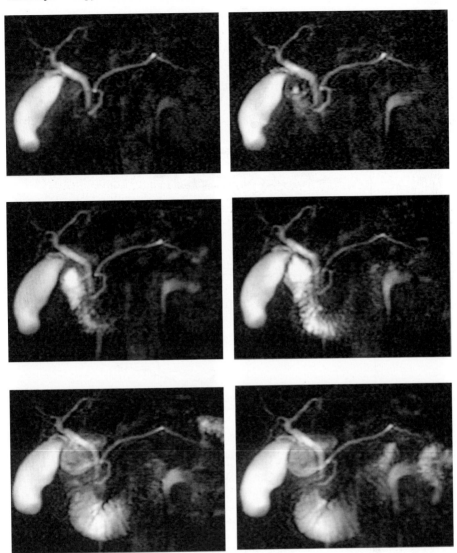

Figure 2. Dynamic secretin magnetic resonance pancreatography (MRP) in a normal subject. A Pancreatogram is obtained at baseline and every 30 seconds after secretin injection: note the duodenal filling and the changes in main pancreatic duct (MPD) diameter. (Images courtesy of C.Matos, MD.)

strable MPD stone or stricture, endoscopic manipulations of the pancreas remain largely experimental.

Pain Management

The aim of endotherapy in painful CP is to decompress the MPD, similar to the aim of surgical drainage procedures that have been performed for many years.

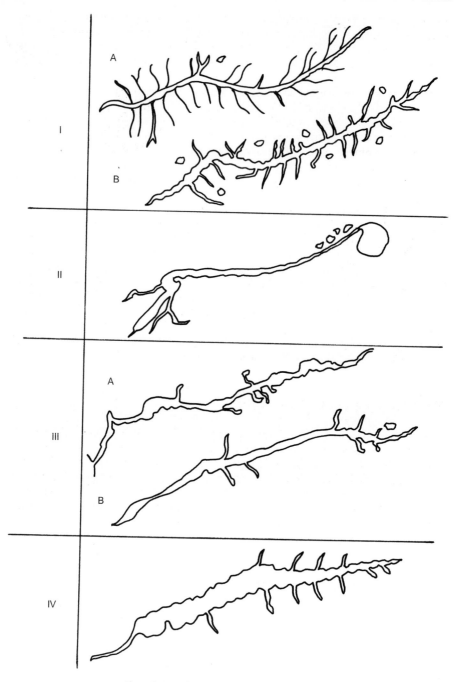

Figure 3. Morphological classification of CP.

Another goal of MPD drainage might be slowing the evolution of atrophy and pancreatic insufficiency by decreasing the chronic ischaemia process in the pancreas, and improving steatorrhea by restoring the residual flow of pancreatic juice to the duodenum. Currently, the single major indication for endoscopic treatment remains the elective treatment of pain. The rationale for proposing an endoscopic approach as a first-choice treatment before surgery includes the fact that ductal decompression is able to ensure pain control, that it may avoid resection and that this technique of MPD drainage provides the simultaneous delivery of pancreatic juice and bile into the duodenum.

The development of endotherapy for CP around the world has been much slower than that of endotherapy for biliary diseases for several reasons: the rarity of the disease, the heterogeneity of its morphological presentation, the technical requirements (lithotriptor with precise X-ray focusing, medical, surgical and radiological experience in the team, sophisticated accessories) and perhaps also the medical-social approach to patients with alcohol-related diseases.

Although we performed the first endoscopic pancreatic sphincterotomy 20 years ago [18] in a patient presenting with chronic pancreatitis and an impacted calcified stone at the level of the papilla, most developments of endotherapy for CP started only 10 years ago [10,19,20], with the availability of extracorporeal shock wave lithotripsy (ESWL) which provides millimetric disintegration of calcified calculi in nearly all cases and facilitates their extraction. Many centres are presently involved in the endoscopic management of CP, with good immediate technical results and data are now available for the long-term follow-up that can be compared with surgical series [21–26] (Table 1).

Methodology for Endotherapy

The endoscopic treatment of CP has to be guided by the morphological information obtained before ERCP, by various imaging techniques (plain film, MRCP or spiral CT) as described above. For patients with mild or moderate CP in the Cambridge classification (type IA or B in our classification (Figure 3), it is an open question whether any decompression would be beneficial for a patient presenting with acute relapsing clinical attacks of pancreatitis. Only controlled trials will give the answer on the long-term effectiveness of pancreatic sphincterotomy as the treatment for the earliest stage of primary CP. We think that the treatment

Table 1. Technical results and complications

Author	n	Complete stone clearance (%)	Adequate MPD drainage (%)	Complications (%)
Cremer (21)	76	ND	94	5
Delhaye (20)	123	59	90	9
Sauerbruch (19)	24	42	94	8
Binmoeller (35)	93	ND	88	6
Smits (36)	51	70	ND	18
Ponchon (23)	33	ND	85	30
Dumonceau (25)	70	50	ND	13
Bittencourt (24)	119	82	91	4
Total	589	65	90	9

of these patients remains currently experimental. It is possible that the routine use of DSMRP might help, in the near future, to select those patients with the highest probability of benefit from endoscopic therapy. For patients with type II CP, pseudocyst without gross abnormality of the MPD, one must be prepared to perform a cyst duodenostomy or a cyst gastrostomy after having recognized the bulging of the cyst against the upper gastrointestinal tract. If the cyst is of a relatively suitable size (< 5 cm) and is in contact with the MPD, an endoscopic pancreatic sphincterotomy (EPS) combined with nasopancreatic drain placement is often sufficient to achieve cyst resolution.

Extracorporeal Shock Wave Lithotripsy (ESWL)

Since most patients referred with severe chronic pancreatitis of types III to V have embedded calculi obstructing the MPD, the principle in these cases is to remove stones and treat strictures if necessary. If calcified stones are present, ESWL may be performed as the first procedure before sphincterotomy. Good quality plain films of the pancreatic area taken in left and right oblique position are mandatory to decide on this preliminary treatment (Figure 4). Without previous ESWL, deep cannulation of the MPD fails in 50% of these patients. On the other hand, ESWL is usually not necessary for patients with radiolucent stones. These "protein plugs" are usually friable and can be extracted immediately after sphincterotomy (27) or they are spontaneously eliminated if they are small.

It is of major importance to use a lithotriptor with a focusing system including two X-ray generators. Ultrasound localisation of stones lacks precision and efficacy. The high quality of the fluoroscopy obtained in two axes at a 45° angula-

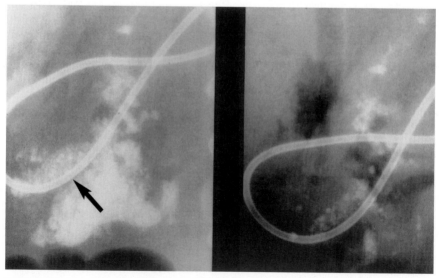

Figure 4. Plain films before and after extracorporeal shockwave lithotripsy (ESWL) and removal of stone fragments.

tion (Lithostar, Siemens, Erlangen, Germany) is mandatory for small calculi and for stones of less calcified density. This is the key point for reaching a 99% success of disintegration. Analgesia using midazolam and meperidine (pethidine) is usually sufficient to perform the procedure but general anaesthesia is sometimes necessary for less compliant patients and, in these cases, ESWL and therapeutic ERCP may be performed consecutively. During ESWL, one hundred shock waves per minute are delivered at an electric power of 19 kV during sessions of about 30 minutes with a mean required number of 1500 shocks/stone. The quality of fragmentation is evaluated by fluoroscopic control. Multiple or very large stones sometimes require repeated ESWL sessions.

Recently, a Japanese group (28) applied ESWL without subsequent endoscopic approach in 32 patients with MPD stones. Complete disintegration was obtained in all cases with further ductal clearance in 24 patients, without the need for endoscopic extraction. Pain relief was obtained in 79% of the patients after a mean period of 44 months. Although this option is probably limited to patients without associated stricture, it deserves further investigations as a first-line treatment for such patients.

Endoscopic Pancreatic Sphincterotomy (EPS)

EPS is the cornerstone technique of pancreatic endoscopy, which finally provides access to the MPD (29). The aim of EPS in chronic pancreatitis is not only to decrease the pancreatic duct pressure but mainly to facilitate the extraction of calculi. The EPS is performed at the major papilla for most of the patients and at the minor papilla for patients having a pancreas divisum anatomy but also for those having a "dominant" dorsal duct in whom therapeutic access to the MPD is much easier through the accessory papilla.

The pancreatic sphincterotomy may be done directly by inserting a papillotome (most often over a guide wire) into the pancreatic duct and directing the cut (using pure cutting current to avoid further fibrosis) between 11 and 10 o'clock positions. This has the potential limitation of further difficult access to the bile duct and, mainly, of difficult evaluation of the extent of the pancreatic cut. Therefore, EPS is usually performed in two steps: first biliary papillotomy and then pancreatic septotomy. Endoscopic biliary sphincterotomy (EBS) as the first approach may also have the advantage of avoiding the rare biliary complications that may occur after primary pancreatic sphincterotomy: some patients present with jaundice the day after EPS, probably due to oedema occurring at the level of the biliary sphincter. After biliary sphincterotomy, the pancreatic orifice is usually seen at 5 o'clock on the margins of the sphincterotomy. Its orifice can often be better visualised by sucking a little air in the duodenum, inducing its transient opening. When deep cannulation of the MPD has been achieved, pancreatic sphincterotomy or "septotomy" is performed using pure cutting current. The cut is done with the distal part of the cutting wire, at 12 o'clock, over a length of 5 to 8 mm (depending on the diameter of the MPD) to create the largest possible access.

For minor papilla sphincterotomy, a similar technique is used. The access to the duct is, however, sometimes more difficult, requiring the use of a special catheter (cannula, needle, Wilson-Cook) or the help of a hydrophilic guide wire

(Terumo). In very difficult cases, the technique of pancreatic rendez-vous can be used to gain access to the minor papilla (30).

EPS is sometimes the single endoscopic technique required in cases with pancreatic stones impacted at the papilla or when there are relatively small floating stones or protein plugs in the MPD that can pass spontaneously to the duodenum. These patients are unusual and, most often, sphincterotomy has to be followed by stone fragment removal, stenting, or both.

Extraction of Pancreatic Calculi

The ability to remove a stone is related to its size, degree of impaction and the presence of a downstream stricture. Most often stones are very hard and impacted into the wall of the MPD or the entrance of secondary ducts. Therefore, ESWL is often mandatory prior to any attempt at extraction. It provides a millimetric fragmentation of the stones making the extraction much easier.

For stone fragment extraction, we usually use first a small dormia basket. It is passed opened into the pancreatic duct. When the stones are visible on the plain film, a good trick is to introduce the dormia basket without contrast medium injection. The localisation of the residual fragments is easier and the basket can be "fiddled" at the level of the fragments to trap them. Another trick is to pass the basket opened into the duct, turning it on its axis in the sheath, and perfusing the sheath with saline: we call this "rotation perfusion", useful for elimination of small fragments. Finally, slightly inflated balloon catheters may be used in some cases but these are of limited help in the pancreas.

If multiple sessions of endoscopy are necessary, a nasopancreatic catheter is left in place between the sessions, perfused with saline or drained according to the presence or not of an associated stenosis. This can also be used as a clinical indication for the need of further pancreatic stenting. Indeed, if a patient tolerates, without pain, the perfusion of a nasopancreatic catheter, this is highly suggestive of the absence of significant stricture. On the contrary, if perfusion of the nasopancreatic catheter is painful it has to be placed on drainage and further stone extraction and/or stenting must be considered (29).

Pancreatic Stenting

Pancreatic stenting will ultimately be required in about 60% of patients with advanced chronic pancreatitis. Stent implantation is decided on clinical (see above) and morphological criteria, especially the presence of an MPD stricture in the head of the pancreas with up-stream dilatation. The methods of insertion include EPS followed by bougienage (up to 11 Fr). If dilatation is difficult, a nasopancreatic catheter can be left in place for 24 hours, which makes further dilation easier. Only large calibre (10 Fr) stents are used in this indication; their design is adapted to the pancreatic duct morphology (Figure 5). Usually, after stenting, disappearance of pain correlates with the reduction in MPD size and is observed in a large majority of the cases (Tables 1–3). However, if plastic stents are able to relieve MPD stricture and to induce symptomatic improvement, their ability to maintain patency of the stricture and to maintain the patient free of

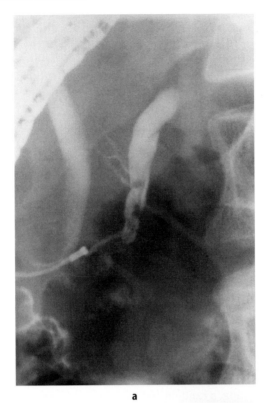

a

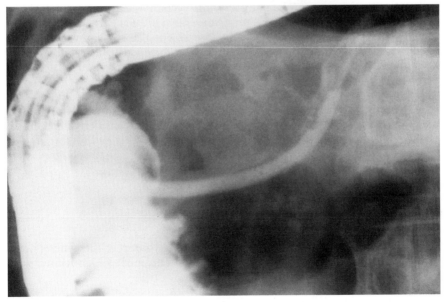

b

Figure 5. Type IV chronic pancreatitis with distal MPD stricture (**a**) requiring the placement of a 10-Fr stent (**b**).

Table 2. Pain relief after extracorporeal shock wave lithotripsy (ESWL) plus endoscopic pancreatic sphincterotomy (EPS) plus stenting

Authors	Patients (n)	Immediate (%)	Late (%)	Years	Surgery (%)
Cremer (21)	76→64	94	94	3.1	15
Delhaye (20)	107→88	100	85	1.2	8
Binmoeller (35)	93→69	(74)	87	4.9	26
Smits (36)	51→49	ND	82	2.8	12
Ponchon (23)	33→23	74	52	1.0	14
Bittencourt (24)	119→69	91	86	5.3	14
Total	479→362	89	85	3.2	15

Table 3. ESWL plus EPS (stenting excluded)

Author	n	Immediate pain relief (%)	n	Late pain relief (%)	Years follow-up	Surgery (%)
Sauerbruch (19)	24	ND	24	50	2	8
Dumonceau (25)	70	95	46	54	5	5

symptoms after removal is only observed in a minority of patients after prolonged stenting. Therefore, stenting requires a careful follow-up and the stent has to be exchanged either systematically (every 6 to 12 months) or "on demand" in compliant patients when a pain relapse occurs. This can be done on an ambulatory basis. At that time however, we have to choose with the patient between elective bypass surgery and repeated stent exchanges. Especially in these patients who require stenting, a randomised trial against surgery would be ideal to define the best life long therapy (31), taking also into account the evolution of exocrine and endocrine functions. However, the achievement of such a trial is difficult not only because of the low frequency of the disease but also some physicians refer patients to highly specialised centres specifically for endoscopic treatment and are not willing to consider random surgical decompression as a first attempt at pain relief.

Currently, it seems established that in severe chronic pancreatitis, endoscopic MPD drainage can provide long-term pain relief with a minimal complication rate (Table 1), especially as far as major complications are considered. It could be considered as a first approach to painful severe pancreatitis and further studies will better define those patients who could benefit from elective surgery after initial endotherapy.

Endoscopic Cystoenterostomy

Endoscopic cystoenterostomy must be considered as a part of the general management of severe chronic pancreatitis (32–34) and must be associated with ductal decompression if required.

There is increasing experience with endoscopic drainage of cysts complicating chronic pancreatitis and longer follow-up data are available (Figure 6). The drainage can be transmural or transpapillary if the cyst is communicating with the pancreatic duct and is not clearly adjacent to the stomach or duodenum

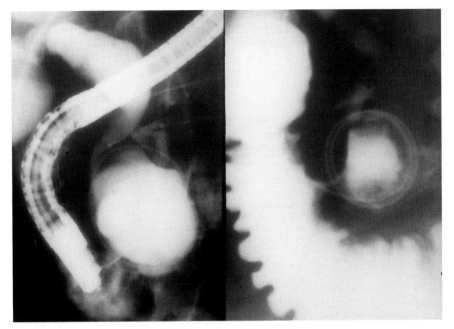

Figure 6. Endoscopic cystoduodenostomy.

(35,36). It has been suggested (37,38) that, when the cyst is accessible by the transpapillary route, this approach should be considered first. This seems reasonable except in the presence of ductal disruption occurring in the setting of severe chronic pancreatitis (39) where both transmural drainage (to drain the residual secretion of the distal pancreas) and transpapillary MPD decompression (to avoid relapse of the collection) are often required. It appears from these cumulative data that the endoscopic approach can be considered for pseudocysts adjacent to the upper GI tract and/or communicating with the MPD, offering a definitive treatment in 65% to 93% of the cases. This is discussed further in the following chapter.

Conclusion

The indications for endoscopic management for chronic pancreatitis are strictly limited to the severe types of pancreatitis where a ductal obstruction is morphologically demonstrated. This technique has gained success over the recent years and allows, with minimal complications, the avoidance or postponement of surgery, the indications for which might become better defined and the patient more carefully selected in the future. Endotherapy has the major advantage that it may be repeated without an increase in morbidity. It can be proposed relatively early in the course of the disease, when pain is of recent onset and morphological lesions of the MPD are demonstrated. It must be considered as an iterative treatment which can be adapted to the successive problems occurring along the course of a chronic disease. It is highly probable that, with the development of non-invasive techniques such as MRCP, it will become unethical to perform ERCP just for imaging the biliary and pancreatic ducts and pancreatic endotherapy will become the only reason to require endoscopic access to the pancreas.

References

1. Amman RW, Akovbiantz A, Largiader F, Schueler G (1984) Course and outcome of chronic pancreatitis. Gastroenterology 86:820–828.
2. Sahel J, Sarles H (1984) Chronic calcifying pancreatitis and obstructive pancreatitis: two entities. In: Gyr KE, Singer MV, Sarles H (eds) Pancreatitis, concepts and classification. Excerpta Medica, Amsterdam, pp 47–49.
3. Worning H (1990) Incidence and prevalence of chronic pancreatitis. In: Beger H, Büchler M, Ditschuneit H (eds) Chronic pancreatitis. Springer, Berlin Heidelberg New York pp 8–14.
4. Le Bodic L, Bignon JD, Raguenes O et al. (1996) The hereditary pancreatitis gene maps to long arm of chromosome 7. Hum Mal Genet 5:549–554.
5. Whitcomb DC, Preston RA, Aston CE et al. (1996) A gene for hereditary pancreatitis maps to chromosome 7q35. Gastroenterology 110:1975–1980.
6. Multigner L, Sarles H, Lombardo D, De Caro A (1985) Pancreatic stone protein II. Implication in stone formation during the course of chronic alcoholic pancreatitis. Gastroenterology 89:387–391.
7. Klöppel G (1990) Focal necrosis: primary event in the pathogenesis of chronic pancreatitis? In: Beger H, Büchler M, Ditschuneit H (eds) Chronic pancreatitis. Springer, Berlin Heidelberg New York, pp 71–76.
8. Van Laethem JL, Robberecht P, Resibois A, Devière J (1996) Transforming growth factor beta promotes development of fibrosis after repeated courses of acute pancreatitis in mice. Gastroenterology 110:576–582.
9. Amman RW, Heitz PU, Klöppel G (1996) Course of alcoholic chronic pancreatitis. A prospective clinico-morphological long-term study. Gastroenterology 111:224–231
10. Cremer M, Devière J, Delhaye M, Vandermeeren A, Baize M (1990) Non-surgical management of severe chronic pancreatitis. Scand J Gastroenterol 25 (Suppl 175):77–84.
11. Kasugai T, Kuno N, Kizu M (1972) Endoscopic pancreatocholangiography. II. The pathological endoscopic pancreatocholangiogram. Gastroenterology 63:227–234.
12. Cremer M, Toussaint J, Hermanus A, Deltenre M, De Toeuf J, Engelhom L (1976) Les pancréatites primitives: classification sur base de la pancréatographie endoscopique. Acta Gastroentero Belg 39:522–546.
13. Axon ATR, Classen M, Cotton P, Cremer M (1984) Pancreatography in chronic pancreatitis: international definition. Gut 25:1107–1112.
14. Reinhold C, Bret PM (1996) Current status of MR cholangiopancreatography. AJR 166:1285–1295.
15. Matos C, Metens Th, Devière J et al. (1997) Pancreatic duct: morphological and functional evaluation by dynamic secretin magnetic resonance pancreatography. Radiology 203:435–444.
16. Lehman G, Sherman S (1995) Pancreas divisum. Diagnosis, clinical significance and management alternatives. Gastrointest. Endosc Clin North Am 5:145–170.
17. Smith MT, Sherman S, Ikenberry SO, Hawes RH, Lehman GA (1996) Alterations in pancreatic ductal morphology following polyethylene pancreatic stent therapy. Gastrointest Endosc 44:268–275.
18. Cremer M (1977) Abstract of the Third International Symposium on Endoscopy. Brussels, February 1977.
19. Sauerbruch T, Holl J, Sackmann M, Paumgartner G (1989) Extracorporeal shock wave lithotripsy for pancreatic duct stones. Gut 30:1406–1440.
20. Delhaye M, Vandermeeren A, Baize M, Cremer M (1992) Extracorporeal shock wave lithotripsy of pancreatic calculi. Gastroenterology 102:610–620.
21. Cremer M, Devière J, Delhaye M, Baize M, Vandermeeren A (1991) Stenting in severe chronic pancreatitis: results of medium-term follow-up in 76 patients. Endoscopy 23:171–176.
22. Smits ME, Rauws EAJ, Tytgat GNJ, Huitbregtse K (1996) Endoscopic treatment of pancreatic stones in patients with chronic pancreatitis. Gastrointest Endosc 43:556–560.
23. Ponchon T, Bory RH, Hedelius F et al. (1995) Endoscopic stenting for pain relief in chronic pancreatitis: results of a standardized protocol. Gastrointest Endosc 42:452–456.

24. Bittencourt PL, Delhaye M, Devière J et al. (1996) Immediate and long-term results of pancreatic ductal drainage in severe painful chronic pancreatitis. Gut 39:A99.

25. Dumonceau JM, Devière J, Le Moine O, Delhaye M, Van Gansbeke D, Cremer M (1996) Endoscopic drainage in chronic pancreatitis associated with ductal stones: long-term results. Gastrointest Endosc 43:547–555.

26. Costamagna G, Gabbrielli A, Multimagni M et al. (1996) Endoscopic pancreatic sphincterotomy (EPS): is this a safe procedure? Results in 128 EPS. Gastroenterology 110:A383.

27. Schneider MU, Lux G (1985) Floating pancreatic duct concrements in chronic pancreatitis. Pain relief by endoscopic removal. Endoscopy 17:8–10.

28. Sohara H, Hoshino M, Hayakawa T et al. (1996) Single application extracorporeal shock wave lithotripsy is the first choice for patients with pancreatic duct stones. Am J Gastroenterol 91:1388–1394.

29. Devière J, Cremer M (1996) Techniques of ERCP. Universa Press, Wetteren, Belgium.

30. Ghattas G, Devière J, Blancas JM, Baize M, Cremer M (1992) Pancreatic rendez-vous. Gastrointest Endosc 38:590–594.

31. Lehman GA, Sherman S (1996) Pancreatic stones: to treat or not to treat? Gastrointest Endosc 43:625–626.

32. Cremer M, Devière J, Engelholm J (1989) Endoscopic management of cysts and pseudocysts in chronic pancreatitis. A 7-years experience. Gastrointest Endosc 35:1–9.

33. Kozarek RA, Brayko CM, Harlan J, Sanowsky RA, Cintora I, Kovac A (1985) Endoscopic drainage of pancreatic pseudocyst. Gastrointest Endosc 31:322–325.

34. Grimm HT, Meyer WH, Nam V, Soenhendra N (1989) New modalities for treating chronic pancreatitis. Endoscopy 21:70–74.

35. Binmoeller KF, Seifert H, Walter A, Soehendra N (1995) Transpapillary and transmural drainage of pancreatic pseudocysts. Gastrointest Endosc 42:219–224.

36. Smits ME, Rauws EA, Tytgat GN, Huibregste K (1995) The efficacy of endoscopic treatment of pancreatic pseudocysts. Gastrointest Endosc 42:202–207.

37. Catalano MF, Geenen JE, Schmalz MJ, Johnson GK, Dean RS, Hogan WJ (1995) Treatment of pancreatic pseudocysts with ductal communications by transpapillary pancreatic duct endoprosthesis. Gastrointest Endosc 42:214–218.

38. Barthet M, Sahel J, Bodiou-Bertei C, Bernard JP (1995) Endoscopic transpapillary drainage of pancreatic pseudocysts. Gastrointest Endosc 42:208–213.

39. Devière J, Bueso H, Baize M et al. (1995) Complete disruption of the main pancreatic duct: endoscopic management. Gastrointest Endosc 42:445–451.

18 Endoscopic Treatment in Chronic Pancreatitis

R. Laugier and C. Renou

Endoscopic treatment of chronic pancreatitis (CP) has drawn benefits from endoscopic procedures which have mainly been described for the main bile duct. This endoscopic therapy reproduces all the surgical methods which are used by the surgeon with the exception of resection of the pancreas.

The main goals of conservative surgery and as a consequence of these endoscopic procedures are:

- to drain and decompress the main bile duct and/or main pancreatic duct,
- to extract stones, either directly or after destruction from the main pancreatic duct,
- to drain cysts into the digestive tract.

Some of these procedures have in common the decrease of ductal and possibly pancreatic tissue pressure, considered as the major factor in the pathogenesis of pain in CP. These procedures are developing throughout Europe and the USA as well as Japan and are more and more commonly named "pancreatic endotherapy".

Main Pancreatic Duct Drainage

Duct drainage and stenting have been discussed fully in the preceding chapter and will be reviewed only briefly here.

Technique

The easiest way of draining the main pancreatic duct (MPD) into the duodenum is pancreatic papillotomy. This technique, associated or not with the biliary sphincterotomy, has been described first by Siegel (1), as easily feasible and safe in a fibrous pancreas as is often the case in CP.

Endoscopic pancreatic sphincterotomy (EPS) alone, decreases the pressure in the MPD when this is regularly dilated from the papilla up to the tail. In fact, this situation appears to be present in only a few cases. In the large majority of cases, EPS is only the first step of a more complex procedure, endotherapy, and includes dilatation and stenting of strictures, as well as stone fragmentation.

Once EPS has been performed, the strictures have to be catheterised using a guide wire. Several sizes, shapes, diameters and materials are now available for achieving such catheterisation (a metallic Teflon coated hydrophilic guide wire is often helpful), (2). The stricture itself may be dilated, either with a bougienage technique or with a hydraulic inflatable balloon, which allows larger diameter dilatation (6 or even 8 mm instead of 4 mm with a 12 Fr dilator (3).

The newly dilated stenosis is usually stented with an endoprosthesis, for maintaining the dilatation throughout time. Stents are routinely made of plastic from 7 to 12 Fr in diameter, and with a length adapted to the position of the strictures on the MPD. Cremer et al. (2) have reported the use of self-expandable metallic mesh stents for treating those stenosis in the long term.

In some cases of CP, in patients with pancreas divisum, or with "predominant duct of Santorini", all these manoeuvres are easily performed at the level of the accessory papilla. Technical design in these cases is identical. The overall technical success rate reported by Burdick and others (4) is 95%.

Results

Immediate results of stenting are excellent while immediate complications are negligible. No mortality has been so far reported. Stent drainage of the MPD provides early pain relief in 75–94% of patients (2,5). This is a further argument supporting the role of high ductal pressure in the pathogenesis of pain. By contrast, the failure of stent decompression to relieve pain in a few patients is consistent with the multifactorial aetiology of pain in CP (6).

Early complications of stenting include acute pancreatitis, which some authors believe could be avoided after EPS by stent insertion itself (5,7), pain exacerbation, stent erosion of the contralateral duodenal wall, and stent migration (either upstream, within the MPD or downstream, into the digestive tract) (7). The most common problems result from stent occlusion: lapse of time and ductal consequences. Large discrepancies exist in the definition of stent occlusion: on a clinical standpoint, Huibregtse et al. (7) reported no case of complete pancreatic stent occlusion during a 2–3 years follow-up period; by contrast Cremer et al. (2) found the mean stent patency to be around 12 months. When a standardised method is used to detect patency, such as a water column test, occlusion occurs at 6 weeks in 50% of cases and is always present after 9 weeks (8). In our personal experience, stent occlusion may develop rapidly in some cases (3–5 months). The precise mechanism of occlusion, which is not yet fully understood, probably includes bacterial colonisation, and the quantitative amount of residual pancreatic secretion, explaining in our view, longer stent patency in advanced cases of CP, in which pancreatic secretion has almost completely vanished. Stent occlusion has been reported to be either asymptomatic or associated with recurrent symptoms or even with pancreatic abscess formation (5). We therefore favour systematic stent exchange every 4 months or at the first recurrence of pain.

If it is now widely accepted that pancreatic stenting is an efficient short- or medium-term treatment, data on the long-term outcome are scarce. In a retrospective study, Binmoeller et al. (5) found that 87% of patients ($n = 69$) who responded to stent drainage sustained clinical improvement during a mean follow-up of 4.9 years. Identical results are reported by other groups (2,4).

The presence of a stent in the pancreatic duct has been found to induce subsequent ductal alterations simulating those of CP (9). Histological evaluation revealed essentially inflammatory, reversible lesions which are consistent with the absence of significant residual changes from prestenting appearance after stent removal (10,11). Secondary ductal alterations, pseudocyst formation and/or infection or enlargement have also been described after stent occlusion; such complications resolved with stent exchange (9). In our view, undiagnosed stent occlusion appears to be a true deleterious factor in the course of the disease: it is why we have adopted the attitude of the systematic stent exchange at 4 months or the immediate exchange after the first symptomatic recurrence.

Indications

Such a stenting non-surgical attitude has to be now considered as feasible, with no mortality rate and very low morbidity; thanks to clinical follow-up, it has been proven to be efficient, even in the relatively long-term. However, up to now no demonstration exists that endoscopic therapy is less costly and provides patients with better results than diversion surgery.

We have nevertheless demonstrated that in patients with painful CP, without MPD dilatation (thus unsuitable for diversion surgery), endoscopic stenting was an effective alternative to resection surgery with a mean follow-up of 24 months (personal results, Int J Pancreatol (in press)). Better anatomical results of stricture treatment were obtained with large balloon dilatation than with only the bougienage technique.

The use of metal mesh stents, which can be compared to a "true prosthetic endoscopic pancreaticoduodenostomy" has not been accepted by most endoscopists, who refuse to introduce an inextirpable stent within the MPD for a benign disease (2).

Main Bile Duct Drainage

Biliary obstruction occurs in more than 10% of patients with CP, due to fibrosis of the pancreatic head. It can result in repetitive colicky pain, biochemical cholestasis, jaundice or even secondary biliary cirrhosis. Endoscopic stenting of biliary strictures is easily feasible after biliary endoscopic sphincterotomy; it may be a real benefit in some acute situations. Biliary stenting has been performed in CP with either one, two or three plastic 10-Fr stents or with self-expandable metal stents. Complications of plastic stents are migration (within bile duct or in the digestive tract) and, of course, obstruction. The latter requires regular stent exchange programmed or on demand. So far, results obtained with a single plastic stent are acceptable clinically and anatomically in less than 30% of patients (12). Our own results using two 10-Fr stents seem, up to now, fairly good with more than 3 years follow-up on a small group of patients. Devière et al. (13) have reported the results obtained in 20 patients treated with metal stents: only two patients developed recurrent biliary obstruction (at 3 and 6 months). According to the fact that some patients also developed duodenal stenosis, the non-surgical management of biliary strictures due to CP, although technically feasible, has not so far a proven advantage over surgery.

Pancreatic Stone Extraction

Drainage of the MPD into the duodenum is improved by EPS, dilatation and maintenance of strictures with stents, but stones, floating or fixed within the lumen, may suppress the beneficial effects of other drainage attempts. It has rapidly become apparent that stone removal should be included in pancreatic endotherapy. After EPS, stones can be extracted only when the size of the MPD downstream allows their passage: they can be extracted after mechanical fragmentation with a dormia basket, following the same procedure as that used for biliary stones (1,7,15,16,17).

This procedure is often technically difficult because stones generally form upstream to a stricture and/or are often impacted in the duct. Thus, fragmentation of stones by other ways than dormia basket has developed. Already in 1987, Sauerbrüch et al. (18) reported the first clinical results concerning the use of extracorporeal shock wave lithotripsy (18). The same group later reported good clinical results on a larger cohort of patients (19,20) with longer follow-up. Other groups rapidly followed this experience with the same type of machine (21,22,23,24) or with piezoelectric shock wave (25,26). This is the kind of machine which is used in our institution. Extracorporeal shock wave lithotripsy seems to have completely replaced intracorporeal lithotripsy using laser beam and miniscopes as proposed by Neuhaus et al. (27) or Renner (28). We are currently testing the efficacy of an intracorporeal hydroelectric shock wave lithotriptor with the help of a miniscope.

So far, the largest series of patients reported after medium-term follow-up originate from Brussels (24) and Amsterdam (29,30). Extracorporeal shock wave lithotripsy included in a complete pancreatic endotherapy (EPS, stenting and dilatation) provides stable and good results in 79–89% of patients (see previous chapter). Complications were infrequent (9%): bouts of pain, mild acute pancreatitis or one exceptional case of guide wire fracture (31). From all these experiences, relief of pain is correlated with the quality of pancreatic drainage, while clinical relapse appears in most of the cases, associated with recurrence of calculi. More than 200 cases have been reported as successful at long-term follow-up.

Cyst Drainage

A cyst cavity has to be drained into the digestive tract: this can be obtained either directly as a result of a cyst-gastrostomy or to a cyst-duodenostomy, or indirectly, through the ductal system and the papilla.

Indirect Transpapillary Drainage

A prerequisite of this technique is to demonstrate the patency of the cysto-ductal communication. This is easily documented by retrograde pancreatography when contrast medium leaves the pancreatic ductal system to fill the cyst cavity. Once such communication has been documented, one can introduce selectively a guide wire into the MPD to cannulate this communication with the tip of the guide wire. According to the diameter of the pancreatic duct and of the cyst to be drained, an EPS may be required. The guide wire having been introduced deeply into the cyst, the communication may be dilated (using either the bougienage technique or a hydraulic inflatable balloon). Finally, a double pigtail endoprosthesis has to be introduced through the papilla into the cyst. It has to keep this communication open until there is complete cyst healing. The duration of stenting has to be adapted to the cyst evaluation, by ultrasonography or computed tomography (CT).

This elegant technique, first described by Huibregtse et al. (7), has to be attempted first, before other approaches in our opinion, because it has a very low risk and thus is safe. It gives excellent results in all series in which such cases are included (7,32–39). The recurrence rate is usually less than 15% of all cases.

As for stricture stenting, the most frequent complication associated with cyst recurrence or infection is due to occlusion of the stent; this is why a relatively short period of stenting seems desirable. The major problem of this technique lies in the fact that it is not always feasible: strictures or stones between the papilla and the communication have to be treated first; above all, it must be pointed out that communication between the cyst and the ductal system has to be present and finally selectively catheterised. We can estimate from our personal experience and from the literature that this technique is feasible in only 30–40% of cysts that are treated endoscopically.

Cyst Drainage into the Stomach or the Duodenum

This appears technically easier for most endoscopists. This technique requires a clear bulging of the cyst into the digestive tract and ultrasonography or CT to demonstrate that the cysto-digestive distance is less than 10 mm when this anatomical condition is present. Thus, cysts of the tail exceptionally give access to an endoscopic direct drainage! At the point of maximal cyst bulging, access is obtained with a diathermy needle or a special device adapted to that specific purpose. We have, as have other groups, developed a diathermy needle which allows removal of the diathermic part of the device and to keep the catheter deep inside the cyst. Thus, after aspiration of some part of the cyst content (for biochemical and bacteriological analysis), cyst opacification becomes feasible; thereafter, another guide-wire is introduced within the cyst over which a durable duodenostomy (or gastrostomy) is performed. There is a general tendency to decrease the size of the endoscopically created communications to a few millimetres and provide them with one or two double pigtail endoprostheses, in order to keep the communication opened until the complete healing of the cyst. The technical success rate appears better for cysto-duodenostomy than for cystogastrostomy, which is consequently associated with higher complication rates (13,33,34,39–42).

The two main complications are haemorrhage and perforation: the latter only seems to be a significant risk when bulging is not clearly present, while the first risk is very difficult to predict. The use of endosonography has been recently emphasised for minimising as much as possible these two risks (43,44). In our experience, endosonography is not only useful for predicting risk but also for choosing the best point to be punctured and for extending indications to some cysts which do not bulge into the duodenum although the distance between the walls is less than 5 mm (45). Cyst relapse rate seems to be lower than 20% for cysto-gastrostomy and less than 10% for cysto-duodenostomy (32–42). Very similar figures are noted after surgical treatment.

Conclusion

Endotherapy nowadays is becoming a reality: more and more endoscopic centres are developing their own experience; it is no longer a matter of extreme speciali-sation. Nonetheless, among treatments which have been developed and have been proven to be feasible, one can distinguish between those which appear as a clear-cut improvement in the large majority of cases with lower morbidity than surgery and similar results, such as from cyst drainage, pancreatic duct drainage and stone clearance, which are endoscopically feasible for relieving pain as surgery does, but which still need more precise evaluation of long-term results and costs. Finally, endoscopic treatment of chronic cholestasis during CP seems up to now of very modest interest if not completely negligible.

References

1. Siegel JM (1980) Endoscopic approach to pancreatic sphincterotomy. In: Syllabus: current controversies in gastroenterology. Gastroenterology.
2. Cremer M, Devière J, Delhaye M, Baize M, Vandermeeren A (1991) Stenting in severe chronic pancreatitis: results of medium-term follow-up in 76 patients. Endoscopy 23:171–176.
3. Fuji T, Amano H, Harima K (1985) Pancreatic sphincterotomy and pancreatic endoprosthesis. Endoscopy 17:69–72.
4. Burdick JS, Hogan W (1991) Chronic pancreatitis: selection of patients for endoscopic therapy. Endoscopy 23:155–160.
5. Binmoeller KF, Jue P, Seifert H, Nam WC, Izbicki J, Soehendra N (1995). Endoscopic pancreatic stent drainage in chronic pancreatitis and a dominant stricture: long-term results. Endoscopy 27:638–644.
6. Karanjia ND, Reber HA (1990) The cause and management of the pain of chronic pancreatitis. Gastroenterol Clin North Am 19:895–904.
7. Huibregtse K, Schneider B, Vrij AH, Tytgat GNJ (1988). Endoscopic pancreatic drainage in chronic pancreatitis. Gastrointest Endosc 34:9–15.
8. Ikenberry SO, Sherman S, Smith M, Lehman GA (1994) The occlusion rate of pancreatic stents. Gastrointest Endosc 40:611–613.
9. Kozarek RA (1990) Pancreatic stents can induce ductal changes consistent with chronic pancreatitis. Gastrointest Endosc 36:93–95.
10. Alvarez C, Robert M, Sherman S, Reber HA (1994) Histologic changes after stenting of the pancreatic duct. Arch Surg 129:765–768.
11. Derfus GA, Geenen JE, Hogan WJ (1990) Effect of endoscopic pancreatic duct stent placement on pancreatic ductal morphology. Gastrointest Endosc 36:206A.
12. Devière J, Devaere S, Baize M, Cremer M (1990) Endoscopic biliary drainage in chronic pancreatitis. Gastroenterology 98:96–100.
13. Devière J, Cremer M, Baize M, Love J, Sugai B, Vandermeeren A (1994) Management of common bile duct stricture caused by chronic pancreatitis with metal mesh self-expandable stents. Gut 35:122–126.
14. Aranha GV, Prinz RA, Freeark RJ, Grenlee HB (1984) The spectrum of biliary tract obstruction from chronic pancreatitis. Arch Surg 119:595–600.
15. Fuji T, Amano H, Ohmura R, Ariyama S, Aibe T, Takemoto T (1989) Endoscopic pancreatic sphincterotomy. Technique and evaluation. Endoscopy 21:27–30.
16. Siegel JH, Pullano WE, Safrany L (1989) Endoscopic therapy for acquired pancreatitis: effective long-term management. 2:168–169.

17. Schneider MU, Lux C (1985). Floating pancreatic duct concrements in chronic pancreatitis. Endoscopy 17:8-10.
18. Sauerbruch T, Holl J, Sackmann M, Werner R, Wotzke R, Paumgartner G (1987) Disintegration of a pancreatitic duct stone with extracorporeal shockwaves in a patient with chronic pancreatitis. Endoscopy 19:207-208.
19. Sauerbruch T, Holl J, Sackmann M, Paumgartner G (1989) Extra-corporeal shockwave lithotripsy of pancreatic stones. Gut 30:1406-1411.
20. Sauerbruch T, Holl J, Sackmann M, Paumgartner G (1992) Extra-corporeal shock wave lithotripsy of pancreatic stones in patients with chronic pancreatitis and pain. Gut 33:969-972.
21. Neuhaus H (1991) Fragmentation of pancreatic stones by extracorporeal shock wave lithotripsy. Endoscopy 23:161-165.
22. Den Toom R, Nijs HG, Van Blankenstein M, Schroder FH, Jeekel J, Terpstra OT (1991) Extracorporeal shock wave lithotripsy of pancreatic duct stones. Am J Gastroenterol 86:1033-1036.
23. Delhaye M, Vandermeeren A, Gabbrielli A, Cremer M (1990) Lithotripsy and endoscopy for pancreatic calculi: the first 104 patients. Gastroenterology 98:A216.
24. Delhaye M, Vandermeeren A, Baize M, Cremer M (1992) Extracorporeal shock wave lithotripsy of pancreatic calculi. Gastroenterology 102:610-620.
25. Kerzel W, Ell C, Schneider HT, Matek W, Heyder N, Hahn EG (1989) Extracorporeal piezo-electric shock wave lithotripsy of multiple pancreatic duct stones under ultrasonographic control. Endoscopy 21:229-231.
26. Robert JY, Bretagne JF, Darnault P et al. (1993) Endoscopic treatment and extracorporeal lithotripsy in chronic calcifying pancreatitis. Gastroenterol Clin Biol 17:797-803.
27. Neuhaus H, Hoffmann W, Classen M (1992) Laser lithotripsy of pancreatic and biliary stones via 3.4 mm and 3.7 mm miniscopes: first clinical results. Endoscopy 24:208-215.
28. Renner I (1991) Laser fragmentation of pancreatic stones. Endoscopy 23:166-170.
29. Dumonceau JM, Devière J, Le Moine O et al. (1996) Endoscopic pancreatic drainage in chronic pancreatitis associated with ductal stones: long-term results. Gastrointest Endosc 43:547-555.
30. Smits M, Rauws E, Tytgat G, Huibregtse K (1996) Endoscopic treatment of pancreatic stones in patients with chronic pancreatitis. Gastrointest Endosc 43:556-560.
31. Heineman M, Mann R, Boeckl O (1993) An unusual complication in attempted non-surgical treatment of pancreatic bile duct stones. Endoscopy 25:248-250.
32. Spinelli P, Meroni E, Prada A (1988) Endoscopic treatment of a pancreatic pseudocyst by naso cystic tube. Endoscopy 20:27-29.
33. Bejanin H, Liguory C, Ink O et al. (1993) Drainage endoscopique des pseudo kystes du pancreas. Gastroenterol Clin Biol 17:804-810.
34. Dohmoto M, Rupp KD (1992) Endoscopic drainage of pancreatic pseudocysts. Surg Endosc 6:118-124.
35. Kozarek RA, Ball TJ, Patterson DJ, Freeny PC, Ryan JA, Traverso LW (1991) Endoscopic transpapillary therapy for disrupted pancreatic duct and peripancreatic fluid collections. Gastroenterology 100:1367-1370.
36. Smits M, Rauws E, Tytgat G, Huibregtse K (1995) The efficacy of endoscopic treatment of pancreatic pseudocysts. Gastrointest Endosc 42:202-207.
37. Barthet M, Sahel J, Bodiou-Bertei C, Bernard JP (1995) Endoscopic transpapillary drainage of pancreatic pseudocysts. Gastrointest Endosc 42:208-213.
38. Catalano M, Geenen J, Schmalz M, Johnson G, Dean R, Hogan W (1995) Treatment of pancreatic pseudocysts with ductal communication by transpapillary pancreatic duct endoprosthesis. Gastrointest Endosc 42:214-218.
39. Binmoeller K, Seifert H, Walter A, Soehendra N (1995) Transpapillary and transmural drainage of pancreatic pseudocysts. Gastrointest Endosc 42:219-224.
40. Kozarek RA, Brayko CM, Harlan J, Sanowki RA, Cintoria I (1985) Endoscopic drainage of pancreatic pseudocysts. Gastrointest Endosc 31:322-328.
41. Cremer M, Devière J, Engelholm L (1989) Endoscopic management of cyst and pseudocysts in chronic pancreatitis: long-term follow-up after 7 years experience. Gastrointest Endosc 35:1-9.
42. Sahel J (1991) Endoscopic drainage of pancreatic cysts. Endoscopy 23:181-184.
43. Grimm H, Binmoeller K, Soehendra N (1992) Endosonography-guided drainage of a pancreatic pseudocyst. Gastrointest Endosc 38:170-174.
44. Fockens R, Johnson T, Van Dullemen R, Huitbregtse K, Tytgat G. Endosonography is a prerequisite before endoscopic drainage of pancreatic pseudocyst. Dig Dis Week 3641A.
45. Gerolami R, Giovannini M, Laugier R (1997) Endoscopic drainage of pancreatic pseudocysts guided by endosonography. Endoscopy 29:106-108.

19 Enzyme Therapy in Chronic Pancreatitis

P. Layer and J. Keller

A typical feature of chronic pancreatitis is progressive impairment of pancreatic enzyme output with resulting maldigestion of macronutrients. It has been demonstrated by us and others that in chronic pancreatitis of alcoholic aetiology, most patients devolop malabsorption in the second decade following the first onset of symptoms, although more rapid courses occur (1,2,3). In chronic pancreatitis of idiopathic origin, the mean latency between onset of symptomatic disease and pancreatic insufficiency is 20 to 30 years (3).

The late manifestation of pancreatic exocrine insufficiency in the course of the disease is explained by the reserve secretory capacity of the gland which is able to compensate for destruction of up to 90–95% of the exocrine parenchymal tissue before steatorrhoea occurs (2,4,5). However, besides duodenal enzyme output, other mechanisms are important for the development of luminal maldigestion. In particular, survival of enzymatic activity within the intestinal lumen during duodenoileal transit of chyme determines the duration of enzymatic digestion availability and is therefore another key factor controlling the degree and site of macronutrient breakdown (6–9).

Lipid Maldigestion

The manifestation of lipid malabsorption in chronic pancreatitis is a result of several mechanisms which all contribute to the earlier development of steatorrhoea compared with malabsorption of other nutrients. Impaired pancreatic lipase activity cannot be compensated for sufficiently by other mechanisms for the following reasons.

First, small intestinal fat digestion is mainly caused by the combined effects of pancreatic lipase and its cofactors, in particular colipase and bile acids. The intestinal mucosa does not express triglyceride-digesting enzyme systems, and luminal lipolytic activity secreted by extrapancreatic sources, in particular lingual and gastric lipase, cannot replace lipid digestion by pancreatic lipase (2,4,10–14). By contrast, starch digestion, although delayed, can reach nearly 80% of normal levels by the action of salivary amylase and by brush-border oligosaccharidases even in the absence of pancreatic amylase activity (6). Similarly, protein is effectively hydrolised by gastric proteases and protein digestion is continued by intestinal mucosal peptidases so that even under experimental conditions of virtually complete loss of luminal pancreatic proteolytic activity, protein digestion is partly maintained (15).

Second, in alcoholic chronic pancreatitis with progressive pancreatic insufficiency, impairment of lipase synthesis and/or secretion occurs earlier and more severely compared with other digestive enzymes within the same patient (1,2,5).

Third, pancreatic bicarbonate secretion which serves to protect pancreatic enzymes against denaturation by gastric acid is diminished in exocrine pancreatic insufficiency. In severe exocrine pancreatic insufficiency and decreased bicarbonate secretion, intraduodenal pH falls below 4, particularly in the late postprandial period (16). Lipase is more sensitive to acid destruction than other enzymes (2,16). Since bile acids are also denatured by low intraduodenal pH, lipid absorption is compromised further.

Fourth, we have shown that in humans, intraluminal degradation rates of the major enzymes differ widely due to stability differences against inactivating mechanisms (7). Moreover, disappearance rates of enzymatic activities and immunoreactivities of the same enzymes are non-parallel (7). Thus, lipase activity decreases rapidly during small intestinal transit: in the absence of its substrate, most of its activity is lost already in the proximal intestine, and only small quantities are delivered to the terminal ileum (7,17). In the presence of triglycerides, the stability of the lipase molecule appears to be enhanced both *in vitro* and *in vivo* (15,18,19). By contrast, approximately 60% of trypsin and chymotrypsin activities secreted reach the mid-jejunum, and between 20% and 30% reach the terminal ileum (7,17). It is intriguing that during small intestinal transit, trypsin activity is preserved to a higher degree than its immunoreactivity, which suggests that structural integrity of the trypsin molecule may not be essential for its proteolytic activity (7). Pancreatic amylase has greater stability because it is partly resistant against proteolysis, and most of its duodenal activity reaches the terminal ileum (7,17,20). The main mechanism causing luminal loss of enzymatic activity within the small intestine is proteolytic degradation. There is strong evidence that chymotrypsin is a major catalyst of lipase degradation (17,21). In consequence, combined inactivation of the major pancreatic proteases including trypsin and chymotrypsin dramatically increases the survival of lipase activity during human duodenoileal transit (17) and decreases fat malabsorption by 80% (19,22). In essence, lipase degradation within the human small intestinal lumen occurs more rapidly than destruction of other enzymes due to its greater instability against proteolysis. Therefore, lipase is available for a shorter period of time for digestive action during small intestinal transit both in healthy individuals (7,17,19) and in patients with exocrine pancreatic insufficiency (23).

The digestive role of pancreatic lipase can be summarised as follows: compared with other key pancreatic enzymes such as trypsin, chymotrypsin or amylase, its luminal digestive action is hardly compensated by non-pancreatic mechanisms; its pancreatic synthesis and secretion is impaired more rapidly, and its intraluminal survival is shorter. These properties are the basis of the crucial role of lipase and its adequate substitution in the pathophysiology and treatment of exocrine pancreatic insufficiency. As a result, steatorrhoea (often associated with malabsorption of the lipid-soluble vitamins A, D, E and K) is the most important digestive malfunction: in general, it is more severe and occurs several years before clinical malabsorption of protein or starch. The latter only develop late, if at all, in the course of progressive pancreatic insufficiency (5).

Regulatory Effects of Nutrient Malabsorption

Manifest malabsorption is rarely present in the early stages of chronic pancreatitis, yet, even within the first 5–10 years of the disease, enzyme output decreases by 60–90% (1). While the remaining secretory capacity still prevents maldigestion, there is evidence that the site of peak digestion and absorption shifts from the duodenum to the distal small intestine and increased amounts of nutrients are delivered to the ileum compared with the physiological malabsorption observed in response to a standard meal ingested by healthy subjects (8,24,25). Nutrient exposure of the ileal lumen causes marked changes in pancreatic secretion: water and digestive enzyme outputs are inhibited, and their ratios are partly modulated (26–28); moreover, gastric secretion, gastric emptying and small intestinal transit are influenced (3,26,28–32). In chronic pancreatitis uncorrected maldigestion causes acceleration of gastric emptying and small intestinal transit (26–30,33).

These effects probably contribute to the symptoms of patients who have no overt malabsorption, and they might explain the pain-relieving effects of enzyme supplementation reported by some of these patients.

Physiology and Pathophysiology of Enzyme Replacement

Treatment of malabsorption in exocrine pancreatic insufficiency requires delivery of sufficient enzymatic activity into the duodenal lumen simultaneously with the meal (4,34). To prevent lipid malabsorption, intraduodenal lipase activity has to reach or exceed a mean threshold of about 40–60 U/ml in postprandial chyme throughout the digestive period (14,24,35). As a result, therapeutic enzyme administration must match this level to effectively treat steatorrhoea in pancreatic insufficiency, which means that for digestion of a regular meal 25 000–50 000 U of lipase are required intraduodenally (5,13,23).

However, with substitution therapy the following problems arise: in unprotected pancreatic enzyme preparations nearly all lipase activity is destroyed by gastric acid, whereas the sturdier proteases survive gastric transit significantly better (16,36). In addition, supplemented lipase is also inactivated by proteolysis in patients with chronic pancreatitis (23), similar to the fate of endogenously secreted lipase in healthy subjects (17). Hence it is necessary to ingest approximately 5–10-fold more lipase than required in the duodenal lumen. The efficacy of enzyme preparations is increased by inhibitors of gastric acid secretion (H_2-blockers or proton pump inhibitors) (34,37,38).

Enteric coating of tablets or capsules prevents acidic denaturation of enzymes. However, such preparations are not emptied from the stomach during the digestive period (39–42). During the fed period, solid particles are liquified by the grinding forces of the "antral mill" which decrease their particle size to below 1–2 mm; duodenal passage of particles exceeding this threshold is prevented by the pylorus (43,44). Resistant particles including acid-resistant tablets or capsules which cannot be reduced in size during the digestive period are retained within the stomach until the subsequent fasting period and are then emptied by phase III of the interdigestive migrating motor complex (39–41). This leads to a dissociation of duodenal delivery of nutrients and enzymes.

Consequently, newer preparations encapsulate pancreatin within acid-resistant, enteric-coated microspheres (micropellets or microtablets) which mix with the meal intragastrically but do not expose their enzyme content, and are emptied into the duodenum together with the meal. Their enzymatic activity is released in the intestine at pH 6. Intraluminal measurements suggest that > 60% of the lipase activity reaches the duodenum (23). The superior efficacy of enteric-coated micropellet preparations compared with conventional pancreatin extracts has been shown in controlled studies (45,46). Dose-response studies suggest that with these preparations, 20–30 kU of lipase per meal markedly reduce steatorrhea (45).

Enzyme release from pancreatin microspheres may take several minutes after their entrance into the intestinal milieu and therefore occurs as far distal as the mid-jejunum, which may cause a distal shift of lipid digestion and absorption (23,47). The physicochemical properties of the coating are determinants for the efficacy of enzyme treatment therapy and likely more important than their lipase content; they might explain treatment failures with individual enzyme preparations (48).

Therapeutic Standards

Enteric-coated pancreatin microspheres are at present standard therapy for the majority of patients with exocrine pancreatic insufficiency. To treat steatorrhea to < 15 g of fat per 24 hours, at least 25–50 kU of lipase per meal at four or five meals per day need to be administered, but even larger doses may be necessary. As outlined above, several mechanisms may interact to diminish the lipolytic action of enzyme supplementation. Effects of treatment should be controlled by clinical signs, in particular body weight and consistency of faeces. If treatment is ineffective even in response to increased dosage, the diet should be modified with redistribution of the overall nutrient intake into five or six (smaller) meals (5). Medium-chain triglycerides (MCT) as replacement of dietary fat have an unpleasant taste and do not improve lipid absorption; we do not recommend them. If the combination of increased enzyme supplementation and decreased meal sizes does not improve symptoms and/or steatorrhoea, the compliance of the patient should be ascertained by estimating faecal chymotrypsin.

In the compliant patient, further increases of pancreatin doses in response to (partial) treatment failures are controversial. In particular, ultra-high dosage has been reported to cause colonic wall alterations in patients with cystic fibrosis (50,51). Although there is no evidence that similar complications may occur in chronic pancreatitis, we avoid continued administration of more than 75 kU of lipase per meal in refractory cases. Instead, we recommend testing of alternative approaches: thus, additional administration of gastric acid secretion inhibitors (H_2-blockers, proton pump inhibitors) may have remarkable effects in refractory patients (5,34), including children with cystic fibrosis (37,38).

Occasionally, particularly after previous gastrointestinal resections, intestinal infections with *Giardia lamblia*, bacterial overgrowth, blind loop syndrome or other intestinal absorption disorders may further compromise absorption and require specific medical or surgical intervention (Figure 1). Patients with gastric resections and/or a gastroenterostomy should be treated with pancreatin granule or powder preparations. Achlorhydric patients or patients on long-term acid-

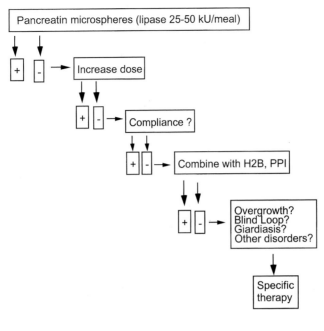

+ success
- failure

H2B: Histamine H_2 receptor antagonist
PPI: proton pump inhibitor

Figure 1. Algorithm for enzyme treatment of pancreatic exocrine insufficiency.

suppressing medication are treated with conventional unprotected pancreatin preparations.

Enzymes for Pain Therapy

Pancreatic enzyme treatment has also been proposed for treatment of pain in chronic pancreatitis even without malabsorption (52), with the rationale that a protease-dependent, negative feedback mechanism contributes both to the physiological regulation of pancreatic secretion in humans and to the pathogenesis of pain. Several, although not all, studies have provided evidence that under certain experimental conditions feedback regulation may occur (17,53–58). Therefore, it has been hypothesised that in chronic pancreatitis decreased intraduodenal protease activities may induce unphysiological stimulation of the residual pancreatic parenchyma, increase intraductal pressure proximal to intrapancreatic stenoses, and cause pain. Administration of proteases should in time decrease secretion, intraductal pressure, and pain (2,5). However, the feedback loop is induced only under extreme experimental conditions (17,55–58); moreover, administration of commercially available pancreatin extracts stimulate rather than suppress enzyme output in humans (59,60).

Therapeutic studies have also reported contradictory results. Whereas several controlled trials have found pain relief in a subset of responders (55,59,61), there was no effect in other studies including a large multicentre trial (62,63). Possibly, effects of enzymes other than feedback suppression of pancreatic function are responsible for the pain-relieving effects in individual patients, such as correcting unphysiological ileal brake mechanisms on motor and secretory functions in response to increased ileal nutrient delivery as discussed above (13,24,26,28–31,35).

New Developments

Due to major theoretical and practical advances within the past two decades, most patients with pancreatic insufficiency can now be treated satisfactorily. Further developments will aim to improve both ease and success of enzyme administration, particularly in refractory patients. Currently, a major therapeutic breakthrough might be expected from different lines of research.

Timing

Efficacy of porcine pancreatin micropellets can be further improved by optimising the timing of luminal enzyme delivery and release. Observations in patients with chronic pancreatitis suggest that fat digestion is increased following administration of pancreatin microspheres whose size is adjusted to that required for physiological prandial gastric emptying of solid nutrients, compared with microspheres of conventional size (23,64). Moreover, reduced protease contents of pancreatin preparations appear to increase luminal lipase survival and lipid absorption (17,22,65). Whether such modifications further decrease steatorrhoea under practical conditions is unclear.

Alternative Lipases

In the treatment of exocrine pancreatic insufficiency acidic and proteolytic degradation of endogenous and pancreatin lipase is a major limiting factor. In contrast to animal pancreatic lipases, certain bacterial and fungal lipases have additional pH optima in acidic milieu (66) and are resistant against acid proteolytic destruction. Commercially available fungal lipases improve steatorrhea, but are not superior to pancreatin preparations (66–69), possibly due to decreased activity in the presence of bile acids.

Under physiological conditions, lingual and gastric lipase activities probably contribute little to cumulative intestinal lipolytic activity in humans (2,10–13,70,71), but there is evidence that in certain patients with pancreatic insufficiency, gastric lipase outputs may be increased (11,12,72,73). Potential advantages of gastric lipase include its greater acid and protease stabilities, and it is therefore conceivable that the use of animal or bioengineered human gastric lipase preparations (74) may find a role in future enzyme replacement concepts.

Presumably, a variety of lipase preparations will be available for future treatment of pancreatic insufficiency. Thus, future utilisation of superior microbial sources (75) and/or molecular biological approaches (76) may provide more effective solutions.

Conclusion

New developments need to be scrutinised for potential long-term adverse effects. An ideal replacement therapy should restore the physiological situation in the lumen characterised by maximal digestion in the proximal gut and subsequent rapid decrease of lipolytic activity and digestion (9,13). Damage to the gastric and/or distal intestinal mucosa, by excessive luminal enzymatic activities in conjunction with unphysiologically increased generation of lipid digestion products, must be excluded.

Acknowledgement

The authors' studies cited in this chapter were supported by the German Research Foundation (DFG grants La 483/5–3 and 2–6).

References

1. DiMagno EP, Malagelada JR, Go VLW (1975) Relationship between alcoholism and pancreatic insufficiency. NY Acad Sci 252:200–207.
2. DiMagno EP, Layer P (1993) Human exocrine pancreatic enzyme secretion. In: Go VLW et al. (eds): The pancreas: biology, pathobiology, and diseases, 2nd edn. Raven Press, New York, pp 275–300.
3. Layer P, Yamamoto H, Kalthoff L, Clain JE, Bakken LJ, DiMagno EP (1994) The different courses of early- and late-onset idiopathic and alcoholic chronic pancreatitis. Gastroenterology 107:1481–1487.
4. DiMagno EP, Go VLW, Summerskill WHJ (1973) Relations between pancreatic enzyme outputs and malabsorption in severe pancreatic insufficiency. N Engl J Med 288:813–815.
5. DiMagno EP, Clain JE, Layer P (1993) Chronic pancreatitis. In: Go VLW et al. (eds): The pancreas: biology, pathobiology, and diseases, 2nd edn. Raven Press, New York, pp 665–706.
6. Layer P, Zinsmeister AR, DiMagno EP (1986) Effects of decreasing intraluminal amylase activity on starch digestion and postprandial gastrointestinal function in humans. Gastroenterology 91:41–48.
7. Layer P, Go VLW, DiMagno EP (1986) Fate of pancreatic enzymes during aboral small intestinal transit in humans. Am J Physiol 251:G475–G480.
8. Keller J, Rünzi M, Goebell H, Layer P (1997) Duodenal and ileal nutrient deliveries regulate human intestinal motor and pancreatic responses to a meal. Am J Physiol 272:G632–G637.
9. Layer P, von der Ohe MR, Holst JJ et al. (1997) Altered postprandial motility in chronic pancreatitis: role of malabsorption. Gastroenterology 112:1624–1634.
10. Sternby B, Holtmann G, Kelly DG, DiMagno EP (1990) Effect of gastric or duodenal nutrient infusion on gastric and pancreatic lipase secretion. Gastroenterology 102:A292
11. Hamosh M (1990) Lingual and gastric lipases. Nutrition 6:421–428.
12. Gargouri Y, Pieroni G, Riviere C et al. (1986) Importance of human gastric lipase for intestinal lipolysis: an *in vitro* study. Biochem Biophys Acta 879:419–423.
13. Layer P, Holtmann G (1994) Pancreatic enzymes in chronic pancreatitis (state-of-the-art). Int J Pancreatol 15:1–11.
14. Carriere F, Barrowman JA, Verger R, Laugier R (1993) Secretion and contribution to lipolysis of gastric and pancreatic lipases during a test meal in humans. Gastroenterology 105:876–888.
15. Layer P, Baumann J, Hellmann C, von der Ohe M, Gröger G, Goebell H (1990) Effect of luminal protease inhibition on prandial nutrient digestion during small intestinal chyme transit. Pancreas 5:718.

16. DiMagno EP, Malagelada JR, Go VLW, Moertel CG (1977) Fate of orally ingested enzymes in pancreatic insufficiency: comparison of two dosage schedules. N Engl J Med 296:1318–1322.

17. Layer P, Jansen JBMJ, Cherian L, Lamers CBHW, Goebell H (1990) Feedback regulation of human pancreatic secretion: effects of protease inhibition on duodenal delivery and small intestinal transit of pancreatic enzymes. Gastroenterology 98:1311–1319.

18. Kelly DG, Sternby B, DiMagno EP (1991) How to protect human pancreatic enzyme activities in frozen duodenal juice. Gastroenterology 100:189–195.

19. Holtmann G, Kelly DG, Sandberg RJ, Bentley KJ, Magocsi L, DiMagno EP (1991) Is the survival of human lipolytic activity (LA) during aboral transit affected by the amount of calories, nutrient, chymotrypsin (CT) or bile acid (BA) entering the duodenum? Gastroenterology 100:A276.

20. Granger M, Abadie B, Marchis-Mouren G (1975) Limited action of trypsin on porcine pancreatic amylase: characterization of the fragments. FEBS Lett 56:189–193.

21. Thiruvengadam R, DiMagno EP (1988) Inactivation of human lipase by proteases. Am J Physiol 255:G476–481.

22. Layer P, Hellmann C, Baumann J, von der Ohe M, Gröger G, Goebell H (1990) Modulation of physiologic fat malabsorption in humans. Digestion 46:153.

23. Layer P, von der Ohe M, Gröger G, Dicke D, Goebell H (1992) Luminal availability and digestive efficacy of substituted enzymes in pancreatic insufficiency. Pancreas 7:745

24. Stephen AM, Haddad AC, Phillips SF (1983) Passage of carbohydrate into the colon. Gastroenterology 85:589–595.

25. Levitt MD, Hirsh P, Fetzer CA, Sheahan M, Levine AS (1987) H_2 excretion after ingestion of complex carbohydrates. Gastroenterology 92:383–389.

26. Layer P, Peschel S, Schlesinger T, Goebell H (1990) Human pancreatic secretion and intestinal motility: effects of ileal nutrient perfusion. Am J Physiol 258:G196–G201.

27. Jain NK, Boivin M, Zinsmeister AR, DiMagno EP (1991) The ileum and carbohydrate mediated feedback regulation of postprandial pancreaticobiliary secretion in normal humans. Pancreas 6:495–505.

28. Layer P, Schlesinger T, Goebell H (1993) Modulation of periodic interdigestive gastrointestinal motor and pancreatic function by the ileum. Pancreas 8:426–432.

29. Read NW, McFarlane A, Kinsman RJ et al. (1984) Effect of infusion of nutrient solutions into the ileum on gastrointestinal transit and plasma levels of neurotensin and enteroglucagon. Gastroenterology 86:274–280.

30. Spiller RC, Trotman IF, Higgins BE et al. (1984) The ileal brake: inhibition of jejunal motility after ileal fat perfusion in man. Gut 25:365–374.

31. Jain NK, Boivin M, Zinsmeister AR, Brown ML, Malagelada JR, DiMagno EP (1989) Effect of perfusing carbohydrates and amylase inhibitor into the ileum on gastrointestinal hormones and gastric emptying of homogenized meal. Gastroenterology 96:377–387.

32. Layer P, Holst JJ, Grandt D, Goebell H (1995) Ileal release of glucagon-like-1 peptide (GLP-1): association with inhibition of gastric acid secretion in humans. Dig Dis Sci 40:1074–1082.

33. Layer P, von der Ohe M, Gröger G, Grandt D, Rünzi M, Goebell H (1995) Late postprandial motility changes in chronic pancreatitis: pathogenetic role of malabsorption. Gastroenterology 108:A368.

34. Regan PT, Malagelada JR, DiMagno EP, Glanzman SL, Go VLW (1977) Comparative effects of antacids, cimetidine, and enteric coating on the therapeutic response to oral enzymes in severe pancreatic insufficiency. N Engl J Med 297:854–858.

35. Layer P, Ohe MR, Grandt D et al. (1997) Altered postprandial motility in chronic pancreatitis: role of malabsorption. Gastroenterology (in press).

36. Heizer WD, Cleaveland CR, Iber FL (1965) Gastric inactivation of pancreatic supplements. Bull Johns Hopkins Hosp 116:261–270.

37. Carroccio A, Pardo F, Montalto G et al. (1992) Use of famotidine in severe exocrine pancreatic insufficiency with persistent maldigestion on enzymatic replacement therapy. Dig Dis Sci 37:1441–1446.

38. Heijerman HG, Lamers CB, Bakker W (1991) Omeprazole enhances the efficacy of pancreatin (pancrease) in cystic fibrosis. Ann Intern Med 114:200–210.

39. Goebell H, Klotz U, Nehlsen B, Layer P (1993) Oroileal transit of slow release 5-ASA. Gut 34:669–675.

40. Code CF, Schlegel JF (1973) The gastrointestinal interdigestive housekeeper: motor correlates of the interdigestive myoelectric complex of the dog. In: Daniel EE (ed) Proc 4th Int Symp on GI Motility. Mitchell Press, Vancouver, pp 631–634.

41. Schlegel JF, Code CF (1975) The gastric peristalsis of the interdigestive housekeeper. In: Vantrappen G (ed) Proc 5th Int Symp on GI Motility. Typoff Press, Leuven, pp 321.
42. Layer P, Gröger G, Dicke D, von der Ohe M, Goebell H (1992) Enzyme pellet size and luminal nutrient digestion in pancreatic insufficiency. Digestion 52:100.
43. Meyer JH, Ohashi H, Jehn D, Thomson JB (1981) Size of liver particles emptied from the human stomach. Gastroenterology 80:1489–1496
44. Meyer JH, Elashoff J, Porter-Fink V, Dressman J, Amidon GL (1988) Human postprandial gastric emptying of 1-3-millimeter spheres. Gastroenterology 94:1315–1325.
45. Kölbel C, Layer P, Hotz J, Goebell H (1986) Der Einfluss eines säuregeschützten, mikroverkapselten Pankreatinpräparats auf die pankreatogene Steatorrhö. Med Klin 81:85–86.
46. Lankisch PG, Lembcke B, Göke B, Creutzfeldt W (1983) Therapie der pankreatogenen Steatorrheo: Bietet der Säureschutz für Pankreasenzyme Vorteile? Verh Dtsch Ges Inn Med 89:864–867.
47. Dutta SK, Rubin J, Harvey J (1983) Comparative evaluation of the therapeutic efficacy of a pH-sensitive enteric-coated pancreatic enzyme preparation with conventional pancreatic enzyme therapy in the treatment of exocrine pancreatic insufficiency. Gastroenterology 84:476–482.
48. Hendeles L, Dorf A, Stecenko A, Weinberger M (1990) Treatment failure after substitution of generic pancrelipase capsules. Correlation with *in vitro* lipase activity. JAMA 263:2459–2461.
49. Caliari S, Benini L, Sembenini C, Gregori B, Carnielli V, Vantini I (1996) Medium-chain triglyceride absorption in patients with pancreatic insufficiency. Scand J Gastroenterol 31:90–94.
50. FitzSimmons SC, Burkhart GA, Borowitz D et al. (1997) High-dose pancreatic enzyme supplements and fibrising colonopathy in children with cystic fibrosis. N Engl J Med 336:1283–1289.
51. MacSweeney EJ, Oades PJ, Buchdahl R, Rosenthal M, Bush A (1995) Relation of thickening of colon wall to pancreatic-enzyme treatment in cystic fibrosis. Lancet 345:752–756.
52. Ihse I, Lilja P, Lundquist I (1977) Feedback regulation of pancreatic enzyme secretion by intestinal trypsin in man. Digestion 15:303–308.
53. Krawisz BR, Miller LJ, DiMagno EP, Go VLW (1980) In the absence of nutrient pancreatic-biliary secretions in the jejunum do not exert feedback control of human pancreatic or gastric function. J Lab Clin Med 95:13–18.
54. Hotz J, Ho SB, Go VLW, DiMagno EP (1983) Short-term inhibition of duodenal tryptic activity does not affect human pancreatic, biliary or gastric function. J Lab Clin Med 101:488–495.
55. Slaff J, Jacobson D, Tillmann CR, Curington C, Toskes PP (1984) Protease-specific suppression of pancreatic exocrine secretion. Gastroenterology 87:44–52.
56. Owyang C, Louie DS, Tatus D (1986) Feedback regulation of pancreatic enzyme secretion. Suppression of cholecystokinin release by trypsin. J Clin Invest 77:2042–2047.
57. Owyang C, May D, Louie DS (1986) Trypsin suppression of pancreatic enzyme secretion. Differential effect on cholecystokinin release and the enteropancreatic reflex. Gastroenterology 91:637–643.
58. Adler G, Reinshagen M, Koop I et al. (1989) Differential effects of atropine and a cholecystokinin receptor antagonist on pancreatic secretion. Gastroenterology 96:1158–1164.
59. Mössner J, Stange JH, Ewald M, Kestel W, Fischbach W (1991) Influence of exogenous application of pancreatic extract on endogenous pancreatic enzyme secretion. Pancreas 6:637–644.
60. Mössner J, Wresky HP, Kestel W, Zeeh J, Regner U, Fischbach W (1989) Influence of treatment with pancreatic extracts on pancreatic enzyme secretion. Gut 30:1143–1149.
61. Isaksson F, Ihse I (1983) Pain reduction by an oral pancreatic enzyme preparation in chronic pancreatitis. Dig Dis Sci 28:97–102.
62. Halgreen H, Thorsgaard Pedersen N, Worning H (1986) Symptomatic effect of pancreatic enzyme therapy in patients with chronic pancreatitis. Scand J Gastroenterol 21:104–108.
63. Mössner J, Secknus R, Meyer J, Niederau C, Adler G (1992) Treatment of pain with pancreatic extracts in chronic pancreatitis: results of a prospective placebo-controlled multicenter trial. Digestion 53:54–66.
64. Kühnelt P, Mundlos S, Adler G (1991) Einfluss der Pelletgrösse eines Pankreasenzympräparates auf die duodenale lipolytische Aktivität. Z Gastroenterol 29:417–421.
65. Layer P, von der Ohe M, Gröger G, Cherian L, Rolle K, Goebell H (1992) Intraluminal proteolytic degradation of lipase and fat malabsorption in pancreatin-treated pancreatic insufficiency. Pancreas 7:745.
66. Zentler Munro PL, Assoufi BA, Balasubramanian K et al. (1992) Therapeutic potential and clinical efficacy of acid-resistant fungal lipase in the treatment of pancreatic steatorrhoea due to cystic fibrosis. Pancreas 7:311–319.

67. Schneider MU, Knoll-Ruzicka ML, Domschke S, Heptner G, Domschke W (1985) Pancreatic enzyme replacement therapy: comparative effects of conventional and enteric-coated microspheric pancreatin and acid-stable fungal enzyme preparations on steatorrhea in chronic pancreatitis. Hepatogastroenterology 32:97–102.

68. Griffin SM, Alderson D, Farndon JR (1989) Acid resistant lipse as replacement therapy in chronic pancreatic exocrine insufficiency: a study in dogs. Gut 30:1012–1015.

69. Moreau J, Bousson M, Saint Marc Girardin MF, Pignal F, Bommelaer G, Ribet A (1988) Comparison of fungal lipase and pancreatic lipase in exocrine pancreatic insufficiency in man. Study of their *in vitro* properties and intraduodenal bioavailability. Gastroenterol Clin Biol 12:787–792.

70. Carriere F, Barrowman JA, Verger R, Laugier R (1993) Secretion and contribution to lipolysis of gastric and pancreatic lipases during a test meal in humans. Gastroenterology 105:876–888.

71. Abrams CK, Hamosh M, Dutta SK, Hubbard VS, Hamosh P (1987) Role of nonpancreatic lipolytic activity in exocrine pancreatic insufficiency. Gastroenterology 92:125–129.

72. Balasubramanian K, Zentler Munro PL, Batten JC, Northfield TC (1992) Increased intragastric acid-resistant lipase activity and lipolysis in pancreatic steatorrhoea due to cystic fibrosis. Pancreas 7:305–310.

73. Borel P, Armand M, Senft M, Andre M, Lafont H, Lairon D (1991) Gastric lipase: evidence of an adaptive response to dietary fat in the rabbit. Gastroenterology 100:1582–1589.

74. Bodmer MW, Angal S, Yarranton GT et al. (1987) Molecular cloning of a human gastric lipase and expression of the enzyme in yeast. Biochim Biophys Acta 909:237–244.

75. Suzuki A, Mizomutu A, Metzger A, Rerknimitr R, Sarr MG, DiMagno EP (1996) Can small amounts of lipolytic activity correct pancreatic steatorrhea and is this related to diet? Gastroenterology 110:A433.

76. Maeda H, Danel C, Crystal RG (1994) Adenovirus-mediated transfer of human lipase complementary DNA to the gallbladder. Gastroenterology 107:231–235.

20 Surgery in Chronic Pancreatitis

J.R. Izbicki, C. Bloechle, J.C. Limmer and W.T. Knoefel

Surgical treatment of chronic pancreatitis remains a major challenge. Most distressing for the patient and his relatives is the finding that, following the trauma and hazards of an operation, relief of symptoms, especially severe pain, has not been achieved. To the surgeon it is no less disturbing to realise that despite technical perfection, a time-consuming procedure has not benefited the patient as expected. Thus, the following main issues have to be considered carefully when surgical treatment of a patient suffering from chronic pancreatitis is planned.

First, the natural course of the disease must be weighted against any therapeutic intervention. Alternative treatment options such as endoscopic intervention and extracorporeal shock wave lithotripsy or the combination of the two should be considered. Second, there has to be proper patient selection including adequate indications and timing for any surgical intervention. Furthermore, the surgeon and the patient must define precisely what they expect as the outcome of an operation. Finally, the ideal procedure for a given individual must be chosen from a variety of operations described for surgical management of chronic pancreatitis. The rationale of an operation should be based on the pathogenesis of pain in chronic pancreatitis for which different hypotheses are proposed (1–3).

Based on studies on the natural history of chronic pancreatitis by Ammann and associates (4), it was hypothesised that eventually most patients will become pain free with progressive "burning out" of the pancreas. Therefore, a conservative approach has been proposed. However, a recently published study based on a larger population and observing a longer follow-up showed that reduction of pain did not occur in more than 50% of the patients while the disease progressed (5). The socioeconomic burden of the disease is closely related to recurrent disabling attacks of pain which cause periodic sick-leave and frequent hospitalisation (5). Considering the impact of the "burning out" process on the patient and society, therapeutic nihilism may not be the appropriate approach.

Whether surgery is superior to other treatments, and if so, which procedure, remains uncertain. Therefore all patients undergoing surgery for chronic pancreatitis should be assessed carefully before operation and during follow-up. This assessment should include examination of exocrine and endocrine pancreatic function, as well as proper estimation of pain intensity and quality of life (6,7).

Table 1. Therapeutic aims of surgery for chronic pancreatitis

1. Pain relief
2. Management of pancreatitis-associated complications of adjacent organs
3. Preservation of exocrine and endocrine pancreatic function
4. Social and occupational rehabilitation
5. Improvement of quality of life

Table 2. Indications for surgical intervention in chronic pancreatitis

1. Intractable pain of pancreatic origin
2. Pancreatitis-associated complications of adjacent organs
   Distal common bile duct obstruction
   Duodenal stenosis
   Segmental portal hypertension (?)
3. Pancreatic pseudocysts with ductal pathology which cannot be permanently managed by endoscopic interventions
4. Internal pancreatic fistula and pancreatic ascites
5. Pancreatic malignancy is not ruled out despite extensive diagnostic work-up
6. Progressive deterioration of the patient

Therapeutic Aims and Indications

Pain relief, management of pancreatitis-associated complications of adjacent organs, preservation of endocrine and exocrine function, as well as social and occupational rehabilitation are the aims of any therapeutic intervention in chronic pancreatitis. The ultimate goal, however, is the improvement of the patient's quality of life (Table 1).

Against this background intractable pain of pancreatic origin represents the most important indication for surgical intervention. Surgery is also indicated to treat complications related to adjacent organs such as distal common bile duct stenosis and segmental duodenal obstruction, pancreatic pseudocysts in conjunction with ductal pathology, and internal pancreatic fistula not amenable to conservative management (5,8–11). Segmental portal hypertension as an indication for surgery is controversial (12–17). Furthermore progressive decline and severe problems associated with enteral nutrition also present an indication for surgery. Occasionally, the inability to exclude pancreatic cancer despite broad diagnostic work-up requires an operation (18,19). The ideal surgical treatment concept should address all these problems (Table 2).

Recently, Nealon and Thompson (20) have drawn attention to the impact of timing of surgery on the natural course of chronic pancreatitis. In a two-part study including a large non-randomised, prospective investigation and a small randomised prospective trial, early operative drainage before the development of significant functional impairment was shown to delay progressive loss of pancreatic function.

Pathogenesis of Pain

Intraductal and Intraparenchymatous Hypertension

The assumption that pain in chronic pancreatitis is caused by ductal and/or parenchymatous hypertension is based upon three main observations. First, a considerable number of patients present with ductal dilatation as verified by per-cutaneous or endoscopic ultrasonography, computed tomography, and endo-scopic retrograde pancreatography. Second, several investigators have measured increased pancreatic ductal and parenchymatous pressures in patients suffering from chronic pancreatitis (1,21–23). Increased intrapancreatic pressures were shown to correlate with pain intensity (24,25). In experimental studies the image of a retroperitoneal compartment syndrome has been drawn to express the changes going along with intrapancreatic hypertension. In the presence of intra-pancreatic hypertension, reduced pancreatic blood flow and decreased intra-pancreatic pH-values were observed, especially following stimulation of exocrine pancreatic secretion (26). Finally, surgical decompression of ductal hyper-tension alleviates pain at least temporarily (19,27–29). The rationale of drainage procedure is based upon these observations.

Perineural Infiltration

An alternative hypothesis of the pathogenesis of pancreatic pain views chronic pancreatitis as a recurrent inflammatory process caused by defective healing after acute pancreatitis (3,30). Inflammatory masses develop featuring an increase of extracellular matrix and a decrease of pancreatic parenchyma. Concomitant peri-neural invasion of inflammatory cells causing the loss of perineural barrier func-tion have been observed (2). On this basis, resection has been favoured in the surgical treatment concept of chronic pancreatitis (16,31).

Surgical Procedures

Reflecting the hypotheses of pain origin in chronic pancreatitis – ductal hyper-tension (1) and perineural inflammation (2) – surgery for chronic pancreatitis is based on two main principles, i.e. drainage and resection. A variety of different procedures has been proposed emphasising one or the other.

In approximately two-thirds of patients with chronic pancreatitis ductal dilata-tion allows for a drainage procedure such as the Partington and Rochelle modification of a longitudinal pancreaticojejunostomy originally described by Puestow and Gillesby (29,32). In the remaining patients resection of different extent has been advocated (33–36). Irrespective of the width of the Wirsung duct approximately 90–95% of patients suffering from chronic pancreatitis that are being referred to surgery present with a problem located in the head of the pan-creas, i.e. proximal ductal alterations and/or the development of an inflammatory mass. Thus the head of the pancreas has been referred to as the pacemaker of the disease and frequently generates complications of adjacent organs, i.e. distal common bile duct stenosis and duodenal obstruction (16,37–39). In these patients, partial pancreatoduodenectomy, known as the Whipple procedure, represents the most commonly employed operative procedure. The sacrifice of otherwise undiseased organs, i.e. the distal stomach, duodenum, and common bile duct, is the major disadvantage of this procedure.

Duodenum-preserving resections of the pancreatic head, first introduced by Beger (40) and later described by Frey as a modification of the Partington and Rochelle procedure (41), have been promoted during the past decade. Duodenum-preserving resection of the head of the pancreas (31,40), includes subtotal resection of the pancreatic head following transection of the pancreas above the portal vein (Figure 1a). Even in the case of distal common bile duct stenosis or segmental duodenal obstruction, extensive resection will allow for decompression, while gastroduodenal passage and common bile duct continuity are preserved (37,42). Identification of the intrapancreatic course of the distal bile duct is facilitated by insertion of a metal probe into the duct through a proximal choledochotomy (43). The body of the pancreas is drained by an end-to-end or end-to-side pancreatojejunostomy using a Roux-en-Y loop. The same jejunal loop drains the resection cavity by an anastomosis to the rim of the resection cavity of the pancreatic head (Figure 1b).

A modified procedure communicated by Frey (23,41) combines a longitudinal pancreaticojejunostomy according to Partington and Rochelle (44) with a limited local excision of the pancreatic head (Figure 2a). This extended drainage procedure refrains from pancreatic transection above the portal vein. For reconstruction a longitudinal pancreatojejunostomy is employed to drain the resection cavity of the head, body, and tail of the pancreas (Figure 2b).

Most recently another extended drainage procedure has been described addressing the rare entity of sclerosing ductal pancreatitis referred to as small duct disease with maximal Wirsungian duct diameter < 3 mm (45). This operation features the longitudinal V-shaped excision of the ventral aspect of the pancreas combined with a longitudinal pancreatojejunostomy sewn to the edge of the organ. With this new procedure the role of distal pancreatectomy, which has until now been indicated only in sclerosing chronic pancreatitis limited to the pancreatic corpus and tail (36), will further be diminished.

Results of Surgery

In patients with ductal dilatation, i.e. ductal diameter > 7 mm, pain relief is achieved in 60–80% of cases by employing a traditional drainage procedure, i.e. Partington and Rochelle's longitudinal pancreaticojejunostomy (27,28). The advantage of this drainage operation is its low mortality and morbidity rates and the preservation of pancreatic function (Table 3). However, 20–40% of patients will not benefit from this kind of drainage operation (27–29). This has been the main argument in favour of classical resection procedures, such as partial pancreatoduodenectomy according to Whipple and lately pylorus-preserving pancreatoduodenectomy (PPPD) according to Longmire and Traverso. Even though these resections are nowadays performed with an acceptable mortality rate, they are still burdened by higher morbidity rates and a significant loss of pancreatic exocrine and endocrine function (Table 3).

Duodenum-preserving resection of the head of the pancreas has been shown to offer both reliable pain relief and the advantage of low mortality and acceptable morbidity with preservation of endocrine and exocrine function (9,31,37, 39,46,47). An alternative to duodenum-preserving pancreatic head resection has been extended drainage as described by Frey, which achieves substantial pain relief in 80–90% of patients (9,23,47). As depicted from data reported in the literature and recently shown by a prospective randomised trial, the results of the

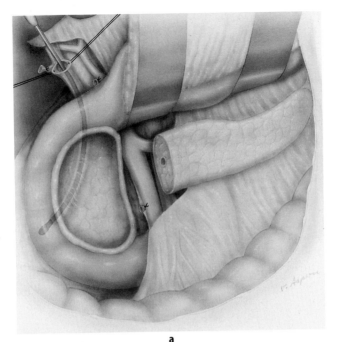

a

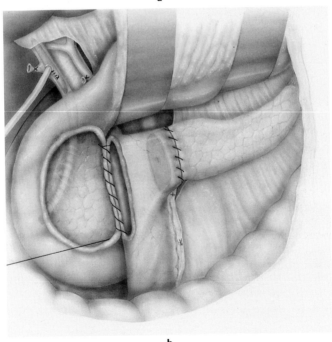

b

Figure 1. a Duodenum-preserving resection of the head of the pancreas as described by Beger. Through a proximal choledochotomy, a metal probe is inserted into the duodenum. **b** Reconstruction with an end-to-end pancreaticojejunostomy with the corpus and a side-to-side pancreatojejunostomy to the resection cavity of the pancreatic head. (Reprinted with permission of JP Lippincott-Raven.)

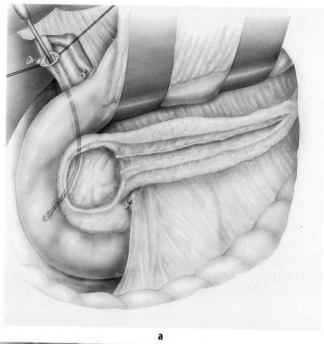

a

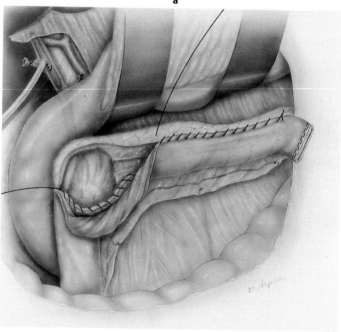

b

Figure 2. a Extended drainage operation including limited local excision of the pancreatic head as described by Frey. Through a proximal choledochotomy, a metal probe is inserted into the duodenum. **b** Reconstruction with a longitudinal side-to-side pancreaticojejunostomy. (Reprinted with permission of JP Lippincott-Raven.)

extended drainage operation of Frey, in terms of pain relief and management of pancreatitis-associated complications of adjacent organs, match the outcome achieved by Whipple resection (18,48), PPPD (16,49,50), and the Beger procedure (9,23,37,39,46,47). Within an intermediate follow-up period, preservation of pancreatic function, social and occupational rehabilitation, and improvement of quality of life were also shown to be more or less the same after the Frey and the Beger operations (9,47). However, the Frey procedure, which is technically easier, can be performed with significantly lower morbidity (Table 3). Preliminary results of our prospective randomised study comparing the Frey procedure with PPPD, which is currently being performed by the authors, confirm these findings (Tables 4–6).

Discussion

Current therapeutic options in operative treatment of chronic pancreatitis mainly address the symptoms and eventually evolving complications of the disease. A special problem is the presence of severe ductal alterations proximally to the papilla of Vater in the pancreatic head and the development of an inflammatory mass in the head of the pancreas, which has been discussed as the pacemaker of the disease (37). For patients with coexisting complications of adjacent organs partial pancreatoduodenectomy according to Whipple or PPPD according to Longmire and Traverso represent the most commonly employed surgical procedure. While it provides complete pain relief in up to 80% of patients (18), the procedure is burdened by high late morbidity and mortality rates (18,51–53). The removal of healthy adjacent organs seems not to be warranted in this benign disease.

On the other hand drainage procedures supposedly carry a lower morbidity and mortality rate, but fail to provide complete long-term pain relief in up to 60% of patients (54–56). Furthermore pancreatitis-associated complications of adjacent organs such as distal common bile duct obstruction and duodenal stenosis require additional bypass procedures (57,58), and carcinoma cannot definitively be ruled out (19).

Modern surgical treatment options such as Beger's duodenum-preserving resection of the head of the pancreas and Frey's extended drainage procedure, which combines longitudinal pancreaticojejunostomy with limited local pancreatic head excision, achieve reliable pain relief and allow definitive management of pancreatitis-associated complications of adjacent organs (40,41). The Beger procedure has been compared in a randomised trial with the classical Whipple procedure showing an advantage of the duodenum-preserving pancreatic head resection with regard to pancreatic function and occupational rehabilitation (48). In a randomised comparison between the Beger procedure and PPPD the former was concluded to be superior in terms of pain alleviation (16). This finding, however, is somewhat puzzling, as the extent of resection in both operations is similar. Thus it is difficult to understand why the preservation of the gastroduodenal passage and common bile duct continuity should cause better pain relief.

The experience with the modified technique described by Frey has so far been limited to the reports from the instituion where the procedure originated (23,41) and the authors' experience (9,47). It has been considered to be easier with regard

Table 3. Results of surgical drainage and resection for chronic pancreatitis

	Partington–Rochelle procedure			Frey procedure		Beger procedure			
	Prinz (27) (n = 86)	Adams (28) (n = 62)	Bassi (61) (n = 261)	Frey (23) (n = 50)	Izbicki (47) (n = 36)[a]	Büchler (39) (n = 298)	Büchler (16) (n = 20)[a]	Izbicki (47) (n = 38)[a]	Klempa (48) (n = 22)[a]
Pain relief or substantial alleviation	80%	65%	77%	75%	93%	88%	75%	95%	70%
Hospital morbidity	21%	6%	12%	22%	22%	29%	15%	32%	55%
Hospital mortality	0%	0%	0.3%	0%	0%	1%	0%	0%	5%
Late mortality	3%	0%	15%	4%	0%	9%	0%	3%	5%
Endocrine insufficiency	50%	23%	11%	11%	3%	2%	–	5%	10%
Exocrine insufficiency	34%	34%	–	11%	3%	–	–	5%	20%
Increase of body weight	–	–	–	64%	78%	81%	88%	89%	80%
Occupational rehabilitation	–	27%	–	32%	68%	63%	80%	74%	75%
Follow-up period (years)	1–24	3–17	5–25	2–9	0.5–4	1–22	0.5	0.5–4	3–5.5

Table 3. (*Continued*)

	Longmire–Traverso procedure (PPPD)			Whipple procedure	
	Büchler (16) (n = 20)[a]	Martin (49) (n = 45)	Stapleton (50) (n = 45)	Klempa (48) (n = 21)[a]	Saeger (18) (n = 111)
Pain relief or substantial alleviation	40%	93%	80%	67%	79%
Hospital morbidity	20%	36%	47%	57%	10%
Hospital mortality	0%	2%	0%	0%	1%
Late mortality	0%	2%	7%	5%	10%
Endocrine insufficiency	–	48%	37%	29%	39%
Exocrine insufficiency	–	79%	80%	95%	40%
Increase of body weight	67%	75%	100%	29%	77%
Occupational rehabilitation	67%	–	–	48%	66%
Follow-up period (years)	0.5	0.5–1.0	2–12	3–5.5	0.5–16

[a] Prospective randomised study.

Table 4. Management of pancreatitis-associated complications of adjacent organs: results of our randomised study comparing Beger's and Frey's operation[a]

	Preoperative		Follow-up[b]	
	Beger	Frey	Beger	Frey
Duodenal stenosis	4/38	3/36	0/38	0/36
Distal common bile duct stenosis	17/38	20/36	2/38[a]	2/36[a]

[a] Following Beger's operation one patient needed endoscopic drainage, in the remaining three patients reoperations were necessary.
[b] Median follow-up: 30 months (range: 6–48 months)

Table 5. Pain assessment – Results of our randomised study comparing Beger's and Frey's operation

	Beger's operation ($n = 38$)		Frey's operation ($n = 36$)	
Criterion	Preoperative (median)	Follow-up (median)	Preoperative (median)	Follow-up (median)
Visual pain analogue scale	80	12 ($P < 0.001$)	75	16 ($P < 0.001$)
Frequency of pain attacks	75	0 ($P < 0.001$)	75	0 ($P < 0.001$)
Pain medication	15	0 ($P < 0.001$)	17	0 ($P < 0.001$)
Inability to work	75	0 ($P < 0.001$)	75	0 ($P < 0.001$)
Pain score	61.25	3 ($P < 0.001$)	60.5	4 ($P < 0.001$)

Preoperative values are compared with follow-up values during a median follow-up of 30 months (range: 6–48 months): Wilcoxon rank-test.

Table 6. Quality of life – Results of our randomised study comparing Beger's and Frey's operation

	Beger ($n = 38$)		Frey ($n = 36$)	
Functional scale	Preoperative (median)	Follow-up (median)	Preoperative (median)	Follow-up (median)
Physical status	40.0	100 ($P < 0.01$)	40.0	100 ($P < 0.01$)
Working ability	50.0	100 ($P < 0.01$)	50.0	100 ($P < 0.01$)
Cognitive functioning	50.0	66.7 (ns)	50.0	66.7 (ns)
Emotional functioning	25.0	83.3 ($P < 0.01$)	33.3	91.7 ($P < 0.01$)
Global quality of life	33.3	83.3 ($P < 0.01$)	16.7	83.3 ($P < 0.01$)

Preoperative values are compared with follow-up values during a median follow-up of 30 months (range: 6–48 months): Wilcoxon rank-test.

to technical feasibility than Beger's procedure, in which resection is more extensive. Furthermore definitive control of associated complications involving adjacent organs has also been claimed to be provided by Frey's procedure (59). To evaluate the efficacy of both techniques of duodenum-preserving resection of the head of the pancreas, a prospective randomised trial was conducted (9).

While mortality rates were zero for both techniques, postoperative morbidity was significantly lower in patients who had undergone Frey's procedure (22% versus Beger group 32%). Both procedures provided permanent control of problems arising from associated complications of adjacent organs in the majority of patients. Furthermore, both techniques equally allowed histological verification of the diagnosis in the mass in the head of the pancreas. Thus none of the patients

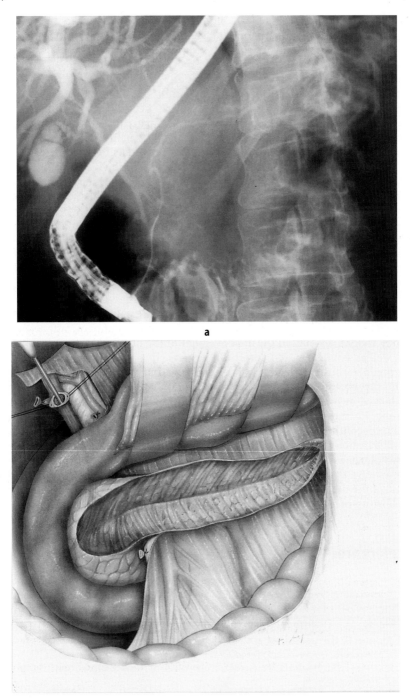

a

b

Figure 3. a Endoscopic retrograde cholangiopancreatography showing small duct disease with a Wirsungian ductal diameter of 2 mm in diffuse sclerosing chronic pancreatitis. **b** Longitudinal V-shaped excision of the ventral pancreas for diffuse sclerosing pancreatitis with narrowing of the main pancreatic duct. Through a proximal choledochotomy, a metal probe is inserted into the duodenum. (Reprinted with permission of JP Lippincott-Raven.)

with histopathological diagnosis of chronic pancreatitis turned out to have pancreatic carcinoma during follow-up. On the other hand pancreatic carcinoma was detected at operation in six patients despite extensive diagnostic work-up. This diagnostic problem, which has been reported previously (18,19), must be considered as another major drawback of any conservative treatment modality. Identification of pancreatic carcinoma while digging out the pancreatic head might be a problem since tumour spillage can occur. This risk must be weighed against the benefits of the procedure in 90% of patients without carcinoma.

In studies on chronic pancreatitis, analysis of pain has so far been done by rather gross scales (5,40,41). To quantify pain intensity more distinctly a pain score comprising a visual analogue scale of pain, frequency of pain attacks and pain-related sick-leave, as well as analgesic medication has recently been suggested (7). Pain, however, reflects only one aspect of sensitive and functional aspects of day-to-day living. Assessment of the quality of life by standardised psychometric measures, first introduced in the evaluation of outcome in cancer treatment (60), seems to be mandatory in evaluation of therapeutic strategies in chronic pancreatitis. Recently we have used the EORTC core quality of life questionnaire for patients with chronic pancreatitis (6,7). Further evaluation of the pancreatic cancer module described in Chapter 40, to determine its utility in chronic pancreatitis, is planned. Both procedures proved equally effective with regard to complete pain relief. In both groups the patients' overall quality of life increased considerably. Relief of symptoms, especially of pain, fatigue, and loss of body weight, accounted for improvement of the physical status, working ability, as well as emotional and social functioning. In the majority of patients neither procedure caused deterioration of exocrine and endocrine pancreatic function. This favourable result is reflected by the fact that occupational rehabilitation was achieved in 74% of patients in the Beger group and in 69% of patients in the Frey group. Furthermore, 69% of patients with chronic pancreatitis of alcoholic origin have discontinued drinking.

It has, however, to be mentioned, that the follow-up data of this study reflect only short-term results, i.e. within a median follow-up of 2.5 years. In order to determine the long-term efficacy of both procedures and to recommend either one of the duodenum-preserving resections of the head of the pancreas a longer follow-up of at least 5 years will be necessary.

References

1. Ebbehoj N, Svendsen LB, Madsen P (1984) Pancreatic tissue pressure in chronic obstructive pancreatitis. Scand J Gastroenterol 19:1066–1068.
2. Bockmann DE, Buechler M, Malfertheimer P, Beger HG (1988) Analysis of nerves in chronic pancreatitis. Gastroenterology 94:1459–1469.
3. Kloeppel G, Maillet B (1993) Pathology of acute and chronic pancreatitis. Pancreas 8:659–670.
4. Ammann RW, Akovbiantz A, Largiader F, Schueler G (1984) Course and outcome of chronic pancreatitis. Gastroenterology 86:820–828.
5. Lankisch PG, Happe-Loehr A, Otto J, Creutzfeldt W (1993) Natural course in chronic pancreatitis. Digestion 54:148–155.
6. Frey CF, Pitt HA, Prinz RA (1996) A plea for uniform reporting of patient outcome in chronic pancreatitis. Arch Surg 131:233–234.
7. Bloechle C, Izbicki JR, Knoefel WT, Kuechler T, Broelsch CE (1995) Quality of life in chronic pancreatitis: results after duodenum-preserving resection of the head of the pancreas. Pancreas 11:77–85.

8. Warshaw AL (1984) Pain in chronic pancreatitis: patients, patience, and the impatient surgeon. Gastroenterology 86:987–989.
9. Izbicki JR, Bloechle C, Knoefel WT, Kuechler T, Binmoeller KF, Broelsch CE (1995) Duodenum-preserving resections of the head of the pancreas in chronic pancreatitis. A prospective randomized trial. Ann Surg 221:350–358.
10. Taylor SM, Adams DB, Andersson MC (1991) Duodenal stricture: a complication of chronic fibrocalcific pancreatitis. South Med J 84:338–341.
11. Izbicki JR, Wilker DK, Waldner H, Rueff FL, Schweiberer L (1989) Thoracic manifestations of internal pancreatic fistulas: report of five cases. Am J Gastroenterol 84:265–271.
12. Warshaw AL, Jin G, Ottinger LW (1987) Recognition and clinical implications of mesenteric and portal vein obstruction in chronic pancreatitis. Arch Surg 122:410–415.
13. Frey CF, Suzuki M, Isaji S (1990) Treatment of chronic pancreatitis complicated by obstruction of the common bile duct or duodenum. World J Surg 14:59–69.
14. Bernades P, Baetz A, Lévy P, Belghiti J, Menu Y, Fékété F (1992) Splenic and portal venous obstruction in chronic pancreatitis. Dig Dis Sci 37:340–346.
15. Little AG, Moossa AR (1981) Gastrointestinal hemorrhage from left-sided portal hypertension. Am J Surg 141:153–158.
16. Büchler M, Friess H, Mueller MW, Wheatley AM, Beger HG (1995) Randomized trial of duodenum preserving pancreatic head resection versus pylorus preserving Whipple in chronic pancreatitis. Am J Surg 169:65–70.
17. Bloechle C, Busch C, Tesch C et al. (1997) Prospective randomized study of drainage and resection on non-occlusive segmental portal hypertension in chronic pancreatitis. Br J Surg 84:477–482.
18. Saeger HD, Schwall G, Trede M (1993) Standard Whipple in chronic pancreatitis. In: Beger HG, Buechler M, Malfertheimer P (eds) Standards in pancreatic surgery. Springer, Berlin Heidelberg New York, pp 385–391.
19. White TT, Hart MJ (1979) Pancreaticojejunostomy versus resection in the treatment of chronic pancreatitis. Am J Surg 138:129–134.
20. Nealon WH, Thompson JC (1993) Progressive loss of pancreatic function in chronic pancreatitis is delayed by main pancreatic duct decompression. Ann Surg 217:458–468.
21. Bradley EL (1982) Pancreatic duct pressure in chronic pancreatitis. Am J Surg 144:313–316.
22. Ebbehoj N, Borly J, Madsen P, Svendsen LB (1990) Pancreatic tissue pressure and pain in chronic pancreatitis. Pancreas 4:556–558.
23. Frey CF, Amikura K (1994) Local resection of the head of the pancreas combined with longitudinal pancreaticojejunostomy in the management of patients with chronic pancreatitis. Ann Surg 220:492–507.
24. Frey CF (1990) Why and when to drain the pancreatic ductal system. In: Beger HG, Buechler MW, Ditschuneit H, Malfertheiner P (eds) Chronic pancreatitis. Springer, Berlin Heidelberg New York, pp 415–425.
25. Limmer JC, Knoefel WT, Bloechle C, Izbicki JR (1996) Correlation between intraductal and intraparenchymatous pancreatic pressure and pain in chronic pancreatitis. Int J Pancreatol 19:237 (abstract).
26. Karanjia ND, Widdison AL, Leung F, Alvarez C, Lutrin FJ, Reber HA (1994) Compartment syndrome in experimental chronic obstructive pancreatitis: effect of decompressing the main pancreatic duct. Br J Surg 81:259–264.
27. Prinz RA, Greenlee HB (1981) Pancreatic duct drainage in 100 patients with chronic pancreatitis. Ann Surg 194:313–320.
28. Adams DB, Ford MC, Anderson MC (1994) Outcome after lateral pancreaticojejunostomy for chronic pancreatitis. Ann Surg 219:481–489.
29. Markowitz JS, Rattner DW, Warshaw AL (1994) Failure of symptomatic relief after panreatico-jejunal decompression for chronic pancreatitis. Arch Surg 129:374–380.
30. Keith RG, Keshavjee SH, Kerenyi NR (1985) Neuropathology of chronic pancreatitis in humans. Can J Surg 28:207–211.
31. Beger HG, Buechler M, Bittner R, Oettinger W, Roscher R (1989) Duodenum-preserving resection of the head of the pancreas in severe chronic pancreatitis. Ann Surg 209:273–278.
32. Puestow CB, Gillesby WJ (1958) Retrograde surgical drainage of pancreas for chronic pancreatitis. Arch Surg 76:898–906.
33. Whipple AO (1946) Radical surgery for certain cases of pancreatic fibrosis associated with calcareous deposits. Ann Surg 124:991–1006.
34. Frey CF, Child CG, Fry W (1976) Pancreatectomy for chronic pancreatitis. Ann Surg 184:403–413.

35. Traverso LW, Longmire WP (1978) Preservation of the pylorus in pancreaticoduodenectomy. Surg Gynecol Obstet 146:959–962.
36. Sawyer R, Frey CF (1994) Is there still a role for distal pancreatectomy in surgery for chronic pancreatitis? Am J Surg 168:6–9.
37. Beger HG, Buechler M (1990) Duodenum-preserving resection of the head of the pancreas in chronic pancreatitis with inflammatory mass in the head. World J Surg 14:83–87.
38. Büchler M, Malfertheiner P, Friess H, Beger HG (1993) Chronic pancreatitis with inflammatory mass in the head of the pancreas: a special entity? In: Beger HG, Buechler M, Ditschuneit H, Malfertheiner P (eds) Chronic pancreatitis. Springer, Berlin Heidelberg New York, pp 41–46.
39. Büchler MW, Friess H, Bittner R et al. (1997) Duodenum-preserving pancreatic head resection: long-term results. J Gastrointest Surg 1:13–19.
40. Beger HG, Krautzberger W, Bittner R, Buechler M, Limmer J (1985) Duodenum-preserving resection of the head of the pancreas in patients with severe chronic pancreatitis. Surgery 97:467–473.
41. Frey CF, Smith GJ (1987) Description and rationale of a new operation for chronic pancreatitis. Pancreas 2:701–707.
42. Izbicki JR, Bloechle C, Knoefel WT et al (1994) Complications of adjacent organs in chronic pancreatitis managed by duodenum-preserving resection of the head of the pancreas. Br J Surg 81:1351–1355.
43. Wilker DK, Izbicki JR, Knoefel WT, Geissler K, Schweiberer L (1990) Duodenum-preserving resection of the head of the pancreas in treatment of chronic pancreatitis. Am J Gastroenterol 85:1000–1004.
44. Partington PF, Rochelle RE (1960) Modified Puestow procedure for retrograde drainage of the pancreatic duct. Ann Surg 152:1037–1042.
45. Izbicki JR, Bloechle C, Broering DC, Kuechler T, Broelsch CE (1997) Longitudinal V-shaped excision of the ventral pancreas for small duct disease in severe chronic pancreatitis. Ann Surg (in press).
46. Buechler M, Friess H, Isenmann R, Bittner R, Beger HG (1993) Duodenum-preserving resection of the head of the pancreas: the Ulm experience. In: Beger HG, Büchler M, Malfertheimer P (eds) Standards in pancreatic surgery. Springer, Berlin Heidelberg New York, pp 436–449.
47. Izbicki JR, Bloechle C, Knoefel WT, Binmoeller KF, Soehendra N, Broelsch CE (1997) Drainage versus Resektion in der chirurgischen Therapie der chronischen Kopfpankreatitis: eine randomisierte Studie. Chirurgie 68:369–377.
48. Klempa I, Spatny M, Menzel J et al. (1995) Pankreasfunktion und Lebensqualität nach Pankreaskopfresektion bei der chronischen Pankreatitis. Chirurgie 66:350–359.
49. Martin RF, Rossi RL, Leslie KA (1996) Long-term results of pylorus-preserving pancreatoduodenectomy for chronic pancreatitis. Arch Surg 131:247–252.
50. Stapleton GN, Williamson RCN (1996) Proximal pancreatoduodenectomy for chronic pancreatitis. Br J Surg 83:1433–1440.
51. Trede M, Schwall G, Saeger HD (1990) Survival after pancreatoduodenectomy. Ann Surg 211:447–458.
52. Trede M, Schwall G (1988) The complications of pancreatectomy. Ann Surg 207:39–47.
53. Jalleh RP, Williamson RC (1992) Pancreatic exocrine and endocrine function after operations for chronic pancreatitis. Ann Surg 216:656–662.
54. Bradley EL (1987) Long-term results of pancreatojejunostomy in patients with chronic pancreatitis. Am J Surg 153:207–213.
55. Greenlee HB, Prinz RA, Aranha GV (1990) Long-term results of side-to-side pancreaticojejunostomy. World J Surg 14:70–76.
56. Frey CF, Suzuki M, Isaji S, Zhu Y (1989) Pancreatic resection for chronic pancreatitis. Surg Clin North Am 69:499–528.
57. Warshaw AL (1985) Conservation of pancreatic tissue by combined gastric, biliary, and pancreatic duct drainage for pain from chronic pancreatitis. Am J Surg 149:563–569.
58. Prinz RA, Aranha GV, Greenlee HB (1985) Combined pancreatic duct and upper gastrointestinal and biliary tract drainage in chronic pancreatitis. Arch Surg 120:361–366.
59. Frey CF, Leary BF (1993) Local resection of the head of the pancreas combined with longitudinal pancreaticojejunostomy: an update. In: Beger HG, Buechler M, Malfertheiler P (eds) Standards in pancreatic surgery. Springer, Berlin Heidelberg New York, pp 471–482.
60. Schipper H (1983) Why measure quality of life? Can Med Assoc J 128:1367–1369.
61. Bassi C, Falconi M, Caldiron E et al. (1997) Surgical drainage and bypass. In: Izbicki JR, Binmoeller KF, Soehendra N (eds) Chronic pancreatitis: an interdisciplinary approach. De Gruyter, Berlin, pp 127–133.

21 Pain Relief in Chronic Pancreatitis

Å. Andrén-Sandberg and J. Axelson

Pain is the cardinal symptom of chronic pancreatitis (1), and is, together with the usual accompanying alcoholism, the most difficult symptom to treat. For some patients with chronic pancreatitis pain is so severe that all their waking hours are devoted to pain control and the quality of life is low in every respect. As patients with chronic pancreatitis at the best can be symptom free, but never cured, the management of symptoms should be of prime concern in most pancreatitic patients. The pattern of pain changes with time, typically being recurrent and intermittent in the initial stages of the disease. Later it usually becomes persistent, but the characterstics of the pain may vary not only between patients but also in the same person from time to time (2).

Obstruction of the pancreatic duct seems to be a major factor in the pathogenesis of chronic pancreatitis, leading to increased ductal or interstitial pressure with local ischaemia and acidosis which generates pain. However, the relationship between morphological changes, ductal pressures and pain is very variable, and other factors must be implicated (3). Autodigestion with tissue necrosis and both pancreatic and peripancreatic inflammation in the earlier stages changes the focal release and uptake of mediators in the peptidergic nerves and could be an important cause of pain. The increased pressure from pseudocysts and other masses may contribute as well. Recently there has been evidence that there is scarring of the nerves in chronic pancreatitis with damage of the perineural sheet, which allows access of inflammatory mediators such as substance P and CGRP (calcitonin gene-related peptide) to the unprotected nerves (4). For the doctor caring for these patients, pain control is obviously a challenge where all the different options may be needed, including surgery.

Surgical Drainage Procedures

Surgical decompression of the obstructed main pancreatic duct is the gold standard against which other therapies should be measured (5). Drainage operations are today most often carried out as a side-to-side pancreaticojejunostomy which is clearly less hazardous than resections and which preserves pancreatic parenchyma. The procedures are based on the concept that ductal obstruction leads to distension and that this in turn gives rise to pain. Accordingly, any measure which improves drainage, either by improving flow into the duodenum or by allowing flow into the jejunum or stomach, might be expected to relieve pain. A technique for intraoperative as well as percutaneous measurement of pancreatic fluid pressure has been developed by Danish investigators. They found a close correlation between tissue pressure and pain in patients who underwent drainage operations for chronic pancreatitis. Postoperative reduction in pressure was followed by relief of pain whereas in patients with recurrent pain the pressure rose again (6). However, there are also a number of studies casting doubt on the relationship between pain in chronic pancreatitis and intrapancreatic pressure (7). One problem with the evaluation of the results of the operations is the different definitions of pain relief and the different follow-ups (8), but in spite of this it is obvious that not all patients will be pain free after technically well-performed drainage operations (7). It is widely accepted that the prospects for pain relief are poor if the pancreatic duct is not dilated, but even so, not all patients will experience pain relief (9,10). About 30% of patients with chronic pancreatitis fail to obtain long-lasting relief of pain (9,11).

For a long time a longitudinal pancreaticojejunostomy according to Partington and Rochelle, i.e. the duct of Wirsung opened from tail of pancreas to the duodenum and anastomosed to the side of the jejunum, has been one of the techniques that has been used most often (12). However, from the current literature it can only be stated that if obstructed parts of the pancreatic duct are left undrained the operation will fail to relieve pain, but provided this is not the case there is little evidence to favour one operative drainage procedure rather than another.

Pancreatic Resections

In the German-speaking countries pancreatic resections have been favoured during the past decade for pain relief in chronic pancreatitis, especially in patients with normal-sized ducts and masses of the head of the pancreas. In this setting, resection of the head, body, or tail regions of the pancreas with removal of varying amounts of parenchyma has been practised. These resections provide reasonably effective pain relief, but attendant immediate postoperative morbidity and long-term morbidity from insulin-dependent diabetes mellitus and post-gastrectomy sequelae detract significantly from the overall quality of life. Distal pancreatectomy has a very limited role in management of pain, and this procedure is associated with a good outcome only in patients with non-dilated pancreatic duct or pseudocyst involving the tail of the pancreas (13).

According to German authors, nearly 30% of patients with chronic pancreatitis develop inflammatory enlargement of the pancreatic head with subsequent obstruction of the pancreatic duct, and sometimes also of the common bile duct and duodenum. In these cases a pancreaticoduodenectomy, "Whipple procedure", has been the procedure of choice for a long time, despite an increase in the incidence of diabetes from about 20% preoperatively to about 60% in the years that follow (14). However, the long-term mortality rate and quality of life after this procedure in patients with chronic pancreatitis has not been encouraging, and in some studies disappointing (5).

To avoid these problems, the original type of pancreaticoduodenectomy has been substituted by the pylorus-preserving pancreaticoduodenectomy (PPPD) and the "Beger procedure". The techniques of standard ("Whipple") and pylorus-perserving resection are basically the same, except for the treatment of the antrum, pylorus and duodenum. The latter procedure, made popular by Traverso and Longmire (15), hoped to preserve normal gastric function and give unimpaired nutrition and prevent bile reflux gastritis. The more conservative procedure of Beger (16) resects the pancreatic head pathology but preserves all extrapancreatic organs including the duodenum. There has been one randomised trial comparing these two procedures (17) showing after 6 months follow-up that patients operated on according to Beger exhibited less pain. Moreover, they had a better preservation of insulin secretion and glucose tolerance, and more stable weight. These data suggest that in chronic pancreatitis as little as possible of extrapancreatic organs should be removed, which seems logical. However, the limited number of patients reported and lack of long-term follow-up preclude any definite conclusions as yet concerning the exact method to be recommended.

It should also be mentioned that there are numerous variations of the previously mentioned operations, the most interesting described by Frey in 1978 (18,19). He combined a coring out of the pancreatic head with a lateral pancreaticojejunostomy. In his own series of patients the pain relief after 5 years follow-up was complete or improved in 87% of cases, which is at least as good as any other procedure described so far. There is also one randomised series of patients comparing the techniques of Beger and Frey (20) where no difference in decrease of pain was found but there was less postoperative morbidity after the Frey method. However, long follow-up of a more substantial series of patients operated upon by independent surgeons is still lacking, which makes this method a good alternative at the present time.

Endoscopic Procedures

If decompression of the pancreatic duct is all that is needed in a majority of the patients with chronic pancreatitis it is tempting to try endoscopic procedures that are less demanding for both the patient and the doctor. However, it should be remembered that surgical sphincterotomy and sphincteroplasty already have proved to be less efficient (21,22), and that these procedures are hardly ever used nowadays. This might be due to the fact that it is unusual to find uniform dilatation of the pancreatic duct system resulting from localised obstruction at the orifice of the main duct (10,23). More recently, however, a number of endoscopic series have evolved that suggest an acceptable complication rate, particularly if undertaken in conjunction with stent placement or stone extraction.

Endocscopic stone extraction has been tried with and without mechanical lithotripsy, extracorporeal shockwave lithotripsy (ESWL), laser lithotripsy and with or without leaving of a stent through the pancreatic duct orifice. Placement of an endoprosthesis in the pancreatic duct is reported to give pain reduction in obstructive chronic pancreatitis (24) but stent occlusion and migration appear to be relatively common. With all modalities taken together it is usual to find a report of 80–90% complete stone clearance and good immediate pain relief (25). However, the long-term results in a larger series are not impressive so far. In a Belgian study Delhaye et al. (26) reported 123 patients, of whom only 60% experienced complete or partial pain relief during 14 months follow-up. Whether this is a good result – 60% pain free after a cheap procedure with few complications compared with open surgery – or a bad result – only 60% pain free patients compared with the usual 80–90% after operations according to Beger or PPPD – can be discussed. So far there has not been any randomised study to compare endoscopic and surgical procedures, and as long as the endoscopists have not yet put the final touches to their techniques or defined the indications for the procedures, it may not be fair to make randomised trials.

At present the endoscopic approach to patients with chronic pancreatitis is still "promising". It seems to be more useful in preventing relapsing attacks of pancreatitis as opposed to helping those with chronic pain (27), and maybe it can be used as an adjunct to choose the right patients for lateral pancreaticojejunostomy: if the patient is doing well with a stent, that has to be removed and changed at certain intervals, he will probably also do well with open surgery. However, it must be remembered that chronic pancreatitis is not the same as stones in the pancreatic duct, to be compared with symptomatic bile duct stones or ureterolithiasis, but is a disease primarily of the pancreatic parenchym a. Therefore it is unlikely that endoscopy could be a good alternative for more than a minority of these patients. But if this subset of patients can be well defined, great progress may have been made in the management of chronic pancreatitis.

Procedures Directed Against Nerves

Pain relief in patients with chronic pancreatitis can also be provided by means of simpler procedures directed against the afferent nerves that carry the painful stimuli from the diseased pancreas to the brain. The sympathetic innervation of the pancreas, including the nerves mediating pain, leaves from cells in the tractus intermediolateralis in the spinal cord from Th5 to Th11. The sympathetic fibers are led to the sympathetic chain and further by the nervus splanchnicus major (from Th5 to Th10) and one or more nervi splanchnici minor (from Th9 to Th11) to synapses in prevertebral abdominal plexi, passing first through the celiac ganglion. The postganglionic fibres pass along the arteries of the liver and spleen and the superior mesenteric artery into pancreatic tissue. Some sympathetic axons run directly to the pancreas without intra-abdominal synapses, mainly from the lower portion of the sympathetic chain (which may partly explain the limitation of pain control after surgical celiacectomy). From a theoretical point of view the pain can be inhibited by cutting the nerve fibres anywhere along these paths. The procedure most often tried is chemical blockage of the celiac ganglion, and a newer alternative is thoracoscopic splanchnicectomy.

Coeliac Ganglion Block

The coeliac block can be done during laparotomy (not taken into account here) or percutaneously, usually from the back. The placement of the injection can be done simply by using anatomical landmarks or by checking the position by fluoroscopy, scout X-ray films, ultrasonography, computed tomography, or angiography. A nerve block with 25 ml of 50% alcohol on each side should be preceded by a positive diagnostic block with long-acting local anaesthesia, carried out at least one day earlier. The method aims at blockage of the splanchnic nerves before they reach the coeliac plexus rather than blockage of more than part of the celiac plexus itself. There are several different ways to acertain that the needle tips and the fluid injected, respectively, are in the right place. The site of the needle can be documented with scout films (27). Theoretically more appealing, is to guide the injections of local anaesthetics (and later neurolytic agents) with fluoroscopy and contrast media in the injected fluid (28,29).

In a critical review Sharfman and Walsh in 1990 (30) analysed data from 15 series published from 1964 to 1983, including 480 patients, on coeliac plexus blocking in pancreatic patients. At least a satisfactory response to the procedure was reported in 87% of the patients. The authors claimed, however, that there were major deficiencies in the reporting of the results. In our practice the results of celiac block have been rather unpredictable, and as the pain tended to recur after about 3 months (10) we think that the indication for this procedure in chronic pancreatitis is at present limited.

Thoracoscopic Splanchnicectomy

As the sympathetic pain fibres are led via the sympathetic chain the stimulus can also be broken inside the thoracic cavity where the chain runs just subpleurally in a wave-like manner over each rib in the posterior part of the mediastinum and is easily seen at thoracoscopy (Figure 1). Thoracoscopic splachnicectomy can be performed bilaterally under general anaesthesia with double-lumen endotracheal intubation, making single lung ventilation possible. We have used only two ports on each side: one optical cannula (10.0 mm) and another 5.5-mm operating cannula. A small hole in the pleura on each side of a splanchnic nerve, 10 mm from the sympathetic chain, is burnt with the hook and the nerves are then cut off completely so that the ends are seen to be well retracted from each other. In uncomplicated cases the patient can be discharged from the hospital the day after the operation.

After a median follow-up time of 18 months the relief of pain stayed stable from the first postoperative week. All but one of the patients had clearly reduced pain, but only about 20% of the patients reported immediate complete pain relief. It is concluded that thoracoscopic splanchnicectomy appears as a promising and relatively simple treatment for severe chronic pancreatic pain (31). However, in all these patients the effect remains difficult to assess due to preoperative addiction to alcohol and strong analgesics, and thus it seems that the results in our prospectively followed group of patients would have been better if the patients had not been on strong drugs for a long time, and if the duration of the pain had been limited.

Conservative Treatment

Analgesic drugs are still the most commonly adopted method for pain relief, such as paracetamol, dextropropoxiphene, prednisolone, non-steroidal anti-inflammatory drugs, tricyclic antidepressants or narcotic analgesic drugs given orally or rectally, and opioids given subcutaneously or intrathecally (10). A problem is that due to the chronic nature of the pain many patients subsequently become addicted to narcotics. A major concept in prescription is therefore to

218

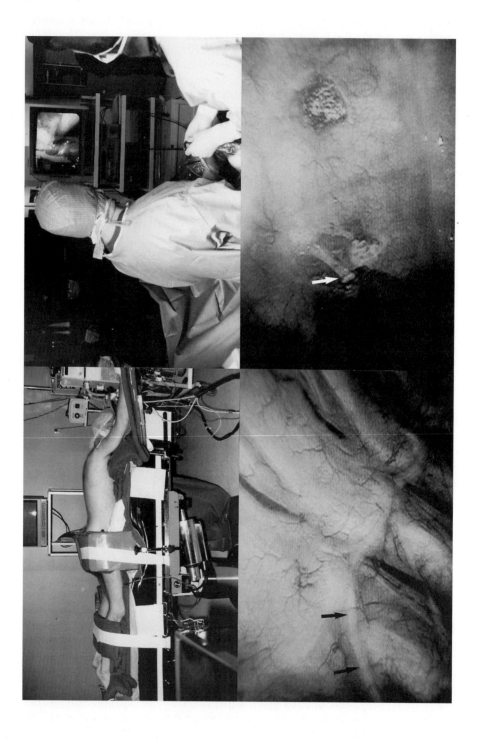

divide the analgesic treatment into three stages (32), the principal agent in each stage being paracetamol, dextropropoxiphen and morphine, and never to proceed to the next step without minute consideration of the short- and long-term effects of the escalation.

Enzymes

There are four studies supporting the pain-relieving effect of oral enzyme preparations in a proportion of patients with chronic pancreatitis (33–36). Thus, it might be worthwhile to give patients a therapeutic trial of enzyme supplements for 1–2 months, provided that a preparation known to increase intraduodenal trypsin activity is used (37).

Personal Experience

Compared with the published data from the large series of patients with chronic pancreatitis both from Europe and the USA the Scandinavian material regarding surgical interventions is always very small. In Lund hardly any patients have been subjected to resection for pain in chronic pancreatitis during the past 15 years – at the same time there have been some resections due to the suspicion of malignancy where the final diagnosis was chronic pancreatitis – and less than 10% of those presenting with morphological characteristics of chronic pancreatitis will ever have a lateral pancreaticojejunostomy. Our rate of major operations is therefore comparatively very low, but it seems that our patients are not doing any worse than those in other reviewed series (1,38).

We believe that the principal prerequisite to keep the surgical frequency low is to have a good personal contact with the patient on a regular basis, and to try to reach an agreement for cooperation between the chosen doctor and the patient. This may be hard if the patient is a drug addict or has severe alcoholic problems, but in such cases it makes no difference which medical or surgical management method is chosen, as the end result will be just as bad. However, if the patient has confidence in the doctor's management overall he or she will be able to withstand more pain without escalating the analgesics, and the treatment can be seen from a long-term perspective. Therefore, we think that continuity in the patient–doctor relationship is of the utmost importance in these patients.

It must be admitted that in Scandinavia the number of patients with chronic pancreatitis may be lower than, for example, in Germany. We very seldom see patients with a mass in the head of the pancreas, few of our patients have very severe pain and most of them are still working. On the other hand it is more

Figure 1. Aspects of the technique for thoracoscopic splanchnicectomy. Upper left: the patient is placed prone, with support beneath the epigastric and upper sternal regions to enable respiratory excursion of the chest walls. Upper right: a standard laparoscopy equipment was used. Lower left: inside the thoracic cavity the sympathetic chain (*arrows*) runs just subpleurally in a wave-like manner over each rib in the posterior part of the mediastinum. Lower right: the nerves are transected one by one along the sympathetic trunck. Each nerve is lifted up (*arrow*) and burnt with the diathermy hook. This is repeated down to the costophrenic recess.

Table 1. Pain relief after thoracoscopic splanchnicectomy as evaluated by a visual analogue scale

	Cancer			Chronic pancreatitis		
	n	Mean (SD)	Median	n	Mean (SD)	Median
Preoperatively	22	8 (1)	8	20	8 (2)	7
After 1 week	22	4 (1)	3	20	3 (3)	2
After 1 month	19	4 (2)	2	20	3 (3)	3
After 3 months	14	3 (1)	2	20	3 (2)	3
After 6 months	6	3 (2)	2	20	4 (2)	3
After 12 months	1	4	4	20	3 (2)	3
After 18 months	–			16	3 (2)	3
After 24 months	–			14	3 (2)	3

common to have a lower grade of pain over a long period of time, making a regular prescription of non-opioid analgesics necessary. We have found that it is wise to have an established relationship between the patient and the surgeon – not only with the general practitioner or gastroenterologist – for a long time before surgery. Maybe the patient's knowledge that he can have a pain-relieving operation quickly if really needed may postpone the operation.

However, there are also patients that certainly need surgical intervention. We think that a borderline is crossed if the patient needs morphine on a regular basis. After a renewed work-up of the patient to avoid missing a pancreatic pseudocyst, a duodenal ulcer, gallbladder disease or other extrapancreatic pathological process, we see thoracoscopic splanchnicectomy as a first choice in most cases as the results are good enough and the procedure does not preclude other interventions later on if needed. If pain relief is not achieved, open surgery would be considered where, if the right prerequisites are present, a longitudinal pancreaticojejunostomy would be the first choice.

Towards the Year 2000

Patients with established chronic pancreatitis do not present with a uniform pattern for the stage of the disease (early or late), the extrapancreatic, secondary symptomatology or the morphological features. This also influences the pattern of pain and the outcome of the attempts of management not only of the symptoms but of the patient as a whole.

A stepwise escalation of pain-relieving drugs also seems to be the first cornerstone in the future, together with information aimed at involvement of the patients in the treatment. However, it may be wise to consider alternative methods rather than to cross the borderline to narcotics. Today thoracoscopic splanchnicectomy seems to be a good option, but its precise role will be better defined in the next few years. In patients with morphological signs of pancreatic disease, such as strictures of the main pancreatic duct near to the duodenum, possible to treat with surgical means, an endoscopically placed stent may be tried. However, the place of this procedure in the armament against pain in chronic pancreatitis must be more carefully evaluated and compared with the present options, if possible in randomised studies. If the stenting proves to be successful, a surgical drainage procedure should be considered as a more lasting procedure, i.e. a procedure that usually gives pain relief for several years provided alcohol abuse is suspended (9).

Surgery in patients with severe pain due to chronic pancreatitis can be performed with low morbidity and without mortality today. However, the indications for section are still not defined versus drainage operations and therefore this type of surgery should, if possible, be performed only in centres dedicated to the scientific follow-up of all patients – operated and not operated upon – for at least 5 years (8).

It is obvious that long-term results in chronic pancreatitis come from an appraisal of the individual's situation, and that the treatment must be tailored to the patient as well as to the disease. The prognosis also depends on the attitude of the patient and may depend more on drinking habits than on the medical and surgical management.

References

1. Lankisch PG (1993) Natural course in chronic pancreatitis. Pain, exocrine and endocrine pancreatic insufficiency and prognosis of the disease. Digestion 54:148–55.
2. Ihse I (1990) Pancreatic pain: causes, diagnosis, and treatment. Acta Chir Scand 156:257–259.
3. Leahy AL, Carter DC (1991) Pain and chronic pancreatitis. Eur J Gastroenterol Hepatol 3:425–433.
4. Bockman DE, Büchler M, Malfertheiner P, Beger HG (1988) Analysis of nerves in chronic pancreatitis. Gastroenterology 94:1459–1469.
5. Eckhauser FE, Knol JA, Mulholland MW, Colletti LM (1996) Pancreatic surgery. Curr Opin Gastroenterol 12:448–456.
6. Ebbehöj N, Borly L, Bulow J, Grönvall Rasmusson S, Madsen P (1990) Evaluation of pancreatic tissue fluid pressure and pain in chronic pancreatitis: a longitudinal study. Scand J Gastroenterol 25:462–466.
7. Carter DC (1993) Surgical procedures in chronic pancreatitis. In: Tred M, Carter DC (eds) Surgery of the pancreas. Churchill Livingstone, Edinburgh, pp 309–319.
8. Lankisch PG, Andrén-Sandberg Å (1993) Standards for the diagnosis of chronic pancreatitis and for the evaluation of treatment. Int J Pancreatol 14:205–212.
9. Holmberg JT, Isaksson G, Ihse I (1985) Long-term results in pancreaticojejunostomy in chronic pancreatitis. Surg Gynecol Obstet 160:339–346.
10. Ihse I, Borch K, Larsson J (1990) Chronic pancreatitis: results of operations for relief of pain. World J Surg 14:53–58.
11. Prinz RA, Aranha GV, Greenlee HB (1986) Redrainage of the pancreatic duct in chronic pancreatitis. Am J Surg 151:150–156.
12. Andrén-Sandberg Å, Hafström A (1996) Partington-Rochelle: when to drain the pancreatic duct and why. Dig Surg 13:109–112.
13. Rattner DW, del Castillo F, Warshaw AL (1996) Pitfalls of distal pancreatectomy for relief of pain in chronic pancreatitis. Am J Surg 171:142–146.
14. Rossi RL, Rothschild J, Braasch JW, Munson JL, ReMine SG (1987) Pancreatoduodenectomy in the management of chronic pancreatitis. Arch Surg 122: 416–420.
15. Traverso LW, Longmire WP (1978) Preserving of the pylorus in pancreaticduodenectomy. Surg Gynecol Obstet 146:959–962.
16. Beger HG, Krautzberger W, Bittner R, Büchler M (1989) Duodenum-preserving resection of the head of the pancreas in severe pancreatitis. Surg Gynecol Obstet 209:273–276.
17. Büchler MW, Friess H, Müller MW, Wheatley AM, Beger HG (1995) Randomized trial of duodenum-preserving pancreatic head resection versus pylorus-preserving Whipple in chronic pancreatitis. Am J Surg 169:65–70.
18. Frey CF, Smith GJ (1987) Description and rationale of a new operation for chronic pancreatitis. Pancreas 2:701–707.
19. Frey CF, Amikura K (1994) Local resection of the head of the pancreas combined with longitudinal pancreatojejunostomy in the management of patients with chronic pancreatitis. Ann Surg 220:492–507.

20. Izbicki JR, Bloechle C, Knoefel WT, Kuechler T, Binmoeller KF, Broelsch CE (1995) Duodenum-preserving resection of the head of the pancreas in chronic pancreatitis: a prospective, randomized trial. Ann Surg 221:350–358.

21. Dreiling DA, Greenstein RJ (1979) State of the art: the sphincter of Oddi, sphincterotomy and biliopancreatic disease. Am J Gatroenterology 72:665–670.

22. Bagley FH, Brasch JW, Taylor RH, Warren KW (1981) Sphincterotomy or sphincteroplasty in the treatment of pathologically mild chronic pancreatitis. Am J Surg 141:418–421.

23. Moossa AR (1987) Surgical treatment of chronic pancreatitis: an overview. Br J Surg 74:661–667.

24. Burdich SJ, Hogan WJ (1991) Chronic pancreatitis: selection of patients for endoscopic therapy. Endoscopy 23:155–160.

25. Martin RF, Hanson BL, Bosco JJ et al. (1995) Combined modality treatment of symptomatic pancreatic duct lithiasis. Arch Surg 130:375–380.

26. Delhaye M, Vandermeeren A, Baize M, Cremer M (1992) Extracorporeal shock-wave lithotripsy of pancreatic calculi. Gastroenterology 102:610–620.

27. Kozarek RA (1993) Endoscopic therapy in chronic pancreatitis. In: Beger HG, Büchler M, Malfertheiner P (eds) Standards in pancreatic surgery. Springer Berlin Heidelberg New York, pp 332–346.

28. Bengtsson M, Löfström JB (1990) Nerve block in pancreatic pain. Acta Chir Scand 156:285–291.

29. Hegedüs V (1979) Relief of pancreatic pain by radiography-guided block. AJR 133:1101–1103.

30. Jackson SH, Jacobs JB (1969) A radiographic approach to celiac ganglion block. Radiology 92:1372–1373.

31. Sharfman WH, Walsh TD (1990) Has the analgesic efficacy of neurolytic celiac plexus block been demonstrated in pancreatic cancer pain? Pain 41:267–271.

32. Andrén-Sandberg Å, Zoucas E, Lillo-Gil R, Gyllstedt E, Ihse I (1996) Thoracoscopic splanchnicectomy for chronic, severe pancreatic pain. Semin Laparosc Surg 3:29–33.   .

33. Hollender LF, Laugner B (1993) Pain-relieving procedures in chronic pancreatitis. In: Trede M, Carter DC (eds) Surgery of the pancreas. Churchill Livingstone, Edinburgh, pp 349–357.

34. Isaksson G, Ihse I (1983) Pain reduction by an oral pancreatic enzyme preparation in chronic pancreatitis. Dig Dis Sci 28:97–102.

35. Slaff J, Jacobson D, Tillman CR, Curington C, Toskes P (1984) Protease-specific suppression of pancreatic secretion. Gastroenterology 87:45–52.

36. Rämö OJ, Poulakkainen PA, Seppälä K, Schröder TM (1989) Self-administration of enzyme substitution in the treatment of exocrine pancreatic insufficiency. Scand J Gastroenterol 24:688–692.

37. Malesci A, Gaia E, Fioretta A, Bocchia P, Ciravegna G, Cantor P, Vantini I (1995) No effect of long-term treatment with pancreatic extracts on recurrent abdominal pain in patients with chronic pancreatitis. Scand J Gastroenterol 30:392–398.

38. Ihse I, Permert J (1990) Enzyme therapy and pancreatic pain. Acta Chir Scand 156:281–283.

39. Amman RW (1993) Quality control following surgery for chronic pancreatitis. In: Beger HG, Büchler M, Malfertheiner P (eds) Standards in pancreatic surgery. Springer Berlin Heidelberg New York, pp 496–508.

22 The Lithostathine/PAP Family

J.-C. Dagorn

Lithostathine and the pancreatitis-associated protein (PAP) belong to the same family of proteins. Several research groups have contributed independently to the description of these proteins, starting from different tissues and different species including human, rat, mouse, dog and cow. Therefore, several names have appeared in the literature for each protein. Identities were discovered later, when cDNA sequences had been obtained and submitted to data banks for comparison. As a result, there is presently no consensus on the nomenclature of the family. Before entering into a description of structural and functional properties of the proteins, the duplications will be recapitulated through a brief historical perspective.

Concerning lithostathines, the first member to be reported was actually named the pancreatic stone protein (PSP) (1), because it was the major protein constituent of calcium carbonate stones characteristic of chronic pancreatitis. It was later shown that PSP was in fact a secretory protein present in normal pancreatic juice. Because it was an inhibitor of calcium carbonate crystal growth (2), its name was changed to lithostathine (3). The same protein was found expressed in regenerating islets (but not in quiescent islets) by the group of Okamoto (4) and was named Reg protein. Finally, Gross et al. (5) described in human pancreatic extracts the pancreatic thread protein (PTP), which is a fragment of lithostathine. Hence, lithostathine/PSP, Reg and PTP are the same protein.

Concerning PAPs, the first description of a pancreatitis-associated protein was made in the rat pancreas (6). It was independently found in the pituitary and named p23 (7). More recently, the group of Bréchot (8) localised the protein to hepatocarcinoma cells, intestine and pancreas and named it HIP.

For the sake of clarity, in this chapter lithostathine will be used for lithostathine/PSP/Reg/PTP, and PAP for PAP/p23/HIP.

Protein Structure

Lithostathine

One of the two human lithostathines (lithostathine 1) is the only protein of the lithostathine/PAP family for which thorough structural information is available. Sequence of the cDNA revealed that the preprotein comprised 166 amino acids, including a signal peptide of 22 amino acids. The mature protein has a protein backbone of 144 amino acids. However, SDS-PAGE analysis of lithostathine purified from pancreatic juice revealed four bands, corresponding to apparent molecular weights (Mr) ranging from 16 to 21 kDa (lithostathines S2 to S5) (9). Those isoforms were attributed to glycosylation. A single glycosylation site was found, on a threonine in position 5. Structure of the glycan was established (10). Progressive loss of sugars from the glycan tree accounts for the different Mr observed. That loss involving sialic acids also accounts for differences in pI observed for the four secretory forms of lithostathine.

One of the major secretory isoforms (lithostathine S3) could be purified to homogeneity. It was crystallised and submitted to X-ray analysis in order to establish its three-dimensional structure with a resolution of 1.55 Å (11). The carboxy-terminal end of the protein showed a tight globular structure maintained by three disulphide bridges, with three helices and six β strands. By contrast, the N-terminal peptide, up to position 13, remained very flexible.

An Arg-Ile bond, at position 11–12 of that peptide was found to have particular importance. Located near the junction of the flexible and globular parts of the molecule, it is highly susceptible to trypsin-like hydrolysis that generates a shorter form called lithostathine S1 (Mr 14 kDa) and the N-terminal undecapeptide. In fact, most juice samples contain some lithostathine S1 in addition to lithostathine S2-5, usually 2–10% depending on the conditions of juice collection. In the case of uncontrolled activation of juice, that proportion may be much higher.

At neutral pH, lithostathine S2-5 is soluble up to a concentration of several mg/ml, but whether it is monomeric or oligomeric in juice is unknown. Contrary to lithostathine S2-5, the S1 form is soluble at acidic pH only; around neutrality, it will aggregate and eventually form fibrils. Those fibrils were the material from which the pancreatic thread protein was described and PTP is in fact the S1 form of lithostathine. In pancreatic stones, lithostathine was also found under the S1 form (PSP).

PAP

The primary structure of PAP was obtained from the sequence of its cDNA (12). The major difference with lithostathine is a five amino acid insertion and lack of glycosylation. Therefore, PAP appears on SDS-PAGE as a single band with a Mr of 17 000. The three-dimensional structure of PAP is not yet reported. It is probably similar to that of lithostathine because the relative positions of the six cysteines are the same and the N-terminal undecapeptide is also easily released by very mild trypsin hydrolysis.

Other Homologies

Lithostathine/PAP sequences were compared with sequences available in data banks. The most interesting finding was a significant homology with calcium-dependent lectins. Amino acid clusters corresponding to the consensus carbohydrate recognition domain (CRD) could be localised and the proteins were classified as a new family among the lectin superfamily (group VII of free CRD lectins) (13). However, crystallographic data on lithostathine showed that the three-dimensional organisation of the CRD was peculiar, compared with other lectins, which may explain why the corresponding carbohydrate ligands, if any, remain unknown.

Gene Structure and Organization

Molecular analysis of the lithostathine/PAP genes and search for additional members of the family was conducted in human, rat and mouse. Two lithostathines and one PAP have been described so far in humans (14), whereas two additional PAPs were reported in rats and mice (15–16). In all cases, the genes have a similar organisation, in six exons and five introns and are located to the same chromosomal cluster. In humans, the three genes are located within 95 kilobases on chromosome 2 (2p12) (14).

Significant homology was observed among nucleotide sequences of the coding regions, which extended to the promoter regions of the genes. Analysis of homologies among protein sequences deduced from nucleotide sequences revealed important similarities among the proteins. In humans, for instance, lithostathine 2 and PAP show respectively 85% and 63% amino acid identities with lithostathine 1. Altogether, these data suggest that members of the lithostathine/PAP family derived from a single ancestor gene. As a consequence, it is possible that these proteins share functional properties, structural variations accounting for different specificities.

Expression in Physiological and Pathological Conditions

Most studies were conducted on lithostathine 1 and PAP1 because the other members of the family were described only recently and appropriate molecular tools were not always available.

Tissue Distribution

Lithostathine 1 and PAP1 are present in various tissues. The two proteins are often coexpressed, although not with the same intensities. Their expression can be constitutive or become significant only after induction.

The site of most abundant lithostathine 1 synthesis is the exocrine pancreas. The protein is expressed in acinar cells and accounts for about 5% of secretory protein. It is not found in duct cells. Lithostathine 1 is not expressed in quiescent pancreatic islets. However, its expression is induced during islet regeneration (17). Lithostathine 1 is also expressed to significant levels in Paneth cells of the intestine (18), and in the kidney, in epithelial cells from the ascending limb of the Henle's loop and proximal tubule (19). Discrete expression was also observed in the normal brain (20).

PAP1 is constitutively expressed in Paneth cells and some goblet cells of the small intestine, with a gradient from duodenum to jejunum (21). It is also present in pituitary cells (7) and luminal epithelial cells of the uterus (22). In normal pancreas, PAP1 is absent from duct cells and barely detectable in acinar cells. When the pancreas is submitted to a stress, such as during acute pancreatitis, PAP1 expression increases rapidly and can reach several hundred times the basal expression (23).

Regulation of Expression

Changes in lithostathine 1 expression were reported in various diseases. An increase was observed during pancreatic inflammation (12–24) and in brain (20), also possibly in relation with inflammation, because the protein was found associated with the protein tangles characteristic of Alzheimer's disease and Down syndrome. The most spectacular overexpression was reported in islets during regeneration (17). There is one example of down-regulation: in patients with chronic calcifying pancreatitis and in alcoholics without evidence of pancreatic disease, lithostathine 1 expression in pancreas was decreased by 60% (12–26). Variations in PAP1 expression are often rapid and important. The most remarkable change occurs in pancreas after induction of acute experimental pancreatitis (23). Maximum increase in mRNA concentration, which can reach 400 times, is observed after 24 hours. At the end of the acute phase, return to normal takes 2–4 days to be completed. PAP1 expression can also be affected by physiological stimuli. In the intestine, expression is very low in the starving rat and increases dramatically upon feeding (27). In the uterus, PAP1 expression is maximum during oestrus and absent from the immature rat uterus (22). It could be induced by oestrogen in oophorectomized animals.

These findings suggest that the promoters of the gene family contain peculiar domains that allow rapid and strong expression, especially in response to stress. The only promoter of the family whose topology has been analysed in detail is the promoter of rat PAP1. Stepwise deletions of the promoter region were inserted upstream from a reporter gene and transfected into cell lines of pancreatic and non-pancreatic origins. Elements conferring pancreas-specific expression, and TNFα and IL-6 response were localised (28,29). This provided a structural basis for the behaviour of PAP1 as an acute phase reactant. It also allowed an understanding of why PAP1 was expressed in hepatocarcinoma cells and not in hepatocytes, after demonstration that cancerous cells had lost the suppressor controlling tissue-specific expression (30).

Function of Lithostathine and PAP

Like many biological fluids, normal pancreatic juice is supersaturated with $CaCO_3$. Because lithostathine was found to be specifically associated with $CaCO_3$ stones, the protein was suspected of participating in the control of $CaCO_3$ crystal growth in juice. *In vitro* studies demonstrated that the S2–5 forms of lithostathine 1 inhibited crystal growth (2) and morphological studies on crystals gave indications on the molecular mechanism of inhibition (31). The S1 form had lost its activity, possibly because it was not soluble at neutral pH. Lithostathine 1 was shown to be the only pancreatic protein with inhibitory capacity. Also, presence of lithostathine in kidney tubules, where $CaCO_3$ supersaturation has been demonstrated, suggests that it may help stabilise primitive urine (19). The protein might therefore be involved in the control of urinary lithogenesis, since epitaxial growth of calcium oxalate crystals onto $CaCO_3$ crystals was observed (32). However, expression of lithostathine in tissues where there is apparently no need for such activity suggests that the protein may have additional functions. A role in the promotion of islet regeneration was proposed (17), but remains a matter of debate (33). Lithostathine S1 was also found to be mitogenic for pancreatic β cells and ductal cell lines, suggesting a paracrine effect (34).

PAP1, more than lithostathine 1, has an expression pattern typical of a stress protein, although originating as a secretory protein. Regarding pancreatic expression, its activity should therefore be sought within the secretory pathway, in the ducts or in the intestine, but no report on that subject is presently available. On the other hand, it was recently reported that PAP1 could induce the adhesion of hepatocytes and bind to extracellular matrix proteins (35). The lectin domain of the protein might be involved, as suggested by experiments showing that PAP1 could induce bacterial aggregation (27). Additional information is clearly required before unifying hypotheses on lithostathine 1 and PAP1 functions can be put forward.

Clinical Relevance of Lithostathine 1 and PAP1

Lithostathine and Chronic Calcifying Pancreatitis (CCP)

Chronic calcifying pancreatitis is characterised by the occurrence in pancreatic ducts of protein plugs that undergo secondary calcification. Lithostathine involvement in the disease was suggested because it could inhibit $CaCO_3$ crystal growth (2) and was also the major protein constituent of stones (1). Demonstration that pancreatic expression of the protein was decreased to the same extent in patients with CCP and in chronic alcoholics without pancreatic disease (25) indicated that underexpression of the protein was not the *primum movens* of the disease. However, it might be a determinant in its development. In conditions where a trypsin-like activity would appear in pancreatic juice, the lithostathine S1 form would be rapidly produced. That form is insoluble and aggregates in the form of fibrils. It might constitute the primary plugs, in agreement with the finding of lithostathine 1 as the almost exclusive protein constituent of stones. A similar mechanism might occur in hereditary pancreatitis, characterised by large protein plugs with peripheral calcification. In that disease, a mutation in the cationic trypsinogen gene conferring resistance of cationic trypsin to the pancreatic secretory trypsin inhibitor has been described (36) and lithostathine seems to be the main constituent of the protein plugs (J.P. Bernard, personal communication).

The PAP1 Promoter

Analysis of the PAP1 gene promoter suggested that it might be of potential interest in the development of new therapeutic strategies. This promoter allows a low level of gene expression in pancreas and strong stimulation in response to pancreatic injury (23). If the expression of a given protein could be beneficial to the damaged pancreas, it might be of therapeutic benefit to deliver its gene to the pancreas, under the control of the PAP1 promoter. The gene would be silent in normal conditions and become overexpressed in response to a stress. This was attempted by inserting into the adenovirus genome a construct with the chloramphenicol acetyl transferase (CAT) gene as reporter, under the control of the PAP1 promoter. The recombinant virus was injected in rats and expression of the CAT gene was monitored (37). In normal conditions, low expression was observed in the exocrine pancreas and background expression was observed in other tissues. Upon induction of pancreatitis, no stimulation was observed except in pancreas where it was severe. Hence, addressing to the pancreas exogenous genes that need to be expressed in response to stress is possible.

Serum Assay of PAP1

Demonstration that PAP1 induction was correlated with the severity of pancreatic injury (38) suggested that PAP1 might be a marker of pancreatic damage. PAP1 being a secretory protein, it should leak into blood with the enzymes that are presently monitored during acute pancreatitis (e.g. amylase, lipase). However, unlike the enzymes, PAP1 levels synthesised by the healthy pancreas are very low. It should therefore be a more specific marker of the disease.

Several applications have been reported. In the follow-up of acute pancreatitis, serum PAP1 concentrations were shown to increase during development of the

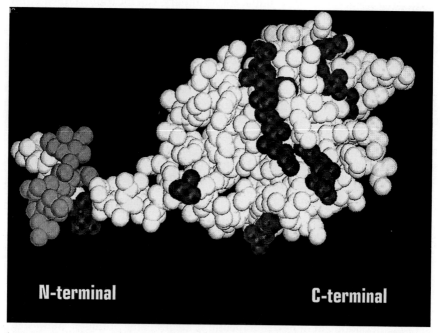

Figure 1. Ball and stick representation of human lithostathine, obtained by X-ray crystallography (11). The N-terminal end of the molecule protrudes from the globular C-terminal moiety. The Arg_{11}-Ile_{12} bond forms a hinge between the two regions, which may explain why it is easily split to generate the S1 form of lithostathine. Flexibility of the N-terminal peptide requires low-temperature crystallography to stabilize its structure and allow data collection. *Dark balls* represent acidic amino acids; they form a patch on the outside of the C-terminal portion of lithostathine, whose negative charges could be involved in binding to calcium ions on the surface of $CaCO_3$ crystals. *Grey balls* represent sugars, borne by the N-terminal peptide. Sequence homology between lithostathine and PAP suggests that their three-dimensional structures are similar.

acute phase and decrease during recovery, allowing prediction of the evolution of the disease (39). However, selection at admission of patients with mild acute pancreatitis on the basis of normal serum PAP1, also observed in the previous study, was not confirmed when the more sensitive commercial assay was used (40). Monitoring serum PAP1 was also found helpful in the follow-up of patients with pancreatic transplantation as a marker of graft rejection (41). In celiac disease, patients in the florid phase had elevated serum PAP1 and that level decreased to normal after the disease had been controlled by gluten-free diet (42). Whether elevated serum PAP reflected pancreatic damage associated with the disease or the intestinal damage *per se* is unknown. Finally, a pilot study showed that PAP1 assay in newborns might be useful for neonatal screening of cystic fibrosis (43). In that disease, the pancreas is already damaged *in utero*. PAP1 synthesis is triggered before birth and cystic fibrosis newborns have elevated blood PAP1.

Conclusion

The lithostathine/PAP family comprises three to five members, depending on the species. All of them are secretory proteins. They are localised in various tissues, the pancreas and the intestinal tract being the major sites of expression. Knowledge of their function(s) is limited. However, because their expression is often enhanced in stress conditions, they might participate in important regulatory or defence pathways.

References

1. De Caro A, Lohse G, Sarles H (1979) Characterization of a protein isolated from pancreatic calculi of men suffering from chronic calcifying pancreatitis. Biochim Biophys Acta 87:1176–1182.
2. Bernard JP, Adrich Z, Montalto G et al. (1992) Inhibition of nucleation and growth of calcium carbonate by lithostathine. Gastroenterology 103:1277–1284.
3. Sarles H, Dagorn JC, Giorgi D, Bernard JP (1990) Renaming pancreatic stone protein as lithostathine. Gastroenterology 99:900–901.
4. Terazono K, Yamamoto H, Takasawa S et al. (1988) A novel gene activated in regenerating islets. J Biol Chem 263:2111–2114.
5. Gross J, Carlson RJ, Brauer AW, Margolies MN, Warshaw AL, Wands JR (1985) Isolation, characterization and distribution of an unusual pancreatic human secretory protein. J Clin Invest 76:2115–2126.
6. Keim V, Rohr G, Stockert HG, Haberich FJ (1984) An additional secretory protein in the rat pancreas. Digestion 29:242–249.
7. Katsumata N, Chakraborty C, Myal Y, et al. (1995) Molecular cloning and expression of peptide 23, a growth hormone-releasing hormone-inducible pituitary protein. Endocrinology 136:1332–1339.
8. Lasserre C, Christa L, Simon MT, Vernier P, Bréchot C (1992) A novel gene (HIP) in human primary liver cancer. Cancer Res 52:5089–5095.
9. Montalto G, Bonicel J, Multigner L, Rovery M, Sarles H, De Caro A (1986) Partial amino acid sequence of human pancreatic stone protein, a novel pancreatic secretory protein. Biochem J 238:227–232.
10. De Reggi M, Capon C, Gharib B, Wieruszeski JM, Michel R, Fournet B (1995) The glycan moiety of human pancreatic lithostathine. Eur J Biochem 230:503–510.
11. Bertrand JA, Pignol D, Bernard JP, Verdier JM, Dagorn JC, Fontecilla-Camps JC (1996) Crystal structure of human lithostathine, the pancreatic inhibitor of stone formation. EMBO J 15:2678–2684.

12. Orelle B, Keim V, Masciotra L, Dagorn JC, Iovanna JL (1992) Human pancreatitis-associated protein. Messenger RNA cloning and expression in pancreatic diseases. J Clin Invest 90:2284–2291.

13. Dusetti NJ, Frigerio JM, Keim V, Dagorn JC, Iovanna JL. (1993) Structural organization of the gene encoding the rat pancreatitis-associated protein. Analysis of its evolutionary history reveals an ancient divergence from the other carbohydrate-recognition domain-containing proteins. J Biol Chem 268:14470–14475.

14. Miyashita H, Nakagawara K, Mori M et al. (1995) Human REG family genes are tandemly ordered in a 95-kilobase region of chromosome 2p12. FEBS Lett 377:429–433.

15. Narushima Y, Unno M, Nakagawara K et al. (1997) Structure, chromosomal localization and expression of mouse genes encoding type III Reg, Reg IIIα, Reg IIIβ, RegIIIγ. Gene 185:159–168.

16. Stephanova E, Tissir F, Dusetti NJ, Iovanna JL, Szpirer J, Szpirer C (1996) The rat genes encoding the pancreatitis-associated protein I, II and III (PAP1, PAP2, PAP3) and the lithostathine/pancreatic stone protein/regeneration protein (Reg) colocalize at 4q33 → q34. Cytogenet Cell Genet 72:83–85.

17. Unno M, Itoh T, Watanabe T et al. (1992) Islet Beta-cell regeneration and *reg* genes. Adv Exp Med Biol 321:61–66.

18. Lechene de la Porte P, De Caro A, Lafont H, Sarles H (1986) Immunocytochemical localization of pancreatic stone protein in the human digestive tract. Pancreas 1:301–308.

19. Verdier JM, Dussol B, Casanova P et al. (1992) Evidence that human kidney produces a protein similar to lithostathine, the pancreatic inhibitor of $CaCO_3$ crystal growth. Eur J Clin Invest 22:469–474.

20. Ozturk M, de la Monte S, Gross J, Wands JR (1989) Elevated levels of an exocrine pancreatic secretory protein in Alzheimer's disease brain. Proc Natl Acad Sci USA 86:419–423.

21. Masciotra L, Lechene de la Porte P, Frigerio JM, Dusetti NJ, Dagorn JC, Iovanna JL (1995) Immunohistochemical localization of pancreatitis-associated protein in human small intestine. Dig Dis Sci 40:519–524.

22. Chakraborty C, Vrontakis M, Molnar P et al. (1995) Expression of pituitary peptide 23 in the rat uterus: regulation by estradiol. Mol Cell Endocrinol 108:149–154.

23. Iovanna JL, Orelle B, Keim V, Dagorn JC (1991) Messenger RNA sequence and expression of rat pancreatitis-associated protein, a lectin-related protein overexpressed during acute pancreatitis. J Biol Chem 266:24664–24669.

24. Giorgi D, Bernard JP, Rouquier S, Iovanna J, Sarles H, Dagorn JC (1989) Secretory pancreatic stone protein messenger RNA: nucleotide sequence and expression in chronic calcifying pancreatitis. J Clin Invest 84:100–106.

25. Bernard JP, Barthet M, Gharib B et al. (1995) Quantification of human lithostathine by high performance liquid chromatography. Gut 36:630–636.

26. Mariani A, Mezzi G, Malesci A (1995) Purification and assay of secretory lithostathine in human pancreatic juice by fast protein liquid chromatography. Gut 36:622–629.

27. Iovanna JL, Keim V, Bosshard A et al. (1993) PAP, a pancreatic secretory protein induced during acute pancreatitis, is expressed in rat intestine. Am J Physiol 265:G611–G618.

28. Dusetti NJ, Ortiz EM, Dagorn JC, Iovanna JL (1995) Identification of a transcriptional regulatory region in the rat pancreatitis-associated protein 1 (PAP1) gene that confers tissue specificity Biochem J 311:643–647.

29. Dusetti NJ, Ortiz EM, Mallo GV, Dagorn JC, Iovanna JL (1995) Pancreatitis associated protein 1 (PAP1), an acute phase protein induced by cytokines. Identification of two functional interleukin-6 response elements in the rat PAP1 promoter region. J Biol Chem 270:22417–22421.

30. Dusetti NJ, Montalto G, Ortiz EM, Masciotra L, Dagorn JC, Iovanna JL (1996) Mechanism of PAP I gene induction during hepatocarcinogenesis: clinical implications. Br J Cancer 74:1767–1775.

31. Geider S, Baronnet A, Cerini C et al. (1996) Pancreatic lithostathine as a calcite habit modifier. J Biol Chem 271:26302–26306.

32. Geider S, Dussol B, Nitsche S et al. (1996) Calcium carbonate crystals promote calcium oxalate crystallization by heterogenous or epitaxial nucleation: possible involvement in the control of urinary lithogenesis. Calcif Tissue Int 59:33–37.

33. Smith FE, Bonner-Weir S, Leahy JL et al. (1994) Pancreatic Reg/pancreatic stone protein (PSP) gene expression does not correlate with beta-cell growth and regeneration in rats. Diabetologia 37:994–999.

34. Zenilman ME, Magnuson TH, Swinson K, Egan J, Perfetti R, Shuldiner AR (1996) Pancreatic thread protein is mitogenic to pancreatic-derived cells in culture. Gastroenterology 110:1208–1214.

35. Christa L, Carnot F, Simon MT et al. (1996) HIP/PAP is an adhesive protein expressed in hepato-carcinoma, normal Paneth and pancreatic cells. Am J Physiol 271:G993–1002.

36. Whitcomb DC, Gorry MC, Preton RA et al. (1996) Hereditary pancreatitis is caused by a mutation in the cationic trypsinogen gene. Hum Genet 14:141–145.

37. Dusetti NJ, Vasseur S, Ortiz EM, Romeo H, Dagorn JC, Iovanna JL (1997) The pancreatitis-associated protein 1 promoter allows targeting to the pancreas of a foreign gene whose expression is up-regulated during pancreatic inflammation. J Biol Chem 272:5800–5804.

38. Keim V, Willemer, Iovanna JL, Adler G, Dagorn JC (1994) Rat pancreatitis-associated protein is expressed in relation to the severity of experimental acute pancreatitis. Pancreas 9:606–612.

39. Iovanna JL, Keim V, Nordback I et al. (1994) Serum levels of pancreatitis-associated protein as indicators of the course of acute pancreatitis. Gastroenterology 106:728–734.

40. Kemppainen E, Sand J, Puolakkainen P et al. (1996) Pancreatitis-associated protein as an early marker of acute pancreatitis. Gut 39:675–678.

41. van der Pijl JW, Boonstra JG, Barthellemy S et al. (1997) Pancreatitis-associated protein: a putative marker for pancreas graft rejection. Transplantation 63:995–1003.

42. Carroccio A, Iovanna JL, Iacono G et al. (1997) Pancreatitis-associated protein in patients with coeliac disease. Serum levels and immunocytochemical localization in small intestine. Digestion 58:98–103.

43. Iovanna JL, Férec C, Sarles J, Dagorn JC (1994) The pancreatitis-associated protein (PAP). A new candidate for neonatal screening of cystic fibrosis. CR Acad Sci III 317:561–564.

Section 4

Endocrine–Exocrine Reactions

23 Diabetes Mellitus and Exocrine Pancreatic Disease

P.D. Hardt and H.-U. Kloer

The exocrine and endocrine pancreas are linked very closely anatomically and physiologically. It has been well recognised in the past that pathological conditions in the exocrine tissue can cause impairment of endocrine function and vice versa. Pancreatic diseases which might cause diabetes mellitus include acute and chronic pancreatitis (including the malnutrition-related tropical forms), pancreatic surgery, haemochromatosis, cystic fibrosis and pancreatic cancer. Impairment of exocrine function and pancreatic morphology in diabetic patients is frequent and well known. Several "classical" theories have been postulated to explain exocrine damage in diabetics. Atrophy of exocrine tissue might be due to a lack of trophic insulin, pancreatic fibrosis could be a result of angiopathy, or neuropathy could lead to impaired exocrine regulation. However, these theories did not fully explain the situation and some newer findings have to be taken into consideration.

Definition, Prevalence and Pathophysiological Concepts in Diabetes Mellitus

Definition and Prevalence

Diabetes mellitus is a syndrome of impaired glucose metabolism. It is characterised by a "chronic and substantial elevation of the circulating glucose concentration as a minimal defining characteristic" (1) and can be caused by different pathological conditions and aetiologies. The main clinical classes are insulin-dependent diabetes mellitus (IDDM), 15–25% of cases and non-insulin-dependent diabetes mellitus (NIDDM), which is present in 75–85% (2). There is a high variation in the prevalence of diabetes mellitus between different ethnic groups which is reported to be 0–50% (3). In Western countries the prevalence of NIDDM is about 5–7% (4,5). There seems to have been an increase in incidence and an increase in age during the last decades: 8% of persons aged 65 years are reported to have diabetes mellitus compared with 17% of those between 65 and 74 years (6).

Pathophysiological Concepts

In about 90% of patients IDDM is believed to be due to autoimmune destruction of the β cells, which might develop because of an interaction of inherited disposition and environmental factors. Suspect gene loci are the human leucocyte antigen class II gene and the insulin gene (7). Environmental factors include neonatal exposure to cow's milk protein (8) and nitrosamine exposure (9), autoimmunity might develop because of impaired HLA-expression induced by viral infections (10). IDDM can also be found in pancreatic disease (pancreatic cancer, pancreatitis, surgery) and in other endocrine diseases (acromegaly, Cushing's syndrome). NIDDM is a heterogeneous syndrome. Genetic factors are more important than in IDDM (e.g. glucokinase mutations in maturity onset diabetes of the young). A factor of great importance is obesity (thrifty genotype theory) (11), another environmental factor seems to be malnutrition *in utero* (thrifty phenotype theory) (12). Different conditions might result in insulin resistance of muscle and liver, glucose toxicity and a β cell defect. Other circumstances which can cause NIDDM include diabetogenic drugs, pregnancy, endocrine and pancreatic disease.

Changes of the Exocrine Pancreas in Diabetes Mellitus

Morphological Changes

In diabetic patients, the pancreas is smaller than in healthy controls, mainly due to involution of exocrine parenchyma (13). Acinar fibrosis and pancreatic atrophy have been reported in maturity-onset diabetics (14). Atrophy including diminution of pancreatic size, fatty infiltration, fibrosis and loss of acinar cells were described in juvenile-onset diabetes (15). The changes in exocrine tissue seem to be more pronounced in IDDM and they correlate inversely with C peptide concentrations in NIDDM (13). About 50% of diabetics are reported to have pancreatic fibrosis, and pathological findings of exocrine tissue are twice as frequent as in controls (16).

Functional Changes

Impaired exocrine pancreatic function in IDDM has been reported by different investigators, most of them performing the secretin-pancreozymin test. Impairment of exocrine secretion was reported in 43–80% (Table 1). There seems to be no correlation between the degree of exocrine insufficiency and the duration of the diabetes (21).

Table 1. Impaired exocrine secretion in IDDM

Author	Year of publication	n	% Impaired function
Pollard et al. (17)	1943	13	61.5
Chey et al. (18)	1963	47	55
Vacca et al. (19)	1964	22	73
Frier et al. (20)	1976	20	80
Lankisch et al. (21)	1982	53	43

Table 2. Impaired exocrine function in NIDDM

Author	Year of publication	n	% Impaired function
Chey et al. (18)	1963	13	15.4
Vacca et al. (19)	1964	33	73

Table 3. Faecal concentrations of elastase 1 and chymotrypsin in diabetics (Hardt et al. unpublished data)

Test	n	Impaired function	Insufficiency
Elastase 1	128	46.1% ($< 200\ \mu g/g$)	28.9% ($< 100\ \mu g/g$)
Chymotrypsin	124	44.7% ($< 6\ U/g$)	21.1% ($< 3\ U/g$)

Table 4. Faecal elastase 1 (E1) concentrations in IDDM, NIDDM, healthy controls and non-pancreatic gastrointestinal disease (NPGD) (Hardt et al. unpublished data)

	n	Mean age	E1 $< 200\ \mu g/g$	E1 $< 100\ \mu g/g$
IDDM	39	50.2 years	74.1%	43.6%
NIDDM	77	63.8 years	36.4%	19.5%
Controls	78		2.6%	
NPGD	68		16.2%	

Information about exocrine function in NIDDM is contradictory. While some authors found almost normal function (22), exocrine insufficiency was described by others (Table 2).

Our group has investigated exocrine pancreatic function in diabetics by indirect tests: 128 diabetic patients (83 men mean age 59.6 years) were asked to fill out a questionnaire and their stool samples were analysed for faecal elastase 1 (E1) and chymotrypsin concentrations. Impairment of exocrine function was present in similar members bychymotrypsin and elastase 1 measurements (Tables 3 and 4).

Another recently performed study investigated 436 diabetic patients from general practitioners (Wagner et al, unpublished data). Impaired exocrine function (E1 $< 200\ \mu g/g$) was found in 59% of IDDM ($n = 87$) and in 59% of NIDDM patients ($n = 349$). Exocrine insufficiency (E1 $< 100\ \mu g/g$) was reported in 40% and 43%. According to these data and the literature, there can be no doubt that pancreatic exocrine changes and diabetes mellitus occur very often in the same patients. The results for IDDM patients correspond well with those reported in the literature as mentioned above. Exocrine dysfunction in NIDDM seems to be less frequent than in IDDM but is much more common than in controls and non-pancreatic gastrointestinal disease.

Pathophysiological Concepts for Exocrine Dysfunction in Diabetes Mellitus

The following hypotheses have been discussed in the past to explain these findings:

- Insulin has a trophic effect on pancreatic acinar tissue (23), and its lack might cause pancreatic atrophy.
- Islet hormones have regulatory functions for exocrine tissue; these might be impaired in diabetes (24).
- Autonomic neuropathy might lead to impaired enteropancreatic reflexes and exocrine dysfunction (25).
- Diabetic angiopathy might cause arterial lesions and lead to pancreatic fibrosis and exocrine atrophy (16,19).
- Elevated levels of other islet hormones, resulting from changes in the islets of Langerhans, might lead to depression of exocrine function. Chronic glucagon elevation – as found in diabetes – can contribute to atrophy and exocrine dysfunction (26–28). Somatostatin, which inhibits exocrine secretion, is elevated in streptozotocin-diabetic rats (29).
- Diabetic acidosis might induce mild pancreatitis (30).

All these concepts do not give a satisfactory explanation for the very frequent changes of the exocrine pancreas in diabetes: if insulin deficiency were the main reason for exocrine dysfunction in diabetes mellitus, why do not all IDDM patients suffer from it? How should exocrine dysfunction be explained in NIDDM in the absence of autonomic neuropathy? If angiopathy was the main reason, why are the changes independent of the duration of diabetes?

Other pathogenic concepts try to explain combined exocrine and endocrine disorders as a result of one pathological process affecting the organ as a whole or a primary process in the exocrine tissue. Viral infections might lead to destruction of exocrine and endocrine tissue simultaneously (31). Autoimmune disease could affect the whole gland. Autoantibodies against exocrine tissue (anti-cytokeratin-autoantibodies) have been reported in diabetics: autoimmune aggression towards islets might be started by exocrine disease (32,33). Islet cell antibody 69 (ICA69), which was believed to be islet-specific, is also expressed in the exocrine pancreas and exocrine tissue might be involved in the autoimmune disease (34). TGFβ1 overexpression can induce pancreatitis in an animal model and can trigger diabetes mellitus together with TNFα (35). Regenerating gene (*reg*) product, known to correlate with changes in β cell mass and function, is primarily a product of the exocrine pancreas (36). Exocrine disease could lead to altered *reg* expression and cause changes in endocrine function. TGFα and gastrin might regulate pancreatic differentiation. Impairment could lead to chronic pancreatitis and diabetes (37).

Pancreatitis-Induced Diabetes (Type III Diabetes)

Pancreatic disease can induce diabetes mellitus. In acute pancreatitis temporary hyperglycaemia can be observed in about 50% of patients, persisting diabetes may affect 1–15% (38,39). In chronic pancreatitis about 60% of patients are reported to have diabetes, 30% to be insulin-dependent (48). Total pancreatectomy leads to IDDM, whereas in distal pancreatectomy 40–50% develop diabetes. Haemochromatosis may lead to diabetes in 50–60% of cases and diabetes occurs in 2–13% of patients with cystic fibrosis (41). However, pancreatic disease is believed to be responsible for diabetes only in about 0.5–1.15% of cases (42,43).

Nevertheless it must be taken into consideration that diabetes secondary to chronic pancreatitis could be more common, which could explain the frequent finding of exocrine insufficiency when diabetics are investigated. Chey et al. (18) commented about their findings that "It is also possible that some of the diabetics are actually patients with chronic pancreatitis. It is this that we would emphasize" (18).

It is not easy to find data about the prevalence of chronic pancreatitis and data are conflicting. However, the prevalence might be as high as 6–13% in non-selected autopsies (44,45). If only 6% had chronic pancreatitis and only 40% of those developed diabetes, we still would have to expect many more "type III" diabetics than commonly believed. Another argument for frequent type III diabetes is the very frequent changes seen on pancreatograms in diabetics, which resemble those found in chronic pancreatitis (46).

Cholelithiasis/Microlithiasis: a Possible Link Between Obesity, Chronic Obstructive Pancreatitis and Diabetes?

We would like to suggest another concept, which could explain the development of chronic pancreatitis and diabetes in a certain population of patients: papillary fibrosis due to repeated passage of stones may cause chronic obstructive pancreatitis which might lead to exocrine dysfunction, impaired glucose tolerance and diabetes.

Since the observations of Opie (47), cholelithiasis is well accepted in the pathogenesis of acute pancreatitis. Cholelithiasis might impair the function of the papilla of Vater by repeated passage of stones or microcalculi which could lead to chronic pancreatitis. This is believed to be a rare event (48); however, we found impaired exocrine function as measured by faecal elastase 1 and chymotrypsin concentrations in 30% of patients with cholelithiasis (n = 121; Hardt et al. unpublished data). Cholelithiasis is frequent in obesity and it might be frequent in diabetics, but data are conflicting. According to Clarke there is no evidence of increased risk of gallstones in diabetes, although an increased fasting volume and poor contraction of the gallbladder is established (49). In one study of 137 autopsies of diabetics and 1319 controls, the prevalence of gallstones was nearly the same (28.4 versus 22.7) (50). Another study compared 1259 autopsies of diabetics to 28 799 controls and found an increased risk of gallstones in diabetics (30.2 versus 11.6) (51). In our own series (n = 128) we found cholelithiasis in 33% of diabetic patients, another group reported 43% in NIDDM (52). So if there is an increased risk of gallstones, especially in obese diabetics, and cholelithiasis can lead to sphincter of Oddi dysfunction or papillary fibrosis, this might lead to chronic pancreatitis and diabetes in some patients.

Conclusions

Morphological and functional changes of the exocrine pancreas are very frequent in diabetics and "classical" theories do not give a satisfactory explanation of these findings. Epidemiological and morphological data suggest that type III diabetes is much more common than believed so far. Exocrine tissue might be involved in autoimmune mechanisms which can lead to β cell destruction. Cholelithiasis might contribute to the development of obstructive pancreatitis and diabetes mellitus.

References

1. Keen H, Barnes DJ (1997) The diagnosis and classification of diabetes mellitus and impaired glucose tolerance. In: Pickup JC, Williams G (eds) Textbook of diabetes, 2nd edn, Blackwell Scientific, Oxford, pp 2.1–2.10.
2. Gatling W, Mullee M, Hill R (1988) General characteristics of a community-based diabetic population. Pract Diabetes 5:104–107.
3. King H, Rewers M (1993) WHO ad hoc diabetes reporting group: global estimates for prevalence of diabetes mellitus and IGT in adults. Diabetes Care 16:157–177.
4. Gatling W, Houston AC, Hill RD (1985) An epidemiological survey: the prevalence of diabetes mellitus in a typical English community. J R Coll Phys Lond 4:248–250.
5. Neill AHW, Gatling W, Mather HM et al. (1987) The Oxford Community Diabetes Study: evidence for an increase in the prevalence of known diabetes in Great Britain. Diabetic Med 4:539–543.
6. Bennett PH (1984) Diabetes in the elderly: diagnosis and epidemiology. Geriatrics 39:37–41.
7. Atkinson MA, Maclaren NK (1994) The pathogenesis of insulin-dependent diabetes mellitus. N Engl J Med 331:1428–1436.
8. Borch-Johnson K, Mandrup-Poulsen T, Zachau-Christiansen B et al. (1984) Relation between breast-feeding and incidence rates of insulin-dependent diabetes mellitus. Lancet II:1083–1086.
9. Dahlquist GG, Blom LG, Persson L-A, Sandstrom AIM, Wall SGI (1990) Dietary factors and the risk of developing insulin-dependent diabetes in childhood. Br Med J 300:1302–1306.
10. Foulis AK (1997) Histology of the islet in insulin-dependent diabetes mellitus: a possible sequence of events. In: Pickup JC, Williams G (eds) Textbook of diabetes, 2nd edn, Blackwell Scientific, Oxford, pp 15.24–15.29.
11. Neel JV (1962) Diabetes mellitus: a thrifty genotype rendered detrimental by "progress"? Am J Hum Genet 14:353–362.
12. Hales CN, Barker DJP (1992) Type 2 (non-insulin dependent) diabetes mellitus; the thrifty phenotype hypothesis. Diabetologia 35:559–601.
13. Gilbeau J, Poncelet V, Libon E, Deruc G, Heller FR (1992) The density, contour and thickness of the pancreas in diabetics. AJR 159:527–531.
14. Lazarus SS, Volk BW (1961) Pancreas in maturity-onset diabetes. Arch Pathol 71:44.
15. Gepts W (1965) Pathology of the pancreas in juvenile diabetes. Diabetes 14:619–633.
16. Warren S, LeCompte PM (1952) The pathology of diabetes mellitus. Lea and Febiger, Philadelphia.
17. Pollard H, Miller L, Brewer W (1943) External secretion of the pancreas and diabetes (study of secretin test). Am J Dig Dis 10:20.
18. Chey WY, Shay H, Shuman CR (1963) External pancreatic secretion in diabetes mellitus. Ann Intern Med 59:812–821.
19. Vacca JB, Henke WJ, Knight WA (1964) The exocrine pancreas in diabetes mellitus. Ann Intern Med 61:242–247.
20. Frier BM, Saunders JHB, Wormsley, KG Bouchier IAD (1976) Exocrine pancreatic function in juvenile-onset diabetes mellitus. Gut 17:685–691.
21. Lankisch PG, Manthey G, Otto J, Talaulicar M, Willms B, Creutzfeldt W (1982) Exocrine pancreatic function in insulin-dependent diabetes mellitus. Digestion 25:210–216.
22. Gröger G, Layer P (1995) Exocrine pancreatic function in diabetes mellitus. Eur J Gastroenterol Hepatol 7:740–746.
23. Williams JA, Goldfine ID (1985) The insulin-pancreatic acinar axis. Diabetes 34:980–986.
24. Henderson JR (1969) Why are the islets of Langerhans? Lancet II:469–470.
25. El Ne Wihi H, Dooley CP, Saad C et al. (1988) Impaired exocrine pancreatic function in diabetics with diarrhoea and peripheral neuropathy. Dig Dis Sci 33:705–710.
26. Lazarus SS, Volk BW (1958) The effect of protracted glucagon administration on blood glucose and on pancreatic morphology. Endocrinology 63:359–371.
27. Dyck WP, Rudick J, Hoexter B, Janowitz HD (1969) Influence of glucagon on pancreatic exocrine secretion. Gastroenterology 56:531–537.

28. Unger RH, Aguilar-Parada E, Müller WA, Eisentraut AM (1970) Studies of pancreatic alpha cell function in normal and diabetic subjects. J Clin Invest 49:837–848.

29. Patel JY, Weir GC (1976) Increased somatostatin content of islets from streptozotocin-diabetic rats. Clin Endocrinol 5:191–194.

30. Tully GT, Lowenthal JJ (1958) The diabetic coma of acute pancreatitis. Ann Intern Med 48:310.

31. Gamble DR, Taylor KW, Cumming H (1973) Coxsackie viruses and diabetes mellitus. Br Med J IV:260–262.

32. Kobayashi T, Nakanishi K, Sugimoto T, Murase T, Kosaka K (1988) Histopathological changes of the pancreas in islet cell antibodies (ICA)-positive subjects before and after the clinical onset of insulin-dependent diabetes mellitus. Diabetes 37:24A (abstract).

33. Kobayashi T, Nakanishi K, Kajio H et al. (1990) Pancreatic cytokeratin: an antigen of pancreatic exocrine cell autoantibodies in type 1 (insulin-dependent) diabetes mellitus. Diabetologia 33:363–370.

34. Mally IM, Cirulli V, Hayek A, Otonkosky T (1996) ICA 69 is expressed equally in the human endocrine and exocrine pancreas. Diabetologica 39:474–480.

35. Sanvito F, Nicols A, Herrera P-J et al. (1995) TGF-β1 overexpression in murine pancreas induces chronic pancreatitis and, together with TNF-α, triggers insulin-dependent diabetes. Biochem Biophys Res Commun 217:1279–1286.

36. Perfitti R, Egan JM, Zenilman ME, Shuldiner AR (1996) Differential expression of *reg*-I and *reg* II genes during aging in normal mouse. J Gerontol 51:B308–315.

37. Kore M (1993) Islet growth factors: curing diabetes and preventing chronic pancreatitis? (editorial). J Clin Invest 92:1113–1114.

38. Warren KW, Fallis LS, Barron J (1950) Acute pancreatitis and diabetes. Ann Surg 132:1003–1010.

39. Scuro LA, Angnelini G, Cavallini G, Vantini I (1984) The late outcome of acute pancreatitis. In: Gyr KL, Singer MV, Sarles H (eds) Pancreatitis: concepts and classification. Excerpta Medica, Amsterdam; pp 403–408.

40. Larsen S (1993) Diabetes secondary to chronic pancreatitis. Dan Med Bull 40:153–162.

41. Ching CK, Rhodes JM (1997) Diabetes mellitus and pancreatic disease. In: Pickup J, Williams G (eds) Textbook of diabetes. Blackwell Scientific, Oxford, pp 24.1–24.12.

42. Alberti KGMM (1988) Diabetes secondary to pancreatopathy: an example of brittle diabetes. In: Tiengo A, Alberti KGMM, DelPrato S, Vranic M (eds) Diabetes secondary to pancreatopathy. International Congress Series 762. Excerpta Medica, Amsterdam; pp 7–20.

43. Günther O (1961) Zur Ätiologie des Diabetes mellitus. Akademie-Verlag, Berlin.

44. Doerr W (1964) Pathogenese der akuten und chronischen Pankreatitis. Verh Dtsch Ges Inn Med 70:718–758.

45. Olsen TS (1978) The incidence and clinical relevance of chronic inflammation in the pancreas in autopsie material. Acta Pathol Microbiol Scand [A] 86:361.

46. Nakanishi K, Kobayashi T, Miyashita H et al. (1994) Exocrine pancreatic ductograms in insulin-dependent diabetes mellitus. Am J Gastroenterol 89:762–766.

47. Opie EL (1901) The etiology of acute hemorraghic pancreatitis. Bull Johns Hopkins Hosp 12:182–192.

48. Büchler MW, Uhl W, Malfertheiner P (1996) Pankreaserkrankungen. Karger, Basel.

49. Clarke BF (1997) Gastrointestinal disorders in diabetes mellitus. In: Pickup JC, Williams G (eds) Textbook of diabetes, 2nd edn, Blackwell Scientific, Oxford, pp 61.1–61.14.

50. Feldmann M, Feldmann M Jr (1954) The incidence of cholelithiasis, cholesterosis and liver disease in diabetes mellitus. Diabetes NY3:305.

51. Lieber MM (1952) The incidence of gallstones and their correlation with other disease. Ann Surg 135:394.

52. Goldstein ME, Schein CJ (1963) The significance of biliary tract disease in the diabetic: its unique features. Am J Gastroenterol 39:630.

24 The Role of Islet Amyloid Polypeptide (IAPP) in the Diabetes and Anorexia of Pancreatic Cancer

U. Arnelo, J. Larsson and J. Permert

Carcinoma of the exocrine pancreas is today the fifth leading cause of cancer death in Western society, with an age-adjusted mortality rate of about 7–9/100 000 in Europe and the USA (57,66). The outcome of the disease is still grim, and has just marginally improved compared with the early part of this century (78). In fact, pancreatic cancer has one of the lowest survival rates of all cancer sites (47), with a 5-year survival of less than 3% (57,78).

Several different factors contribute to the poor prognosis of pancreatic cancer and late diagnosis is of major importance. Other factors that are likely to contribute to the extremely high mortality may be related to the biology of pancreatic adenocarcinomas. Severe, early weight loss, cachexia and metabolic complications such as diabetes are important characteristics of pancreatic cancer. These symptoms are not related to tumour size or to the stage of the disease (34). In fact, metabolic alterations such as diabetes, anorexia and weight loss have been reported as first symptoms of very small pancreatic cancer tumours (58) Metabolic and nutritional complications rather than widespread carcinomatosis are the direct cause of death in many of these patients (33). These facts indicate that pancreatic adenocarcinomas may exert specific metabolic effects that contribute to the severe cachexia and to the associated metabolic disorders, and may influence the poor outcome of the disease.

Islet amyloid polypeptide (IAPP) was first isolated from the amyloid associated with a human insulinoma (74,75) and was subsequently isolated from pancreatic amyloid from patients with non-insulin-dependent diabetes mellitus (NIDDM) (22). It is a 37 amino acid peptide, expressed as pre-pro-IAPP from the gene located on chromosome 12, and is mainly produced by the pancreatic B cells (76). The peptide is stored in the same secretory granules as insulin and is released in parallel with insulin under normal conditions, including feeding (3,14,41,64). The concentration of IAPP in plasma is normally about 10% that of insulin and increases two to fourfold following a glucose load or food intake (1,3,4,12,14,64,67). Although several biological effects of IAPP have been demonstrated, its physiological role has not been established. Marked elevations of plasma IAPP concentration have been reported in weight-losing pancreatic cancer patients with associated diabetes (63). In other types of malignancies as well as in patients with NIDDM, however, circulating concentrations of IAPP have been reported to be normal or just slightly elevated (63,67).

Diabetes in Patients with Pancreatic Cancer

Altered glucose metabolism in a patient with pancreatic adenocarcinoma was first reported in 1833 by Bright, who described a patient who developed symptoms of diabetes mellitus 6 months before he became jaundiced and died of a pancreatic carcinoma (86). Newly diagnosed diabetes or instability in previously known and well-controlled diabetes has been reported as a characteristic of pancreatic cancer (33).

Two different hypotheses have been proposed to explain this association. One hypothesis suggests that diabetes is a predisposing factor of aetiologic significance for pancreatic cancer, while the other suggests that the high incidence of diabetes is an effect of the pancreatic tumour. In support of the first hypothesis, a number of epidemiological investigations have commented on an increased risk for pancreatic cancer in persons previously diagnosed as diabetic. Maddox (39) reported 15 cases of cancer death, as opposed to only 1.62 cases expected, in a long-term follow-up cohort study from Sydney between 1932 and 1947. This finding was supported by Kessler (37), Regazzino et al. (65) and more recently by Cuzik and Babiker (23), who found evidence of an increased risk of pancreatic cancer in diabetic patients. However, when those patients who developed cancer within a year of onset of diabetes are excluded, the evidence becomes weaker. Morris and Nabarro (55) found an increase in pancreatic cancer in diabetics but not in those with long-standing diabetes, and some other recent studies have reported similar findings (21,38,77,79). Some have even reported a decreased risk in long-term diabetics (49,77,79). Recent epidemiological reports have concluded that even though diabetes occurs in a high frequency in pancreatic cancer, diabetes is not a risk factor for pancreatic cancer in the sense that risk factors are generally understood to operate (11,32).

Disparate incidences of impaired glucose tolerance and diabetes have previously been reported in pancreatic cancer patients. A summary of the pertinent literature is shown in Table 1. Impaired glucose tolerance or diabetes was found in 74% of the pancreatic cancer patients in a prospective study that we performed in 50 consecutive patients with pancreatic cancer. In this study we found that 26% of the patients were symptomatic diabetics requiring insulin treatment. This corresponds well to the incidence reported from the previous prospective studies that used diagnostic criteria for diabetes and impaired glucose tolerance comparable to the WHO criteria and to the incidence in more recent studies (Table 1). A large case—control study from Italy, (32) reported that 23% of the patients with pancreatic cancer were symptomatic diabetics at the time of the tumour diagnosis and this frequency was significantly higher compared with the control group and to what could be expected. From this study the authors concluded that there now is evidence to state that diabetes is a consequence of the tumour and not a risk factor for pancreatic cancer.

In our studies the diabetic state in the diabetic patients, as assessed by glucose tolerance and tissue insulin sensitivity, improved after tumour removal by subtotal pancreatectomy, despite a marked reduction in insulin secretion postoperatively (Figure 1) (61,62). Similar findings of an improved glucose metabolism after removal of the pancreatic tumour were also reported from an Italian study (26). Taken together, these findings do not support the hypothesis that the diabetic state in pancreatic cancer is caused by destruction of B cells by the tumour (8). In contrast, the results indicate that a diabetogenic factor produced by pan-

Table 1. Review of literature

Author	Patients with abnormal carbohydrate metabolism	Type of study and diagnostic criteria
Bell (7)	20% (146/743)	Retrospective. Glycosuria or abnormal blood sugar
Green et al. (31)	45% (93/209)	Retrospective. FBS > 6.7 mM or glucosuria
Clark et al. (19)	15% (10/65)	Retrospective. Symptomatic diabetes
Birnbaum et al. (9)	47% (29/63)	Retrospective. FBS > 6.7 mM
Murphy et al. (56)	51% (127/251)	Retrospective. FBS > 7.2 mM symptomatic diabetes, or glucosuria
Karmody et al. (36)	20% (53/265)	Retrospective. FBS > 7.2 mM
Sperti et al. (72)	47% (82/174)	Prospective. Diabetic OGTT or FBS
Schwartz et al. (69)	81% (26/32)	Prospective. OGTT[a] or symptomatic diabetes
Cersosimo et al. (15)	67% (7/11)	Prospective. OGTT[b]
Berkowitz et al. (8)	61% (11/18)	Prospective. OGTT
Del Favero et al. (24)	76% (32/42)	Prospective. Fasting hyperglycaemia
Permert et al. (62)	74% (37/50)	Prospective. OGTT[c]
Gullo et al. (32)	23% (164/720)	Retrospective. Symptomatic diabetes[b]

[a] According to criteria of American Diabetes Association.
[b] According to National diabetes data group.
[c] According to WHO criteria.
OGTT, oral glucose tolerance test; FBS, fasting blood sugar.

creatic adenocarcinomas may be directly or indirectly responsible for the high frequency of diabetes in these patients. The improvement in glucose metabolism seen postoperatively also demonstrates that preservation of some pancreatic tissue is of clinical importance to prevent the development of postoperative diabetes. Islet tissue preservation is also likely to benefit those patients who are diabetic preoperatively, because diabetes may improve or disappear after tumour removal.

Role of IAPP in Diabetes

IAPP is the major constituent of the amyloid that occurs in more than 90% of NIDDM patients (77) and therefore a role for this peptide in the development

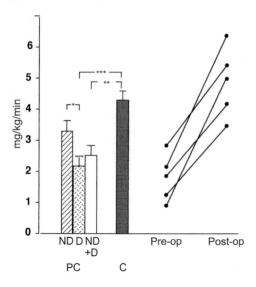

Figure 1. The glucose metabolic rate at an insulin infusion level of 1.0 mU/kg per minute. Left: pancreatic cancer (PC, $n = 16$) and controls (C, $n = 7$); the pancreatic cancer patients were subgrouped into diabetic (D, $n = 11$) and non-diabetic (ND, $n = 6$). Right: pancreatic cancer patients ($n = 5$) investigated before (pre op) and 3 months after (post op) subtotal pancreatectomy. Mean ± SE. *$P < 0.05$, **$P < 0.01$, ***$P < 0.001$.

of NIDDM has been suggested. An aetiological role of IAPP in the development of NIDDM was further suggested by initial studies in which pharmacological doses of IAPP were found to inhibit glycogen synthesis *in vitro*, and to cause impaired glucose tolerance *in vivo* (40,71). A number of subsequent studies using different models have demonstrated an effect of IAPP on glucose metabolism in several species (13,28,29,35,50,51,59,73,74,81,82,85). One previous study demonstrated a dose-responsive reduction in peripheral glucose utilisation in the dog in response to human IAPP (71). However, the effect was only significant at a dose of 25 μg/kg per hour ($\approx$ 108 pmol/kg per minute), a dose that results in plasma concentrations that are 15–50 times higher than the highest concentrations observed in diabetic patients with pancreatic cancer. In all these studies, the levels of IAPP investigated were far above the physiological range.

We performed an experiment in order to evaluate whether or not chronically elevated circulating IAPP, at concentrations similar to those seen in pancreatic cancer patients, is sufficient to cause the insulin resistance that is frequently seen in these patients (4). In this experiment we could not demonstrate an effect of IAPP on glucose metabolic capacity studied with the hyperinsulinaemic euglycaemic clamp technique. At IAPP doses that were in the range of the doses used in our experiment, short-term studies of IAPP on glucose metabolism have likewise failed to demonstrate effects (28,71,82). The results of these and other studies demonstrate that IAPP does have effects on peripheral glucose metabolism, but only at markedly supraphysiological concentrations.

The lack of effect on glucose disposal at IAPP plasma concentrations that were sufficient to cause other metabolic effects and in the range of what is observed in pancreatic cancer patients suggests that IAPP on its own does not account for the insulin resistance that accompanies pancreatic cancer. Indeed, the physiological importance of IAPP in peripheral glucose metabolism is still controversial.

Role of IAPP in Anorexia

Accumulating evidence from several animal studies in rats and mice suggest that IAPP may be of importance as a regulator of food intake (1–5,10,16–18,42–46, 52–54). While effects of IAPP on glucose metabolism are observed only at very high concentrations, an effect on food intake has been demonstrated at concentrations that are in the range of what has been observed at least during pathophysiological conditions in humans (2). When the effect of IAPP on food intake is compared with the effect of the most studied prototypic satiating peptide, cholecystokinin (CCK), it is clear that on an equimolar basis IAPP inhibits food intake more potently (1,42).

We and others have demonstrated that, in rats, IAPP potently inhibits food intake when administered systematically either acutely (1,3,18), or chronically (2,4). In one study we administered IAPP subcutaneously for 7 days to rats by an osmotic minipump at doses that produce circulating plasma concentrations similar to the plasma levels seen in patients with pancreatic cancer. We found that IAPP, at these concentrations, produced a dose-dependent reduction of food intake (Figure 2). The effect was transient but remained throughout the experiment in rats that received the highest infusion rate. Analysis of the meal pattern revealed that the reduction in food intake was caused by a reduction in the numbers of meals whereas the size of the individual meals was unaffected (2). This and other experiments suggested that effects of IAPP on food intake are specific and not caused by malaise or other non-specific effects (2,13,17,42).

The mechanisms by which IAPP suppresses food intake are not clarified. The most likely way of action is that IAPP acts as an endocrine factor which is released from the pancreatic islets into the circulation after ingestion of nutrients. The satiating effect is then mediated through a distant target organ. The two most likely candidates are the CNS and/or the stomach.

Several pieces of evidence suggest that IAPP may act in the brain to suppress food intake. Exogenous IAPP inhibits food intake when administered intra-

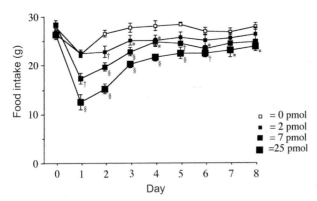

Figure 2. Effects of islet amyloid polypeptide (IAPP) infusion on daily food intake. IAPP was administered subcutaneously to rats fed *ad libitum* by osmotic minipumps at 0 (*open squares*), 2 (*small filled squares*), 7 (*medium filled squares*), and 25 (*large filled squares*) pmol/kg per minute for 8 days, $n = 8$ per dose. Day 0 denotes the day before insertion of the pump. Values are means ± SE. $*P < 0.05$, $†P < 0.01$, $§P < 0.001$.

hypothalamically to rats (5,16,17), and intracerebroventricularly to mice (52) and rats (10). Furthermore, high-affinity binding sites for IAPP have been demonstrated in the lamina terminals and area postrema, areas that have been implicated in control of feeding behaviour (70). Because these regions are not protected by the blood–brain barrier (BBB), they could be reached by circulating IAPP (70). For other peptides, such as insulin, specific transport processes across the BBB have been described (60,68). One study indicated that peripherally administered ^{125}I-IAPP gains access to the mouse brain, but it remains to be determined whether circulating IAPP is actively transported across the BBB into other brain regions (6). Finally, another study suggests that IAPP may be synthesised in the hypothalamus (16).

Recent evidence from a limited number of rat experiments suggests that the effect of IAPP on food intake could be secondary to inhibition of gastric emptying (20,30,82,83). Young et al. (82) showed that subcutaneous bolus injections of IAPP potently delayed gastric emptying at doses that produced plasma concentrations that were approximately three times higher than those observed in fasting rats. The same group has reported that IAPP on a molar basis was a more potent inhibitor of gastric emptying compared with a large number of normally secreted peptides that have a documented effect on gastric emptying (30).

In conclusion, it is not likely that IAPP on its own is responsible for the diabetes that occurs in the majority of pancreatic cancer patients. However, it cannot be ruled out that IAPP may contribute to this type of diabetes, together with other alterations in islet cell secretion that are observed in these patients. On the other hand, it is likely that IAPP could contribute to the anorexia and cachexia in pancreatic cancer patients, in particular since IAPP not only produces a reduction in food intake, but also dose-dependently affects body weight gain (2).

References

1. Arnelo U, Blevins JE, Larsson J et al. (1996) Effects of acute and chronic infusion of islet amyloid polypeptide on food intake in rats. Scand J Gastroenterol 31:83–89.
2. Arnelo U, Permert J, Adrian TE, Larsson J, Westermark P, Reidelberger RD (1996) Chronic infusion of islet amyloid polypeptide causes anorexia in rats. Am J Physiol 271:R1654–R1659.
3. Arnelo U, Reidelberger RD, Adrian TE, Larsson J, Westermark P, Permert J (1996) Islet amyloid polypeptide: a physiological regulator of satiety? Digestion 57:217 (abstract).
4. Arnelo U, Permert J, Larsson J, Reidelberger RD, Arnelo C, Adrian TE (1997) Chronic low dose islet amyloid polypeptide infusion reduces food intake but does not influence glucose metabolism in unrestrained conscious rats: Studies using a novel aortic catheterization technique. Endocrinology 138:4081–4085.
5. Balasubramaniam A, Renugopalakrishnan V, Stein M, Fischer JE, Chance WT (1991) Syntheses, structures and anorectic effects of human and rat amylin. Peptides 12:919–924.
6. Banks WA, Kastin AJ, Maness LM, Huang W, Jaspan JB (1995) Permeability of the blood–brain barrier to amylin. Life Sci 57:1993–2001.
7. Bell ET (1957) Carcinoma of the pancreas II. The relation of carcinoma of the pancreas to diabetes mellitus. Am J Pathol 33:499–523.
8. Berkowitz D, Greenberg L Glassman S (1963) The intravenous tolbutamide test as a diagnostic aid in carcinoma of the pancreas. Am J Med Sci 243:150–154.
9. Birnbaum D, Kleeberg J (1958) Carcinoma of the pancreas: a clinical study based on 84 cases. Ann Intern Med 48:1171–1184.
10. Bouali SM, Wimalawansa SJ, Jolicoeur FB (1995) In vivo central actions of rat amylin. Regul Pept 56:167–174.

11. Boyle P, Hsieh CC, Maisonneuve P et al. (1989) Epidemiology of pancreatic cancer. Int J Pancreatol 5:327–346.
12. Bretherton-Watt D, Gilbey S, Ghatei MA, Beacham J, Bloom SR (1990) Lack of effect of amylin amide on carbohydrate metabolism in man. Diabetologia 33:115–117.
13. Bretherton-Watt D, Gilbey SG, Ghatei MA, Beacham J, Macrae AD, Bloom SR (1992) Very high concentrations of islet amyloid polypeptide are necessary to alter the insulin response to intravenous glucose in man. J Clin Endocrinol Metab 74:1032–1035.
14. Butler PC, Chou J, Carter WB et al. (1990) Effects of meal ingestion on plasma amylin concentration in NIDDM and nondiabetic humans. Diabetes 39:752–756.
15. Cersosimo E, Pisters P, Pesola G, McDermott K, Bajorunas D, Brennan MF (1991) Insulin secretion and action in patients with pancreatic cancer. Cancer 67:468–493.
16. Chance WT, Balasubramaniam A, Zhang FS, Wimalawansa SJ, Fischer JE (1991) Anorexia following the intrahypothalamic administration of amylin. Brain Res 539:352–354.
17. Chance WT, Balasubramaniam A, Chen X, Fischer JE (1992) Test of adipsia and conditioned taste aversion following intrahypothalamic injection of amylin. Peptides 13: 961–964.
18. Chance WT, Balasubramaniam A, Stallion A, Fischer JE (1993) Anorexia following the systemic injection of amylin. Brain Res 607:185–188.
19. Clark CG, Mitchell PEG (1961) Diabetes and primary cancer of the pancreas. Br Med J II:1259–1262.
20. Clementi G, Caruso A, Cutuli VMC, de Bernardis E, Prato A, Amico-roxas M (1996) Amylin given by central or peripheral routes decreases gastric emptying and intestinal transit in the rat. Experientia 52:677–679.
21. Conrath S (1986) The use of epidemiology, scientific data, and regulatory authority to determine risk factors in cancer of some organs of the digestive systems. Regul Toxicol Pharmacol 38:435–441.
22. Cooper GJS, Willis AC, Clark A, Turner RC, Sim SB, Reid KBM (1987) Purification and characterization of a peptide from amyloid-rich pancreases of type 2 diabetic patients. Proc Natl Acad Sci USA 84:8628–8632.
23. Cuzick J, Babiker AG (1989) Pancreatic cancer, alcohol, diabetes mellitus and gallbladder disease. Int J Cancer 43:415–421.
24. Del Favero G, Fogar P, Meggiato T, et al. (1992) C-peptide pattern in patients with pancreatic cancer. Digestion 52:77.
25. Faith MB, Bierman HR (1985) Glucose tolerance in cancer of the pancreas. Proc Ann Meet Am Assoc Cancer Res 26:1.
26. Fogar P, Pasquali C, Basso D et al. (1994) Diabetes mellitus in pancreatic cancer follow-up. Anticancer Res 14:2827–2930.
27. Fox JN, Frier BM, Armitage M, Ashby JP (1985) Abnormal insulin secretion in carcinoma of the pancreas: response to glucagon stimulation. Diabetes Med 2:113–116.
28. Frontoni S, Choi SB, Banduch D, Rosetti L (1991) In vivo insulin resistance induced by amylin primarily through inhibition of insulin-stimulated glucogen synthesis in skeletal muscle. Diabetes 40:568–573.
29. Fürnsinn C, Nowotny P, Roden M et al. (1993) Insulin resistance caused by amylin in conscious rats is independent of induced hypocalcemia and fades during long-term exposure. Acta Endocrinol 129:360–365.
30. Gedulin BR, Jodka CM, Green DL, Young AA (1996) Comparison of 21 peptides on inhibition of gastric emptying in conscious rats. Gastroenterology 110:A668.
31. Green RC Jr, Bagenstoss AH, Sprague RG (1958) Diabetes mellitus in association with primary carcinoma of the pancreas. Diabetes 7:308–311.
32. Gullo L, Pezzilli R, Morselli-Labate AM (1994) Diabetes and the risk of pancreatic cancer. N Eng J Med 331:81–84.
33. Inagami J, Rodriguez V, Bodey GP (1974) Causes of death in cancer patients. Cancer 33:568–573.
34. Ingelfinger FJ (1946) The diagnosis of cancer of the pancreas. N Engl J Med 235:653–661.
35. Johnson KH, O'Brien TD, Jordan K, Betsholtz C, Westermark P (1990) The putative hormone islet amyloid polypeptide (IAPP) induces impaired glucose tolerance in cats. Biochem Biophys Res Commun 167:507–513.
36. Karmody AJ, Kyle J (1969) The association between carcinoma of the pancreas and diabetes mellitus. Br J Surg 56:362–364.
37. Kessler II (1970) Cancer mortality among diabetics. J Natl Cancer Inst 44:673–686.
38. Klöppel G, Bommer G, Commandeur G, Heitz PH (1978) The endocrine pancreas in chronic pancreatitis. Virchows Arch 377:157–174.
39. Lancaster HD, Maddox JK (1958) Diabetic mortality in Australia. Aust Ann Med 7:145–150.

40. Leighton B, Cooper GJS (1988) Pancreatic amylin and calcitonin gene-related peptide cause resistance to insulin in skeletal muscle *in vitro*. Nature 335:632–635.
41. Lukinius A, Wilander E, Westermark GT, Engström U, Westermark P (1989) Co-localization of islet amyloid polypeptide and insulin and the B cell secretory granules of the human pancreatic islets. Diabetologia 32:240–244.
42. Lutz TA, Del Prete E, Scharrer E (1994) Reduction in food intake in rats by intraperitoneal injection of low doses of amylin. Physiol Behav 55:891–895.
43. Lutz TA, Del Prete E, Scharrer E (1995) Subdiaphragmatic vagotomy does not influence the anorectic effect of amylin. Peptides 16:457–462.
44. Lutz TA, Geary N, Szabady MM, Del Prete E, Scharrer E (1995) Amylin decreases meal size in rats. Physiol Behav 58:1197–1202.
45. Lutz TA, Del Prete E, Szabady MM, Scharrer E (1995) Circadian anorectic effects of peripherally administered amylin in rats. Z Ernährungswiss (Eur J Nutr) 34:214–219.
46. Lutz TA, Del Prete E, Szabady MM, Scharrer E (1996) Attenuation of the anorectic effects of glucagon, cholecystokinin, and bombesin by the amylin receptor antagonist CGRP(8–37). Peptides 17:119–124.
47. Malt RA (1983) Treatment of pancreatic cancer. JAMA 250:1433–1437.
48. McKiddie MT, Burchanan KD, McBain GC, Bell G (1969) The insulin response to glucose in patients with pancreatic disease. Postgrad Med J 45:726–728.
49. Mills PK, Beeson WL, Abbey DE, Fraser GE, Phillips RL (1988) Dietary habits and past medical history as related to fatal pancreas cancer risk among adventists. Cancer 61:2578–2585.
50. Mitsukawa T, Takemura J, Nakazato M et al. (1992) Effects of aging on plasma islet amyloid polypeptide basal level and response to oral glucose load. Diabetes Res Clin Pract 15:131–134.
51. Molina JM, Cooper GJS, Leighton B, Olefsky JM (1990) Induction of insulin resistance in vivo by amylin and calcitonin gene-related peptide. Diabetes 39:260–265.
52. Morley JE, Flood JF (1991) Amylin decreases food intake in mice. Peptides 12:865–869.
53. Morley JE, Morley PMK, Flood JF (1993) Anorectic effects of amylin in rats over the life span. Pharmacol Biochem Behav 44:577–580.
54. Morley JE, Flood JF, Horowitz M, Morley PMK, Walter MJ (1994) Modulation of food intake by peripherally administered amylin. Am J Physiol 267:R178–R184.
55. Morris DV, Nabarro JD (1984) Pancreatic cancer and diabetes mellitus. Diabetic Med 1:119–121.
56. Murphy R, Smith FH (1963) Abnormal carbohydrate metabolism in pancreatic carcinoma. Med Clin North Am 47:397–405.
57. National Cancer Institute (1991) Annual cancer statistics review 1973–1988. Department of Health and Human Service, Bethesda, NIH publication No 91–2789.
58. Ozaki H (1992) Improvement of pancreatic cancer treatment. From the Japanese Experience in the 1980s. Int J Pancreatol 12:5–9.
59. Panagiotidis G, Salehi AA, Westermark P, Lundquist I (1992) Homologous islet amyloid polypeptide: effects on plasma levels of glucagon, insulin and glucose in the mouse. Diabetes Res Clin Practice 18:167–171.
60. Pardridge WM (1986) Receptor-mediated peptide transport through the blood–brain barrier. Endocrine Rev 7:314–330.
61. Permert J, Adrian TE, Jacobsson P, Jorfelt L, Fruin AB, Larsson J (1993) Is profound peripheral insulin resistance in patients with pancreatic cancer caused by a tumor-associated factor? Am J Surg 165:61–66.
62. Permert J, Ihse I, Jorfelt L, von Schenck, Arnquist HJ, Larsson J (1993) Improved glucose metabolism after subtotal pancreatectomy for pancreatic cancer. Br J Surg 80:1047–1050.
63. Permert J, Larsson J, Westermark GT et al. (1994) Islet amyloid polypeptide in patients with pancreatic cancer patients and diabetes. N Engl J Med 330:313–318.
64. Pieber TR, Roitelman J, Lee Y, Luskey KL, Stein DT (1994) Direct plasma radioimmunoassay for rat amylin-(1–37): concentrations with acquired and genetic obesity. Am J Physiol 267:E156–E164.
65. Regazzino M, Melton LJ, Chu CP, Palumbo PJ (1982) Subsequent cancer risk in the incidence cohort of Rochester, Minnesota, residents with diabetes mellitus J Chron Dis 35:13–19.
66. Rosewicz S, Wiedenmann B (1997) Pancreatic carcinoma. Lancet 349:485–489.
67. Sanke T, Hanabusa Y, Nakano C et al. (1991) Plasma islet amyloid polypeptide (amylin) levels and their responses to oral glucose in Type 2 (non-insulin-dependent) diabetic patients. Diabetologia 34:129–132.
68. Schwartz MW, Bergman RN, Kahn SE et al. (1991) Evidence for entry of plasma insulin into cerebrospinal fluid through an intermediate compartment in dogs. J Clin Invest 88:1272–1281.

69. Schwartz SS, Ziedler A, Moossa AR, Kuku SF, Rubenstein AH (1978) A prospective study of glucose tolerance, insulin, C-peptide, and glucagon responses in patients with pancreatic carcinoma. Am J Dig Dis 23:1107–1114.

70. Sexton PM, Paxinos G, Kenney MA, Wookey PJ, Beaumont K (1994) In vitro autoradiographic localization of amylin binding sites in rat brain. Neuroscience 62:553–567.

71. Sowa R, Sanke T, Hirayama J et al. (1990) Islet amyloid polypeptide amide causes peripheral insulin resistance in vivo in dogs. Diabetologia 33:118–120.

71a. Sperti C, Pasquali C, Behboo R, Isoardi R, Cappellazzo F, Pedrazzoli S (1992) Diabetes and pancreatic cancer. Digestion 52:123.

72. Wang M-W, Carlo P, Rink TJ, Young AA (1991) Amylin is more potent and more effective than glucagon in raising plasma glucose concentration in fasted, anesthetized rats. Biochem Biophys Res Commun 181:1288–1293.

73. Wang M-W, Carlo P, Fineman M, Rink TJ, Young AA (1992) Induction of acute hyperglycemia, hyperlactemia and hypocalcemia in fed and fasted BALB/c mice by intravenous amylin injection. Endocrine Res 18:321–332.

74. Westermark P, Wernstedt C, Wilander E, Sletten K (1986) A novel peptide in the calcitonin gene-related family as an amyloid fibril protein in the endocrine pancreas. Biochem Biophys Res Commun 140:827–831.

75. Westermark P, Wernstedt C, Wilander E, Hayden DW, O'Brien TD, Johnson KH (1987) Amyloid fibrils in human insulinoma and islets of Langerhans of the diabetic cat are derived from a neuropeptide-like protein also present in normal islet cells. Proc Natl Acad Sci USA 84:3881–3885.

76. Westermark P, Johnson KH, O'Brien TD, Betsholtz C (1992) Islet amyloid polypeptide: a novel controversy in diabetic research. Diabetologia 35:297–303.

77. Whittemore AS, Paffenberg RS, Anderson K, Halpern J (1983) Early precursors of pancreatic cancer in college men. J Chron Dis 36:251–256.

78. Williamson RCN (1988) Pancreatic cancer: the greatest oncological challenge. Br Med J 296:445–446.

79. Wydner EL, Mabuchi K, Maruchi N (1973) Epidemiology of cancer of the pancreas. J Natl Cancer Inst 50:645–667.

80. Young AA, Cooper GJS, Carlo P, Rink TJ, Wang M-W (1993) Response to intravenous injection of amylin and glucagon in fasted, fed, and hypoglycemic rats. Am J Physiol 264:E943–E950.

81. Young AA, Rink TJ, Wang M-W (1993) Dose response characteristics for the hyperglycemic, hyperlactemic, hypotensive and hypocalcemic actions of amylin and calcitonin gene-related peptide-I (CGRPa) in the fasted, anesthetized rat. Life Sci 52:1717–1726.

82. Young AA, Gedulin B, Vine W, Percy A, Rink TJ (1995) Gastric emptying is accelerated in diabetic BB rats and is slowed by subcutaneous injections of amylin. Diabetologia 38:642–648.

83. Young AA, Gedulin B, Rink TJ (1996) Dose-responses for the slowing of gastric emptying in a rodent model by glucagon-like peptide (7–36) NH$_2$, amylin, cholecystokinin, and other possible regulators of nutrient uptake. Metab Clin Exp 45:1–3.

84. Young DA, Deems RO, Deacon RW, McIntosh RH, Foley JE (1990) Effects of amylin on glucose metabolism and glycogenolysis in vivo and in vitro. Am J Physiol 259:E457–E461.

85. Zimmerman B (1954) Editorial. Diabetes and gross lesions of the pancreas. J Clin Endocrinol Metab 14:481–483.

25 Endocrine Tumours of the Pancreas

D. Al-Musawi and R.C.N. Williamson

Endocrine (neuroendocrine, islet-cell) tumours of the pancreas are being recognised with increasing frequency because of improvements in imaging and peptide radioimmunoassay. They were originally described as APUDomas because it was thought that they had a common origin from neural crest cells with the ability to perform amine precursor uptake and decarboxylation. This theory has since been disproved, and it has been proposed that the neuroendocrine and mucosal endocrine cells are derived from a common bipotential cell.

The islets of Langerhans contain at least five cell types: β cells which produce insulin, α cells which produce glucagon, γ cells which produce somatostatin, F cells which produce pancreatic polypeptide and enterochromaffin cells which produce serotonin. These cells have the potential to synthesise more than one hormone and also "ectopic" hormones that are not usually found in the pancreas, such as gastrin, adrenocorticotropin, vasoactive intestinal peptide and growth hormone.

Although many pancreatic endocrine tumours are multihormonal, one peptide generally predominates and is responsible for producing a clinical syndrome. Other tumours are full of peptide hormones but are functionally inactive. These neoplasms present widely variable and sometimes dramatic clinical syndromes. They run an unpredictable course, and only curative resection has been shown to alter the outcome of the disease (1). Palliative treatments including chemotherapy, hepatic artery embolisation/chemoembolisation or somatostatin analogue therapy can sometimes prolong symptom-free survival (2).

Incidence

Pancreatic endocrine tumours are rare, with an incidence of less than 1 per 100 000 population per year. Insulinomas are the commonest variant and account for up to 50%, whilst gastrinomas account for 20% and the rarer functioning tumours only 5%; the remaining 25% are non-functioning tumours. Approximately one quarter of islet cell tumours are associated with the multiple endocrine neoplasia type I (MEN-I) syndrome, and nearly half of these are malignant. The remaining three-quarters are sporadic, of which 70% are malignant.

Pathology

The islet-cell lesion may be one of the following: (1) generalised hyperplasia, (2) discrete adenoma, (3) generalised adenomatosis, (4) carcinoma. In MEN-I these lesions may be associated with similar lesions in the anterior pituitary (16%) and parathyroid (80%) glands.

There is a slight disposition for islet-cell tumours to arise within the body and the tail of the pancreas, correlating with a greater islet-cell concentration in these locations, though some recent series have shown that non-functioning tumours favour the head (2,3). There are reports of an association with pancreatitis secondary to ductal obstruction by the tumour (4,5). Most of these tumours are solid, but they can occasionally be cystic. Among 30 patients with cystic tumours of the pancreas in one series, only two were neuroendocrine (6).

In the common types of slow-growing tumour, malignancy cannot be established histologically. The only indisputable sign of malignancy is invasion of adjacent organs or metastatic spread to regional lymph nodes or the liver. Lengthy follow-up is required to establish the benign nature of the lesion because metastasis may appear some years after removal of primary tumour.

General Clinical Features and Diagnosis

The clinical presentation of the secretory tumours depends on the type and amount of hormone produced. They usually present early when average tumour size is 1–3 cm. The diagnosis is based on the demonstration of elevated circulating levels of the relevant hormone. Non-functioning tumours tend to present late with locally advanced or metastatic disease because they lack the features of an endocrine syndrome. Their presenting features resemble those of "ordinary" pancreatic cancer and include jaundice, pain, weight loss, palpable mass and haemorrhage (2). Occasionally pancreatitis is the first signal of the presence of the tumour. Unlike exocrine carcinoma which tends to cause chronic obstructive pancreatitis, endocrine tumours generally present with recurrent acute pancreatitis (5). Confirmation of the diagnosis can be provided by histopathological and immunohistochemical analysis of a resection specimen or a biopsy of a liver metastasis.

Insulinoma

Insulinomas have been reported in all age groups. At least 75% are solitary and benign. Malignancy occurs in about 10% of cases. The remaining 15% are multifocal lesions either in the form of adenomatosis, nesidioblastosis or islet-cell hyperplasia. In Rothmund's large multicentre series of 396 patients with benign insulinomas, tumours were equally distributed throughout the pancreatic head, body and tail (7). Although size alone does not always correlate with the severity of symptoms, malignant insulinomas are usually larger than benign lesions and approximately one-third have metastasised at the time of initial diagnosis (8).

The symptoms of neuroglycopenia (i.e. cerebral glucose deprivation) are bizarre behaviour, memory loss or unconsciousness. Patients may be mistakenly treated for psychiatric illness. In Stefanini's study of 1067 patients with insulinomas (8), 92% described non-specific neurological symptoms such as apathy, behavioural disturbances or seizures. Many patients are overweight because eating can relieve their symptoms.

Diagnosis

The classic Whipple's triad is present in most cases and comprises hypoglycaemic attacks produced by fasting, blood glucose below 2 mmol/l during the attacks, and relief of symptoms by administration of glucose. The most useful diagnostic test is the demonstration of fasting hypoglycaemia in the presence of an inappropriately high level of insulin. Most patients develop hypoglycaemia within 24 hours of fasting and almost all within 72 hours. On blood sampling a ratio of plasma insulin to glucose greater than 0.3 is diagnostic. This test was accurate in 98.3% of 396 patients reported by Rothmund (7). Proinsulin, which constitutes more than 25% of total insulin, can also be measured; levels greater than 40% suggest a malignant tumour. Measurement of plasma C-peptide (endogenous flanking peptide of insulin) is helpful since it is not elevated in psychiatric patients who are self-administering exogenous insulin. Drugs that release insulin (tolbutamide, glucagon, calcium, arginine, leucine) were used in the past as a provocative test. They are now obselete (9).

Imaging and Localisation

Preoperative

As over 50% of insulinomas are less than 1.5 cm, ultrasonography and computed tomography fail to detect at least half of them. Selective arteriography is currently the best localisation procedure (10), with a sensitivity approaching 100% in our own experience (10). Most of these tumours are hypervascular (Figure 1), producing a tumour "blush" (on angiography) and enhancing very quickly on computed tomography with intravenous contrast. Percutaneous transhepatic portal venous sampling is a highly invasive procedure but may be considered when arteriography is inconclusive or in patients with MEN-I. A more useful technique is selective arterial injection of calcium (which stimulates insulin production from the tumour) followed by sequential hepatic or peripheral venous sampling. This technique was found to be highly accurate in a small series reported recently (11). Both endoscopic and laparoscopic ultrasonography are currently being evaluated as alternative methods for localisation of islet-cell tumours, but further experience is needed.

Intraoperative

In about 10% of cases, the tumour is so small or deeply located that it cannot easily be found by operative examination of the pancreas. Intraoperative ultrasonography (IOUS) is a useful modality in such circumstances. When IOUS is

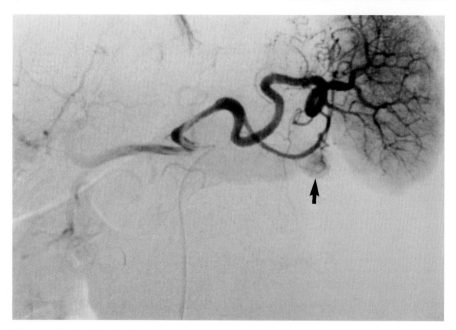

Figure 1. Selective digital subtraction angiogram of the splenic artery showing a tumour blush in the tail of pancreas due to insulinoma. (Reproduced by courtesy of Dr James Jackson, Department of Radiology, Hammersmith Hospital.)

combined with skilled surgical exploration, the sensitivity improves greatly, possibly to 100% (12). This fact will probably make accurate preoperative localisation less important in the future as surgeons become more experienced with the use of the ultrasound probe and technology improves. On IOUS, 90% of islet-cell tumours appear hypoechoic. It also helps to determine the relationship of the tumour to the pancreatic duct, bile duct and blood vessels and to identify liver metastases.

Treatment

The ideal treatment is surgical excision of all tumour tissue. Patients awaiting operation may benefit from diazoxide therapy, which suppresses insulin release from normal islet β cells and from insulinoma cells. A full laparotomy is required, in particular examining the liver for metastasis. The pancreas is fully exposed to permit direct inspection and bimanual palpation. The head is mobilised by an extended Kocher manoeuvre; the body and the tail are inspected by opening the lesser sac along the avascular plane of the transverse colon. To examine the posterior surface of the left pancreas, the peritoneum along the lower (and if necessary upper) border is incised to allow gentle mobilisation of the gland (13). Insulinomas are darkish in colour and are palpable in at least 90% of cases. As multiple insulinomas occur in 10% of patients, a thorough search should continue after finding a single tumour.

In general, adenomas should be enucleated to preserve the maximum of normal pancreatic parenchyma. After enucleation the residual cavity should be inspected. If it is superficial, it may be closed or left open with a drain nearby, but if it is deep or there is an obvious ductal leak, a Roux-en-Y loop of jejunum should be anastomosed to the margins of the cavity. When the insulinoma is deep-seated in the body or the tail of the pancreas, distal conservative (spleen-preserving) pancreatectomy is an appropriate alternative. Insulinomas in the head are best enucleated because pancreatoduodenectomy is a major undertaking for a benign tumour. Only 2 of 72 patients at the Mayo clinic (14), and only 5% of 366 patients in a French series required such resection (15).

If the insulinoma cannot be detected after careful palpation and the use of IOUS, other options must be considered, such as biopsy of any suspicious area of parenchyma and/or selective catheterisation and sampling from the draining veins. There is little indication for blind distal pancreatectomy unless the angiogram is highly suggestive. Intraoperative monitoring of blood glucose is often done as a means of determining if the tumour has been excised, but it is not very reliable. For islet-cell hyperplasia, nesidioblastosis, or multiple benign adenomas, distal subtotal pancreatectomy usually decreases insulin levels sufficiently for medical management to be effective. For metastatic insulinoma, resection of both the primary and secondary lesions is warranted if technically possible; otherwise, diazoxide or octreotide may help to control symptoms.

Gastrinoma

Gastrinomas are the second commonest functioning tumour of the pancreas. They account for 1 in 1000 cases of duodenal ulcer disease. The association of virulent peptic ulcer disease and islet-cell tumour was first made in 1955 by Zollinger and Ellison. Gastrinomas are usually small tumours less than 2 cm in diameter. Although most are pancreatic in origin, 20–40% arise from the duodenum where they may sometimes be multiple and tiny (microadenomas). Other less common primary sites for gastrinomas include the stomach, jejunum, liver and ovary. Primary lymph node gastrinomas have been described, but many of these are likely to represent metastases from occult duodenal or pancreatic carcinomas. Gastrinomas occur in both sporadic (75%) and familial (25%) forms, the familial type being associated with MEN-I. These familial tumours are usually multiple and only 30% are malignant, whereas sporadic gastrinomas are usually unifocal and over 60% are malignant. Previously at least half of all gastrinomas had metastasised by the time of diagnosis, but now, with the frequent use of radioimmunoassay, small solitary tumours are being found at an earlier stage. Approximately 90% of gastrinomas occur in the gastrinoma triangle which is bounded by the junction of cystic duct and common bile duct superiorly, the junction of the second and third parts of the duodenum inferiorly, and the junction of the neck and body of the pancreas medially.

Zollinger–Ellison syndrome is dominated by gastric acid hypersecretion, which causes severe multiple peptic ulcers. The ulcers are usually duodenal, but may occur in the oesophagus, stomach and jejunum. Ulcer symptoms are often refractory to large doses of antacids or standard doses of H_2 blocking agents. Complications such as haemorrhage, perforation and obstruction are common.

Diarrhoea and steatorrhoea are due to acid inactivation of pancreatic lipase and small bowel mucosal damage.

Diagnosis

The diagnosis of gastrinoma syndrome requires the demonstration of elevated fasting serum gastrin levels while the patient is not taking antacids, H_2 receptor antagonists or proton pump inhibitors and in the presence of high basal gastric acid secretion. Patients with gastrinoma usually have serum gastrin levels exceeding 500 pg/ml. Grossly elevated gastrin levels (> 5000 pg/ml) or the presence of chains of human chorionic gonadotropin in the serum usually indicate malignancy (16).

Gastrinoma can be differentiated from other causes of hypergastrinaemia by performing a secretin stimulation test. Secretin is a potent stimulant of gastrin release from gastrinomas but has little effect on other types of hypergastrinaemia such as gastric outlet obstruction, retained antrum after a Billroth II gastrectomy and the rare condition of G cell hyperplasia. Serum calcium should be measured routinely in all patients with gastrinoma to exclude associated hyperparathyroidism.

Imaging and Localisation

Preoperative

Preoperative ultrasonography and CT have a low yield (20–30% sensitive) in patients with primary gastrinoma, reflecting the small size and the extrapancreatic location of the tumour (17), but CT can detect hepatic and nodal metastases. Radiolabelled octreotide scans help to define the extent of the tumour (Figure 2). These scans are performed by injection of tyrosine-3-octreotide (synthetic derivative of somatostatin) labelled with [^{123}I] which will accumulate in the primary islet-cell tumour and its metastases if they contain somatostatin receptors. In one study, high levels of somatostatin receptors were found in four of five gastrinomas, two of five insulinomas and a high proportion of carcinoid tumours (18).

Selective angiography remains the investigation of choice. It is less sensitive for gastrinoma than insulinoma, probably because gastrinomas tend to be less vascular and less likely to blush. Recently, pharmacoangiography has been used by selective intra-arterial injection of secretin combined with peripheral venous sampling to measure the level of gastrin. Doppman and colleagues (19) used this technique in 17 patients and found it the most sensitive test for localising gastrinomas, making transhepatic portal venous sampling obsolete.

Contrast-enhanced colour Doppler ultrasonography is a rapidly advancing field in oncoradiology (20). Injected microbubbles are used to cross the pulmonary capillaries and produce a useful systemic Doppler ultrasound enhancement of the tumour neovascularity. As neuroendocrine tumours are usually hypervascular, contrast-enhanced US has been successful in the localisation of small pancreatic islet-cell tumours and also in assessing liver metastases. It can

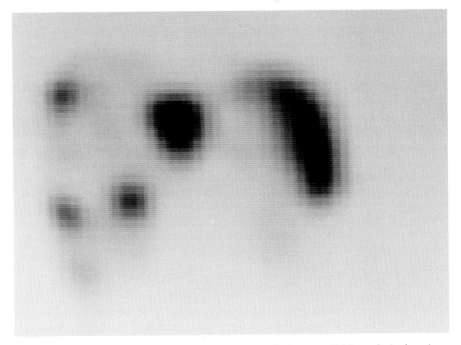

Figure 2. Indium-labelled octreotide scan demonstrating multiple areas of high uptake in the epigastrium and right lobe of liver due to non-functioning neuroendocrine tumour of the head of pancreas with liver metastases.

detect pancreatic gastrinomas as small as 5 mm that have been missed by computed tomography.

Intraoperative

IOUS is best in pancreatic tumours, for which 100% sensitivity has been claimed when combined with surgical palpation (21). Intraoperative endoscopy with transillumination of the duodenal wall can help to detect duodenal gastrinomas. Any uncertainties in the duodenum can be resolved by duodenotomy and bidigital palpation of the wall.

Treatment

Sporadic gastrinoma

The optimal curative treatment of gastrinoma is surgical excision. Failure to image the gastrinoma should certainly not preclude explorative laparotomy because many of these lesions can be found by an experienced surgeon (12). Adequate exposure of the pancreas is required, as for insulinoma. All suspicious lesions should be biopsied and sent for frozen section. IOUS is helpful to locate intrapancreatic tumours and determine their relationship to the pancreatic duct. The mucosal surface of the duodenum must be carefully palpated for micro-adenomas through a duodenotomy in the second part of the duodenum. Small gastrinomas detected in this fashion can simply be enucleated. Tumours in the pancreas are usually enucleated or excised locally with or without Roux loop cover (13). Again, as for insulinoma, distal conservative pancreatectomy is indicated for deeper lesions in the body or tail. For deep lesions in the head of pancreas and for multiple duodenal adenomas, pancreatoduodenectomy should be considered in fit patients, especially if adjacent lymph nodes are involved confirming the malignant nature of the tumour. Whipple's resection may be preferred to pylorus-preserving procedures because the duodenal bulb is often deformed from recurrent peptic ulcers.

Patients who respond poorly to antisecretory drugs and have either no tumour or multifocal disease at exploration should only be treated by total gastrectomy to prevent life-threatening peptic ulcer complications. As gastrinomas are located more in the head, blind distal pancreatectomy for occult tumour is not justified.

Familial Gastrinoma (MEN-I)

MEN-I patients with associated islet-cell tumours present a dilemma to the surgeon because they usually have multiple pancreatic and duodenal adenomas. We recommend a thorough attempt at preoperative localisation and an exploratory laparotomy on patients with no evidence of liver metastasis. The duodenal mucosa should be scrutinised and the pancreas examined in detail for multiple lesions. Patients with hyperparathyroidism should have parathyroidectomy before gastrinoma surgery to stabilise blood calcium levels.

Metastatic Gastrinoma

Gastric acid hypersecretion can usually be controlled by a proton pump inhibitor. Thus some patients with metastatic gastrinomas may remain symptom-free until late in the course of the disease, while others require treatment for painful or enlarging metastatic lesions. Results with chemotherapy for liver metastases have not been encouraging. Streptozotocin, 5-fluorouracil and doxorubicin have been the only drugs with therapeutic efficiency. Hepatic artery ligation or embolisation for metastatic gastrinoma has not been adequately evaluated. Hepatic artery embolisation combined with chemotherapy (chemoembolisation) has been successfully used in 50% of patients (22). Palliative surgical debulking may help to control the Zollinger–Ellison syndrome. As somatostatin reduces gastrin levels and gastric acid secretion, its synthetic analogue octreotide may also be effective in relieving symptoms.

Other Functioning Tumours

VIPoma

VIPomas secrete vasoactive intestinal polypeptide (VIP). Ninety per cent are located in the pancreas and 20% of these are multifocal. The remaining 10% are extrapancreatic in sites such as the adrenal medulla or paraganglionic tissue, and these are especially common in children. Approximately half of VIPomas are malignant. These tumours present with watery diarrhoea, hypokalaemia and achlorhydria (WDHA syndrome). The diarrhoea is profuse, with an average of 5 l/day (pancreatic cholera), and it results in massive faecal loss of potassium and bicarbonate; there is severe hypokalaemia and metabolic acidosis. As the half-life of VIP is only 2 minutes, the diagnosis can be confirmed by the finding of elevated plasma peptide histidine methionine (PHM), produced from the per-pro-VIP molecule in a more stable form. Since most VIPomas exceed 3 cm in diameter and are solitary, localisation by scanning and selective angiography is not difficult.

The definitive treatment of VIPoma is surgical excision following adequate fluid and electrolyte replacement. Glucocorticoids or octreotide offer good symptomatic control for diarrhoea. Surgical options include enucleation or distal pancreatectomy. Blind pancreatic resection is probably unwarranted since islet-cell hyperplasia is an unproven cause of the syndrome (23). Surgical debulking of metastatic disease provides effective palliation. The average survival of patients with malignant VIPoma syndrome is approximately 12 months.

Glucagonoma

Glucagonomas are rare α cell tumours of the pancreatic islet and are responsible for the characteristic syndrome of migratory necrolytic dermatitis, weight loss, diabetes mellitus, deep venous thrombosis, anaemia and hypoalbuminaemia. The age range is 20–70 years, and the tumour is commonest in women. Glucagonomas are usually found in the body and tail of pancreas and rarely affect the head. By the time of diagnosis they tend to be large and have often metastasised to the liver, lymph nodes, adrenals or vertebrae. The diagnosis is confirmed by finding an elevated plasma glucagon level.

Definitive surgical treatment is indicated in nearly every case, good palliation being achieved by subtotal removal of tumour. When the tumour is still localised to the pancreas, surgical resection can completely reverse the clinical manifestations of the syndrome and result in a lasting cure. Perioperative management includes hyperalimentation and prophylactic low molecular weight heparin. Non-surgical palliative options include selective arterial embolisation, chemotherapy and octreotide therapy. Streptozotocin plus 5-fluorouracil can reduce both tumour size and circulatory glucagon levels. Octreotide normalises serum glucagon, improves skin rash, and promotes weight gain but has no effect on tumour size. Sporadic case reports of liver transplantation for hepatic metastases (following removal of the primary glucagonoma) are available with a variable survival benefit (24,25).

Somatostatinoma

Somatostatinomas are similarly rare (γ cell) tumours, characterised by diabetes mellitus, diarrhoea, steatorrhoea and gastric hypochlorhydria. Most of them are large and readily demonstrated by CT; half the patients have hepatic metastases at diagnosis. Confirmation of the diagnosis can be made by finding an elevated somatostatin level in the plasma.

Small somatostatin-rich periampullary tumours have been reported in patients with von Recklinghausen's disease. These duodenal lesions usually present early because of local effects, do not cause a typical "syndrome" and are associated with a normal plasma level of somatostatin. The treatment of choice is surgical excision whenever possible. Combined chemotherapy including streptozotocin is the best non-operative treatment for unresectable tumours.

Non-functioning Tumours

These tumours account for 15–41% of pancreatic endocrine tumours and are not associated with a recognisable hormonal syndrome. Many of them are located in the head of the pancreas (2,3) and are malignant (3). They are usually solid tumours, but cystic forms have occasionally been reported (26). They are identical histologically to functioning tumours but differ in their clinical course and outcome. Lacking the features of an endocrine syndrome, they seldom present until there is advanced local disease or distant metastases.

The presenting features are those of mass effect, including pain, weight loss and a palpable mass. Obstructive jaundice is not uncommon, but sometimes liver function is well preserved despite a large tumour in the pancreatic head. Distortion of the duodenal loop may cause vomiting. Bleeding into the gastrointestinal tract or peritoneal cavity is an occasional feature, likewise recurrent acute pancreatitis. The gut hormone profile is normal except for an occasional elevation in pancreatic polypeptide (2). The neuroendocrine origin is confirmed by immunohistochemical analysis of the tumour tissue, which is positive for chromogranin and neuron-specific enolase.

The localisation procedures of choice are contrast-enhanced CT and selective angiography. Radiological features in favour of these tumours (as opposed to typical pancreatic adenocarcinoma) are an unusually large size, calcification within the tumour and hypervascularity. Non-functioning neuroendocrine neoplasia should be suspected in a patient with a large pancreatic tumour who has not lost much weight or who presents with a mass in the head of pancreas with minimal jaundice. Angiography will show a tumour blush in 70–80% of such cases (2), and a similar impression can be gained from the contrast-enhanced CT scan.

Surgical resection is probably the best treatment, whether curative or palliative, but it should not be performed if there is serious risk because these patients may have prolonged survival with non-operative treatment. Operative excision has the added benefits of preventing life-threatening haemorrhage and relieving pain. Although these tumours are seldom curable by radical excision, many patients will remain symptom-free for several years (2). Unlike pancreatic exocrine carcinomas, non-functioning endocrine malignancies many respond favourably to adjuvant chemotherapy. The 5-year survival is about 15% (9).

References

1. O'Shea D, Bloom SR, Williamson RCN (1996) Endocrine tumours. In: McCulloch P, Kingsnorth A (eds) Management of gastrointestinal cancer. BMJ Publishing, London, pp 300–320.
2. Cheslyn-Curtis S, Sitaram V, Williamson RCN (1993) Management of non-functioning neuroendocrine tumours of the pancreas. Br J Surg 80:625–762.

3. Eckhauser FE, Cheung PS, Vinik AI, Strodel WE, Lioyd RV, Thompson NW (1986) Non-functioning malignant neuroendocrine tumors of the pancreas. Surgery 100:978.

4. Simpson WF, Adams DB, Metcalf JS, Anderson MC (1988) Non-functioning pancreatic neuroendocrine tumors presenting as pancreatitis: report of four cases. Pancreas 3:223–231.

5. Mao C, Howard JM (1996) Pancreatitis associated with neuroendocrine (islet cell) tumours of the pancreas. Am J Surg 171:562–564.

6. Zanow J, Gellert K, Benhidjeb T, Muller JM (1996) Cystic tumours of the pancreas. Chirurgil 67:719–124.

7. Rothmund M, Angelini L, Brunt M, Farndon JR, Geelhoed G, Grama D (1990) Surgery for benign insulinoma: an international review. World J Surg 14:393–399.

8. Stefanini P, Carboni M, Patrassi N, Basoli A (1974) Beta-islet cell tumors of the pancreas: results of a study on 1067 cases. Surgery 75:597–609.

9. Reber HA, Way LW (1995) Pancreas. In: Way LW (ed) Current surgical diagnosis and treatment. Appleton and Lange, Connecticut, pp 558–584.

10. Geoghegan JG, Jackson JE, Lewis MPN et al. (1994) Localisation and surgical management of insulinoma. Br J Surg 81:1025–1028.

11. Doppman JL, Miller DL, Chang R, Shawker TH, Gordon P, Norton JA (1994) Insulinomas: localisation with selective intra-arterial injection of calcium. Radiology 178:237–241.

12. Norton JA, Cromack DT, Shawker TH et al. (1987) Intra-operative ultrasonographic localisation of islet cell tumors (a prospective comparison to palpation). Ann Surg 207:160–168.

13. Aldridge MC, Williamson RCN (1993) Surgery of endocrine tumours of the pancreas. In: Lynn J, Bloom SR (eds) Surgical endocrinology, Butterworth-Heinemann, Oxford, pp 503–520.

14. van Heerden JA, Edis JA, Service FJ (1979) The surgical aspects of insulinomas. Ann Surg 189:677–682.

15. Boissel P, Proye C (1985) Les tumeurs endocrines du pancreas. Paris, Masson.

16. Way LW (1995) Zollinger–Ellison syndrome. In: Way LW (ed) Current surgical diagnosis and treatment. Appleton and Lange, Connecticut, pp 474–476.

17. Wise SR, Johnson J, Sparks J, Carey LC, Ellison EC (1989) Gastrinoma: the predictive value of pre-operative localisation. Surgery 106:1087–1093.

18. Reubi JC, Maurer R, von Werder K et al. (1987) Somatostatin receptors in human endocrine tumors. Cancer Res 47:551–558.

19. Doppman JL, Miller DL, Chang R et al. (1990) Gastrinomas: localisation by means of selective intra-arterial injection of secretin. Radiology 174:25–29.

20. Cosgrove DO, Blomley MJK (1997) Evaluation of tumours using echo-enhancing agents. In: Goldberg BB (ed). Ultrasound contrast agents, Martin Dunitz, London, pp 159–168.

21. Norton JA, Doppman JL, Collen JL et al. (1986) Prospective study of gastrinoma localisation and resection in patients with Zollinger–Ellison syndrome. Ann Surg 204:468–479.

22. Moertel CG, May GR, Martin JK et al. (1985) Sequential hepatic artery occlusion (HAO) and chemotherapy for metastatic carcinoid tumour and islet cell tumor (ICT). Proc Am Soc Clin Oncol 4:80(abstract).

23. Moossa AR, Stabile BE (1996) Vipoma. In: Cuschieri A, Giles GR, Moossa AR (eds) Essential surgical practice 3rd edn, Butterworth-Heinemann Ltd, Oxford, pp 1274–1275.

24. Anthubar M, Jauch K, Briegel J, Groh J (1996) Results of liver transplantation for gastroenteropancreatic tumor metastases. World J Surg 20:73–76.

25. Alsina AE, Bartus S, Hull D, Rosson R, Schweizer RT (1990) Liver transplant for metastatic neuroendocrine tumour. J Clin Gastroenterol 12:533–537.

26. Lapeyrie H, Loizon P, Chapuis H et al. (1989) Non-functioning or silent endocrine tumours of the pancreas. Apropos of a case of cystic form. Ann Chir 43:302–305.

Section 5

Pancreatic Cancer

26 Molecular Basis of Pancreatic Cancer: Strategies for Genetic Diagnosis and Therapy

F.C. McCormick and N.R. Lemoine

Cancer is essentially a genetic disease, and tumour progression occurs as a multistep process with the accumulation of multiple genetic abnormalities that lead to an unstable malignant genotype. The molecular biology of pancreatic cancer is still poorly understood, though recently significant progress has been made with the identification of at least four genes involved in tumorigenesis. The genetic profile of pancreatic cancer not only involves proto-oncogene activation, and loss of tumour suppressor gene function but also derangement of the signal transduction systems for growth factors and their receptors.

Knowledge of the molecular biology of pancreatic cancer is becoming of increasing value for diagnosis. In the future, it is hoped that such knowledge will be exploited to provide a basis for the development of novel approaches to determine prognosis, and develop new therapeutic and screening strategies.

Molecular Biology of Pancreatic Adenocarcinoma

Tumour Suppressor Genes

p53

Mutation of the p53 gene is probably the most common genetic event in human malignancy. This gene encodes a 53 kDa nuclear phosphoprotein that can interact with cellular and viral proteins to regulate transcription and it can directly bind DNA, both specifically and non-specifically, to act as a transcription factor. This gene is involved in the cell cycle, apoptosis, DNA repair and synthesis, cell differentiation and genomic plasticity and its activity is affected by the cellular environment and the physical conformation of its protein.

Mutation of just one p53 allele leads to a dominant negative effect, causing unregulated cellular proliferation (1,2) and as mutant p53 is more stable than wild-type it has a longer half-life and tends to accumulate in neoplastic tissue where it can be visualised by immunohistochemistry (3). At least 50% of pancreatic cancers show allelic loss (deletion of one copy of the gene) at the p53 locus 17p13 (4).

There is a broad range of mutations seen in p53 and these have provided clear evidence for carcinogen fingerprinting. From examination of this spectrum of mutations, it may be possible to identify specific mutagens. The frequency and range of p53 mutations may act as an indicator of carcinogen exposure and this could prove useful in assessing human cancer risk.

Experimental studies have shown that while inactivation of the p53 tumour suppressor gene is insufficient to cause pancreatic cancer in transgenic mice (5), cooperation between activated KRAS and inactivated p53 have been noted in a number of models producing cellular transformation with enhanced metastases (6,7).

p16 (CDKN2/MTS1/p16^{INK4})

This tumour suppressor gene is located on chromosome 9p21 (8) and is critical to cell cycle control. During the cell cycle, the cell must pass through an important checkpoint, the restriction point, to progress to G1 phase. This requires activation of CDK4 by cyclin D1. The CDK4/cyclin D1 complex participates in phosphorylation of the retinoblastoma gene product pRb. This enables free E_2F to dissociate from hypophosphorylated Rb/E_2F complex, enabling progression through the G1/S transition phase of the cell cycle. p16 prevents Rb phosphorylation by inactivating the CDK4/cyclin D1 complex thus inhibiting progression through the cell cycle. It is inactivated in approximately 80% of pancreatic carcinomas, either by mutation of one allele and deletion of the other or alternatively by homozygous deletion of both alleles (9,10). Also, aberrations of the p16 gene have been found in the germline of certain patients with pancreatic carcinoma associated with familial melanoma (11,12).

The deleted fragment commonly includes the candidate suppressor gene p15, which lies at a closely adjacent locus and hence it is possible that this gene is also important in the pathogenesis of pancreatic cancer.

SMAD4 (DPC4-deleted in pancreatic carcinoma, locus 4)

This gene is located on chromosome 18q21.1 and has 11 exons. There is allelic loss at chromosome 18q in approximately 90% of pancreatic carcinomas and approximately 30% of pancreatic tumours are found to have homozygous deletions at 18q21.1 (13,14). The 3′ end of the gene is highly conserved and reports of mutations within this region support the idea that the C-terminal region is important for tumour suppressor function (13). Exons 1, 2 and 11 bear great sequence similarity to the *Drosophila melanogaster* protein Mad (Mothers against dpp) and the *Caenorhabditas elegans* proteins sma-2, sma-3 and sma-4. These proteins form part of the post-receptor transforming growth factor beta (TGFβ) signalling pathway and it is suggested that SMAD4-induced tumour suppression acts along a TGFβ-like signalling pathway. SMAD4 has been found to be responsive to both TGFβ and TGFβ-superfamily growth factors such as BMP2 and BMP4 (15,16). Data suggest that whilst SMAD4 appears to contribute to the carcinogenesis of sporadic pancreatic carcinoma, it is not involved in the tumorigenesis of head and neck and breast cancers.

Oncogenes

Kras

The RAS oncogene family consists of three human genes NRAS, KRAS and HRAS and these are the most frequently mutated dominant oncogenes in human neoplasia (17). These genes encode small GTP-binding proteins that are involved in signal transduction. They participate in signalling for a variety of cellular functions including cellular differentiation, cell cycle progression, cytoskeletal organisation and protein transport and secretion. Activation occurs by the binding of GTP via a guanine nucleotide exchange factor triggered by tyrosine kinase receptors. The return to the resting state by intrinsic GTPase activity is enhanced by GTPase-activating proteins (GAPs). Point mutations reduce the ability of the KRAS protein to respond to GAPs. The bound GTP fails to hydrolyse, causing the gene to be perpetually locked into the active conformation so leading to continuous transmission of growth signal to the nucleus. Signal transduction systems from a variety of growth factor receptors overexpressed in pancreatic carcinoma converge on the RAS protein, producing further growth stimulation.

KRAS mutations are the commonest genetic event described in pancreatic carcinoma and are found in up to 85% of advanced cases of ductal adenocarcinoma (18–20). This is an exceptionally high frequency compared with other tumours. Mutations in the NRAS and HRAS are uncommon. The spectrum of RAS mutations is suggestive of multiple carcinogen involvement or errors in the DNA repair mechanism rather than causation by a single, specific mutagen. However, there is similarity between the G to A transition commonly seen in pancreatic and colorectal cancer and those induced by alkylating agents, suggesting possible involvement of dietary genotoxins.

The pattern of KRAS mutations has been reported to be markedly different in Japanese compared with Europeans and there appears to be regional variation within Europe (21), raising the possibility of ethnic and/or environmental differences. By correlating all these genetic findings with epidemiology, it may be possible to identify geographical or ethnic differences in the pathogenesis of this disease as well as identifying specific genotoxic substances.

Other Genes

DCC (Deleted in Colorectal Carcinoma)

Whilst there is allelic loss at chromosome 18q in approximately 90% of pancreatic carcinomas, inactivation of the SMAD4 gene only accounts for approximately half of those, suggesting further tumour suppressor genes may be targeted by 18q losses. The DCC gene is a complex gene consisting of 29 exons spanning 1.4 megabases and it is situated on chromosome 18q close to DPC4. Initial reports suggested abnormalities in the expression of the DCC gene in pancreatic cancer (22,23) though subsequent data suggested that deletion of the DCC locus is uncommon (24). Definitive sequence analysis of this large gene has not been carried out in pancreatic carcinoma.

BRCA2

This is one of the genes responsible for predisposition to male and female breast cancer within a small subset of patients (25,26). Pancreatic carcinoma develops in a significant number of members of male and female breast cancer families (27,28) and recent data have suggested that this gene may also be involved in a subgroup of patients with pancreatic carcinoma (29).

APC (Adenomatous Polyposis Coli Gene)

This gene is located at chromosome 5q21 and was first identified in patients with familial adenomatous polyposis (30). At present there is a discrepancy of results between Western groups that have found no evidence of gene mutations or loss of protein expression of the APC gene (31,32) and those of some Japanese authors who reported inactivating mutations in a small number of cases, predicting a truncation of the gene product (33). The significance of this discrepancy has not been explained yet and whether it represents some form of ethnic variation remains to be seen.

Microsatellite Instability (MSI)

Microsatellites are short repetitive sequences of DNA scattered throughout the genome. These vary between individuals and have a relatively low inherent mutational rate. MSI has been seen in several tumours including colorectal and gastric tumours but the presence of MSI in pancreatic cancer is controversial. In the literature, Japanese studies tend to support the presence of MSI in pancreatic cancer (34) whilst most Western groups find this to be a rare phenomenon (35). This apparent geographical variation raises the possibility of ethnic differences.

Early Intraductal Neoplastic Change

Investigation into human neoplasia shows that most epithelial malignancies progress through several precursor lesions and recent studies have suggested that this is also true for pancreatic cancer. Several ductal lesions may be seen in association with pancreatic carcinoma. These include squamous metaplasia, flat and papillary ductal hyperplasia with or without cellular atypia, ductular complexes, ulcer-associated cell lineage (UACL) and carcinoma-in-situ. Many of these lesions are found not only in pancreatic adenocarcinoma but also in the ageing pancreas and chronic pancreatitis, and it is debatable whether these are potentially precursor lesions or are merely changes secondary to tumour obstruction. Carcinoma-in-situ is rarely found in the absence of invasive tumour.

Recently, there has been substantial success in the identification of genetic abnormalities within some ductal lesions, predominantly involving KRAS and p16 (36–38). This has been aided by the use of microdissection of the ductal epithelium of interest, possibly utilising micromanipulators, lasers or glues. However, the current classification of ductal lesions is inadequate and misleading. In practice, there appears to be a spectrum of histological abnormalities within the pancreatic ductal system, where one or more features may be seen together. Therefore, in an attempt to determine precursor lesions, it is of the utmost importance to assess accurately the histological features present before interpreting the associated molecular biological changes.

KRAS and p16 mutations, identical to those found in invasive pancreatic carcinoma, have been found in non-dysplastic, hyperplastic ductal lesions showing both papillary and non-papillary morphology, as well as in dysplastic ductal lesions (38). This is a very strong argument to consider these changes as precursor lesions. However, KRAS mutations have also been found in ductal lesions of the normal pancreas and should not be considered as a marker for preneoplastic change alone (39). In fact, activated RAS appears to induce growth arrest in both human and rodent cell lines (40,41) and additional molecular events appear to be necessary, such as the inactivation of either p53 or p16.

As approximately 25% of pancreatic ductal adenocarcinomas retain the wild-type KRAS, there must be alternative neoplastic pathways, that may also be seen within the preneoplastic ductal lesions.

Growth Factors and their Receptors

Carcinogenesis requires loss of control of the cell cycle coupled with derangement of cell activation and the latter includes deregulation of growth factor expression and cell-signal transduction. There is overexpression of several growth factor receptor-ligand families and these appear to participate in aberrant autocrine and paracrine pathways so contributing to pancreatic tumour cell growth. Some of these changes also occur in chronic pancreatitis suggesting that overexpression of these receptor-ligand systems in itself is not sufficient to produce malignant transformation, but in combination with other genetic abnormalities may lead to a distinct growth advantage. Further discussion of growth factors is found in Chapter 28.

Cytogenetics

Data on the cytogenetic abnormalities of pancreatic carcinoma indicate that there is a wide variety of karyotypic abnormalities, most of which are complex and include numerical and structural abnormalities (42).

The most frequent findings are whole chromosomal gains in chromosomes 20 and 7, and whole chromosomal losses in chromosomes 18, 13, 12, 17 and 6. The most frequent loss of alleles occurs on chromosomal arms 1p, 9p, 17p and 18q with less common losses observed at 3p, 6p, 6q, 8p, 10p, 12q, 13q, 18p, 21q and 22q.

In summary, our knowledge of the cellular and molecular genetic basis of pancreatic cancer has increased dramatically over the past decade, aided principally by advances in laboratory techniques. The challenge now is to harness and translate this knowledge into various strategies for improving diagnostic capabilities, aiding screening and developing therapeutic regimes in order to benefit those who are affected or at risk of this disease.

Diagnostic and Therapeutic Strategies

Diagnosis

Pancreatic carcinoma is commonly a silent disease that usually presents at a late stage. To aid diagnosis and staging, imaging modalities such as computed tomography, abdominal ultrasonography, angiography, magnetic resonance imaging (MRI) and endoscopic retrograde cholangiopancreatography (ERCP) are required. Ideally, early stage diagnosis could improve the appalling prognosis of this tumour but there are severe limitations in visualising small lesions (presently 1 cm or less) and reliable screening by imaging techniques is presently not possible.

Sometimes the definitive diagnosis of pancreatic carcinoma has to be determined from differential diagnoses including chronic pancreatitis. This may require the assistance of cytodiagnosis and includes biochemical and cytological analysis of pure pancreatic juice and brushings taken at ERCP, percutaneous needle biopsies of pancreas, as well as serum and stool samples. The biochemical studies involve analysis of multiple assays of tumour-associated antigens including CA 19.9, DU-PAN-2, CA 125, CA 50 and CA 242. These appear to bear some relationship to resectability of tumour and prognosis but are relatively imprecise (43–45).

Exploitation of the frequent and highly specific features of malignant pancreatic cells such as the high frequency of KRAS, TP53 and p16 mutations has enabled the development of several new approaches to diagnosis and presently these are adjuncts to conventional techniques. Mutations of oncogenes and tumour suppressor genes in material may be detected by simple and sensitive PCR-based assays and several reports indicate good correlation of positive results with a histologically proven diagnosis of pancreatic cancer (46,47). KRAS mutations may be detected not only in body fluids but also in stool samples (48) and recently it has been reported that tumour cells carrying KRAS mutations can be detected in the peripheral blood of patients with pancreatic cancer, even when there are no clinically identifiable metastases (49,50).

Accumulation of mutant p53 can be detected very easily by immunochemical assays which can be used to detect cells in body fluids. Also, detection of anti-p53 antibodies in the blood has been suggested as a potential screening test (51).

Inactivation of the p16 gene appears to occur almost exclusively in pancreatic carcinoma and not in other gastrointestinal tract carcinomas, and hence it may be possible to detect mutations of this gene by multiple genetic assays which could help to localise the origin of the shed neoplastic cells. However, as previously described, gene mutations may be found in cases with non-invasive tumour and so interpretation of these mutations should be considered in the context of other findings.

It is hoped that further advances in our knowledge of the genetic events of pancreatic cancer, including identification of those events associated with the earliest stages of neoplasia and preneoplasia coupled with advances in technology, will enable pancreatic cancer to be diagnosed in the future, at an early and treatable stage. Also, identification of the responsible gene(s) should allow counselling and even preventative intervention in families with an inherited site-specific predisposition to pancreatic cancer.

Therapeutic Potentials

Gene therapy is defined as the transfer and expression of exogenous genetic material into human cells to produce a therapeutic response. In theory, the malignant nature of tumour cells may be rendered benign by correcting the relevant genetic abnormalities by somatic gene therapy. However, this is a rather simplistic view and correction of a single mutant oncogene or restoration of the function of a solitary tumour suppressor gene may be inadequate to reverse the malignant phenotype. An alternative method is to target and selectively destroy the malignant cells.

The main problem of these techniques is the difficulty in achieving efficient and targeted gene delivery *in vivo* whilst avoiding or at least minimising harm to normal cells. The "bystander effect" is seen in a mixed population of cells that includes cells showing successful gene transfer and other cells that are unaffected. The expression and subsequent effects of the gene transfer (for example, cell death) may be seen not only in the expressing cells, but also within the adjacent non-expressing cells, and this is extremely useful where transduction efficiency is poor.

Germline and Somatic Gene Therapy

In theory, gene therapy could be applied to germ cells, but this is presently considered to be ethically unacceptable and so permanent correction of familial cancer predisposition syndromes by gene transfer into germ cells (usually ova) cannot be considered (52,53). However, genetic intervention in the form of *in vitro* fertilisation and preimplantation diagnosis is routinely carried out for familial genetic diseases such as cystic fibrosis and Duchenne muscular dystrophy (53–55). This strategy could be used in the prevention of cancer in cases of inherited cancer predisposition syndromes at an intermediate stage when the disease still involves only a single genetic abnormality rather than at the multigene stage seen in established cancer. For example, in patients with familial adenomatous polyposis caused by "loss of function" mutations in the APC gene, the introduction of a normal gene into the intestinal epithelial cells by intraluminal delivery of liposome-complexed DNA has led to temporary restoration of functional gene expression (56).

It is recognised that up to 5% of cases of pancreatic cancer have a hereditary component and may occur as part of multisite syndromes such as familial atypical multiple mole melanoma syndrome (57) and ataxia telangiectasia (58). In the future, strategies could be applied to treat individuals known to carry a specific genetic abnormality predisposing to pancreatic cancer development.

Somatic gene therapy involves the insertion of genes into the diploid cells of an individual, but the genetic material will not be passed on to the subject's progeny. There are four major approaches to genetic intervention for cancer therapy and all have advantages and disadvantages. These are outlined below.

Replacement or Augmentation of Tumour Suppressor Gene Function

Mutational inactivation of several tumour suppressor genes frequently occurs in pancreatic carcinoma, and these are potential targets for genetic intervention to replace tumour suppressor function. TP53 is found mutated in approximately half of pancreatic carcinomas. It is involved in cell cycle arrest and apoptosis in response to DNA damage. Restoration of function by transferring wild-type TP53 into tumour cells expressing mutant p53 can cause phenotypic reversion of transformed cells *in vivo* and *in vitro* (59,60).

However, approximately 35% of pancreatic cancer cases show no p53 gene abnormalities and even in cases with mutations there can be significant intra-tumoral heterogeneity of expression. Also, there is some evidence of an alternative mechanism of p53 inactivation that has been found in the upregulated expression of the MDM2 gene product in about 60% of pancreatic cancers and cell lines (61).

p16 is another tumour suppressor gene that is abnormal in approximately 80% of pancreatic cancer cases. It has recently been shown that ectopic expression of p16[INK4] can block entry into S phase of the cell cycle induced by RAS onco-gene and/or the c-*myc* oncogenes, provided there is functional retinoblastoma protein (62). As most pancreatic cancers have normal RB1 genes there is potential for a p16[INK4] replacement strategy in this disease.

SMAD4 is a candidate tumour suppressor gene which presently requires more detailed investigation but may well be another target for gene therapy.

Whilst data suggest that correction of a mutated tumour suppressor gene to the wild type may produce dramatic antitumour effects, it is likely that individual tumour suppressor genes may be important only at specific times in tumour evolution because of the acquisition of other genetic mutations that contribute to tumorigenesis. Also because of the heterogeneous nature of the tumour, there may be separate subclones that have evolved along different pathways (63,64).

Blockade of Dominant Gene Expression

Several strategies may be employed, one of which is the inhibition of dominant gene expression by the "antisense" approach. As gene expression is modulated by naturally occurring antisense interactions there is great interest in the development of antisense technology to target specific cellular transcription and translation (65). All strategies are based on complementary base pairing. Either synthetic oligonucleotides or recombinant genes in reverse orientation are introduced using expression vectors. Most work has used modified oligonucleotides showing increased stability and lipid solubility. Chimaeric oligonucleotides have the modified linkage for only part of the model, either at the 5′ or 3′ end, as intra-cellular degradation is usually due to exonuclease activity (66). Candidates for potential antisense therapies include the KRAS and p53 genes.

Inhibition of the RAS signalling pathway with several independent methods has been shown to modulate critical aspects of RAS-mediated transformation in whole cells (67–69). Three regions of the KRAS mRNA have been targeted in the design of antisense oligonucleotides (70). These were able to produce dose-dependent antiproliferative effects in human pancreatic cancer cell lines although there was generally poor discrimination between the antisense and the control (either sense, mismatched or randomised) oligonucleotides. There was little evidence for reduced KRAS protein levels using Western blot analysis in any of the oligonucleotide-treated cells.

By interfering with the localisation of the mutant gene product, its function may be altered. The active RAS protein must be localised to the cell membrane, and this process requires lipid modification of its carboxy terminus. This may be inhibited by drugs that interfere with HMG CoA reductase or other enzymes involved in the metabolism of cholesterol. Drugs such as lovastatin have been shown to inhibit growth and tumorigenicity of pancreatic cancer cells (71,72).

Antisense technology in its present state is deficient in many areas. A study using antisense oligonucleotides against p53 showed that although there was an antiproliferative effect, there was no evidence that the effect of the oligo-nucleotides was mediated by either an antisense interaction or by regulation of p53 expression (73).

Genetically Directed Enzyme Producing Therapy (GDEPT)

The principle of this method is to take advantage of the transcriptional differences between normal and malignant cells. Transfer of a metabolic suicide gene (a prodrug-activating enzyme) into target cells enables selective gene expression that is directed by a tumour/tissue-specific gene promoter. These enzymes produce cellular susceptibility of the target cells to the toxin metabolised from the subsequently administered prodrug. Several enzymes are commonly used. The herpes simplex virus thymidine kinase (HSV-tk) converts the antiviral agent ganciclovir to potent inhibitors of DNA polymerase α (74). Cytosine deaminase converts 5-fluorocytosine to 5-fluorouracil and further metabolic breakdown products that obstruct DNA and RNA synthesis (75). A variety of gene promoters might be exploited for GDEPT in pancreatic carcinoma and already there have been encouraging results reported with the human HER2 promoter and the CEA promoter (76,77). When the HER2 promoter is fused to the cytosine deaminase gene or HSV thymidine kinase gene and introduced into pancreatic cells *in vitro* or *in vivo* using plasmid and viral vectors, expression of the insert occurs only in the HER2 expressing cancer cells (76). This is very encouraging evidence for the specificity of targeting gene expression, in order to minimise potential toxicity in clinical trials.

The CEA gene is expressed in a variety of adenocarcinomas as well as normal intestinal cells, and is a candidate for the tissue-selective targeting of gene expression. In one study, the CEA promoter was fused to the HSV-tk gene and introduced to the CEA-positive pancreatic cell line BxPc3 using an amphotropic retrovirus (77). When treated with the prodrug ganciclovir, the tumour cells were killed, and the fact that not all the target cells needed to be transduced for significant cytotoxicity to occur suggested a "bystander effect".

Other candidate promoter systems include those of the MUC1 gene, MUC2 gene, MUC4 gene, MUC5 gene (78,79) and those of other up-regulated receptor–ligand systems, especially FGFs and FGFRs (80).

There are many technical obstacles to overcome before GDEPT systems may be considered effective options. More effective delivery systems and improvements in promoter specificity and efficacy need to be developed. Even those cells that are transduced may not exhibit efficient gene expression and a further complication is that tumour cells are genetically unstable, so that potential clones could arise that cease to express the suicide gene.

Immunomodulation Strategies

Understanding the principles of the immune system is critical to the design and engineering of cells to stimulate an effective antitumour response. This requires the activation of several types of immune cell including T cells, B cells, antigen-presenting cells and natural killer cells. As most tumours are not immunogenic they must be genetically modified and methods include engineering tumour cells to either secrete cytokines or to express costimulatory immune molecules on their surface. The effects are often pleiomorphic, either direct with cytolysis or indirect with the recruitment of effector cells to the tumour site.

Systemic cytokine administration is associated with dose-limiting toxicity and therefore attempts to enhance local cytokine secretion have been made by either transfecting tumour-infiltrating lymphocytes or transfecting tumour cells.

Polynucleotide vaccination involves the inoculation of experimental animals with plasmids encoding a variety of proteins. This has been shown to stimulate both antibody and T cell immune responses against these proteins *in vivo* (81,82). These responses are specific and sometimes long-lived and are a means of generating tumour-specific immune reactions. In a murine model an idiotypic DNA vaccination induced low levels of anti-idiotypic antibody in serum (83).

There are several possible candidate antigens for pancreatic carcinoma including underglycosylated mucins which can be recognised by MHC-unrestricted T cells (84). Mutated tumour suppressor genes and oncogenes such as RAS and TP53 represent potential targets for immune recognition and attack stimulated by constructs which direct expression of gene fragments that contain T cell epitopes (85). One method is the use of mutant RAS peptides as a vaccine for specific immunotherapy (86). RAS genes are known to carry mutations at specific sites and as the spectrum is limited it is possible to elicit an antitumour immune response by loading antigen-presenting cells with synthetic RAS peptide. A pilot phase I/II study using this technique has shown that a potentially beneficial immune response develops, even in patients with advanced malignant disease (87).

Other potential targets may include normal proteins that show elevated expression in pancreatic carcinoma such as upregulated growth factor receptors, which may act as a tumour antigen for an immune response. Also, in pancreatic cancer there is re-expression of embryonic antigens, in particular CEA, and this has been used for active adoptive immunotherapy (88).

The question to what extent human tumour cells are immunogenic is still controversial. Advances in our understanding of the costimulatory signals in the regulation of the immune response are encouraging and suggest that immunotherapy may become an important therapeutic device for cancer therapy.

In conclusion, over the past decade our knowledge of molecular biology, coupled with technical advances, has revolutionised our comprehension of cancer. In understanding the molecular and cellular biology of early preneoplastic change within the pancreatic ductal system and of invasive pancreatic carcinoma, it is hoped that new strategies for the diagnosis of early cancer and the amelioration of invasive disease by targeted gene therapy will radically alter the terrible prognosis of this aggressive disease. Also, it is hoped that in the future there may be sensitive and specific screening techniques to detect those genetically at risk of this disease with the ability to offer effective preventative intervention.

References

1. Lane D, Benchimol S (1990) p53: oncogene or anti-oncogene? Genes Dev 4:1–8.
2. Vogelstein B, Kinzler K (1992) p53 function and dysfunction. Cell 70:523–526.
3. Iggo R, Gatter K, Bartek J, Lane DP, Harris AL (1990) Increased expression of mutant forms of p53 oncogene in primary lung cancer. Lancet 335:675–679.
4. Berrozpe G, Schaeffer J, Peinado MA, Real FX, Perucho M (1994) Comparative analysis of mutations in the p53 and K-*ras* genes in pancreas cancer. Int J Cancer 58:185–191.
5. Donehower LA, Harvey M, Slagle BL et al. (1992) Mice deficient for p53 are developmentally normal but are susceptible to spontaneous tumours. Nature 356:215–221.
6. Taylor WR, Eagan SE, Mowat M, Greenberg AH, Wright JA (1992) Evidence for synergistic interactions between *ras*, *myc* and a mutant form of p53 in cellular transformation and tumor dissemination. Oncogene 7:1383–1390.
7. Zambetti GP, Olsen D, Labrow M, Levine AJ (1992) A mutant p53 protein is required for maintenance of the transformed phenotype in cells transformed with p53 plus *ras* cDNAs. Proc Natl Acad Sci USA 89:3953–3956.
8. Kamb A, Gruis NA, Weaver-Feldhaus J et al. (1994) A cell cycle regulator potentially involved in the genesis of many tumor types. Science 264:436–440.
9. Caldas C, Hahn SA, da Costa LT et al. (1994) Frequent somatic mutations and homozygous deletions of the p16 (MTS1) gene in pancreatic adenocarcinoma. Nature Genet 8:27–31.
10. Naumann M, Savitkaia N, Eilert C, Scgramm A, Kalthoff H, Schmiegel W (1996) Frequent codeletions of p16/MTS1 and p15/MTS2 and genetic alterations in p16/MTS1 in pancreatic tumours. Gastroenterology 110:1215–1224.
11. Hussussian CJ, Struewing JP, Goldstein AM et al. (1994) Germline p16 mutations in familial melanoma: Nature Genet 8:15–21.
12. Kamb A, Shattuck-Eidens D, Eeles R et al. (1994) Analysis of the p16 gene (CDNK2) as a candidate for the chromosome 9p melanoma susceptibility locus. Nature Genet 8:23–26.
13. Hahn SA, Schutte M, Hoque AT et al. (1996) DPC4, a candidate tumour suppressor gene at human chromosome 18q21.1 Science 271:350–353.
14. Hahn SA, Hoque AT, Moskaluk CA et al. (1996) Homozygous deletion map at 18q21.1 in pancreatic carcinoma. Cancer Res 56:490–494.
15. Lagna G, Hata A, Hemmati-Brivanlou A, Massague J (1996) Partnership between DPC4 and SMAD proteins in TGF-β signalling pathways. Nature 381:561–562.
16. Massague J (1996) TGFβ signaling: receptors, transducers and Mad proteins. Cell 85:947–950.
17. Bos JL (1989) The *ras* oncogenes in human cancer: a review. Cancer Res 49:4682–4689
18. Grunewald R, Lyons J, Frohlich A et al. (1989) High frequency of Ki-*ras* codon 12 mutation in pancreatic adenocarcinomas. Int J Cancer 43:1037–1041.
19. Hruban RH, Van Mansfeld ADM, Offerhaus GJ et al. (1993) K*ras* oncogene activation in adenocarcinoma of the human pancreas. A study of 82 carcinomas using a combination of mutant-enriched polymerase chain reactions, analysis and allele-specific oligonucleotide hybridization. Am J Pathol 143:545–554.
20. Kalthoff H, Schmiegel W, Roeder C et al. (1993) p53 and K-RAS alterations in pancreatic epithelial cell lesions. Oncogene 8:289–298.
21. Scarpa A, Capelli P, Villanueva A et al. (1994) Pancreatic cancer in Europe: Ki-*ras* gene mutation pattern shows geographical differences. Int J Cancer 57:167–171.
22. Simon B, Weinel R, Hohne M et al. (1994) Frequent alterations of the tumor suppressor genes p53 and DCC in human pancreatic cancer. Gastroenterology 106:1645–1651.
23. Hohne MW, Halatsch M-E, Kahl GF, Weinel RJ (1992) Frequent loss of expression of the potential tumor suppressor gene DCC in ductal pancreatic adenocarcinoma. Cancer Res 52:2616–2619.
24. Barton CM, McKie AB, Hogg A et al. (1995) Abnormalities of the RB1 and DCC tumor suppressor genes: uncommon in human pancreatic cancer. Mol Carcinogen 13:61–69.
25. Wooster R, Neuhausen SL, Mangion J et al. (1994) Localization of a breast cancer susceptibility gene BRCA 2, to chromosome 13q12–13. Science 265:2088–2090.
26. Schutte M, da Costa LT, Hahn SA et al. (1995) Identification by representational difference analysis of a homozygous deletion in pancreatic carcinoma that lies within the BRCA2 region. Proc Natl Acad Sci USA 92:5950–5954.
27. Teng DH, Bogden R, Mitchell J et al. (1996) Low incidence of BRCA2 mutations in breast carcinoma and other cancers. Nature Genet 13:241–244.

28. Phelan CM, Lancaster JM, Tonin P, et al. (1996) Mutational analysis of the BRCA2 gene in 49 site specific breast cancer families. Nature Genet 13:120–122.

29. Wooster R, Bignall G, Lancaster J et al. (1995) Identification of the breast cancer susceptibility gene BRCA2. Nature 378:789–792.

30. Kinzler KW, Nilbert MC, Vogelstein B et al. (1991) Identification of a gene located at chromosome 5q21 that is mutated in colorectal cancers. Science 251:1366–1370.

31. Smith KJ, Johnson KA, Bryan TM et al. (1993) The APC gene product in normal and tumor cells. Proc Natl Acad Sci USA 90:2846–2850.

32. McKie AB, Filipe MI, Lemoine NR (1993) Abnormalities affecting the APC and MCC tumour suppressor gene loci on chromosome 5q occur frequently in gastric cancer but not in pancreatic cancer. Int J Cancer 55:598–603.

33. Horii A, Nakatsuru S, Miyoshi Y et al. (1992) Frequent somatic mutations of the APC gene in human pancreatic cancer. Cancer Res 52:6696–6698.

34. Han H-J, Yanagisawa A, Kato Y, Park J-G, Nakamura Y (1993) Genetic instability in pancreatic cancer and poorly differentiated type of gastric cancer. Cancer Res 53:5087–5089.

35. Hahn SA, Seymour AB, Hogue ATMS et al. (1995) Allotype of pancreatic adenocarcinoma using xenograft enrichment. Cancer Res 55:4670–4675.

36. Yanagisawa A, Ohtake K, Ohashi K et al. (1993) Frequent c-Ki-*ras* oncogene activation in mucous cell hyperplasias of pancreas suffering from chronic inflammation. Cancer Res 53:953–956.

37. DiGiuseppe JA, Hruban RH, Offerhaus GJ, Clement MJ (1994) Detection of K-*ras* mutations in mucinous pancreatic duct hyperplasia from a patient with a family history of pancreatic cancer. Am J Pathol 144:889–895.

38. Moskaluk CA, Hruban RH, Keen SE (1997) p16 and K*ras* gene mutations in the intraductal precursors of human pancreatic adenocarcinoma. Cancer Res 57:2140–2143.

39. Tada M, Ohashi M, Shiratori Y et al. (1996) Analysis of K-*ras* gene mutation in hyperplastic duct cells of the pancreas without pancreatic disease. Gastroenterology 110:227–231.

40. Hicks GG, Egan SE, Greenberg AH, Mowat M (1991) Mutant p53 tumour suppressor alleles release *ras*-induced cell cycle growth arrest. Mol Cell Biol 11:1344–1352.

41. Ridley AJ, Paterson HF, Noble M, Land H (1988) *ras*-mediated cell cycle arrest is altered by nuclear oncogenes to induce Schwann cell transformation. EMBO J 7:1635–1645.

42. Griffin CA, Hruban RH, Morsberger LA et al. (1995) Consistent chromosome abnormalities in adenocarcinoma of the pancreas. Cancer Res 55:2394–2399.

43. Forsmark CE, Lambiase L, Vogel SB (1994) Diagnosis of pancreatic cancer and prediction of unresectability using the tumour-associated antigen CA 19–9. Pancreas 9:731–734.

44. Gentiloni N, Caradonna P, Costamagna G et al. (1995) Pancreatic juice 90K and serum CA19–9 combined determination can discriminate between pancreatic cancer and chronic pancreatitis. Am J Gastroenterol 90:1069–1072.

45. Von Rosen A, Linder S, Hamemberg V, Wiechel KL (1996) Clinical relevance of tumour markers CA19–9 and CA 50 in sera from patients with pancreatic duct carcinoma. Surg Oncol 1:109–113.

46. van Es JM, Polak MM, van den Berg FM et al. (1995) Molecular markers for the diagnostic cytology of neoplasms in the head region of the pancreas: mutation of K-*ras* and overexpression of the p53 protein product. J Clin Pathol 48:218–222.

47. Van Laethem J-L, Vertongen P, Deviere J et al. (1995) Detection of C-Ki-*ras* gene codon 12 mutations from pancreatic duct brushings in the diagnosis of pancreatic tumours. Gut 36:781–787

48. Caldas C, Hahn SA, Hruban RH, Redston MS, Yeo CJ, Kern SE (1994) Detection of K-*ras* mutations in the stool of patients with pancreatic adenocarcinoma and pancreatic ductal hyperplasia. Cancer Res 54:3568–3573.

49. Tada M, Omata M, Kawai S et al. (1993) Detection of *ras* gene mutations in pancreatic juice and peripheral blood of patients with pancreatic adenocarcinoma. Cancer Res 53:2472–2474.

50. Anker P, Lefort F, Vasioukhin V et al. (1997). K-*ras* mutations are found in DNA extracted from the plasma of patients with colorectal cancer. Gastroenterology 112:1114–1120.

51. Marxsen J, Schmiegel W, Roder C et al. (1994) Detection of the anti-p53 antibody-response in malignant and benign pancreatic disease. Br J Cancer 70:1031–1034.

52. Harris JD, Sikora K (1993) Human genetic therapy. Mol Aspects Med 14:455–546.

53. Wivel NA, Walters L (1993) Germline gene modification and disease prevention: some medical and ethical perspectives. Science 262:533–538.

54. Gullick WJ, Handyside A (1994) Pre-implantation diagnosis of inherited predisposition to cancer. Eur J Cancer 30A:2030–2032.

55. Delhanty JD, Handyside AH, Winston RM (1994) Preimplantation diagnosis. Lancet 343:1569–1570.
56. Westbrook CA, Chamura SJ, Arenas RB, Kim SY, Otto G (1994) Human APC expression in rodent colonic epithelium *in vivo* using liposomal gene delivery. Hum Mol Genet 3:2005–2010.
57. Lynch HT, Fusaro L, Furaso R, Lynch J, Smyrk T (1994) Hereditary pancreatic cancer. Pedigree analysis of pancreatic cancer families. Int J Pancreatol 16:210–214.
58. Swift M, Sholman L, Perry M, Chase C (1976) Malignant neoplasms in the families of patients with ataxia telangiectasia. Cancer Res 36:209–215.
59. Takahashi T, Carbone D, Nau MM et al. (1992) Wild-type but not mutant p53 suppresses the growth of human lung cancer cells bearing multiple genetic lesions. Cancer Res 52:2340–2343
60. Cai DW, Mukhopadhyay T, Lui T, Fujiwara T, Roth JA (1993) Stable expression of the wild-type p53 gene in human lung cancer cells after retrovirus-mediated gene transfer. Hum Gene Ther 4:617–624.
61. Ebert M, Yokoyama M, Kobrin MS, Friess H, Buchler MW, Korc K (1994) Increased MDM2 expression and immunoreactivity in human pancreatic adenocarcinoma. Int J Oncol 5:1279–1284.
62. Serrano M, Gomez-Lahoz E, DePintro RA, Beach D, Bar-Sagi D (1995) Inhibition of *ras*-induced proliferation and cellular transformation by p16^{ink4}. Science 267:249–252.
63. Goyette MC, Cho K, Fasching CL et al. (1992) Progression of colorectal cancer is associated with multiple tumour suppressor gene defects but inhibition of tumorigenicity is accomplished by correction of any single defect via chromosome transfer. Mol Cell Biol 12:1387–1395.
64. Vogelstein B, Fearon ER, Kern SE et al. (1989) Allotype of colorectal carcinomas. Science 244:207–211.
65. Murray J, Crockett N (1992) Antisense techniques: an overview. In: Murray J (ed) Antisense RNA and DNA. Wiley Liss, New York, pp 1–49.
66. Spinolo J, Iversen P, Smith L et al. (1992) Antisense p53 oligodeoxynucleotide for systemic human anti-leukemic therapy. Hum Gene Ther 3:2A.
67. James GL, Goldstein JL, Brown MS et al. (1993) Benzodiazepine peptidomimetics: potent inhibitors of *ras* farnesylation in animal cells. Science 260:1937–1942.
68. Kohl NE, Mosser SD, deSolmas SJ et al. (1993) Selective inhibition of *ras*-dependent transformation by a farnesyltransferase inhibitor. Science 260:1934–1937
69. Kohl NE, Wilson FR, Mosser SD et al. (1994) Protein farnesyltransferase inhibitors block the growth of *ras*-dependent tumours in nude mice. Proc Natl Acad Sci USA 91:9141–9145.
70. Carter G, Gilbert C, Lemoine NR (1995) Effects of antisense oligonucleotides targeting the KRAS oncogene in pancreatic cancer cell lines. Int J Oncol 6:1105–1112.
71. Mikulski SM, Viera A, Darzynkiewicz Z, Shogen K (1992) Synergism between a novel amphibian oocyte ribonuclease and lovastatin in inducing cytostatic and cytotoxic effects in human lung and pancreatic carcinoma cell lines. Br J Cancer 66:304–310.
72. Sumi S, Beauchamp RD, Townsend CM et al. (1992) Inhibition of pancreatic adenocarcinoma cell growth by lovastatin. Gastroenterology 103:982–989.
73. Barton CM, Lemoine NR (1995) Antisense oligonucleotides directed against TP53 have antiproliferative effects unrelated to effects on p53 expression. Br J Cancer 71:429–437.
74. Reid R, Mar E-C, Huang E-S, Topal MD (1988) Insertion and extension of acyclic dideoxy and ara nucleotides by herpesviridae, human α and human β polymerases. A unique inhibition mechanism for 9-(1,3-dihydroxy-2-propoxymethyl) guanine triphosphate. J Biol Chem 263:3898–3904.
75. Danielsen S, Kilstrup M, Barilla K, Jochimsen B, Neuhard J (1992) Characterization of *Escherichia coli* codBA operon encoding cytosine permease and cytosine deaminase. Mol Microbiol 6:1334–1344.
76. Harris JD, Gutierrez AA, Hurst HC, Sikora K, Lemoine NR (1994) Gene therapy for cancer using tumour-specific prodrug activation. Gene Ther 1:170–175.
77. Di Maio JM, Clary BM, Via DF, Coveney E, Pappas TN, Lyerly HK (1994) Directed enzyme prodrug gene therapy for pancreatic cancer *in vivo*. Surgery 116:205–213.
78. Balague C, Gambus G, Carrato C et al. (1994) Altered expression of MUC2, MUC4 and MUC5 mucin genes in pancreas tissue and cancer cell lines. Gastroenterology 106:1054–1061.
79. Hollingsworth MA, Strawhecker JM, Caffrey TC, Mack DR (1994) Expression of MUC1, MUC3 and MUC4 mucin mRNAs in human pancreatic and intestinal tumour cell lines. Int J Cancer 57:198–203.
80. Leung HY, Gullick WJ, Lemoine NR (1994) Expression and functional activity of fibroblast growth-factors and their receptors in human pancreatic cancer. Int J Cancer 59:667–675.

81. Ulmer JB, Donnelly JJ, Parker SE et al. (1993) Heterologous protection against influenza by injection of DNA encoding a viral protein. Science 54:1745–1749.

82. Hawkins RE, Winter G, Hamblin TJ, Stevenson FK, Russel SJ (1993) A genetic approach to idiotypic vaccination. J Immunother 4:273–278.

83. Stevenson FK, Zhu D, King CA, Ashworth LJ, Kumar S, Thompsett A (1995) A genetic approach to idiotypic vaccination for B cell lymphoma. Ann N Y Acad Sci 772:212–226.

84. Barnd DL, Lan MS, Metzger RS, Finn OJ (1989) Specific tumour histocompatibility complex-unrestricted recognition of tumour-associated mucins by human cytotoxic cells. Proc Natl Acad Sci USA 86:7159–7163.

85. Schlichtholz B, Legros Y, Gillet D et al. (1992) The immune response to p53 in breast cancer patients is directed against immunodominant epitopes unrelated to the mutational hotspot. Cancer Res 52:6380–6384.

86. Gjertsen MK, Bakka A, Breivik J et al. (1995) Vaccination with mutant *ras* peptides and induction of T-cell responsiveness in pancreatic carcinoma patients carrying the corresponding RAS mutation. Lancet 346:1399–1400.

87. Gjertsen MK, Bakka A, Breivik J et al. (1996) *Ex vivo ras* peptide vaccination in patients with advanced pancreatic cancer: results of a phase I/II study. Int J Cancer 65:450–453.

88. Conry RM, Lobuglio AF, Loechel F et al. (1995) A carcinoembryonic antigen polynucleotide vaccine has *in vivo* antitumour activity. Gene Ther 2:59–65.

27 Metalloproteinases and Stromal Biology in Cancer

James D. Evans, Anthony Kawesha, Paula Ghaneh and John P. Neoptolemos

The normal extracellular matrix (ECM) comprises the basement membrane and interstitial stroma and functions as a supportive framework for parenchymal cells and a physical barrier which regulates the entry of cells into the tissue (35). The integrity of the ECM is carefully controlled but may be disrupted during tissue remodelling or various pathological situations including healing, inflammation and neoplastic disease (54,91,127). In several cancers including carcinoma of the breast and rectum, loss of basement membrane integrity is associated with an increased risk of metastases and a poorer prognosis (13,31). Pancreatic cancer is characterised by a strong desmoplastic reaction with proliferation of interstitial connective tissue (50) in particular type I collagen and fibronectin (63). In addition, however, loss of type IV collagen, the principal constituent of the basement membrane, is frequently observed indicating that proteolytic degradation may be an important feature of the invasive phenotype of pancreatic cancer (51,117).

The process of tumour progression and metastasis involves a number of important interactions between the primary tumour and the ECM, including degradation of the basement membrane and connective tissue stroma followed by invasion of viable tumour cells into lymphatic and vascular channels (intravasation). Once at the distant site, extravasation of tumour cells into the surrounding stroma, matrix degradation and tumour infiltration by new blood vessels (angiogenesis) are fundamental for the successful establishment of distant metastases (55). Four main classes of proteases have been implicated in the proteolytic events upon which tumour invasion is critically dependent (36,53). These are the serine proteases such as urokinase or tissue-type plasminogen activators (uPA, tPA), plasmin and elastase (75) cysteine proteases including cathepsins B and L (104) aspartyl proteases such as cathepsin D and the matrix metalloproteinases (55). Although enzymes from all classes may be involved, the degradation of type IV collagen within the basement membrane is a critical early event in cancer invasion and metastasis suggesting that the matrix metalloproteinases may be of particular importance in tumour progression.

Matrix Metalloproteinases

The matrix metalloproteinases (MMPs) are an expanding family of at least 15 structurally related proteolytic enzymes which collectively are able to degrade all components of the extracellular matrix (ECM) (17). MMPs all contain a zinc ion at the active site and are secreted as proenzymes which require activation in order to exert proteolytic activity (58). In normal tissues, MMPs have an important physiological role in wound healing (126), bone resorption (23) and embryogenesis (9). More recently, MMPs have been implicated in diseases such as rheumatoid arthritis (41) and cancer (55,113).

Classification

MMPs may be classified into four main groups according to substrate specificity (67) (Table 1). MMPs vary according to their spectrum of activity. MMPs 1, 2, 8 and 9 degrade all types of mammalian collagen by a single sequence-specific cleavage which unwinds the helical collagen fibre to produce protein products, which are then susceptible to further processing by other members of the MMP family (60,70). In addition to their collagenolytic activity, MMP2 and MMP9 have gelatinolytic activity and are able to degrade fibronectin, laminin and insoluble elastin (100). Stromelysins 1 and 2 (MMP3, MMP10) have a broader spectrum of activity and degrade ECM proteoglycans, laminin, fibronectin and gelatins (58). Stromelysin 3 (MMP11) has been shown to degrade the serpin α-1 antitrypsin which may potentiate the activity of serine proteases such as urokinase but its preferred substrate remains unknown at present (81). The most recent subgroup of MMPs is the membrane-type or MT-MMPs of which four members have been identified to date (86,96,110,125). As their name implies, they are not secreted but are membrane associated. Their substrates have yet to be clearly established but MT-MMP1 (MMP14) and MT-MMP3 (MMP16) are able to activate pro-MMP2 (96,108). On the basis of sequence homology, however, two enzymes do not fit neatly into the collagenase, stromelysin or gelatinase subgroups. Matrilysin (MMP7 or PUMP1) is a short truncated protease with a similar substrate specificity to the stromelysin subgroup (89) whereas metalloelastase (MMP12) degrades elastin (101). The most recent addition to the MMP family is MMP18 which has some homology to the stromelysins but its precise substrate specificity is unknown (16).

Structure

MMPs contain several distinct domains with considerable sequence homology between different family members (58,106). At the N-terminal end, the first domain is the leader sequence which targets the molecule for secretion and which is removed to produce the proenzyme. The prodomain contains the highly conserved sequence PRCGVPNPD and its cleavage results in the conversion of the proenzyme to the active enzyme. Sanchez-Lopez et al. (92) demonstrated that mutations within this region result in the spontaneous activation of MMPs. The catalytic domain contains conserved histone residues which are thought to represent the zinc-binding domain, crucial for the activity of the enzyme (93). With the exception of MMP7 (PUMP1), all MMPs contain a haemopexin domain which may be involved in the determination of substrate specificity or recognise a cell surface receptor, but its precise function remains unknown. Type IV collagenases/gelatinases (MMPs 2,3,9,10) also contain a cysteine-rich substrate binding region with sequence homology to fibronectin (106).

283

Table 1. Family of matrix metalloproteinases (MMP)

Group	MMP	Synonyms	Transcript size (kb)	Enzyme size (kDa)	Substrate
Collagenases	MMP 1	Type I collagenase or interstitial collagenase	2.0	57S, 52A	Collagen I, II, III, VII, X
	MMP 8	PMN or Neutrophil collagenase			Collagen I, II, III
	MMP 13	Collagenase 3			Collagen I
Gelatinases	MMP 2	Type IV collagenase (72 kDa) or Gelatinase A	2.8	72S	Collagen IV, V, VII, X Fibronectin, gelatins, elastin
	MMP 9	Type IV collagenase (92 kDa) or Gelatinase B	2.8	92S, 66–78A	Collagen I, III, IV, V Gelatins
Stromelysins	MMP 3	Stromelysin 1 or Transin	1.9	60S, 52A	Collagen III, IV, V, gelatins Proteoglycans, laminin Fibronectin
	MMP 10	Stromelysin 2 or Transin 2	1.7	53S, 47A	Collagen III, IV, V, fibronectin Gelatins
	MMP 11	Stromelysin 3	2.4		Serine protease inhibitors
	MMP 7	Putative matrix metalloproteinase (PUMP 1) or matrilysin	1.2	28S, 19A	Gelatin, fibronectin
	MMP 12	Metalloelastase			Elastin, non-fibrillar collagen
	MMP 18	None	2.7	57S	Not defined
Membrane-Bound	MMP 14	MT-MMP 1	4.5	63S	Pro-MMP 2
	MMP 15	MT-MMP 2			Not defined
	MMP 16	MT-MMP 3			Pro-MMP 2
	MMP 17	MT-MMP 4			Not defined

MT-MMP 1–4, membrane-type matrix metalloproteinases 1–4.

Site of Synthesis

The site of MMP production has been studied using immunohistochemistry and *in situ* hybridisation. MMP2 is the most abundantly expressed enzyme in normal tissues where expression is confined to stromal cells (59). MMP7 is expressed in glandular epithelial cells of the gastrointestinal tract and endometrium (90) and MMP9 in haematopoetic cells (46). Several studies in a variety of tissues have demonstrated expression of stromelysins by stromal cells (45,87). Gelatinases may be expressed in tumour cells (19,24) but most studies have reported expression within stromal cells (45,87,128a). As their name implies, MT-MMPs are expressed on tumour cell membranes (96).

Regulation of MMP Activity

MMP activity may be regulated in three ways: by regulation of MMP mRNA transcription and secretion of pro-MMPs, regulation of activation of MMPs or by inhibition by specific tissue inhibitors of the MMPs (TIMPs).

Transcriptional Regulation

In most cell types, MMP genes are not constitutively expressed but may be induced by a variety of agents including growth factors, cytokines, oncogene products or tumour promoters such as the phorbol esters (58). Many growth factors are known to induce the expression of the protein products of the proto-oncogenes c-*fos* and c-*jun* which then bind at specific DNA sequences sites, the TPA response element (TRE) and the activation protein-1 (AP-1) site (95) Brenner et al. (9) demonstrated that TGF-α induces prolonged activation of c-*jun* and collagenase gene expression mediated by the TRE/AP-1 binding site. Platelet-derived growth factor (PDGF) or phorbol esters induce c-*fos* resulting in collagenase and stromelysin gene expression which can be blocked by antisense c-*fos* RNA (49,98). Interleukin-1 (IL-1) modulates transcription of the MMP1 gene mediated by binding to the PEA3 transcription factor upstream of the AP-1 binding site (40). Moreover, IL-1 induces the expression of c-*fos*, c-*jun* and c-*myc* resulting in transcription of MMPs 3, 9 and uPA in human fibroblasts (30,61,124). Overexpression of the epidermal growth factor receptor (EGFR) or its ligands is frequently observed in pancreatic cancer (52), and in oesophageal cancer EGF has been shown to increase production of MMP9 but not MMPs 1, 2 and 3 (102). Kerr et al. (49) showed that TGFβ inhibited stromelysin gene expression. Transfection of the *ras* oncogene induces a metastatic phenotype associated with increased production of MMP9 in NIH/3T3 fibroblasts (114) and MMP2 in bronchial epithelial cells (15).

Regulation of MMP Activation

All MMPs are secreted as inactive proenzymes contained within zymogen granules. The pro-MMP molecule is folded so that cysteine residues within the prodomain form a complex with the zinc molecule thereby inhibiting the action of the enzyme. MMPs can be activated *in vitro* by organomercurial compounds (72,74), mediated by a conformational change in the molecule which disrupts the cysteine–zinc interaction and frees the zinc to participate in proteolytic cleavage

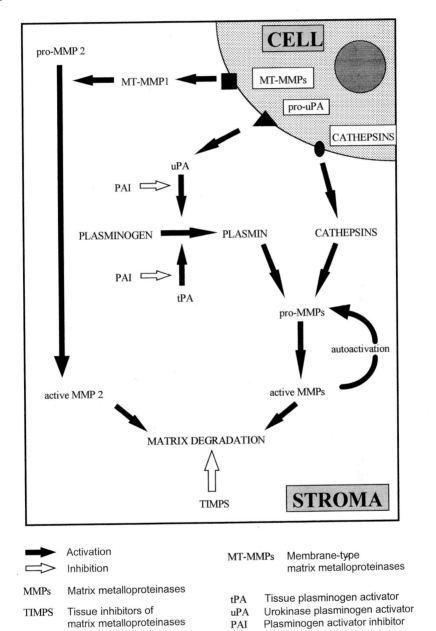

Figure 1. Proposed cascade for activation of matrix metalloproteinases illustrating activation of MMPs by other proteases (cathepsins and plasmin), autoactivation of pro-MMPs by active MMPs and MT-MMP1 and the antagonistic effects of TIMPs on matrix degradation.

of substrate (58). MMP1 and MMP9 are activated by serine proteases such as plasmin, cathepsin G, trypsin and α-chymotrypsin (73,74). A proteolytic cascade has been postulated in which pro-uPA is secreted by tumour cells or tumour stroma and binds to a specific cell surface receptor on tumour cells (88). Once activated, uPA converts plasminogen to plasmin which not only degrades ECM proteins directly but converts procollagenases and prostromelysins to their active forms (43,56,109). Activated members of one MMP family may activate other MMP types (18,94); resulting in a cascade of activation (Figure 1). Membrane-associated MT-MMP1 activates MMP2 produced by stromal fibroblasts (96) whereas tumour cells may promote MMP production by fibroblasts (48). Elevated levels of tPA correlate with survival (26) and inhibitors of uPA have been shown to inhibit invasion *in vitro* (107).

Inhibition by Tissue Inhibitors of Matrix Metalloproteinases (TIMPs)

The biological effect of active MMPs within the ECM is directly regulated by specific tissue inhibitors of the metalloproteinases (TIMPs). Four TIMPs have been described to date (Table 2) (37,99,105,116). Overexpression of MMPs is associated with an increase in the expression of TIMPs (45,128a) but MMPs and TIMPs may be regulated independently of one another (6,39,76).

TIMP1 is a 184 amino acid protein which inhibits pro-MMPs 2 and 9 and activated MMP 1, MMP3 and MMP9 (66,106,121,122,124), stimulates the growth of erythroid precursors and is mitogenic for several normal and malignant cell lines (42). Cells which produce MMPs also synthesise and secrete TIMP1 with the level of expression of each determining the net collagenolytic activity (44,123). TIMP2 is a 194 amino acid protein with 50% sequence homology to TIMP1 (21). TIMP3 shows 40% and 45% sequence homology with TIMP1 and TIMP2 respectively, although the substrate for TIMP3 has not been identified (116). TIMP4 shows 37% sequence homology to TIMP1 and 51% homology to TIMP2 and TIMP3 (37).

TIMPs bind to active MMPs non-covalently in a 1 : 1 stoichiometric manner (12) but demonstrate variable affinity for different MMPs. TIMP1 and TIMP2 preferentially bind to active MMP9 and MMP2 respectively although both TIMPs will also bind to the proforms of each enzyme (21,124). The resultant MMP activity will depend upon the balance between MMPs and TIMPs and small changes in either will lead to a significant alteration in overall proteolytic activity (82). TGFβ induces TIMP1 expression and reduced expression of collagenases and stromelysins in cultured fibroblasts (28).

Table 2. Tissue inhibitors of the metalloproteinases (TIMPs)

TIMP	Transcript-size (kb)	Enzyme size (kDa)	Function
TIMP 1	0.9	28	Inhibits pro-MMP 9 and several activated MMPs
TIMP 2	3.5 and 1.0	21	Inhibits pro-MMP 2 and activated MMP 2
TIMP 3	2.0	21.6	Not defined
TIMP 4	1.4	22	Not defined

MMPS and Cancer

MMP activity has been correlated with tumour invasion and metastases in a number of gastrointestinal tumours. Nomura et al. (71) demonstrated by immunohistochemistry (IHC) the exclusive expression of MT-MMP1 in 28 (61%) and of MMP2 in 14 (30%) of 46 gastric cancers; in 13 (93%) of 14 MMP2-positive cases, MT-MMP1 co-localised to the carcinoma cells and there was a close correlation between MT-MMP1 expression and vascular invasion. Increased gelatinase expression in gastric cancer was associated with higher tumour grade and stage in liver metastases compared with the primary tumour (24,39) whilst TIMP2 expression was inversely related to tumour stage and grade (39).

Colorectal cancers overexpress gelatinases as shown by IHC (33,45) and zymography (78) which may be correlated with tumour stage (24). Yoshimoto et al. (128) demonstrated expression of MMP7 (PUMP1) in colorectal cancer tissue by RT-PCR in 9 (90%) of 10 cases with absent expression in adjacent normal tissue. Overexpression of MMP7 mRNA was reported in 39 (83%) of 47 cases of colorectal cancer which correlated with tumour stage; the highest expression was observed in metastatic liver lesions (64). Stromelysin 3 expression was correlated with tumour stage in colorectal cancer (84) and MMP1 expression was shown to be associated with a poor prognosis (68).

Increased MMP expression has been reported also in carcinomas of the ovary (11), prostate (77), breast (3) lung (10) and head and neck (65). Serum expression of MMP9 has been correlated with lymph node and lung metastasis in rat mammary adenocarcinoma (69) and high serum levels of MMPs 1, 2 and 3 and of TIMPs 1 and 2 have been reported in patients with cancer (2,34).

MMPS and Pancreatic Cancer

Moll et al. (62) demonstrated that the RWP 1 pancreatic cancer cell line expressed collagenolytic activity localised to the basal plasma membrane, an ideal site to concentrate proteolysis for tissue invasion. The SUIT 2 cell line has type 1 collagenolytic activity, due to MMP1 expression (111). Specific MMP expression differs between different pancreatic cancer cell lines (Table 3) although MMP1, MMP2, MMP7, MMP9, TIMP1 and TIMP2 are those most abundantly expressed (8,129,130,131).

Interestingly, the pattern of MMP expression in human pancreatic cancer tissue specimens differs from that reported in cell lines (Table 4). Bramhall et al. (7) reported overexpression of MMP2, MMP3 and TIMP1 in pancreatic and ampullary cancers by immunohistochemistry. Northern analysis demonstrated that MMP2, MMP7, MMP9, TIMP1 and TIMP2 are those most abundantly expressed in pancreatic cancer tissue (8,38) and *in situ* hybridisation demonstrated coexpression of MMP2 and MT-MMP1 in 60% of pancreatic cancers. MMP2 was expressed both in tumour epithelium and within the stroma while MMP7, MT-MMP1, TIMP1 and TIMP2 were located predominantly within tumour epithelium (8). Satoh et al. (97), found that MMP2 expression was higher in invasive ductal adenocarcinoma compared with intraductal neoplasm with the level of expression correlating with the degree of basement membrane disruption. TIMP1 expression was found to have an inverse relationship with the

Table 3. Matrix-metalloproteinases (MMPs) and tissue inhibitors of matrix-metalloproteinases (TIMPs) mRNA expression in pancreatic cancer cell lines

Reference	Cell Line	MMP 1	MMP 2	MMP 3	MMP 7	MMP 9	MMP 10	MMP 11	TIMP 1	TIMP 2
Bramhall et al. (8)	SUIT 2	+	–	+	+	ND	–	–	+	+
	HS766T	–	–	–	–	ND	–	–	+	–
	BxPC3	–	–	–	–	ND	–	–	+	–
	ASPC1	–	–	+	–	ND	–	–	+	+
	CFPaC1	–	–	–	+	ND	–	–	+	–
	CaPan 1	–	–	–	+	ND	–	–	+	–
	CaPan 2	–	–	–	–	ND	–	–	+	–
Taniguchi et al. (111)	SUIT 2	+	ND	ND	+	ND	ND	ND	ND	ND
Moll et al. (62)	RWP 1	+	ND	ND	ND	ND	ND	ND	ND	ND
Zucker et al. (131)	RWP 1	ND	+	ND	ND	+	ND	ND	ND	ND
	RWP 2		+			+				

+, expressed; –, not expressed; ND, not done.

Table 4. Matrix metalloproteinase (MMPs) and tissue inhibitors of matrix metalloproteinases (TIMPs) mRNA expression in pancreatic cancer-tissue

Reference	Number of cases	MMP1 (%)	MMP2 (%)	MMP3 (%)	MMP7 (%)	MMP9 (%)	MMP11 (%)	TIMP1 (%)	TIMP2 (%)
Bramhall et al. (8)	17	0	93	18	88	ND	41	100	53
Gress et al. (38)	8	0	75	0	ND	75	ND	75	75
Sato et al. (96)[a]	16	ND	100	ND	ND	ND	ND	ND	ND
Sato et al. (97)[b]	14	ND	64	ND	ND	ND	ND	ND	ND

[a] Adenocarcinoma of the pancreas.
[b] Intraductal neoplasm of the pancreas.
ND, not done.

presence of lymph node metastases while increased MMP expression was associated with tumour dedifferentiation (5,7).

MMP Inhibitors in the Treatment of Cancer

Given the failure of conventional treatments and the overexpression of MMPs in pancreatic cancer there has been considerable interest in the therapeutic potential of MMP inhibitors.

Pre-clinical Studies

Hoyhtya et al. (47) demonstrated that antibodies to type IV collagenase reduced the invasiveness *in vitro* of metastatic human (A2058) melanoma cells. Transfection of human TIMP1 complementary DNA into the human gastric cancer cell line KKLS resulted in a 70% reduction in metastatic potential compared with TIMP1 non-expressing cells (115). Overexpression of TIMP2 by stable transfection has also been shown to produce a marked reduction in net metalloproteinase activity associated with suppression of tumour invasion (22).

Batimastat (BB-94; British Biotech, Oxford, UK) was one of the first synthetic low molecular weight broad-spectrum inhibitors of the MMP family. BB-94 contains a peptide backbone which binds to MMPs and a hydroxyamic acid group which binds to the catalytically active zinc atom. Nanomolar concentrations of BB-94 inhibit interstitial collagenase, stromelysin and the 72- and 92-kDa type IV collagenases but only weakly inhibit the serine protease plasmin and angiotensin-converting enzyme (ACE), a metalloproteinase (20). BB-94 has been shown to reduce tumour burden and ascitic volume and to prolong the survival of nude mice transplanted with human ovarian carcinoma xenografts. Interestingly, at subsequent autopsy, the tumour was found to be encapsulated in dense stroma with necrosis of some tumour cells (20). Similar results have been reported in a human colorectal ascites xenograft model (120). Batimastat had no cytotoxic effects on tumour cell lines *in vitro* (20). Batimastat was also shown to inhibit locoregional regrowth and metastases of a human breast carcinoma (MDA-MB-435) following resection in athymic nude mice (103).

Wang et al. (118) orthotopically implanted fragments of human colonic carcinoma into 40 athymic nude mice. BB-94 resulted in a reduction in primary tumour burden and a significant reduction in the incidence of local and regional invasion from 12 (67%) of 18 mice in the control group to 7 (35%) of 20 in the treated group. A significant reduction in distant metastases and a prolonged median survival time were also observed in mice treated with BB-94 (118). Chirivi et al. (14) demonstrated a reduction in the number and size of lung metastases in mice given B16-BL6 murine melanoma cells and treated with BB-94 while other studies have demonstrated a reduction in the incidence of lung and liver metastases in two human colorectal cancer models (119) and inhibition of angiogenesis (32,112).

The combination of the synthetic broad spectrum MMP inhibitor CT1746 (Celltech, Slough, UK) and cyclophosphamide has been shown to act synergistically to inhibit the growth and metastasis of the murine Lewis lung carcinoma when compared with either agent used alone (1).

Clinical Trials of MMP Inhibitors

Batimastat was one of the first MMPs to be tested in clinical trials. Some efficacy was found when batimastat was administered intraperitoneally or intrapleurally to patients with malignant ascites or malignant pleural effusions (57,79). Ilomastat (GM 6001; Glycomed, Alameda, California, USA) was another first generation MMPI utilised as a topical agent in patients with corneal ulcerations (32). The major drawback of these early agents was their low solubility necessitating administration by the parenteral route.

More recently, orally bioavailable broad-spectrum MMP inhibitors have been developed and have entered clinical trials. Marimastat (BB-2516; British Biotech) contains a hydroxyamate zinc-binding site. The molecule fits into the active site of the MMPs producing a potent but reversible inhibition of enzyme activity at nanomolar concentrations (4). Marimastat is a broad-spectrum inhibitor active against all major classes of MMPs but has little or no activity against more distantly related metalloproteinases such as encephalase and ACE (4). A phase I study of marimastat (BB-2516) demonstrated that high plasma levels could be achieved following a single oral daily dose of between 25 and 800 mg given to healthy volunteers (25).

A phase II trial of marimastat for the treatment of advanced pancreatic cancer has recently been completed (29). This multicentre study involved over 100 patients with inoperable pancreatic cancer most of whom received 25 mg of marimastat once daily for 28 days with the option to continue treatment in those patients with a radiological (computed tomography) or serological (CA19-9) evidence of disease stabilisation. Patients with irresectable stage II or III disease had a median survival time of 7 months compared with less than 3 months in those with stage IV disease. Patients with stable CT appearances after 28 days of treatment had a median survival time of over 7 months compared with 4 months in those with a progressive CT scan (29). Musculoskeletal pain was the only significant side effect and was time- and dose-dependent, resolving after temporary cessation of treatment with reintroduction of marimastat at a lower dose.

Similar studies in a number of other inoperable solid cancers suggest that marimastat may exert a biological effect on tumour growth. In patients with gastric cancer, a reduction in tumour cellularity with an increase in fibroblastic matrix development was observed in some patients following treatment with marimastat similar to changes observed in experimental models (80). In colorectal cancer 10 (36%) of 28 patients had a fall in serum carcinoembryonic antigen (CEA) (85), while 10 (45%) of 22 patients with ovarian cancer had evidence of disease stabilisation as assessed by serum CA125 levels (83). However, the encouraging data from these studies need to be confirmed. A series of randomised controlled clinical trials in a variety of cancer types comparing marimastat with conventional treatments were commenced at the end of 1996.

Selective MMPIs have been developed on the basis that certain tumours may rely upon a particular class of MMP for invasion. Three orally bioavailable matrix metalloproteinase inhibitors (MMPIs) are believed to be in clinical trials in patients with cancer namely AG3340 (Agouron, London, UK), CGS-27023A (Novartis, London, UK), D5410 (Chiroscience, Cambridge, UK) although no data have been reported to date.

Conclusions

Overexpression of several MMPs has been demonstrated in carcinoma of the pancreas. This expanding family of proteases appears to play a critical role in tumour invasion and metastasis and this has led to the development of specific MMPIs. The preliminary results of clinical trials of MMPIs in pancreatic and other solid cancers are encouraging but need to be confirmed by randomised clinical trials which are in progress. In the future, there is considerable potential to extend the use of these novel agents to the adjuvant setting following macroscopic resection of early pancreatic cancers either alone or in combination with existing chemotherapeutic regimes.

References

1. Anderson IC, Shipp MA, Docherty AJP, Teicher BA (1996) Combination therapy including a gelatinase inhibitor and cytotoxic agent reduces local invasion and metastasis of murine Lewis lung carcinoma. Cancer Res 56:715–710.
2. Baker T, Tickle S, Wasan H, Docherty A, Isenberg D, Waxman J (1994) Serum metalloproteinases and their inhibitors: markers for malignant potential. Br J Cancer 70:506–512.
3. Basset P, Bellocq JP, Wolf C et al. (1990) A novel metalloproteinase gene specifically expressed in stromal cells of breast carcinomas. Nature 348:699–704.
4. Beckett RP, Davison AH, Drummond AH, Huxley P, Whittaker M (1996) Recent advances in matrix metalloproteinase inhibitor research. Drug Dev Today 1:16–26.
5. Bramhall SR, Lemoine N, Stamp G, Donovan IA, Dunn J, Neoptolemos JP (1994) 72 kDa collagenase, stromelysin 1 and tissue inhibitor of metalloproteinase 1 expression in pancreatic cancer. Digestion 55:286 (abstract).
6. Bramhall SR, Lemoine N, Stamp G, Neoptolemos JP (1995) Enhanced expression of matrix metalloproteinases is often unopposed by their inhibitors (tissue inhibitors of metalloproteinases) in pancreatic cancer. Br J Surg 82:707–708.
7. Bramhall SR, Stamp G, Dunn J, Lemoine N, Neoptolemos JP et al. (1996) Expression of collagenase (MMP2), stromelysin (MMP3) and tissue inhibitor of metalloproteinases (TIMP1) in pancreatic and ampullary disease. Br J Cancer 73:972–978.
8. Bramhall SR, Lemoine N, Stamp G, Neoptolemos JP (1997) Imbalance of expression of matrix metalloproteinases (MMPs) and tissue inhibitors of the matrix metalloproteinases (TIMPs) in human pancreatic cancer. J Pathol (in press).
9. Brenner DA, Ohara M, Angel P, Chojkier M, Karin M (1989) Prolonged activation of *jun* and collagenase genes by tumour necrosis factor alpha. Nature 337:661–663.
10. Brown PD, Bloxidge RE, Stuart NSE, Gatter KC, Carmichael J (1993) Association between expression of activated 72-kilodalton gelatinase and tumour spread in non-small cell lung carcinoma. J Natl Cancer Inst 85:574–578.
11. Campo E, Merino MJ, Tavassoli FA, Charonis AS, Stetler-Stevenson WG, Liotta LA (1992) Evaluation of basement membrane components and the 72 kDa type IV collagenase in serous tumours of the ovary. Am J Surg Pathol 16:500–507.
12. Cawston TE, Galloway WA, Mercer E, Murphy G, Reynolds JJ (1981) Purification of rabbit bone inhibitor of collagenase. Biochem J 195:159–165.
13. Charpin C, Lissitzky JC, Jacquemier J et al. (1986) Immunohistochemical detection of laminin in 98 human breast carcinomas: a light and electron microscopic study. Hum Pathol 17:355–365.
14. Chiviri RG, Garofalo A, Crimmin MJ, Hoffman RM (1994) Inhibition of metastatic spread and growth of B16-BL6 murine melanoma by a synthetic matrix metalloproteinase inhibitor. Int J Cancer 58:460–464.
15. Collier IE, Smith J, Kronenberg A et al. (1988) The structure of human skin fibroblast collagenase gene. J Biol Chem 263:10711–10782.
16. Cossins J, Dudgeon TJ, Catlin G, Gearing AJH, Clements JM (1996) Identification of MMP-18, a putative novel human matrix metalloproteinase. Biochem Biophys Res Commun 228: 494–498.

17. Cottam DW, Rees RC (1993) Regulation of matrix metalloproteinases: their role in tumour invasion and metastasis (review). Int J Oncology 2:861–872.

18. Crabbe T, Smith B, O'Connell JP, Docherty A (1994) Human procollagenase A can be activated by matrilysin. FEBS Lett 345:14–16.

19. David L, Nesland J, Holm R et al. (1994) Expression of laminin, collagen IV, fibronectin and type IV collagenase in gastric carcinoma. Cancer 73:518–527.

20. Davies B, Brown PD, Eats N, Crimmin MJ, Balkwill FR (1993) A synthetic matrix metallo-proteinase inhibitor decreases tumour burden and prolongs survival of mice bearing human ovarian carcinoma xenografts. Cancer Res 53:2087–2091.

21. DeClerck Y, Yean TD, Ratzkin BJ, Lu HS, Langley KE (1989) Purification and characterisation of two related but distinct metalloproteinase inhibitors secreted by bovine aortic endothelial cells. J Biol Chem 264:17445–7053.

22. DeClerck Y, Perez N, Shimada H, Boone TC, Langley KE, Taylor SM (1992) Inhibition of invasion and metastasis in cells transfected with an inhibitor of metalloproteinases. Cancer Res 52:701–708.

23. Delaisse JM, Vaes G (1992) Mechanism of mineral solublisation and matrix degradation in osteoclastic bone resorption. In: Rifkin BR, Gay CV (eds) Biology and physiology of the osteoclast. CRC Press, Boca Raton, pp 290–314.

24. D'Errico A, Garbisa S, Liotta L, Astronova V, Stetler-Stevenson W, Grigioni W (1991) Augmentation of type IV collagenase, laminin receptor and Ki67 proliferation antigen associated with human colon, gastric and breast carcinoma progression. Mod Pathol 4: 239–246.

25. Drummond A, Beckett P, Bone et al. (1995) BB-2516: an orally bioavailable matrix metallo-proteinase inhibitor with efficacy in animal cancer models. Proc Am Assoc Cancer Res 36:100 (abstract).

26. Duffy MJ, O'Grady P, Devaney D, O'Siorain L, Fennelly JJ, Lijnen HR (1988) Tissue plasminogen activator, a new prognostic marker in breast cancer. Cancer Res 48:1348–1349.

27. Duffy MJ (1992) The role of proteolytic enzymes in cancer invasion and metastasis. Clin Exp Metastasis 10:145–155.

28. Edwards DR, Murphy G, Reynolds JJ (1987) Transforming growth factor beta modulates the expression of collagenase and metalloproteinase inhibitor. EMBO J 6:1899–1904.

29. Evans JD, Bramhall SR, Carmichael J (1996) A phase II trial of marimastat (BB-2516) in advanced pancreatic cancer. Ann Oncol 7:51 (abstract).

30. Fini ME, Plucinska IM, Mayer AS, Gross RH, Brickerhoff LE (1987) A gene for rabbit synovial cell collagenase: member of a family of MMP that degrade the CT matrix. Biochemistry 26:6156–6165.

31. Forster SJ, Talbot IC, Clayton DG, Critchley DR (1986) Tumour basement membrane laminin in adenocarcinoma of the rectum: An immunohistochemical study of biological and clinical significance. Int J Cancer 37:813–817.

32. Galardy RE, Grobelny D, Foellmer HG, Fernandez LA (1994) Inhibition of angiogenesis by the matrix metalloproteinase inhibitor N-[2R-2-(hydroxomidocarbonymethyl)-4-methyl-pentanoyl)]-L tryptophan methylamide. Cancer Res 54:4715–4718.

33. Gallegos NC, Smales C, Savage FJ, Hembry RM, Boulos PB (1995) The distribution of matrix metalloproteinases and tissue inhibitor of the metalloproteinases in colorectal cancer. Surg Oncol 4:21–29.

34. Garbisa S, Pozzatti R, Muschel RJ et al. (1987) Secretion of type IV collagenolytic protease and metastatic phenotype: induction by transfection with c-Ha-ras but not c-Ha-ras plus Ad2-Ela. Cancer Res 47:1523–1528.

35. Goldfarb RH (1986) Proteolytic enzymes in tumour invasion and degradation of host extra-cellular matrices. In: Honn KV, Powers WE, Sloane BF (eds) Mechanisms of cancer metastasis. Martinus Nijhoff, Boston, pp 341–375.

36. Gottesman M (1990) The role of proteases in cancer. Semin Cancer Biol 1:97–100.

37. Greene J, Wang M, Liu YE, Raymond LA, Rosen C, Shi YE (1996) Molecular cloning and charac-terisation of human tissue inhibitor of metalloproteinase 4. J Biol Chem 271:30375–30380.

38. Gress TM, Muller-Pillasch F, Lerch MM, Freiss H, Buchler M, Alder G (1995) Expression and in situ localisation of genes coding for extracellular matrix proteins and extracellular matrix degrading proteases in pancreatic cancer. Int J Cancer 62:407–413.

39. Grigoni WF, D'Errico A, Fortunato C et al. (1994) Prognosis of gastric carcinoma revealed by interactions between tumour cells and basement membrane. Mod Pathol 7:220–225.

40. Gutman A, Wasylyk B (1990) The collagenase gene promoter contains a TPA and oncogene-responsive unit encompassing the PEA3 and AP-1 binding sites. EMBO J 9:2241–2246.

41. Harris E (1990) Rheumatoid arthritis: pathophysiology and implications for therapy. N Engl J Med 322:1277–1289.

42. Hayakawa T, Yamashita K, Tanzawa K, Uchijima E, Iwata K (1992) Growth-promoting activity of tissue inhibitor of the metalloproteinases-1 (TIMP 1) for a wide range of cells. A possible new growth factor in serum. FEBS Lett 298:29–32.

43. He C, Wilhelm SM, Pentland AP et al. (1989) Tissue cooperation in a proteolytic cascade activating human intestinal collagenase. Proc Natl Acad Sci USA 86:2632–2636.

44. Herron GS, Banda MJ, Clark EJ, Gavrilovic J, Werb Z (1986) Secretion of metalloproteinases by stimulated capillary endothelial cells. J Biol Chem 261:2814–2818.

45. Hewitt RE, Leach IH, Powe DG, Clarke IM, Cawston TE, Turner DR (1991) Distribution of collagenase and tissue inhibitor of the metalloproteinases (TIMP) in colorectal tumours. Int J Cancer 49:666–672.

46. Hibbs M, Hoidal J, Kang A (1987) Expression of a metalloproteinase that degrades native type V collagen and denatured collagens by cultured human alveolar macrophages. J Clin Invest 80:1644–1650.

47. Hoyhtya M, Hujanen E, Turpeenniemi-Hujanen T et al. (1990) Modulation of type IV collagenase activity and invasive behaviour of metastatic human melanoma (A2058) cells in vitro by monoclonal antibodies to type IV collagenase. Int J Cancer 46:282–286.

48. Ito A, Nakajima S, Sasaguri Y, Nagase H, Mori Y (1995) Co-culture of human breast adenocarcinoma MCF-7 cells and human dermal fibroblasts enhances the production of matrix metalloproteinases 1, 2 and 3 in fibroblasts. Br J Cancer 71:1039–1045.

49. Kerr LD, Miller DM, Matrisian LM (1990) TGF-Beta-1 inhibition of transin stromelysin gene expression is mediated through a fos sequence. Cell 61:267–278.

50. Kloppel G (1993) Pathology of non-endocrine pancreas tumours. In: Go LW, DiMagno EP, Gardner HD, Lebenthal E, Reber HA, Scheele GA (eds) The pancreas. Biology, pathobiology and disease. 2nd edn. Raven Press, New York, pp 871–897.

51. Lee CS, Montebello J, Georgiou T, Rode J (1994) Distribution of type IV collagen in pancreatic adenocarcinoma and chronic pancreatitis. Int J Exp Pathol 75:79–83.

52. Lemoine NR, Hughes CM, Barton CM et al. (1992) The epidermal growth factor and its receptors in human pancreatic carcinoma. J Pathol 166:7–12.

53. Liotta LA (1986) Tumour invasion and metastasis: role of the extracellular matrix. Cancer Res 46:1–7.

54. Liotta LA, Tryggvason K, Garbisa S, Hart I, Foltz CM, Shafdie S (1980) Metastatic potential correlates with enzymatic degradation of basement membrane collagen. Nature 284:67–68.

55. Liotta LA, Stetler Stevenson WG (1991) Tumour invasion and metastasis: an imbalance of positive and negative regulation. Cancer Res 51(Suppl):5054–5059.

56. Mackey AR, Corbitt RH, Hartzler JL, Thorgeirsson UP (1990) Basement membrane type IV collagen degradation: evidence for the involvement of a proteolytic cascade independent of metalloproteinases. Cancer Res 50:5997–6001.

57. Macualay V, O'Byrne K, Saunders M et al. (1995) A phase I study of the matrix metalloproteinase inhibitor batimastat (BB-94) in patients with pleural effusions. Br J Cancer 71:11 (abstract).

58. Matrisian LM (1990) Metalloproteinases and their inhibitors in matrix remodelling. Trends Genet 6:121–125.

59. Matrisian LM (1993) Matrix metalloproteinase gene expression. Ann N Y Acad Sci 732:42–50.

60. McCroskery PA, Richards JF, Harris ED (1975) Purification and characterisation of a collagenase extracted from rabbit tumours. Biochem J 152:131–142.

61. Mochan E, Uhl J, Newton R (1986) Interleukin 1 stimulation of synovial cell plasminogen activator production. J Rheumatol 13:15–19.

62. Moll UM, Lane B, Zucker S, Suzuki K, Nagase H (1990) Localisation of collagenase at the basal plasma membrane of a human pancreatic carcinoma cell line. Cancer Res 50:6995–7002.

63. Mollenhauer J, Roether I, Kern HF (1987) Distribution of extracellular matrix proteins in pancreatic ductal adenocarcinoma and its influence on tumour cell proliferation in vitro. Pancreas 2:14–24.

64. Mori M, Barnard GF, Mimori K, Ueo H, Akiyoshi T, Sugimachi K (1995) Overexpression of matrix metalloproteinase 7 mRNA in human colon carcinomas. Cancer 75(Suppl):1516–1519.

65. Muller D, Breathnach R, Engelmann A et al. (1991) Expression of collagenase related metalloproteinase genes in human lung or head and neck tumours. Int J Cancer 48:550–556.

66. Murphy GJP, Reynolds JJ, Werb Z (1985) Biosynthesis of tissue inhibitor of the metalloproteinases by human fibroblasts in culture. J Biol Chem 260:3079–3083.

67. Murphy GJP, Murphy G, Reynolds JJ (1991) The origin of matrix metalloproteinases and their familial relationships. FEBS Lett 289:4–7.

68. Murray G, Duncan M, O'Neil P, Melvin W, Fothergill J (1996) Matrix metalloproteinase 1 is associated with poor prognosis in colorectal carcinomas. Nature Med 2:461–462.

69. Nakajima M, Welch DR, Wynn DM, Tsuruo T, Nicolson GL (1993) Serum and plasma M(r) 92000 progelatinase levels correlate with spontaneous metastasis of rat 13762NF mammary adenocarcinoma. Cancer Res 53:5802–5807.

70. Nethery A, O'Grady RL (1989) Identification of a metalloproteinase co-purifying with rat tumour collagenase and the characteristics of fragments of both enzymes. Biochim Biophys Acta 994:149–160.

71. Nomura H, Sato H, Seiki M, Mai M, Okada Y (1995) Expression of membrane-type matrix metalloproteinase in human gastric carcinomas. Cancer Res 55:3263–3266.

72. Okada Y, Morodomi T, Enghild J et al. (1990) Matrix metalloproteinase 2 from human rheumatoid synovial fibroblasts. Purification and activation of the precursor and enzymic properties. Eur J Biochem 194:721–730.

73. Okada Y, Tsuchiya H, Shimizu H et al. (1990) Induction and stimulation of 92 kDa gelatinase/type IV collagenase production in osteosarcoma and fibrosarcoma cell lines by tumour necrosis factor alpha. Biochem Biophys Res Commun 171:610–617.

74. Okada Y, Gonoji Y, Naka K et al. (1992) Matrix metalloproteinase 9 (92 kDa gelatinase/type IV collagenase) from HT1080 human fibrosarcoma cells. J Biol Chem 267:21712–21719.

75. Ossawski L, Reisch E (1983) Antibodies to plasminogen activator inhibit human tumour metastasis. Cell 35:611–619.

76. Overall CM, Wrana JL, Sodek J (1989) Independent regulation of collagenase, 72 kDa progelatinase, and metalloendoproteinase inhibitor expression in human fibroblasts by transforming growth factor-beta. J Biol Chem 264:1860–1869.

77. Pajouh MS, Nagle RB, Breatynach R, Finch JS, Brawler MK, Bowden GT (1991) Expression of metalloproteinase genes in human prostate cancer. J Cancer Res Clin Oncol 117:144–150.

78. Parsons SL, Watson SA, Collins H, Clarke P, Steele RJC (1996) Colorectal cancers overexpress gelatinases (matrix metalloproteinases 2 and 9). Gastroenterology 110:A574 (abstract).

79. Parsons S, Watson S, Amar S, Steele R (1996) Phase I/II trial of a matrix metalloproteinase inhibitor in patients with malignant ascites. Gastroenterology 110:A575 (abstract)

80. Parsons SL, Watson SA, Griffin NR, Steele RJC (1996) An open phase I/II study of the oral matrix metalloproteinase inhibitor inhibitor marimastat in patients with inoperable gastric cancer. Ann Oncol 7:47 (abstract)

81. Pei D, Majmudar G, Weiss SJ (1994) Hydrolytic inactivation of a breast carcinoma cell-derived serpin by human stromelysin-3. J Biol Chem 269:25849–25855.

82. Ponton A, Coulombe B, Skup D (1991) Decreased expression of tissue inhibitor of the metalloproteinases in metastatic tumour cells leading to increased levels of collagenase activity. Cancer Res 51:2138–2143.

83. Poole C, Adams M, Barley V (1996) A dose-finding study of marimastat, an oral matrix metalloproteinase inhibitor, in patients with advanced ovarian cancer. Ann Oncol 7:68 (abstract)

84. Porte H, Chastre E, Prevot S et al. (1995) Neoplastic progression of human colorectal cancer is associated with overexpression of the stromelysin 3 and NM-40/SPARC genes. Int J Cancer 64:70–75

85. Primrose J, Bleiberg H, Daniel F (1996) A dose-finding study of marimastat, an oral matrix metalloproteinase inhibitor, in patients with advanced colorectal cancer. Ann Oncol 7:35(abstract)

86. Puente XS, Pendas AM, Llano E, Velasco G, Lopez-Otin C (1996) Molecular cloning of a novel membrane-type matrix metalloproteinase from human breast carcinoma. Cancer Res 56:944–949.

87. Pyke C, Ralfkiaer E, Tryggvason K, Dano K (1993) Messenger RNA for two type IV collagenases is located in stromal cells in human colon cancer. Am J Pathol 142:359–364.

88. Pyke C, Kristensen P, Ralfkiaer E et al. (1991) Urokinase-type plasminogen activator is expressed in stromal cells and its receptor in cancer cells are invasive foci in human colon adenocarcinomas. Am J Pathol 138:1059–1067.

89. Quantin B, Murphy G, Breathnach R (1989) Pump-1 cDNA codes for a protein with similar characteristics to those of classical collagenase family members. Biochemistry 28:5325–5334.

90. Rodgers WH, Osteen KG, Matrisian LM, Naevre M, Giudice LC, Gorstein F (1993) Expression and localisation of matrilysin, a matrix metalloproteinase, in human endometrium during the reproductive cycle. Am J Obstet Gynecol 168:253–260.

91.   Salo T, Makela M, Kylmaniemi M, Autio-Harmanainen H, Larjava H (1994) Expression of matrix metalloproteinase 2 and 9 during early wound healing. Lab Invest 70:176–182.

92.   Sanchez-Lopez R, Nicholson R, Gesnel MC, Matrsian LM, Breathnach R (1988) Structure–function relationship in the collagenase family member transin. J Biol Chem 263:11892–11899

93.   Sanchez-Lopez R, Alexander CM, Behrendtsen O, Breathnach R, Werb Z (1993) Role of zinc binding and hemopexin-domain-encoded sequences in the substrate specificity of collagenase and stromelysin-2 as revealed by chimeric proteins. J Biol Chem 268:7238–7247.

94.   Sang QX, Birkedel-Hanson H, Van Wart HE (1995) Proteolytic and non-proteolytic activation of human neutrophil progelatinase. Biochim Biophys Acta 1251:99–108.

95.   Sassone-Corsi P, Lamph WW, Kamps M, Verma IM (1988) Fos-associated cellular p39 is related to nuclear transcription factor AP-1. Cell 54:553–563.

96.   Sato H, Takin T, Okada Y et al. (1994) A matrix metalloproteinase expressed on the surface of invasive tumour cells. Nature 370:61–65.

97.   Satoh K, Ohtani H, Shimosegawa T, Koizumi M, Sawai T, Toyota T (1994) Infrequent stromal expression of gelatinase A and intact basement membrane in intraductal neoplasms of the pancreas. Gastroenterology 107:1488–1495.

98.   Schonthal A, Herrlich P, Rahmsdorf HJ, Ponta H (1988) Requirement for fos gene expression in the activation of collagenase by other oncogenes and phorbol esters. Cell 54:324–334.

99.   Sellers A, Murphy G, Meickle MC, Reynolds JJ (1979) Rabbit bone collagenase inhibitor blocks the activity of other neutral metalloproteinases. Biochem Biophys Res Commun 87:581–587.

100. Senior RM, Griffin GL, Fliszar CJ, Shapiro SD, Goldberg GI, Welgus HG (1991) Human 92- and 72-kilodalton type IV collagenases are elastases. J Biol Chem 266:7870–7875.

101. Shapiro SD, Kobayashi DK, Ley TJ (1993) Cloning and characterisation of a unique elastolytic metalloproteinase produced by human alveolar macrophages. J Biol Chem 268:23824–23829.

102. Shima I, Sasaguri Y, Kasukawa J et al. (1993) Production of matrix metalloproteinase 9 (92 kDa gelatinase) by human oesophageal squamous cell carcinoma in response to epidermal growth factor. Br J Cancer 67:721–727.

103. Sledge GW, Qualali M, Goulet R, Bone EA, Thomas W, Brown PD (1995) Effect of matrix metalloproteinase inhibitor batimastat on breast cancer regrowth and metastasis in athymic mice. J Natl Cancer Res 87:1546–1550.

104. Sloane BF, Dunn JR, Houn KV (1981) Lysosomal cathepsin B: correlation with metastatic potential. Science 212:1151–1153.

105. Stetler-Stevenson WG (1989) Tissue inhibitor of metalloproteinase (TIMP 2). J Biol Chem 264:17374–17378.

106. Stetler-Stevenson WG (1990) Type IV collagenases in tumour invasion and metastasis. Cancer Metastasis Rev 9:289–303.

107. Stonelake PS, Jones CE, Neoptolemos JP, Baker PR (1997) Inhibition of proteinase-mediated basement membrane degradation by human breast cancer cells. Br J Cancer (in press).

108. Strongin A, Collier I, Bannikov G, Marmer BL, Grant GA, Goldberg GI (1995) Mechanism of cell surface activation of 72 kDa type IV collagenase. J Biol Chem 270:5331–5338.

109. Suzuki K, Enghild JJ, Morodomi T, Salveson G, Nagase H (1990) Mechanisms of activation of tissue procollagenase by matrix metalloproteinase 3 (stromelysin). Biochemistry 29:10261–10270.

110. Takino T, Sato H, Shinagawa A, Seiki M (1995) Identification of the second membrane-type matrix metalloproteinase (MT-MMP-2) gene from a human placenta cDNA library. J Biol Chem 270:23013–23020.

111. Taniguchi S, Iwamura T, Katsuki T (1992) Correlation between spontaneous metastatic potential and type 1 collagenolytic activity in a human pancreatic cancer cell line (SUIT 2) and sublines. Clin Exp Metastasis 10:259–266.

112. Taraboloetti G, Garofalo A, Belotti D (1995) Inhibition of angiogenesis and murine hemangioma growth by batimastat, a synthetic inhibitor of matrix metalloproteinases. J Natl Cancer Inst 87:293–298.

113. Tarin D, Hoyt BJ, Evans DJ (1982) Correlation of collagenase secretion with metastatic colonisation potential in naturally occurring murine mammary tumours. Br J Cancer 46:266–278.

114. Thorgeirsson UP, Turpeenniemi-Hujanen T, Williams JE et al. (1985) NIH/3T3 cells transfected with human tumour DNA containing activated ras oncogenes in express the metastatic phenotype in nude mice. Mol Cell Biol 5:259–262.

115. Tsuchiya Y, Satro H, Endo Y et al. (1993) Tissue inhibitor of the metalloproteinase 1 is a negative regulator of the metastatic ability of a human gastric cancer cell line, KKLS in the chick embryo. Cancer Res 53:1397–1402.

116. Uria JA, Ferrando AA, Velasco G, Freije JMP, Lopez-Otin C (1994) Structure and expression in breast tumours of human TIMP 3, a new member of the metalloproteinase inhibitor family. Cancer Res 54:2091–2094.

117. Wang ZH, Manabe T, Ohishio G et al. (1994) Immunohistochemical study of heparin sulphate proteoglycan in adenocarcinomas of the pancreas. Pancreas 9:758–763.

118. Wang X, Fu X, Brown PD, Crimmin MJ, Hoffman RM (1994) Matrix metalloproteinase inhibitor BB-94 (batimastat) inhibits human colon tumour growth and spread in a patient-like orthotopic model in nude mice. Cancer Res 54:4726–4728.

119. Watson SA, Morris TM, Robinson G, Crimmin MJ, Brown PD, Hardcastle JD (1995) Inhibition of organ invasion by the matrix metalloproteinase inhibitor batimastat (BB-94) in two human colon carcinoma metastases models. Cancer Res 55:3629–3633.

120. Watson SA, Morris TM, Parsons SL, Steele RJC, Brown PB (1996) Therapeutic effect of the matrix metalloproteinase inhibitor batimastat in a human colorectal cancer ascites model. Br J Cancer 74:1354–1358.

121. Welgus HG, Stricklin GP (1983) Human skin fibroblast collagenase inhibitor. J Biol Chem 258:12259–12264.

122. Welgus HG, Jeffrey JJ, Eisen AZ, Roswit WT, Stricklin GP (1985) Human skin fibroblast collagenase; interaction with substrate and inhibitor. Collagen Rel Res 5:167–179.

123. Welgus HG, Campbell EJ, Bar-Shavit Z, Senior RM, Teitelbaum SL (1985) Human alveolar macrophages produce a fibroblast-like collagenase and collagenase inhibitor. J Clin Invest 76:219–224.

124. Wilhelm SM, Collier IE, Marmer BL, Eisen AZ, Grant GA, Goldberg GL (1989) SV40 transformed human lung fibroblasts secrete a 92 kDa type IV collagenase which is identical to that secreted by normal human macrophages. J Biol Chem 264:17213–17221.

125. Will H, Hinzman B (1995) cDNA sequence and mRNA tissue distribution of a novel human matrix metalloproteinase with a potential transmembrane segment. Eur J Biochem 231:602–608.

126. Wolf C, Chenard MP, Durand de Grossouvre P, Bellocq JP, Chambon P, Basset P (1992) Breast-cancer-associated stromelysin-3 gene is expressed in basal cell carcinoma and during cutaneous wound healing. J Invest Dermatol 99:870–872.

127. Wysocki AB, Staiano-Coico L, Grinnell F (1993) Wound fluid from chronic leg ulcers contains elevated levels of metalloproteinases MMP-2 and MMP-9. J Invest Dermatol 101:64–68.

128. Yoshimoto M, Itoh F, Yamamoto H, Hinoda Y, Imai K, Yachi A (1993) Expression of MMP 7 (PUMP 1) mRNA in human colorectal cancers. Int J Cancer 54:614–18.

128a. Zeng ZS, Guillem JG (1995) Distinct pattern of matrix metalloproteinase 9 and tissue inhibitor of metalloproteinase 1 mRNA expression in human colorectal cancer and liver metastasis. Br J Cancer 72:575–582.

129. Zucker S, Lysik RM, Wieman J, Wilkie DP, Lane B (1985) Diversity of human pancreatic cancer cell proteinases: role of cell membrane metalloproteinases in collagenolysis and cytolysis. Cancer Res 45:6168–6178.

130. Zucker S, Wieman JM, Lysik RM (1987) Enrichment of collagen and gelatin degrading activities in the plasma cell membranes of human cancer cells. Cancer Res 47:1608–1614.

131. Zucker S, Moll UM, Lysik RM (1990) Extraction of type-IV collagenase/gelatinase from plasma membranes of human cancer cells. Int J Cancer 45:1137–1142.

28 Pancreatic Cancer: Growth Factors and Growth Factor Receptors

H. Friess, P. Büchler, P. Berberat, J. Kleeff, M. Korc and M.W. Büchler

Cancer of the pancreas presently has an incidence of approximately 8 to 10 cases per 100 000 citizens in industrialised European countries (1), an incidence that has been increasing over the past decades (2,3). In the USA the disease presently represents the fourth leading cause of cancer death in men and in women (1,4,5). Approximately 30 000 patients die every year from pancreatic cancer – nearly the same number as are diagnosed – and most of the newly diagnosed patients present with an irresectable tumour (1,5). Therefore, most patients can be offered only palliative surgical treatment, including biliary or enteral bypass operations (3,6,7).

All of the common conservative oncological strategies such as chemotherapy and radiotherapy have not significantly improved the prognosis for pancreatic cancer (8,9,10). Furthermore, other therapeutic options, such as antihormonal therapy using tamoxifen or buserelin (11,12), or application of specific monoclonal anti-pancreatic cancer cell antibodies (13,14), have not led to a significant improvement in survival. Of the few patients who are resectable at the time of diagnosis, most develop metastatic disease or local recurrence after curative surgical intervention within the first or second postoperative year, without having any additional effective therapeutic options for curative or palliative treatment. All these aspects contribute to a dismal prognosis, with an overall survival of 4–6 months following the establishment of the diagnosis and an overall 5-year survival rate of less than 0.4% (4,6,7).

It is still not clear why cancer of the pancreas is such a devastating disease. The mechanisms of its aggressive growth and early metastatic behaviour are poorly understood. First hints of the important role of growth factors and their receptors in the pathogenesis of pancreatic cancer became evident in the late 1980s. The expression pattern of these factors was first studied in human pancreatic carcinoma cell lines (15–18), and these experiments showed overexpression of the epidermal growth factor (EGF) receptor and an increase in EGF mRNA levels. Surprisingly, these cells also produce transforming growth factor alpha (TGFα). Like EGF, this polypeptide is an additional ligand of the EGF receptor (19,20).

Receptor studies have revealed that both EGF and TGFα are able to bind to the EGF receptor. After binding, the ligand–receptor complex is internalised into the cytosol. EGF often gets recycled, in contrast to TGFα, which is rapidly degraded (20). The ligand–receptor interaction underlies a negative regulation pattern (16,18,20). Both growth factors, but especially EGF, induce down-regulation of the EGF receptor (18). However, TGFα has been found to be 10 to 100 times more potent than EGF in enhancing the anchorage-independent growth of human pancreatic cancer cell lines (19).

In light of the fact that pancreatic cancer cells overexpress the EGF receptor and produce its stimulating ligands TGFα and EGF, as well as possessing the ability to recycle EGF, the growth advantage of malignant cells seems obvious. Based on these basic experimental data we started to analyse the role of growth factors and growth factor receptors in human pancreatic cancer.

In this chapter we describe part of the research which we have recently conducted on growth factors and growth factor receptors in pancreatic cancer. Due to space limitations, however, several studies in other growth factor families and their receptors cannot be presented.

EGF Receptor Family and Ligands in Pancreatic Cancer

The epidermal growth factor (EGF) receptor family consists of several members. To this growth factor receptor family belongs the EGF receptor 1, also known as human EGF receptor 1 (HER-1); c-erbB-2 (HER-2) (21,22), c-erbB-3 (HER-3) (23) and c-erbB-4 (HER-4) (24). Sequence analysis of the different domains of this growth factor receptor superfamily revealed homologies between 60% and 83% (25). The EGF receptor is a 170-kDa glycoprotein consisting of three domains. One is an extracellular, ligand-binding domain; the second is a hydrophobic transmembrane domain; and the third is a highly conserved intracellular domain with tyrosine kinase activity (25,26,27). Binding of a ligand to the EGF receptor results in receptor dimerisation and causes increased catalytic activity of the tyrosine kinase, which leads to the phosphorylisation of several intracellular substrates, including phospholipase C-γ, MAP kinase and the *ras* GTPase activating protein (GAP)(26,27).

EGF Receptor and Ligands

Two activating ligands for the EGF receptor – epidermal growth factor (EGF) and transforming growth factor α (TGFα) – can be characterised as the prototypes of a growth factor family which also includes amphiregulin, betacellulin, cripto and heparin-binding EGF (25,28–31).

In order to study the roles of the EGF receptor, EGF and TGFα in human pancreatic cancer, we analysed their patterns of expression in human pancreatic tissue samples. Cell culture experiments revealed that EGF receptor overexpression leads to malignant transformation of these cells. Additionally, these *in vitro* experiments showed that cancer cell proliferation can be enhanced by the presence of EGF and TGFα (32–36).

These cell culture studies gave the first hints that alterations within the EGF receptor family and their ligands might be important for the course and prognosis of tumour diseases *in vivo*. In order to study gene expression, modern molecular biology techniques as well as immunohistochemical analysis of human tumour tissue samples were used. With the latter technique, enhanced protein

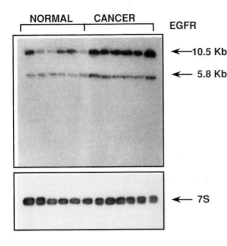

NORMAL   CANCER   EGFR

←—10.5 Kb

←— 5.8 Kb

←— 7S

Figure 1. Northern blot analysis of EGR receptor mRNA expression in the normal pancreas (*NORMAL*) and in pancreatic cancer (*CANCER*). In pancreatic cancer samples a marked overexpression of EGF receptor mRNA was present in comparison with the normal controls. Reproduced from The Journal of Clinical Investigation, 1992; 90: 1352–1360 by copyright permission of The American Society for Clinical Investigation.

levels for EGF receptor, EGF and TGFα in human pancreatic cancers were found (37,38). Using Northern blot analysis and *in situ* hybridisation we showed enhanced expression of the EGF receptor (Figure 1) and EGF and/or TGFα in pancreatic cancer cells. Many cancer cells exhibited concomitant overexpression of the EGF receptor and EGF and/or TGFα, indicating that autocrine and paracrine mechanisms of this receptor–ligand system might play a crucial function in the pathogenesis of pancreatic cancer (37,38). In order to confirm this assumption, immunohistochemical studies in 87 human pancreatic cancer tissues were performed. Patients who had increased levels of the EGF receptor and EGF and/or TGFα died earlier in the postoperative course than patients who did not simultaneously overexpress the EGF receptor with one of its ligands (37). In addition to EGF and TGFα, amphiregulin expression was also enhanced in human pancreatic cancer samples, and its concomitant presence with the EGF receptor was associated with shorter patient survival (39,40).

C-*erb*-B-2

The potential role of the proto-oncogene c-*erb*B-2 (detected in the late 1980's) in tumour pathogenesis of pancreatic cancer was also investigated (41,42). According to sequence analysis, c-*erb*B-2 has structural features in common with other growth factor receptors and close similarity to the EGF receptor. The c-*erb*B-2 gene encodes a transmembrane receptor with a molecular weight of 185 kDa. As with most proto-oncogenes, c-*erb*B-2 can be activated to a transforming oncogene by several mechanisms (25). Single point mutations, which stabilise the dimeric receptor conformation, as well as truncation of the gene, which leads to deletion of the extracellular domain, are able to activate this protein. Most commonly, c-*erb*B-2 signalling is activated by gene amplification leading to an aberrantly high gene expression. Signal transmission of this receptor can also be activated physiologically through binding of specific ligands such as NDF (neu differentiation factor), glial growth factors and heregulin (27,43–46). The

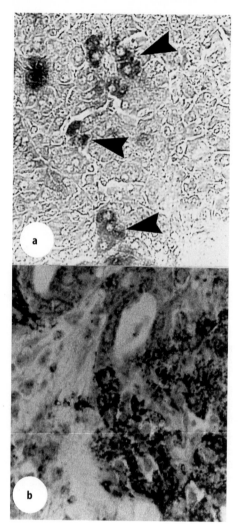

Figure 2. c-erbB2 immunostaining in the normal human pancreas (**a**) and in pancreatic cancer (**b**). In the normal pancreas only a few acinar cells (*arrowheads*) exhibited weak to moderate c-erbB2 immunoreactivity in some areas. In contrast, in pancreatic cancer samples moderate to intense c-erbB2 immunoreactivity was present in the cancer cells.

overexpression of c-*erb*B-2 leads to malignant cell transformation *in vitro* (22,26,44). Of 76 pancreatic cancer samples we investigated, 34 (45%) exhibited increased c-*erb*B-2 immunoreactivity in the pancreatic cancer cells (Figure 2) (42). *In situ* hybridisation and Northern blot analysis indicated that the increase in c-*erb*B-2 immunoreactivity was associated with overexpression of the corresponding mRNA (42). Statistical analysis showed that overexpression of c-*erb*B-2 mRNA in the pancreatic cancer cells was associated with better tumour differentiation (42). In contrast to the EGF receptor, the presence of c-*erb*B-2 was not associated with advanced tumour stage or worse postoperative survival periods. These findings suggest that the activation of c-*erb*B-2 in human pancreatic cancer leads to better differentiation of the cancer cells, which has already been described in studies with cultured human mammary cancer cell lines (46).

C-erbB-3

c-erbB-3 is the third member of the EGF receptor-related family of growth factor receptors (23). The structure of c-erbB-3 protein is closely related to the EGF receptor and the c-erbB-2 receptor. Immunohistochemical studies demonstrated moderate to intense immunoreactivity of c-erbB-3 in human pancreatic cancer cells (47), and Northern blot analysis of c-erbB-3 indicated that pancreatic cancer cells also overexpress this growth factor receptor. In contrast to the normal human pancreas, in which only low levels of c-erbB-3 mRNA are expressed (48), quantitative mRNA analysis demonstrated a sixfold increase in c-erbB-3 mRNA in the pancreatic cancer tissues in comparison with normal controls. In immuno-histochemistry, 47% (27 of 58) of the pancreatic cancer samples exhibited positive immunostaining. Positive immunoreactivity for c-erbB-3 in pancreatic cancer cells was associated with advanced tumour stages and significantly shorter postoperative survival (48). Although the ligand that activates c-erbB-3 has not yet been identified, these findings suggest that overexpression of the EGF receptor and/or c-erbB-3 seems to play an important role in pancreatic cancer progression and patient prognosis (48).

TGF βs and TGF β Receptors

The TGFβ superfamily of cytokines includes TGFβ, activin and the bone morphogenic proteins (BMPs). They elicit a broad range of cellular responses, including the regulation of cell division, cell death and survival, cell differentiation, recognition and specification of developmental fate. They also figure prominently in the control of tissue recycling and repair, in the formation and production of extracellular matrix proteins, and in stimulation of angiogenesis and immunosuppression (49–54). TGFβs inhibit growth in many epithelial cells; however, cell proliferation is not inhibited in all pancreatic carcinoma cell lines by TGFβ1, which represents the prototype of this growth factor family. Meanwhile, it has been shown that the influence of TGFβ on growth of tumour cell lines is dependent on the culture conditions (49,54,55). Therefore, alterations in culture conditions can cause TGFβ to stimulate rather than to inhibit cancer cell growth.

The role of TGFβs in human pancreatic carcinomas was characterised in a recently published study (56). It was demonstrated that all three mammalian TGFβ isoforms; TGFβ1, TGFβ2 and TGFβ3, are overexpressed in many human pancreatic cancer cells in vivo (56). Overexpression of the TGFβs as determined by in situ hybridisation and Northern blot analysis was associated with increased immunoreactivity of the peptides in the pancreatic cancer cells (56). Analysis of the survival data of 60 resected pancreatic cancer patients demonstrated that the presence of TGFβ1, TGFβ2 or TGFβ3 in the pancreatic tumour cells was associated with more aggressive growth and significantly reduced postoperative survival periods (56). These findings indicate that TGFβs may act as growth stimulators in human pancreatic cancer in vivo.

Members of the TGFβ superfamily act through specific cell membrane receptors. Three major TGFβ-binding receptors have been identified during recent years: TGFβ receptor-1, TGFβ receptor-2, and TGFβ receptor-3 (57–60). A combination of biochemical and genetic evidence has shown that the TGFβ family members signal by simultaneously contacting the TGFβ receptor-1 and the TGFβ receptor-2, which has serine/threonine kinase activity (60,61). Both receptors are required for TGFβ signalling in mammalian cells. The type 2 receptor seems to act upstream of the type 1 receptor (51). One major difference between these two receptor types is in their ligand-binding properties. In contrast to the TGFβ receptor-1, the TGFβ receptor-2 recognises TGFβ and activin in the medium (61). This complex consisting of ligand-bound TGFβ receptor-2 is recognised by the TGFβ receptor-1, forming an oligomeric complex, probably a heterotetramer. The BMP receptor system is different, because both receptors seem to have low affinity for the ligand and together achieve high affinity (51,61,62). TGFβ receptor-3, a proteoglycan also known as betaglycan (59), is not directly involved in signal transmission (59). However, the mechanism of signal transduction by these receptors is largely unknown. The signal originated by members of the TGFβ superfamily appears to be transduced by a set of evolutionary conserved proteins, known as SMADs, which upon activation directly translocate to the nucleus, where they may activate transcription (51,61,62).

In the normal human pancreas, all three TGFβ receptors are present (57). Pancreatic cancer cells show overexpression of TGFβ receptor-2 but not of TGFβ receptor-3 (57). *In situ* hybridisation has demonstrated the presence of TGFβ receptor-2 mRNA especially within pancreatic cancer cells but also in the desmoplastic tissue adjacent to the tumour (57). These findings, together with the previous report of TGFβ overexpression in pancreatic cancer cells, suggest that TGFβ might contribute to the neoplastic process and enhance the proliferation of tumour cells in human pancreatic carcinomas through autocrine and/or paracrine activation of the TGFβ receptor-2 (56,57).

aFGF and bFGF

Fibroblast growth factor (FGF) constitutes a third family of growth factors. It includes the two abundant prototypic members, acidic FGF (aFGF) and basic FGF (bFGF), as well as seven additional related proteins (63,64): FGF 3 (int-2); FGF 4, or Kaposi FGF (the gene product of hst); FGF 5; FGF 6; FGF 7 (keratinocyte growth factor); FGF 8 (androgen-induced growth factor); and FGF 9 (63,65–68). aFGF and bFGF are capable of influencing various biological functions, such as cell differentiation, tissue homeostasis, regeneration and repair, cell migration and angiogenesis (66–72). The biological functions of the other members of the FGF family have not yet been studied in detail.

aFGF and bFGF are the prototypes of this growth factor family. aFGF has been detected in nerve tissue, heart, kidney, prostate and liver, whereas bFGF seems to be more ubiquitous in human tissues (64–72). Despite the fact that aFGF and bFGF have no signal peptide sequence and are not secreted, they are highly abundant in the extracellular matrix and basement membranes of a variety of tissues. A common feature of all members of the FGF family is their high affinity for heparin and the structurally related cell surface and extracellular matrix heparan sulphates. aFGF and bFGF bind to specific transmembrane receptors which possess intracellular tyrosine kinase activity and an extracellular domain consisting of two or three immunoglobulin-like regions (68–70). To achieve a biological effect, FGF is dependent on the presence of heparin sulphate proteoglycans, which are found on the cell surface or in the extracellular matrix. The first step in the course of binding to cell surface receptors seems to be the formation of an appropriate FGF–heparin complex. This complex then binds to the cognate FGF receptor to form an active trimolecular complex consisting of the heparin-like molecule, FGF, and the FGF receptor (65,66,71,72). aFGF, bFGF and four high-affinity FGF receptors have already been demonstrated in the normal human pancreas (73). In studies with isolated rat pancreatic acini, it has been shown that aFGF and bFGF can stimulate amylase release, which might have physiological implications in the regulation of the exocrine pancreas (74).

Upon analysing human pancreatic cancer tissue, we found that aFGF and bFGF are overexpressed in a significant number of pancreatic cancers (75). *In situ* hybridisation localised both increased mRNA moieties within the pancreatic cancer cells (75). Tumour cells surrounding areas with chronic pancreatitis-like alterations also exhibited increased expression of aFGF and bFGF mRNA in the pancreatic acinar and ductal cells (75). Overexpression of aFGF and bFGF mRNA was accompanied by increased levels of the corresponding proteins, as demonstrated by intense immunoreactivity for aFGF and bFGF in pancreatic cancer cells and in the desmoplastic tissue surrounding the cancer mass. Furthermore, Western blot analysis revealed 8- and 11-fold increases in aFGF and bFGF levels, respectively, in the cancer samples in comparison with the corresponding levels in the normal samples. Characteristically, cancer samples exhibited a 16.5-kDa and a faint 20-kDa band, as well as several small bands in the molecular weight range of 10–15 kDa of aFGF. These low molecular weight forms could be due to an alternative splicing variant or to degradation products of aFGF (71,76). The significance of these multiple isoforms is not fully understood; however, it is known that alternative splicing in the extracellular domain of these receptors results in altered ligand binding specificities (71,76). Alternative splicing of the intracellular cytoplasmic domain results in isoforms with increased oncogenic potential (71). According to a recent report, low molecular weight forms of FGF 4 have higher receptor affinity and biological activity than FGF 4 itself (71,77). So it seems possible that these forms of aFGF could also achieve biological activity in human pancreatic cancer tissues. In the case of bFGF, a major 18-kDa band and a minor 24-kDa band were visible. In addition, there was a minor 15-kDa bFGF band in the cancer samples. For bFGF it was shown that the alternative spliced isoforms have altered ligand binding or signalling qualities, depending on which region of the gene is spliced (71,76). The 24-kDa protein and other high molecular weight forms of bFGF have been previously described in cell extracts of mammary gland cells, neonatal fibroblasts and hepatocellular tumour cells (78,79,80). It is supposed that these high molecular weight forms of bFGF are transported directly into the nucleus after synthesis in the cytoplasm (81). Also, in the case of the 18-kDa bFGF protein, transport into the nucleus is known to occur after binding to the cell surface receptors and subsequent internalisation into the cytoplasm (63). The histological detection of nuclear bFGF immunoreactivity in pancreatic cancer cells could therefore be caused by nuclear bFGF accumulation from intracellular and/or extracellular sources (63,81).

Summary

Growth factors and growth factor receptors are polypeptides which stimulate cell growth and differentiation. In pancreatic cancer a variety of growth factors:

EGF (37,38), TGFα (37,38), amphiregulin (39,40), betacellulin (82), heparin-binding EGF-like growth factor (83), cripto (84), aFGF (75), bFGF (75), keratinocyte growth factor (85), TGFβs (56), hepatocyte growth factor (86), platelet-derived growth factors (87); and growth factor receptors: EGF receptor (37,38), c-erbB2 (41,42), c-erbB3 (48), FGF-receptor-1 (70), TGFβ receptors (57,88), c-met (86), platelet-derived growth factor receptors (87), have their expression enhanced. The concomitant presence of the EGF receptor and its ligands EGF, TGFα (37,38) and/or amphiregulin (39,40), the presence of c-erbB3 (48), bFGF (75), TGFβs (56) in the pancreatic cancer cells is associated with tumour aggressiveness and shorter survival periods following tumour resection. In addition to these alterations, p53 (89,90) and K-ras (91,92) mutations are frequently present in these tumours. Taken together, the abundance of growth-promoting factors and the disturbance of pathways with proliferation-inhibitory effects may combine to give pancreatic cancer cells a distinct growth advantage which results clinically in rapid tumour progression and poor survival.

Acknowledgement

This study was supported by the SNF Grant 32-39529 awarded by the Swiss National Research Foundation to H.F.

References

1. Parker SL, Tong T, Bolden, S, Wingo PA (1997) Cancer statistics, 1997. Cancer J Clin 47:5–27
2. Silverberg E, Lubera JA (1989) Cancer statistics. Cancer J Clin 3:3–39.
3. Warshaw AL, Femandes-Del Castillo C (1992) Pancreatic carcinoma. N Engl J Med 326: 455–465.
4. Gudjonsson B (1987) Cancer of the pancreas: 50 years of surgery. Cancer 60:2284–2303.
5. National Cancer Institute (1991) Annual cancer statistics review 1973–1988. Department of Health and Human Services, Bethesda (NIH publication no. 91–2789).
6. Büchler M, Ebert M, Beger HG (1993) Grenzen chirurgischen Handelns beim Pankreaskarzinom. Langenbecks Arch Chir Suppl (Kongressbericht):460–464.
7. Friess H, Büchler M, Beglinger C, Krüger M, Beger HG (1993) Low-dose octreotide treatment is not effective in patients with advanced pancreatic cancer. Pancreas 8:540–544.
8. Cullinan SA, Moertel CG, Fleming TR, for the North Central Cancer Treatment Group (1985) A comparison of three chemotherapeutic regimens in the treatment of advanced pancreatic and gastric carcinoma. JAMA 253:2061.
9. Moertel CG, Childs DS, Reitemeier RJ, Colby MY, Holbrook M (1969) Combined 5-fluorouracil and supervoltage radiation therapy of locally unresectable gastrointestinal cancer. Lancet II:865–900.
10. Moertel CG, Frytak S, Hahn RG (1981) Therapy of locally unresectable pancreatic carcinoma: a randomized comparison of high dose (6000 rads) radiation alone, moderate dose radiation (4000 rads) + 5-fluorouracil, and high dose radiation + 5-fluorouracil. The Gastrointestinal Tumor Study Group. Cancer 48:1705.
11. Andrén-Sandberg A (1990) Treatment with an LHRH analogue in patients with advanced pancreatic cancer. Acta Chir Scand 156:549–551.
12. Friess H, Büchler M, Krüger M, Beger HG (1992) Treatment of duct carcinoma of the pancreas with the LH-RH analogue buserelin. Pancreas 7:516–521.
13. Büchler M, Friess H, Schultheiss KH, et al. (1991) A randomized controlled trial of adjuvant immuno-therapy (murine monoclonal antibody 494/32) in resectable pancreatic cancer. Cancer 68:1507–1512.
14. Friess H, Büchler M, Schulz G, Beger HG (1989) Therapie des Pankreaskarzinoms mit dem monoklonalen Antikörper BW 494/32: erste klinische Ergebnisse. Immun Infekt 17:24–26.

15. Glinsmann-Gibson BJ, Korc M (1991) Regulation of transforming growth factor-α mRNA expression in T$_3$M$_4$ human pancreatic carcinoma cells. Pancreas 6:142–149.
16. Korc M, Magun B (1985) Recycling of epidermal growth factor in a human pancreatic carcinoma cell line. Proc Natl Acad Sci USA 82:6172–6175.
17. Korc M, Meltzer P, Trent J (1986) Enhanced expression of epidermal growth factor receptor correlates with alterations of chromosome 7 in human pancreatic cancer. Proc Natl Acad Sci USA 83:5141–5144.
18. Korc M, Finman JE (1989) Attenuated processing of epidermal growth factor in the face of marked degradation of transforming growth factor alpha. J Biol Chem 264:14990–14999.
19. Smith JJ, Derynck R, Korc M (1987) Production of transforming growth factor-α in human pancreatic cancer cells: evidence for a superagonist autocrine cycle. Proc Natl Acad Sci USA 84:7567–7570.
20. Derynck R (1988) Transforming growth factor-alpha. Cell 54:593–595.
21. Coussens L, Yank-Feng TL, Liao YC, et al. (1985) Tyrosine kinase receptor with extensive homology to EGF receptor shares chromosomal location with neu oncogene. Science 230: 1132– 1139.
22. Di Fiore PP, Pierce JH, Kraus MH, et al. (1987) erbB-2 is a potent oncogene when overexpressed in NIH/3T3 cells. Science 237:178–182.
23. Kraus MH, Issing W, Miki T et al. (1989) Isolation and characterization of ERBB3, a third member of the ERBB/epidermal growth factor receptor family: evidence for overexpression in a subset of human mammary tumours. Proc Natl Acad Sci USA 86:9193–9197.
24. Plowman GD, Culouscou JM, Whitney GS, et al. (1993) Ligand specific activation of HER4/p 180erbB4, a fourth member of the epidermal growth factor receptor family. Proc Natl Acad Sci USA 90:1746–1750.
25. Prigent SA, Lemoine NR (1992) The type 1 (EGFR-related) family of growth factor receptors and their ligands. Prog Growth Factor Res 4:1–24.
26. Schlessinger J, Ulrich A (1992) Growth factor signaling by receptor tyrosine kinases. Neuron 9:383–391.
27. Ullrich A, Schlessinger J (1990) Signal transduction by receptors with tyrosine kinase activity. Cell 61:203–212.
28. Shing Y, Christofori G, Hanahan D et al. (1993) Betacellulin: a mitogen from pancreatic beta cell tumors. Science 259:1604–1607.
29. Ciccodicola A, Dono R, Obici S et al. (1989) Molecular characterization of a gene of the "EGF family" expressed in undifferentiated human NTERA2 teratocarcinoma cells. EMBO J 8:1987–1991.
30. Higashiyama S, Abraham JA, Miller J et al. (1991) A heparinbinding growth factor secreted by macrophage-like cells that is related to EGF. Science 251:936–939.
31. Plowman GD, Green JM, McDonald VL et al. (1981) The amphiregulin gene encodes a novel epidermal growth factor-related protein with tumor-inhibitory activity. Mol Cell Biol 10:1969–1981.
32. Aaronson SA (1991) Growth factors and cancer. Science 254:1146–1153.
33. Hendler FJ, Ozanne BW (1984) Human squamous cell lung cancers express increased epidermal growth factor receptors. J Clin Invest 74:647–651.
34. Libermann TA, Nusbaum HR, Razon N et al. (1985) Amplification, enhanced expression, and possible rearrangement of the EGF receptor gene in primary human brain tumors of glial origin. Nature 313:144–147.
35. Neal DE, Marsh C, Bennett MK et al. (1985) Epidermal-growth-factor receptors in human bladder cancer: Comparison of invasive and superficial tumours. Lancet 1:366–368.
36. Sainsbury JR, Farndon JR, Sherbet GV, Harris AL (1985) Epidermal-growth-factor receptors and oestrogen receptors in human breast cancer. Lancet I:364–366.
37. Yamanaka Y, Friess H, Kobrin MS et al. (1993) Coexpression of epidermal growth factor receptor and ligands in human pancreatic cancer is associated with enhanced tumor aggressiveness. Anticancer Res 13:565–570.
38. Korc M, Chandrasekar B, Yamanaka Y et al. (1992) Overexpression of the epidermal growth factor receptor in human pancreatic cancer is associated with concomitant increase in the levels of epidermal growth factor and transforming growth factor alpha. J Clin Invest 90:1352–1360.
39. Ebert M, Yokoyama M, Kobrin MS et al. (1994) Induction and expression of amphiregulin in human pancreatic cancer. Cancer Res 54:3959–3962.
40. Yokoyama M, Ebert M, Funatomi H et al. (1995) Amphiregulin is a potent mitogen in human pancreatic cancer cells: correlation with patients survival. Int J Oncol 6:625–631.

41. Hall PA, Huges CM, Staddon SL (1990) The c-erbB-2 protooncogene in human pancreatic cancer. J Pathol 161:1995–2000.
42. Yamanaka Y, Friess H, Kobrin MS (1993) Overexpression of HER2/neu oncogene in human pancreatic cancer. Hum Pathol 24:1127–1134.
43. Holmes WE, Sliwkowski MX, Akita RW (1992) Identification of heregulin, a specific activator of p 185 *erb*-B2. Science 256:1205–1210.
44. Hudziak RM, Schlessinger J, Ullrich A (1987) Increased expression of the putative growth factor receptor p 185HER2 causes transformation and tumorigenesis of NIH 3T3 cells. Proc Natl Acad Sci USA 84:7159–7163.
45. Marchionni MA, Goodearl ADJ, Chen MS (1993) Glial growth factors are alternatively spliced *erb*B2 ligands expressed in the nervous system. Nature 362:312–318.
46. Peles E, Ben-Levy R, Tzahar E et al. (1993) Cell type-specific interaction of Neu differentiation factor (NDF/heregulin) with Neu/Her-2 suggests complex ligand-receptor relationships. EMBO J 12:961–971.
47. Lemoine NR, Lobresco M, Leung H et al. (1992) The *erb*-B-3 gene in human pancreatic cancer. J Pathol 168:269–273.
48. Friess H, Yamanaka Y, Kobrin MS et al. (1995) Enhanced *erb*B-3 expression in human pancreatic cancer correlates with tumor progression Clin Cancer Res 1:1413–1420.
49. Hebda PA (1988) Stimulatory effects of transforming growth factor-beta and epidermal growth factor on epidermal cell outgrowth from porcine skin explant cultures. J Invest Dermatol 91:440–445.
50. Massague J (1990) The transforming growth factor-β family: Annu Rev Cell Biol 6:597–641.
51. Chen X, Rubock MJ, Whitman M (1996) A transcriptional partner for MAD proteins in TGF-β signalling. Nature 383:691–696.
52. Massague J, Cheifetz S, Laiho M et al. (1992) Transforming growth factor-β: Cancer Surv 12:81–103.
53. Roberts AB, Sporn MG, Assoian RK, Smith JM, Roche NS (1986) Transforming growth factor type-b: Rapid induction of fibrosis and angiogenesis *in vivo* and stimulation of collagen formation *in vitro*: Proc Natl Acad Sci USA 83:4167–4171.
54. Sporn MB, Roberts AB (1992) Transforming growth factor-β: recent progress and new challenges. J Cell Biol 119:1017–1021.
55. Madri JA, Pratt BM, Tucker AM (1988) Phenotypic modulation of endothelial cells by transforming growth factor-β depends upon the composition and organization of the extracellular matrix. J Cell Biol 106:1375–1384.
56. Friess H, Yamanaka Y, Büchler M et al. (1993) Enhanced expression of transforming growth factor-beta isoforms in pancreatic cancer correlates with decreased survival. Gastroenterology 105:1846–1856.
57. Friess H, Yamanaka Y, Büchler M et al. (1993) Enhanced expression of the type II transforming growth factor-beta receptor in human pancreatic cancer cells without alteration of type III receptor expression. Cancer Res. 53:2704–2707.
58. Lin HY, Wang XF, Ng-Eaton E, Weinberg RA, Lodish HF (1992) Expression cloning of the TGF-β type II receptor, a functional transmembrane serine/threonine kinase. Cell 68:775–785.
59. Lopez-Casillas F, Cheifetz S, Doody J et al. (1991) Structure and expression of the membrane proteoglycan betaglycan, a component of the TGF-β receptor system. Cell 67:785–795.
60. Wrana JL, Attisano L, Carcamo J et al. (1992) TGF-β signals through a heteromeric protein kinase receptor complex. Cell 71:1003–1014.
61. Massague J (1996) TGF-β signalling: receptors, transducers, and Mad proteins. Cell 85:947–950.
62. Lagna G, Hata A, Hemmati A, Massague J (1996) Partnership between DPC4 and SMAD proteins in TGF-β signalling pathways. Nature 383:832–836.
63. Bouche G, Gas N, Prats H (1987) Basic fibroblast growth factor enters the nucleolus and stimulates the transcription of ribosomal genes in ABAE cells undergoing G0–G1 transition. Proc Natl Acad Sci USA 84:6770–6774.
64. Burgess WH, Maciag T (1989) The heparin-binding (fibroblast) growth factor family of proteins. Annu Rev Biochem 58:575–606.
65. Folkman J, Klagsbrun M (1987) Angiogenic factors. Science 235:442–447.
66. Gospodarowicz D, Neufeld G, Schweigerer L (1986) Molecular and biological characterization of fibroblast growth factor, an angiogenic factor which also controls the proliferation and differentiation of mesoderm and neuroectoderm derived cells. Cell Diff 19:1–17.
67. Gospodarowicz D, Ferrara N, Schweigerer L, Neufeld G (1987) Structural characterization and biological functions of fibroblast growth factor. Endocrine Rev 8:95–114.
68. Klagsbrun M (1989) The fibroblast growth factor family: structural and biological properties. Prog Growth Factor Res 1:207–235.

69. Givol D, Yayon A (1992) Complexity of FGF receptors: genetic basis for structural diversity and functional specificity. FASEB J 6:3362–3369.
70. Kobrin MS, Yamanaka Y, Friess H, Lopez ME, Korc M (1993) Aberrant expression of the type I fibroblast growth factor receptor in human pancreatic adenocarcinomas. Cancer Res 53:4741–4744.
71. Friesel RE, Maciat T (1995) Molecular mechanisms of angiogenesis: fibroblast growth factor signal transduction. FASEB J 9:919–925.
72. Gomm JJ, Smith J, Ryall GK et al. (1991) Localization of basic fibroblast growth factor and transforming growth factor $\beta1$ in the human mammary gland. Cancer Res 51:4685–4692.
73. Friess H, Kobrin MS, Korc M (1992) Acidic and basic fibroblast growth factors and their receptors are expressed in the human pancreas. Pancreas 7:737 (abstract).
74. Chandrasekar B, Korc M (1992) Binding and biological actions of acidic and basic fibroblast growth factors in isolated rat pancreatic acini. Gastroenterology 102:A725 (abstract).
75. Yamanaka Y, Friess H, Büchler MW et al. (1993) Overexpression of acidic and basic fibroblast growth factors in human pancreatic cancer correlates with advanced tumor stage. Cancer Res 53:5289–5296.
76. Coutts JC, Gallagher JT (1995) Receptor for fibroblast growth factors. Immunol Cell Biol 73:584–589.
77. Bellosta P, Talarico D, Rogers D, Basilico C (1993) Cleavage of K-FGF produces a truncated molecule with increased biological activity and receptor binding affinity. J Cell Biol 121:705–713.
78. Fu Y-M, Spirito P, Yu Z-X et al. (1991) Acidic fibroblast growth factor in the developing rat embryo. J Cell Biol 114:1261–1273.
79. Li S, Shipley GD (1991) Expression of multiple species of basic fibroblast growth factor mRNA and protein in normal and tumor-derived mammary epithelial cells in culture. Cell Growth Differ 2:195–202.
80. Shimoyama Y, Gotoh M, Ino Y et al. (1991) Characterization of high-molecular-mass forms of basic fibroblast growth factor produced by hepatocellular carcinoma cells: possible involvement of basic fibroblast growth factor in hepatocarcinogenesis. Jpn J Cancer Res 82:1263–1270.
81. Bugler B, Amalrie F, Prats H (1991) Alternative initiation of translation determines cytoplasmic or nuclear localization of basic fibroblast growth factor. Mol Cell Biol 11:573–577.
82. Yokoyama M, Funatomi H, Kobrin MS et al. (1995) Betacellulin, a member of the epidermal growth factor family, is overexpressed in human pancreatic cancer. Int J Oncology 7:825–829.
83. Yokayama M, Funatomi H, Hope Ch et al. (1996) Heparin-binding EGF-like growth factor expression and biological action in human pancreatic cancer cells. Int J Oncology 8:289–295.
84. Friess H, Yamanaka Y, Büchler MW et al. (1994) Cripto, a member of the epidermal growth factor family, is overexpressed in human pancreatic cancer and chronic pancreatitis. Int J Cancer 56:668–674.
85. Siddiqui I, Funatomi H, Kobrin MS et al. (1995) Increased expression of keratinocyte growth factor in human pancreatic cancer. Biochem Biophys Res Commun 215:309–315.
86. Ebert M, Yokoyama M, Friess H, Büchler MW, Korc M (1994) Coexpression of the c-met protooncogene and hepatocyte growth factor in human pancreatic cancer. Cancer Res 54:5775–5778.
87. Ebert M, Yokoyama M, Friess H et al. (1995) Induction of platelet-derived growth factor A and B chains and overexpression of their receptors in human pancreatic cancer. Int J Cancer 62:529–535.
88. Baldwin RL, Friess H, Yokoyama M et al. (1996) Attenuated ALK5 Receptor expression in human pancreatic cancer: correlation with resistance to growth inhibition. Int J Cancer 67:283–288.
89. Barton CM, Staddon SL, Hughes CM et al. (1991) Abnormalities of the p53 tumour suppressor gene in human pancreatic cancer. Br J Cancer 64:1076–1082.
90. Casey G, Yamanaka Y, Friess H et al. (1993) p53 mutations are common in pancreatic cancer and are absent in chronic pancreatitis. Cancer Lett 69:151–160.
91. Grünewald K, Lyons J, Fröhlich A et al. (1989) High frequency of Ki-ras codon 12 mutations in pancreatic adenocarcinomas. Int J Cancer 43:1037–1041.
92. Almoguera C, Shibata D, Forrester K et al. (1988) Most human carcinomas of the exocrine pancreas contain mutant c-K-ras genes. Cell 53:549–554.

29 n-3 Polyunsaturated Fatty Acids in the Treatment of Pancreatic Cancer Cachexia

M.D. Barber, J.A. Ross and K.C.H. Fearon

Pancreatic adenocarcinoma is the fifth leading cause of cancer death in the Western world with an incidence of about 10/100 000 person-years (1). Over 95% of patients will die of their disease. The 5-year survival rate is 1.3% with a median survival of 4.1 months (2). More than 80% of cancers are irresectable at diagnosis and even in those patients suitable for surgical resection the 5-year survival rate is less than 25% in the best centres (3).

Numerous studies of radiotherapy and chemotherapeutic agents show little benefit and significant toxicity (4,5). Current trials of combination chemotherapy and radiotherapy tend to concentrate on patients who have already had surgical resection (3). This leaves little in the way of treatment options for the vast majority of patients with irresectable disease. A trial comparing the antimetabolite gemcitabine and the matrix metalloproteinase inhibitor marimastat in these patients is currently recruiting. These new agents have shown some benefits against surrogate disease markers but little objective antitumour activity and they retain the side effects of traditional chemotherapeutic agents (6–10).

Cancer Cachexia

Patients with advanced cancer frequently exhibit progressive weight loss and this is associated with a shorter survival time and reduced quality of life and indeed, some patients appear to die of such severe wasting (11–13). In a recent survey of patients with irresectable pancreatic cancer we found that 85% had unintentionally lost weight by the time of diagnosis and that the median weight loss close to the time of death was almost 25% (14). Clearly in a proportion of these individuals weight loss contributed to their demise.

The term cachexia is derived from the Greek words *kakos*, meaning "bad," and *hexis*, meaning "condition." The syndrome is characterised by anorexia, early satiety, changes in taste perception, weight loss, weakness, anaemia and oedema (15). Cachexia is not exclusive to cancer but is also seen in a variety of inflammatory conditions such as sepsis, acquired immunodeficiency syndrome and rheumatoid arthritis (16–18).

Mechanisms of Cachexia

For loss of weight to occur there is usually a reduction in energy intake or an increase in energy expenditure or a combination of the two. In pancreatic cancer it would appear that both reduced intake and increased expenditure apply (14,19). In uncomplicated starvation there is an adaptation to conserve protein and to reduce energy expenditure. In cancer cachexia these adaptations do not appear to compensate adequately and a situation more akin to the so-called metabolic response to trauma develops with continuing breakdown of body stores and increased energy expenditure (19,20). Numerous changes in nutrient metabolism are seen in weight-losing cancer patients. Insulin resistance, glucose intolerance, increased glucose production and consumption and increased Cori cycle activity have been shown (21–24). A decrease in lipogenesis is seen due to decreased lipoprotein lipase activity (25,26). Protein turnover is elevated and increases further with more advanced disease (27,28).

About 40% of patients with advanced pancreatic cancer display an acute-phase protein response at diagnosis. Close to the time of death this proportion rises to 80% (29). The acute phase protein response is an alteration in the balance of protein production by the liver, usually in response to injury, trauma or infection, in an attempt to aid the prevention of ongoing tissue damage, the eradication of infecting organisms and the activation of repair processes (30). The presence of an acute phase protein response in pancreatic cancer patients, as measured by an elevated serum C-reactive protein level, is strongly associated with shorter survival (29). It has been suggested that an imbalance between the amino acid composition of acute phase proteins and skeletal muscle, the body's labile amino acid reserve, helps drive the accelerated wasting seen during an acute phase response (31).

Overall, these metabolic changes result in a diversion of nutrients away from peripheral tissues and increased expenditure of energy. In the acute situation, such as trauma or infection, the net effect is presumably beneficial in supplying the nutrients and proteins to aid the defence of the body but in a chronic condition such as cancer these changes would appear to be detrimental.

Mediators of Cachexia

There are several obvious causes of anorexia in patients with advanced cancer such as tumour obstruction of the gastrointestinal tract, pain, depression, anxiety, steatorrhoea, constipation, general debility and the effects of treatments such as opiates, radiotherapy and chemotherapy. However, there remain many patients with advanced pancreatic cancer in whom there is no overt cause of reduced food intake. Weight loss begins early in the course of malignant disease and the degree of wasting correlates poorly with the size of the tumour. Thus it would appear that the anorexia and metabolic changes of cachexia are driven by mediators produced by the tumour or by the body in response to the tumour (Figure 1).

Cytokines, including tumour necrosis factor, interleukins 1 and 6, ciliary neurotrophic factor and interferon-gamma have been shown to induce some of the features of cachexia following administration to animals or humans (32–36).

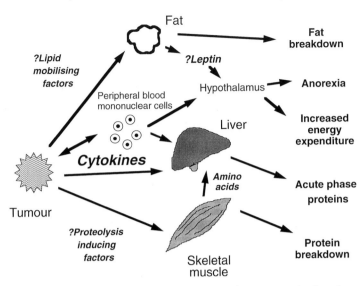

Figure 1. Hypothesis of mechanism of wasting in cancer. The nature and roles of many of the mediators shown remain to be elucidated.

Elevated serum levels of tumour necrosis factor and interleukin-6 and the soluble receptors for tumour necrosis factor have been found in cancer patients and in some instances correlated with severity of disease or weight loss (19,37–41). However, the pattern of symptoms and metabolic changes produced by exogenous cytokines differs from that of classical cachexia and antibody blocking experiments have shown only a limited ability to reverse these changes (42–44). Thus the relevance of cytokines within the circulation may be limited. Increased production of tumour necrosis factor and interleukin-6 by isolated peripheral blood mononuclear cells of patients with cancer has also been observed and is in keeping with a local action for these cytokines (19,45). In pancreatic cancer such enhanced cytokine production correlates well with hypermetabolism and an acute phase response (19). Most of the proinflammatory cytokines, but primarily interleukin-6, have been shown to induce the hepatic acute phase protein response (36,46–48). Cytokines thus are likely to work *in vivo* at a local level through a complex network of interrelationships, they stimulate acute phase protein production and probably also play a wider role in cachexia.

Changes in hormone levels and target-organ sensitivity are also seen in cachexia. In weight-stable patients with pancreatic cancer increased insulin secretion has been found with peripheral insulin resistance (49). However, in trials in which weight-losing patients were included, a markedly reduced insulin response to feeding is seen. Changes in insulin production seem to be unrelated to loss of pancreatic tissue (50–52). Elevated cortisol and glucagon levels have also been described (23,53,54). These changes may be stimulated by cytokines (32,33) and may tend to amplify the acute phase response (30). Infusion of hydrocortisone or cortisol, glucagon and adrenaline in humans produces many of the features of the acute phase response including increased energy expenditure, negative nitrogen balance, C-reactive protein production and glucose intolerance (55,56).

The existence of further proteolytic and lipolytic factors has been suggested (57). The recent characterisation of a 24-kDa glycoprotein found in the urine of cachectic cancer patients (but not those losing weight for other reasons) which causes weight loss through proteolysis when given to mice and appears distinct from known cytokines may represent one of these agents, and may be an important new mediator in the process of cancer cachexia (58,59).

The role of leptin, the recently identified protein produced by adipocytes which regulates food intake and body weight, in cachexia remains to be clarified. The production and end-organ effects of leptin is modulated by cytokines and gluco-corticoids, thus it may be an important mediator in cachectic cancer patients (60,61).

Therapy for Cachexia

The best way to cure cancer cachexia is to cure the cancer; however, this is only an option for the minority of patients. The next most obvious way to treat this phenomenon would be to supplement nutritional intake. However, studies of hyperalimentation in cancer cachexia using enteral or parenteral supplementation have been disappointing with limited weight gain, mainly of water and fat (62–67). Oral supplementation is often limited by anorexia and early satiety but even when a limited increase in calorie and nitrogen intake has been achieved this has not led to significant weight gain or clinical benefit (68).

Numerous other agents have been suggested to be useful in cachexia but none have lived up to their promise. The antiserotoninergic cyproheptadine, pro-kinetic metoclopramide and corticosteroid dexamethasone are said to improve appetite but have not been shown to prevent weight loss. The progestogens medroxyprogesterone acetate and megestrol acetate, the gluconeogenesis inhibitor hydrazine sulphate and psychotropic tetrahydrocannabinol have been shown to produce weight gain in some groups of cachectic patients but where studies of body composition have been performed much of this weight gain can be attributed to the accumulation of water (69–73). While producing some benefits in experimental models, insulin and megestrol acetate have been associated with accelerated tumour growth (74,75) and many of these agents have significant additional side effects.

Polyunsaturated Fatty Acids

Humans are unable to synthesise fatty acids with double bonds more proximal to the methyl end than the ninth carbon atom. Thus there are two families of essential fatty acids: those with the last double bond six or three atoms from this position. The parent of the omega-6 or n-6 fatty acids is linoleic acid (C18:2n–6). This is found in many plant seeds and is elongated and desaturated *in vivo* to form arachidonic acid (C20:4n–6). The parent of the n-3 family is alpha-linolenic acid (C18:3n–3), which is found associated with chloroplasts. Linseed, rapeseed and soybean oils contain some but the richest source, particularly of the longer chain eicosapentaenoic (C20:5n–3) and docosahexaenoic (C22:6n–3) acids is marine algae (76). These algae form the lowest level of the marine food chain and thus n-3 fatty acids are found in appreciable quantities in many marine animals where the high level of desaturation may help keep cell membranes fluid at ocean temperatures (77).

Epidemiology

Interest in polyunsaturated fatty acids in human disease has increased substantially since observations on Greenland Eskimos in the 1970's. The latter showed that, despite a fat and cholesterol intake similar to Western Europe, diseases such as coronary heart disease and cancer were rare (78,79). The major dietary difference between this population and those with a higher incidence of such diseases seemed to be in the type of fat rather than the quantity consumed. The main sources of fat in Greenland Eskimos were fish, seals and whales resulting in a higher consumption of n-3 fatty acids and a lower intake of n-6 and saturated fats (80,81). In the UK n-3 fatty acids make up less than 0.5% of the fats in our diet resulting in levels of less than 1% in the body's lipid pools. In populations such as Eskimos with a high intake, n-3 fatty acids may make up 15% of cholesterol esters and 7% of phospholipids (80,82).

The thrust of initial research was in the cardiovascular field where n-3 fatty acids have been shown to decrease blood viscosity, improve the lipid profile and lower blood pressure (see (76) for review) but since then research has expanded into many fields representing many increasingly prevalent diseases, especially those of an inflammatory nature. Beneficial effects for n-3 fatty acids have now been described in inflammatory bowel disease (83,84), rheumatoid arthritis (85), asthma (86), atopic dermatitis (87), psoriasis (88), models of sepsis (89), postoperative complications (90), organ transplantation (91), schizophrenia (92) and cancer. Indeed, it is tempting to speculate that human metabolism evolved to use a higher ratio of n-3 to n-6 and saturated fatty acids than is currently common in the Western diet.

Biological Activity

Polyunsaturated fatty acids have been shown to have a myriad of biological effects at the tissue, cellular and molecular levels, many of which may have a role in arresting cachexia. The 20 carbon polyunsaturated fatty acids are metabolised by cyclooxygenase into the prostanoids, prostaglandins and thromboxanes, and by 5-lipoxygenase into the leukotrienes. The n-6 fatty acid arachidonic acid is the major precursor for these substances in man and gives rise to the 2-series prostanoids (such as thromboxane A_2 and prostglandin E_2 and I_2) and the 4-series leukotrienes (leukotriene B_4, C_4 etc). Eicosapentaenoic acid is also metabolised by these enzymes into the 3-series prostanoids and 5-series leukotrienes. The balance of prostanoids is a major determinant of the haemostatic state with a reduced coagulative tendency following n-3 fatty acid supplementation. Leukotrienes are involved in regulating inflammatory responses. 5-series leukotrienes are less active and compete with those of the 4-series for binding sites resulting in anti-inflammatory effects (76,77,93–96).

Fish oil supplementation reduces production of the cytokines interleukin-1, interleukin-6 and tumour necrosis factor by mononuclear cells in normal volunteers and this effect is maintained for some weeks after stopping supplementation (97–99). Fish oil also increases the ratio of T suppressor to helper cells, decreases T cell proliferative response to mitogens, decreases delayed hypersensitivity skin response and reduces neutrophil chemotaxis (94,97,98,100).

Polyunsaturated fatty acids influence the activity of a number of receptors and enzymes which have a fundamental role in cellular signalling. When agonists stimulate receptors in the cell membrane they may activate adenylate cyclase or a phospholipase, the second messenger products of which (lipids in the case of phospholipases) influence the actions of cAMP-dependent protein kinase and protein kinase C respectively. It has been shown that n-3 fatty acids influence the effects of adenylate cyclase (57,101), phospholipase A_2 (102), cAMP-dependent protein kinase (103) and protein kinase C (103,104). Eicosapentaenoic acid also binds to membrane voltage-sensitive sodium channels and may alter the conductance of the channel (105), n-3 fatty acids bind to the cytoplasmic glucocorticoid receptor at a site different from the hormone binding site and markedly reduce its affinity for the hormone (106,107).

Peroxisome proliferator-activated receptor α is a gene transcription factor which induces the breakdown of leukotrienes and thus has a role in limiting the duration and extent of inflammation. A variety of polyunsaturated fatty acids including eicosapentaenoic acid and leukotrienes themselves appear to increase the activity of this factor (108,109).

These numerous effects can be seen to overlap in such a way that it is difficult to be sure of the relative role of each factor in any observed change. Early interest in effects on prostanoid metabolism has given way to an emphasis on actions on proinflammatory cytokines but it is likely that the two systems are interrelated and that both of these depend on effects at a molecular level.

Polyunsaturated Fatty Acids in Cancer

Early work using polyunsaturated fatty acids in *in vitro* studies of cancer demonstrated that eicosapentaenoic acid and other polyunsaturated fatty acids would kill or inhibit the growth of many malignant cell lines including those from human lung, breast, prostate (110), pancreatic (111), melanoma (112) and colorectal cancers (113). These effects were achieved at fatty acid concentrations of 10–300 μM. The mechanism for this action seems to be via cell cycle arrest and induction of apoptosis (114). The addition of inhibitors of prostaglandin synthesis inhibitors such as indomethacin had no effect on this cytotoxicity (113,115). However, the addition of the antioxidants vitamin E, superoxide dismutase or glutathione peroxidase and the saturated fatty acid oleic acid inhibited cell death while the prooxidants iron and copper enhanced it (111,115). This would suggest that the cytotoxicity of polyunsaturated fatty acids occurs via their peroxidation rather than any effect on eicosanoids. However, the levels of an indirect measure of lipid peroxidation have not been reliably associated with the degree of cell death suggesting that other factors may be involved (111).

These widespread cytotoxic effects *in vitro* led to much animal work, mostly using tumours implanted into immunocompromised mice. These studies suggested that the growth rates of transplanted human prostate (116), breast (117–122), colon (123,124) and lung (125,126) tumours could be slowed by the administration of eicosapentaenoic acid. Reduced rates of metastases have also been shown (121,127). Doses have varied from about 2 to 20 g eicosapentaenoic acid/kg body weight given with the diet, but most groups started the experimental diet before the implantation of tumours. Again the antitumour effects seem to be inhibited by antioxidants (118,119) and enhanced by iron (118,122).

Tisdale and coworkers (128) have studied a mouse colorectal tumour model in which the animals consistently lose weight with tumour progression. Despite experimental diets not being commenced until the subcutaneously implanted tumours were palpable, tumour growth rate was reduced and weight loss abolished with doses of about 2.5 g eicosapentaenoic acid/kg given with diet or by gavage (129–133). Similar attenuation of weight loss with eicosapentaenoic acid has also been shown in a mouse model using lung cancer cells transfected with interleukin-6 to produce cachexia (134).

Other studies have shown that eicosapentaenoic acid increases the resistance of cultured cells to transformation by radiation and transfection by the Harvey *ras* oncogene *in vitro* (135). Studies in rats administered carcinogens have shown that those fed higher proportions of fish oil containing eicosapentaenoic acid developed fewer tumours and had decreased expression of H-*ras* (in contrast to the findings for n-6 fatty acids) (136–138). Recent epidemiological studies have shown that increasing consumption of fish and fish oil correlates with a decreased risk of colorectal and breast cancer (139–141).

It is difficult to untangle the role of docosahexaenoic acid, the other common long chain n-3 fatty acid, in these findings. This is normally found in relatively high concentrations in the structural lipids of the brain and retina in humans (142). Most of the experiments described in this chapter were performed using mixtures of n-3 fatty acids containing both eicosapentaenoic acid and docosahexaenoic acids. Supplementation of docosahexaenoic acid alone in normal volunteers results in increased levels of both docosahexaenoic and eicosapentaenoic acids in plasma and platelet phospholipids but feeding of eicosapentaenoic acid does not result in any change in docosahexaenoic acid levels suggesting conversion in only one direction *in vivo* (143). In studies comparing the two, docosahexaenoic acid has had similar and in some cases superior effects in inhibiting the growth or killing of tumour cell lines *in vitro* (110,111,126), in reducing the growth rate of tumours and number of metastases in experimental tumours in mice (121) and in reducing the transformation of cultured cells by radiation and transfection (135).

Work on the antineoplastic activity of n-3 fatty acids is extending slowly into the human arena (144,145) but the main drive of our clinical research has been into the anticachectic effects of these agents.

Effects of Eicosapentaenoic Acid on Pancreatic Cancer Cachexia

As mentioned previously, there appears to be a metabolic block to the accretion of lean body mass in cachectic patients, in part attributable to enhanced proinflammatory cytokine release (Figure 1). Moreover, in healthy volunteers fish oil supplementation has been shown to down-regulate production of these cytokines (97).

To test whether supplementation with fish oil could affect the progress of cachexia in patients with advanced pancreatic cancer we conducted a study using Maxepa, a mixed marine triglyceride preparation containing 18%

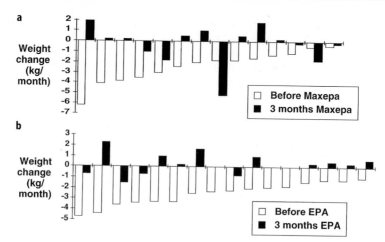

Figure 2. Weight change (kg/month) of patients with irresectable pancreatic carcinoma treated with **a** 12 g Maxepa (*n* = 14) or **b** 6 g EPA (*n* = 16) daily for 3 months.

eicosapentaenoic acid and 12% docosahexaenoic acid. This was given orally at a median dose of 12 g per day (equivalent to 2 g eicosapentaenoic acid per day) to 18 patients with irresectable pancreatic cancer. Before treatment all patients were losing weight at a median rate of 2.9 kg per month. Following 3 months supplementation patients had a median weight gain of 0.2 kg/month with less than half of the patients continuing to lose weight (Figure 2a). There was no change in the percentage of total body water over the time of the study. This regimen also produced a fall in the serum C-reactive protein level suggesting that some of the metabolic abnormalities of pancreatic cancer could be reversed, resulting in the stabilisation of weight (146).

Subsequently we have examined the role of eicosapentaenoic acid alone in reversing cachexia. Twenty-seven patients with irresectable pancreatic cancer were given 6 g per day of 95% pure eicosapentaenoic acid orally after a 4-week dose escalation period. Patients were losing a median of 2.0 kg per month at baseline. After 4 weeks, patients had a median weight gain of 0.75 kg and this effect remained at 3 months with a median weight gain of 0.25 kg per month (Figure 2b). Again there was no change in the percentage total body water over the course of the study confirming that the achievement of weight stability was not due to changes in hydration (147). There were no serious side effects in these studies and median survival was approximately 7 months. In these patients there was a down-regulation of interleukin-6 and tumour necrosis factor production by mononuclear cells and of the acute phase protein response (148,149).

Future Research

These apparently beneficial effects raise the question of the mechanism of action of eicosapentaenoic acid at the tissue, cell and molecular level. Our recent interest has concentrated on the effect of eicosapentaenoic acid on proinflammatory cytokines and the acute phase protein response in cachexia but effects on other potental mediators such as hormones, leptin and new lipolytic and proteolytic factors may eclipse this.

None of the patients in the above studies received any additional nutritional support and it may be that the supply of a nutritional supplement at the same time as fish oil might not only arrest the cachectic process but also reverse it. Also, if larger doses of eicosapentaenoic acid could be delivered it may be possible to reproduce some of the anticancer effects seen *in vitro* and in animal studies. Randomised, controlled studies are required to consolidate these anti-cachectic effects, confirm an effect on survival and reveal any unexpected side effects. Nevertheless, eicosapentaenoic acid would appear to be a well-tolerated, relatively cheap and effective anticachectic agent with the potential to lengthen survival and possibly to slow tumour growth in pancreatic cancer.

References

1. Rosewicz S, Weidenmann B (1997) Pancreatic carcinoma. Lancet 349:485–489.
2. Ahlgren JD (1996) Epidemiology and risk factors in pancreatic cancer. Semin Oncol 23:241–250.
3. Neoptolemos JP, Kerr DJ (1995) Adjuvant therapy for pancreatic cancer. Br J Surg 82:1012–1014.
4. Thomas PRM (1996) Radiotherapy for carcinoma of the pancreas. Semin Oncol 23:213–219.
5. Schnall SF, Macdonald JS. (1996) Chemotherapy of adenocarcinoma of the pancreas. Semin Oncol 23:220–228.
6. Casper ES, Green MR, Kelsen DP et al. (1994) Phase II trial of gemcitabine (2,2´-difluoro-deoxycytidine) in patients with adenocarcinoma of the pancreas. Invest New Drugs 12:29–34.
7. Rothenberg ML, Burris HA, Andersen JS et al. (1995) Gemcitabine: effective palliative therapy for pancreas cancer patients failing 5-FU. Proc Am Soc Clin Oncol 14:198.
8. Moore M, Andersen J, Burris H et al. (1995) A randomised trial of gemcitabine versus 5FU as first-line therapy in advanced pancreatic cancer. Proc Am Soc Clin Oncol 14:199.
9. Anonymous (1996) Biotech's uncertain present. Lancet 347:1497.
10. Carmichael J, Fink U, Russell RCG et al. (1996) Phase II study of gemcitabine in patients with advanced pancreatic cancer. Br J Cancer 73:101–105.
11. Warren S (1935) The immediate causes of death in cancer. Am J Med Sci 184:610–616.
12. DeWys WD, Begg C, Lavin PT et al. (1980) Prognostic effect of weight loss prior to chemo-therapy in cancer patients. Am J Med 69:491–497.
13. Oveson L, Hannibal J, Mortensen EL (1993) The interrelationship of weight loss, dietary intake, and quality of life in ambulatory patients with cancer of the lung, breast, and ovary. Nutr Cancer 19:159–167.
14. Wigmore SJ, Plester CE, Ross JA, Fearon KCH (1997) Contribution of anorexia and hyper-metabolism to weight loss in anicteric patients with pancreatic cancer. Br J Surg 84:196–197.
15. Fearon KCH, Carter DC (1988) Cancer cachexia. Ann Surg 208:1–5.
16. Grunfeld C, Feingold LH (1992) Metabolic disturbances and wasting in the acquired immuno-deficiency syndrome. N Engl J Med 327:329–337.
17. Roubenoff R, Roubenoff RA, Ward LM, Holland SM, Hellman DB (1992) Rheumatoid cachexia: Depletion of lean body mass in rheumatoid arthritis. Possible association with tumor necrosis factor. J Rheumatol 19:1505–1510.
18. Cangiano C, Laviano A, Muscaritoli M, Meguid MM, Cascino A, Fanelli FR (1996) Cancer anorexia: new pathogenic and therapeutic insights. Nutrition 12(Suppl) 1:S48–51.
19. Falconer JS, Fearon KCH, Plester CE, Ross JA, Carter DC (1994) Cytokines, the acute-phase response, and resting energy expenditure in cachectic patients with pancreatic cancer. Ann Surg 219:325–331.
20. Brennan MF (1977) Uncomplicated starvation versus cancer cachexia. Cancer Res 37:2359–2364.
21. Chlebowski RT, Heber D, Block JB (1982) Serial assessment of glucose metabolism in patients with cancer cachexia. Clin Res 30:69A.
22. Edén E, Edström S, Bennegård K, Scherstén T, Lundholm K (1984) Glucose flux in relation to energy expenditure in malnourished patients with and without cancer during periods of fasting and feeding. Cancer Res 44:1718–1724.

23. Holroyde CP, Skutches CL, Boden G, Reichard GA (1984) Glucose metabolism in cachectic patients with colorectal cancer. Cancer Res 44:5910–5913.
24. Shaw JHF, Wolfe RR (1987) Glucose and urea kinetics in patients with early and advanced gastrointestinal cancer: the response to glucose infusion, parenteral feeding, and surgical resection. Surgery 101:181–191.
25. Jeevanandam M, Horowitz GD, Lowry SF, Brennan MF (1986) Cancer cachexia and the rate of whole body lipolysis in man. Metabolism 35:304–310.
26. Vlassara H, Spiegel RJ, San Doval D, Cerami A (1986) Reduced plasma lipoprotein lipase activity in patients with malignancy-associated weight loss. Horm Metabol Res 18:698–703.
27. Fearon KCH, Hansell DT, Preston P et al. (1988) Influence of whole body protein turnover rate on resting energy expenditure in patients with cancer. Cancer Res 48:2590–2595.
28. Melville S, McNurlan MA, Calder AG, Garlick PJ (1990) Increased protein turnover despite normal energy metabolism and responses to feeding in patients with lung cancer. Cancer Res 50:1125–1131.
29. Falconer JS, Fearon KCH, Ross JA et al. (1995) Acute-phase protein response and survival duration of patients with pancreatic cancer. Cancer 75:2077–2082.
30. Baumann H, Gauldie J (1994) The acute phase response. Immunol Today 15:74–80.
31. Reeds PJ, Fjeld CR, Jahoor F (1994) Do the differences between the amino acid compositions of acute-phase and muscle proteins have a bearing on nitrogen loss in traumatic states? J Nutr 124:906–910.
32. Michie HR, Spriggs DR, Manogue KR et al. (1988) Tumor necrosis factor and endotoxin induce similar metabolic responses in human beings. Surgery 104:280–286.
33. Starnes HF, Warren RS, Jeevanandam M et al. (1988) Tumor necrosis factor and the acute metabolic response to tissue injury in man. J Clin Invest 82:1321–1325.
34. Strassmann G, Fong M, Kenney JS, Jacob CO (1992) Evidence for the involvement of interleukin 6 in experimental cancer cachexia. J Clin Invest 89:1681–1684.
35. Hellerstein MK, Meydani SN, Meydani M, Wu K, Dinarello CA (1989) Interleukin-1-induced anorexia in the rat. Influence of prostaglandins. J Clin Invest 84:228–235.
36. Espat NJ, Auffenberg T, Rosenberg JJ et al. (1996) Ciliary neurotrophic factor is catabolic and shares with IL-6 the capacity to induce an acute phase response. Am J Physiol 271:R185–R190.
37. Aderka D, Engelmann H, Hornik V et al. (1991) Increased serum levels of soluble receptors for tumor necrosis factor in cancer patients. Cancer Res 51:5602–5607.
38. Knapp ML, Al-Sheibani S, Riches PG, Hanham IWF, Phillips RH (1991) Hormonal factors associated with weight loss in patients with advanced breast cancer. Ann Clin Biochem 28:480–486.
39. Kurzrock R, Redman J, Cabanillas F, Jones D, Rothberg J, Talpaz M (1993) Serum interleukin-6 levels are elevated in lymphoma patients and correlate with survival in advanced Hodgkin's disease and with B symptoms. Cancer Res 53:2118–2122.
40. Preston T, Fearon KCH, McMillian DC et al. (1995) Effect of ibuprofen on the acute-phase response and protein metabolism in patients with cancer and weight loss. Br J Surg 82:229–234.
41. Staal-van den Brekel AJ, Dentener MA, Schols AMWJ, Buurman WA, Wouters EFM (1995) Increased resting energy expenditure and weight loss are related to a systemic inflammatory response in lung cancer patients. J Clin Oncol 13:2600–2605.
42. Mahoney SM, Beck SA, Tisdale MJ (1988) Comparison of weight loss induced by recombinant tumour necrosis factor with that produced by a cachexia-inducing tumour. Br J Cancer 57:385–389.
43. Langstein HN, Norton JA (1991) Mechanisms of cancer cachexia. Hematol Oncol Clin North Am 5:103–123.
44. McNamara MJ, Alexander HR, Norton JA (1992) Cytokines and their role in the pathophysiology of cancer cachexia. JPEN J Parenter Enteral Nutr 16(Suppl):50S–55S.
45. Aderka D, Fisher S, Levo Y, Holtmann H, Hahn T, Wallach D (1985) Cachectin/tumour-necrosis-factor production by cancer patients. Lancet II:1190.
46. Heinrich PC, Castell JV, Andus T (1990) Interleukin-6 and the acute phase response. Biochem J 265:621–636.
47. Oldenburg HSA, Rogy MA, Lazarus DD et al. (1993) Cachexia and the acute-phase protein response in inflammation are regulated by interleukin-6. Eur J Immunol 23:1889–1894.
48. O'Riordain MG, Ross JA, Fearon KCH (1995) Insulin and counterregulatory hormones influence acute-phase protein production in human hepatocytes. Am J Physiol 269:E323–E330.
49. Gullo L, Ancona D, Pezzilli R, Casadei R, Campione O (1993) Glucose tolerance and insulin secretion in pancreatic cancer. Ital J Gastroenterol 25:487–489.

50. Schwartz SS, Zeidler A, Moosa AR, Kuku SF, Rubenstein AH (1978) A prospective study of glucose tolerance, insulin, C-peptide, and glucagon responses in patients with pancreatic carcinoma. Dig Dis 23:1107–1114.
51. Fox JN, Frier BM, Armitage M, Ashby JP (1985) Abnormal insulin secretion in carcinoma of the pancreas: response to glucagon stimulation. Diabetic Med 2:113–116.
52. Cersosimo E, Pisters PWT, Pesola G, McDermott K, Bajorunas D, Brennan MF (1991) Insulin secretion and action in patients with pancreatic cancer. Cancer 67:486–493.
53. Schaur RJ, Fellier H, Gleispach H, Fink E, Kronberger L (1979) Tumor host relations. I. Increased plasma cortisol in tumor-bearing humans compared with patients with benign surgical disease. J Cancer Res Clin Oncol 93:281–285.
54. Burt ME, Aoki TT, Gorschboth CM, Brennan MF (1983) Peripheral tissue metabolism in cancer-bearing man. Ann Surg 198:685–691.
55. Bessey PQ, Watters JM, Aoki TT, Wilmore DW (1984) Combined hormonal infusion simulates the metabolic response to injury. Ann Surg 200:264–281.
56. Watters JM, Bessey PQ, Dinarello CA, Wolff SM, Wilmore DW (1986) Both inflammatory and endocrine mediators stimulate host responses to sepsis. Arch Surg 121:179–190.
57. Tisdale MJ (1993) Mechanism of lipid mobilisation associated with cancer cachexia: interaction between the polyunsaturated fatty acid, eicosapentaenoic acid, and inhibitory guanine nucleotide-regulatory protein. Prostaglandins Leukot Essent Fatty Acids 48:105–109.
58. McDevitt TM, Todorov PT, Beck SA, Khan SH, Tisdale MJ (1995) Purification and characterisation of a lipid-mobilising factor associated with cachexia-inducing tumors in mice and humans. Cancer Res 55:1458–1463.
59. Todorov P, Cariuk P, McDevitt T, Coles B, Fearon K, Tisdale M (1996) Characterisation of a cancer cachectic factor. Nature 379:739–742.
60. Grunfeld C, Zhao C, Fuller J, Pollock A, Moser A, Freidman J, Feingold KR (1996) Endotoxin and cytokines induce expression of leptin, the ob gene product, in hamsters. A role for leptin in the anorexia of infection. J Clin Invest 97:2152–2157.
61. Schwarz M (1997) Proc Nutr Soc (in press).
62. Nixon DW, Lawson DH, Kutner M et al. (1981) Hyperalimentation of the cancer patient with protein-calorie undernutrition. Cancer Res 41:2038–2045.
63. Cohn SH, Vartsky D, Vaswani AN et al. (1982) Changes in body composition of cancer patients following combined nutritional support. Nutr Cancer 4:107–119.
64. Evans WK, Makuch R, Clamon GH et al. (1985) Limited impact of total parenteral nutrition on nutritional status during treatment for small cell lung cancer. Cancer Res 45:3347–3353.
65. Klein S, Simes J, Blackburn GL (1986) Total parenteral nutrition and cancer clinical trials. Cancer 58:1378–1386.
66. Lipman TO (1991) Clinical trials of nutritional support in cancer. Parenteral and enteral therapy. Hematol Oncol Clin North Am 5:91–102.
67. Ng E-H, Lowry SF (1991) Nutritional support and cancer cachexia. Evolving concepts of mechanisms and adjunctive therapies. Hematol Oncol Clin North Am 5:161–184.
68. Oveson L, Allingstrup L, Hannibal J, Mortensen EL, Hansen OP (1993) Effect of dietary counseling on food intake, body weight, response rate, survival, and quality of life in cancer patients undergoing chemotherapy: a prospective, randomised study. J Clin Oncol 11:2043–2049.
69. Chlebowski RT, Bulcavage L, Grosvenor M et al. (1987) Hydrazine sulphate in cancer patients with weight loss. A placebo-controlled clinical experience. Cancer 59:406–410.
70. McMillan DN, Simpson JM, Preston T et al. (1994) Effect of megestrol acetate on weight loss, body composition and blood screen of gastrointestinal cancer patients. Clin Nutr 13:85–89.
71. Nelson KA, Walsh D, Sheehan FA (1994) The cancer anorexia-cachexia syndrome. J Clin Oncol 12:213–225.
72. Gebbia V, Testa A, Gebbia N (1996) Prospective randomised trial of two dose levels of megestrol acetate in the management of anorexia-cachexia syndrome in patients with metastatic cancer. Br J Cancer 73:1576–1580.
73. Simons JPFHA, Aaronson NK, Vansteenkiste JF et al. (1996) Effects of medroxyprogesterone acetate on appetite, weight, and quality of life in advanced-stage non-hormone-sensitive cancer: A placebo-controlled multicenter study. J Clin Oncol 14:1077–1084.
74. Beck SA, Tisdale MJ (1989) Effect of insulin on weight loss and tumour growth in a cachexia model. Br J Cancer 59:677–681.
75. Beck SA, Tisdale MJ (1990) Effect of megestrol acetate on weight loss induced by tumour necrosis factor α and a cachexia-inducing tumour (MAC16) in NMRI mice. Br J Cancer 62:420–424.
76. Leaf A, Weber PC (1988) Cardiovascular effects of n-3 fatty acids. N Engl J Med 318:549–557.

77. Nordøy A, Dyerberg J (1989) n-3 fatty acids in health and disease. J Intern Med 225(Suppl 1):1–3.
78. Neilsen NH, Hansen JPH (1980) Breast cancer in Greenland: selected epidemiological, clinical, and histological features. J Cancer Res Clin Oncol 98:287–299.
79. Anonymous (1983) Eskimo diets and diseases. Lancet I:1139–1141.
80. Dyerberg J, Bang HO, Hjørne N (1975) Fatty acid composition of the plasma lipids in Greenland Eskimos. Am J Clin Nutr 28:958–966.
81. Bang HO, Dyerberg J, Hjørne N (1976) The composition of food consumed by Greenland Eskimos. Acta Med Scand 200:69–73.
82. Bull NL, Day MJL, Burt R, Buss DH (1983) Individual fatty acids in the British household food supply. Hum Nutr: Appl Nutr 37A:373–377.
83. Lorenz R, Weber PC, Szimnau P, Heldwein W, Strasser T, Loeschke K (1989) Supplementation with n-3 fatty acids from fish oil in chronic inflammatory bowel disease: a randomised, placebo-controlled, double-blind, cross-over trial. J Intern Med 225(Suppl 1):225–232.
84. Belluzzi A, Brignola C, Campieri M, Pera A, Boschi S, Miglioli M (1996) Effect of an enteric-coated fish-oil preparation on relapses in Crohn's disease. N Engl J Med 334:1557–1560.
85. Lau CS, Morley KD, Belch JJF (1993) Effects of fish oil supplementation on non-steroidal anti-inflammatory drug requirement in patients with mild rheumatoid arthritis: a double-blind placebo controlled study. Br J Rheumatol 32:982–989.
86. Arm JP, Horton CE, Eiser NM, Clark TJH, Lee TH (1988) The effects of dietary supplementation with fish oil on asthmatic responses to antigen. J Allergy Clin Immunol 81:183.
87. Bjørneboe A, Søyland E, Bjørneboe G-EA, Rajka G, Drevon CA (1989) Effects of n-3 fatty acid supplement to patients with atopic dermatitis. J Intern Med 225(Suppl 1):233–236.
88. Bittiner SB, Tucker WFG, Cartwright I, Bleehen SS (1988) A double-blind randomised, placebo-controlled trial of fish oil in psoriasis. Lancet I:378–380.
89. Johnson JA, Griswold JA, Muakkassa FF (1993) Essential fatty acids influence survival in sepsis. J Trauma 35:128–131.
90. Kenler AS, Swails WS, Driscoll DF et al. (1996) Early enteral feeding in postsurgical cancer patients. Fish oil structured lipid-based polymeric formula versus a standard polymeric formula. Ann Surg 223:316–333.
91. van der Heide JJH, Bilo HJG, Donker JM, Wilmink JM, Tegzess AM (1993) Effect of dietary fish oil on renal function and rejection in cyclosporine-treated recipients of renal transplants. N Engl J Med 329:769–773.
92. Laugharne JD, Mellor JE, Peet M (1996) Fatty acids and schizophrenia. Lipids 31 (Suppl): S163–S165.
93. Fischer S, Weber PC. Thromboxane A$_3$ (TXA$_3$) is formed in human platelets after dietary eicosapentaenoic acid (C20:5ω3) (1983) Biochem Biophys Res Commun 116:1091–1099.
94. Lee TH, Hoover RL, Williams JD et al. (1985) Effect of dietary enrichment with eicosa-pentaenoic and docosahexaenoic acids on in vitro neutrophil and monocyte leukotriene gener-ation and neutrophil function. N Engl J Med 312:1217–1224.
95. Fitzgerald GA, Braden G, Fitzgerald DJ, Knapp HR (1989) Fish oils in cardiovascular disease. J Intern Med 225 Suppl 1:25–29.
96. Schmitt EB, Dyerberg J (1989) n-3 fatty acids and leukocytes. J Intern Med 225 (Suppl 1):151–158.
97. Endres S, Ghorbani R, Kelley VE et al. (1989) The effect of dietary supplementation with n-3 polyunsaturated fatty acids on the synthesis of interleukin-1 and tumor necrosis factor by mononuclear cells. N Engl J Med 320:265–271.
98. Meydani SN, Lichtenstein AH, Cornwall S et al. (1993) Immunological effects of National Cholesterol Education Panel Step-2 diets with and without fish-derived n-3 fatty acid enrichment. J Clin Invest 92:105–113.
99. Cooper AL, Gibbons L, Horan MA, Little RA, Rothwell NJ (1993) Effect of dietary fish oil supplementation on fever and cytokine production in human volunteers. Clin Nutr 12:321–328.
100. Calder PC (1996) Immunomodulatory and anti-inflammatory effects of n-3 polyunsaturated fatty acids. Proc Nutr Soc 55:737–774.
101. Alam SQ, Ren Y-F, Alam BS (1988) (^{3}H)forskolin- and (^{3}H)dihydroalprenolol-binding sites and adenylate cyclase activity in heart of rats fed diets containing different oils. Lipids 23:207–213.
102. Ballou LR, Cheung WY (1985) Inhibition of human platelet phospholipase A$_2$ activity by unsaturated fatty acids. Proc Natl Acad Sci USA 82:371–375.
103. Speizer LA, Watson MJ, Brunton LL (1991) Differential effects of omega-3 fish oils on protein kinase activities in vitro. Am J Physiol 261:E109–E114.

104. Holian O, Nelson R (1992) Action of long-chain fatty acids on protein kinase C activity: comparison of omega-6 and omega-3 fatty acids. Anticancer Res 12:975–980.

105. Kang JX, Leaf A (1996) Evidence that free polyunsaturated fatty acids modify Na+ channels by directly binding to the channel proteins. Proc Natl Acad Sci USA 93:3542–3546.

106. Vallette G, Vanet A, Sumida C, Nunez EA (1991) Modulatory effects of unsaturated fatty acids on the binding of glucocorticoids to rat liver glucocorticoid receptors. Endocrinology 129:1363–1369.

107. Sumida C, Vallette G, Nunez EA (1993) Interaction of unsaturated fatty acids with rat liver glucocorticoid receptors: studies to localise the site of interaction. Acta Endocrinol 129:348–355.

108. Keller H, Dreyer C, Medin J, Mahfoudi A, Ozato K, Wahli W (1993) Fatty acids and retinoids control lipid metabolism through activation of peroxisome proliferator-activated receptor-retinoid X receptor heterodimers. Proc Natl Acad Sci USA 90:2160–2164.

109. Devchand PR, Keller H, Peters JM, Vazquez M, Gonzalez FJ, Wahli W (1996) The PPARα-leukotriene B4 pathway to inflammation control. Nature 384:39–43.

110. Bégin ME, Ells G, Das UN, Horrobin DF (1986) Differential killing of human carcinoma cells supplemented with n-3 and n-6 polyunsaturated fatty acids. J Natl Cancer Inst 77:1053–1062.

111. Falconer JS, Ross JA, Fearon KCH, Hawkins RA, O'Riordain MG, Carter DC (1994) Effect of eicosapentaenoic acid and other fatty acids on the growth in vitro of human pancreatic cancer cell lines. Br J Cancer 69:826–832.

112. McMillan DN, Murray A, Noble BS, Purasiri P, Heys SD, Eremin O (1994) Differential responses of human solid tumour cells in vitro to essential fatty acids. Eur J Surg Oncol 20:104–105.

113. Mengeaud V, Nano JL, Fournel S, Rampal P (1992) Effects of eicosapentaenoic acid, gamma-linolenic acid and prostaglandin E1 on three human colon carcinoma cell lines. Prostaglandins Leukot Essent Fatty Acids 47:313–319.

114. Lai PBS, Ross JA, Fearon KCH, Anderson JD, Carter DC (1996) Cell cycle arrest and induction of apoptosis in pancreatic cancer cells exposed to eicosapentaenoic acid in vitro. Br J Cancer 74:1375–1383.

115. Bégin ME, Ells G, Horrobin DF (1988) Polyunsaturated fatty acid-induced cytotoxicity against tumour cells and its relationship to lipid peroxidation. J Natl Cancer Inst 80:188–194.

116. Karmali RA, Reichel P, Cohen LA, Terano T, Hirai A, Tamura Y, Yoshida S (1987) The effects of dietary w-3 fatty acids on the DU-145 transplantable human prostatic tumor. Anticancer Res 7:1173–1180.

117. Pritchard GA, Jones DL, Mansel RE (1989) Lipids in breast carcinogenesis. Br J Surg 76:1069–1073.

118. Gonzalez MJ, Schemmel RA, Gray JI, Dugan L, Sheffield LG, Welsch CW (1991) Effect of dietary fat on growth of MCF-7 and MDA-MB231 human breast carcinomas in athymic nude mice: relationship between carcinoma growth and lipid peroxidation product levels. Carcinogenesis 12:1231–1235.

119. Gonzalez MJ, Schemmel RA, Dugan L, Gray JI, Welsch CW (1993) Dietary fish oil inhibits human breast carcinoma growth: a function of increased lipid peroxidation. Lipids 28:827–832.

120. Rose DP, Connolly JM (1993) Effects of dietary omega-3 fatty acids on human breast cancer growth and metastases in nude mice. J Natl Cancer Inst 85:1743–1747.

121. Rose DP, Connolly JM, Rayburn J, Coleman M (1995) Influence of diets containing eicosa-pentaenoic or docosahexaenoic acid on growth and metastasis of breast cancer cells in nude mice. J Natl Cancer Inst 87:587–592.

122. Hardman WE, Barnes CJ, Grant W, Knight CW, Cameron IL (1995) A high fish oil diet sup-plemented with ferric citrate safely inhibits primary and metastatic human breast carcinoma growth in nude mice. Proc Am Assoc Cancer Res 36:114.

123. Sakaguchi M, Imray C, Davis A et al. (1990) Effects of dietary n-3 and saturated fats on growth rates of the human colonic cancer cell lines SW-620 and LS 174T in vivo in relation to tissue and plasma lipids. Anticancer Res 10:1763–1768.

124. Sakaguchi M, Rowley S, Kane N et al. (1990) Reduced tumour growth of the human colonic cancer cell lines COLO-320 and HT-29 in vivo by dietary n-3 lipids. Br J Cancer 62:742–747.

125. de Bravo MG, de Antueno RJ, Toledo J, De Tomás ME, Mercuri OF, Quintans C (1991) Effects of an eicosapentaenoic and docosahexaenoic acid concentrate on a human lung carcinoma grown in nude mice. Lipids 26:866–870.

126. Mæhle L, Eilertsen E, Mollerup S, Schønberg S, Krokan HE, Haugaen A (1995) Effects of n-3 fatty acids during neoplastic progression and comparison of in vitro and in vivo sensitivity of two human tumour cell lines. Br J Cancer 71:691–696.

127. Connolly JM, Rose DP (1996) Suppression of human breast cancer metastases by dietary eicosapentaenoic acid fed as neoadjuvant therapy to nude mice. Proc Am Assoc Cancer Res 37:71.

128. Bibby MC, Double JA, Ali SA, Fearon KCH, Brennan RA, Tisdale MJ (1987) Characterisation of a transplantable adenocarcinoma of the mouse colon producing cachexia in recipient animals. J Natl Cancer Inst 78:539–546.

129. Tisdale MJ, Dhesi JK (1990) Inhibition of weight loss by w-3 fatty acids in an experimental cachexia model. Cancer Res 50:5022–5026.

130. Tisdale MJ, Beck SA (1991) Inhibition of tumour-induced lipolysis *in vitro* and cachexia and tumour growth *in vivo* by eicosapentaenoic acid. Biochem Pharmacol 41:103–107.

131. Beck SA, Smith KL, Tisdale MJ (1991) Anticachectic and antitumour effect of eicosapentaenoic acid and its effect on protein turnover. Cancer Res 51:6089–6093.

132. Hudson EA, Beck SA, Tisdale MJ (1993) Kinetics of the inhibition of tumour growth in mice by eicosapentaenoic acid-reversal by linoleic acid. Biochem Pharmachol 45:2189–2194.

133. Hudson EA, Tisdale MJ (1994) Comparison of the effectiveness of eicosapentaenoic acid administered as either the free acid or ethyl ester as an anticachectic and antitumour agent. Prostaglandins Leukot Essent Fatty Acids 51:141–145.

134. Ohira T, Nishio K, Ohe Y et al. (1996) Improvement by eicosanoids in cancer cachexia induced by LLC-IL6 transplantation. Cancer Res Clin Oncol 122:711–715.

135. Takahashi M, Przetakiewicz M, Ong A, Borek C, Lowenstein JM (1992) Effect of ω3 and ω6 fatty acids on transformation of cultured cells by irradiation and transfection. Cancer Res 52:154–162.

136. Abou-El-Ela SH, Prasse KW, Carroll R, Wade AE, Dharwadkar S, Bunce OR (1988) Eicosanoid synthesis in 7,12-dimethylbenz(a)anthracene-induced mammary carcinomas in Sprague-Dawley rats fed primrose oil, menhaden oil or corn oil diet. Lipids 23:948–954.

137. Reddy BS, Sugie S (1988) Effect of different levels of omega-3 and omega-6 fatty acids on azoxymethane-induced colon carcinogenesis in F344 rats. Cancer Res 48:6642–6647.

138. Karmali RA, Chao C-C, Basu A, Modak M (1989) II. Effect of n-3 and n-6 fatty acids on mammary H-*ras* expression and PGE_2 levels in DMBA-treated rats. Anticancer Res 9:1169–1174.

139. Kaizer L, Boyd NF, Kriukov V, Trichler D (1989) Fish consumption and breast cancer risk: An ecological study. Nutr Cancer 12:61–68.

140. Sasaki S, Horacsek M, Kesteloot H (1993) An ecological study of the relationship between dietary fat intake and breast cancer mortality. Prev Med 22:187–202.

141. Caygill CPJ, Charlett A, Hill MJ (1996) Fat, fish, fish oil and cancer. Br J Cancer 74:159–164.

142. Sardesai VM (1992) The essential fatty acids. Nutr Clin Pract 7:179–186.

143. von Schacky C, Weber PC (1985) Metabolism and effects on platelet function of the purified eicosapentaenoic and docosahexaenoic acids in humans. J Clin Invest 76:2446–2450.

144. Holroyde CP, Skutches CL, Reichard GA (1988) Effects of dietary enrichment with n-3 poly-unsaturated fatty acids in metastatic breast cancer. Proc Am Soc Clin Oncol 7:42.

145. Anti M, Armelao F, Marra G et al. (1994) Effects of different doses of fish oil on rectal cell proliferation in patients with sporadic colonic adenomas. Gastroenterol 107:1709–1718.

146. Wigmore SJ, Ross JA, Falconer JS et al. (1996) The effect of polyunsaturated fatty acids on the progress of cachexia in patients with pancreatic cancer. Nutrition 12(Suppl):S27–S30.

147. Wigmore SJ, Ross JA, Barber MD, Fearon KCH (1997) Phase II trial of high purity eicosa-pentaenoic acid in patients with pancreatic cancer cachexia. Proc Nutr Soc (in press).

148. Wigmore SJ, Fearon KCH, Ross JA, Carter DC (1996) Eicosapentaenoic acid, cytokines and the acute-phase protein response in pancreatic cancer. Br J Surg 83:1649–1650.

149. Wigmore SJ, Fearon KCH, Maingay JP, Ross JA (1997) Down-regulation of the acute-phase response in patients with pancreatic cancer cachexia receiving oral eicosapentaenoic acid is mediated via suppression of interleukin-6. Clin Sci 92:215–221.

30 Anticancer Effects of Essential Fatty Acids

D. Ravichandran and C.D. Johnson

Essential fatty acids (EFAs) consist of two groups of fatty acids (n-6 or omega-6, derived from linoleic acid (LA) and n-3 or omega-3, derived from alpha-linolenic acid (LNA)) that cannot be synthesised *de novo*, and thus must be supplied in the diet. Once supplied, these fatty acids can be elongated and/or desaturated to produce other fatty acids within that omega family (Figure 1). EFAs are important structural constituents of all cellular membranes. Changes in plasma membrane fatty acid composition can affect the fluidity of the membrane and ion or substrate transport into the cells, the activity of membrane-associated enzymes and the functioning of receptors and/or signal transduction processes. EFAs are also the precursors of eicosanoids: prostaglandins, leukotrienes and thromboxanes; and are necessary to maintain the impermeability barrier of the skin and for cholesterol transport and metabolism.

Anticancer Effect of Essential Fatty Acids

EFAs have a wide range of anticancer effects which include a direct growth inhibitory effect on malignant cells and an antimetastatic effect. These are discussed in detail below. In addition they can modify the membrane characteristics of malignant cells to make concurrent chemotherapy more effective (1,2). With regard to an antitumour effect the most important fatty acids are gamma linolenic acid (GLA), an 18 carbon fatty acid with three double bonds of the n-6 family and eicosapentaenoic acid (EPA), a 20 carbon fatty acid of the n-3 family with five double bonds. GLA is present in various seed oils such as that of evening primrose (EPO). Marine animals such as fish are a rich source of EPA and docosahexaenoic acid (DHA).

Effect of EFAs on Tumour Growth

In Vitro Studies

Fatty acids of both EFA groups have a direct cytotoxic (at high concentrations) or growth inhibitory effect (at low concentrations) on malignant cells. In general, fatty acids with three, four or five double bonds, such as GLA and EPA

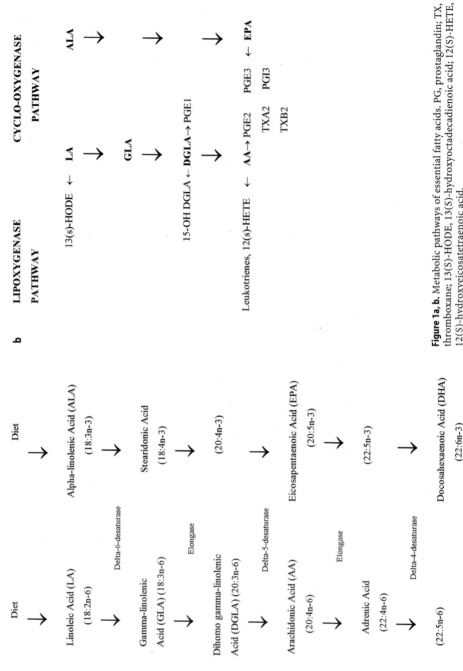

Figure 1a, b. Metabolic pathways of essential fatty acids. PG, prostaglandin; TX, thromboxane; 13(S)-HODE, 13(S)-hydroxyoctadecadienoic acid; 12(S)-HETE, 12(S)-hydroxyeicosatetraenoic acid.

demonstrate best cytotoxicity. This effect is not organ or tissue specific as a variety of malignant cells of both epithelial and non-epithelial origin are susceptible. The effect is concentration dependent and the critical concentration varies between cell types. It is also time dependent and relatively long exposure to the fatty acid (5–7 days) is necessary for growth inhibition at lower concentrations. The sensitivity varies with the degree of differentiation of the tumour, poorly differentiated cell lines responding more slowly than more differentiated cell lines (3). Conventional anticancer drug resistance mechanisms have little influence on the effect of fatty acids; in fact multidrug-resistant variants appear more sensitive than the corresponding non-resistant cells (4). The effect also has a degree of selectivity towards malignant cells. At concentrations that are cytotoxic or severely growth inhibitory to malignant cells, the corresponding non-malignant cells are largely unaffected (5,6). GLA demonstrates good selectivity, EPA is somewhat less selective (7). In addition, tumorigenic cells are more sensitive than the non-tumorigenic cells (8,9).

The antitumour effect is related to modification of the membrane fatty acid composition of the cells (10) and appears to be due to increased free radical production in cancer cells as a result of increased lipid peroxidation (11,12).

Animal Studies

In general EFAs such as EPA and GLA have shown tumour growth inhibitory properties although some EFAs such as LA appear to have tumour-promoting activity. Most studies have used the oil of evening primrose (EPO) as the source of GLA and fish oil as the source of n-3 fatty acids. EPO given parenterally or orally inhibited breast (13–15) and lung cancer (16) growth in rodents. Intraperitoneal injection in malignant ascites was associated with increased survival (17,18). Intra-arterial therapy with GLA (in lipoidol) was effective in a rabbit liver cancer model (19). Others found it difficult to reproduce the *in vitro* growth inhibitory effect in animal models using the same cell lines which were sensitive *in vitro* (20–22).

Fish oil therapy has been associated with the inhibition of growth of a variety of tumours and the effect has been more consistent than with EPO. These include human colonic carcinoma in nude mice (23,24) and breast cancer in a variety of animal models (15,25–28). Prolongation of the DNA replication time (S phase) was seen in fish oil-mediated mammary tumour growth inhibition (29), although the mechanism of this phenomenon remains unclear. Oral EPA and DHA inhibited the growth of human lung and breast carcinomas in mice (30,31). Fish oil inhibited the growth of human prostate tumours in nude mice in comparison with corn oil fed animals, but was ineffective when the tumour burden was increased (32,33).

In summary, EFAs are uniformly and selectively growth inhibitory when added to malignant cells in culture. They also inhibit tumour growth *in vivo*, n-3 EFAs more consistently than n-6.

Human Studies

The number of human studies where fatty acids have been used as anticancer agents is small and the results are variable. In a randomised trial in Dukes' C colorectal carcinoma (34), EPO therapy following surgical resection did not influence survival, but the dose of EPO (3 g/day providing 270 mg GLA) was low. In patients with a variety of malignant tumours, EPO (9–18 grams daily = GLA 810–1620 mg) resulted in clinical improvement and increased survival, especially in hepatocellular cancer (35). However, a subsequent double-blind placebo-controlled trial in primary liver cancer (36) failed to confirm this benefit. Using a different approach, 15 patients with cerebral glioma, a highly malignant CNS tumour, were treated by infusing GLA in the tumour bed following surgical excision (37). Twelve patients remained without obvious recurrence after 16–20 months which was unusual for their tumour grade of III or IV. No toxicity was seen.

In one study with n-3 fatty acids, one partial response was obtained in 12 patients with advanced breast cancer with fish oil therapy (38).

Effect of EFAs on Tumour Metastasis

Tumour metastasis is a complex multistep process. The initial step of detachment and motility follows impaired cell to cell and cell to matrix adhesion. Invasion is facilitated by tissue degradation by enzymes which is accompanied by migration of tumour cells into areas modified by proteolysis. Cell adhesion molecules that are involved in cell–cell and cell–matrix adhesions such as cadherins, catenins and intergrins, proteolytic enzymes including collagenase, other matrix metalloproteinases (MMP) and plasminogen activators play an important part in these events.

EPA treatment *in vitro* reduced the invasiveness of malignant cells and the production of collagenase, and reduced the number of lung metastases produced in mice on iv injection (39). The activity of urokinase, a plasminogen activator, was inhibited by GLA and EPA *in vitro* (40). Prostaglandin E1 derived from DGLA, an immediate metabolite of GLA, appears to inhibit the expression of MMPs (41). GLA increases the E-cadherin and alpha-catenin expression of a variety of human malignant cells *in vitro* (42–43). In contrast to the effect on E-cadherin, hepatocyte growth factor or scatter factor (HGF/SF) is a potent stimulus for tumour cell motility and invasion, and GLA inhibited the HGF/SF stimulated colon cancer cell colony scattering, cell dissociation and invasion in another *in vitro* study (44). GLA also inhibited the invasion potential of a breast cancer cell line *in vitro* although no antimetastatic effect was seen in mice with as diet containing 8% GLA (45).

During the haematogenous phase of the metastatic process, adhesion of tumour cells to the endothelium and subendothelial matrix is a critical event. 12 (s)-Hydroxyeicosatetraenoic acid, 13 (s)-HETE) and 13(s)-hydroxyocadecadienoic acid (13(S)-HODE) are the 12-lipoxygenase and 15-lipoxygenase metabolites of AA and LA respectively (Figure 1). 12(S)-HETE enhances the process of endothelial adhesion while 13(S)-HODE blocks this (46). The balance between the effects of these molecules appears to have an important regulatory effect on the metastatic ability of the cells. One metabolite of GLA, 15-OH-DGLA, is an inhibitor of 12-lipoxygenase activity (47). Inhibition of thromboxane A2 (TXA2) production (which has potent vasoconstricting and platelet aggregatory effect) by EPA and DGLA, and inhibition of angiogenesis by n-3 fatty acids (48) may also contribute towards an antimetastatic effect.

In animal studies corn oil, rich in LA, appears to promote metastasis compared with diets rich in GLA and EPA (30,49). In experimental metastasis models where cancer cells were injected IV, fewer lung metastases were seen with melanoma and breast carcinoma in rodents fed fish oil compared with those fed corn oil (50,51) and with a high alpha-linolenate diet in mice challenged with Yoshida ascites tumour cells (52). Others found that both n-6 and n-3 fatty acids had no influence on the spontaneous metastasis of a rat mammary adenocarcinoma (51,53). In fact, in the study by Adams et al. (51) the group of rats fed a high fish oil diet (20.5%) developed more spontaneous lung metastases than a high corn oil diet group. In humans a low n-6 fatty acid content of breast cancer tissue is associated with a high probability of early metastasis after adjusting for other factors such as histological grade and size (54).

Thus, in summary, EFAs appear to exert a complex effect on tumour metastasis. While GLA and to a lesser extent EPA have shown consistent antimetastatic properties *in vitro*, the results of animal studies have been variable. LA-rich diets enhance metastasis in animal models. Further studies are needed before fatty acids can be considered for use as antimetastatic agents in human cancer.

EFAs as Antitumour Agents in Human Pancreatic Carcinoma

In Vitro Studies

In line with previous studies, EFAs are also growth inhibitory to human pancreatic cancer cell lines *in vitro* (55). In our studies we used the lithium salt of GLA (LiGLA) which is the compound used in animal and clinical studies of pancreatic carcinoma. LiGLA is a water soluble, injectable and relatively pure and stable form of this fatty acid. LiGLA represents a major advance over using EPO as the source of GLA. Two pancreatic cancer cell lines (MIA PaCa2 and Panc 1) were incubated in the presence of this fatty acid for 7 days and the number of live cells at the end of this period was assessed by methyltetrazolium (MTT) assay (56). Human non-malignant fibroblasts were used as control. LiGLA had a dose-dependent growth inhibitory effect on both cancer cell lines (Figure 2). Fifty per cent growth inhibition (IC50) of both cancer cell lines was seen at 10–13 μmol/l. By contrast the growth of fibroblasts was inhibited only at relatively high concentrations (IC50 = 110.8 μmol/l) in keeping with the selectivity noted in other studies. Time course studies showed that the degree of growth inhibition increased with the time of exposure to LiGLA, reaching a maximum after 5–7 days. A lithium effect and non-specific fatty acid effects were excluded by control experiments.

Nude Mice Studies

We have done a series of experiments to study the effect of parenterally administered LiGLA on the growth of human pancreatic carcinoma in nude mice. These studies differ from many previous animal studies in the form of fatty acid used (lithium salt), the route of administration (parenteral as opposed to oral) and,

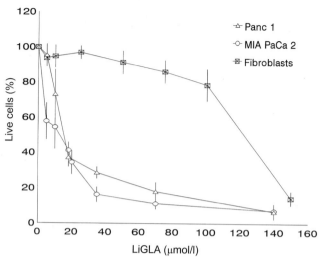

Figure 2. The effect of increasing concentration of the lithium salt of gamma linolenic acid (LiGLA) on the growth of MIA PaCa2 and Panc 1 cell lines and fibroblasts. The growth of cells exposed to LiGLA for 7 days is expressed as a percentage of the growth of cells in the medium-only control wells. The values at each concentration are the means of 3–8 separate observations, each consisting of 4–10 test wells; vertical bars represent standard error of the mean (SEM).

more importantly, in that the treatment was only begun when the tumours were established and growing, rather than at the time of implantation or before, thus mimicking the clinical situation. Pancreatic tumours were produced sub-cutaneously over the left flank in mice using the MIA PaCa2 cell line. This tumour model was characterised by progressive increase in tumour volume without local invasion, distant metastasis or significant loss of host body weight. Once progressive tumour growth was confirmed, the mice were divided into treatment and control groups. LiGLA was administered either intraperitoneally (ip) (at two different doses of 0.5 mg/g or 1 mg/g body weight, given by 10 daily injections dissolved in normal saline), intravenously (iv) (in a galactosomal form, 1 mg/g in 10 daily tail vein injections) or intratumorally (single injection of LiGLA, dose based on tumour volume). Control groups received lithium oleate (for ip and it groups) or blank galactosomes (iv group). Tumour response was assessed from the relative change in the tumour volume compared with the volume at the beginning of therapy.

Intravenous galactosomal LiGLA (and control galactosomes) was well tolerated with no adverse effects. However, ip 1 mg/g LiGLA was quite toxic, and was associated with the development of a chemical peritonitis and death of five animals in the treatment group. Post-mortem examination revealed intraperitoneal adhesions. No significant differences in tumour growth were seen between the treatment and control groups with iv and both ip doses of LiGLA, and there was no significant alteration of the tumour phospholipid fatty acid composition. When the untreated tumours were tested with LiGLA using an *ex vivo* chemosensitivity assay (differential staining cytotoxicity (DiSC) assay) which is a 4-day *in vitro* chemosensitivity test designed to identify the drug sensitivity or resistance of fresh tumour cells (57), the LC90 values for the tumour cells varied from 169 to

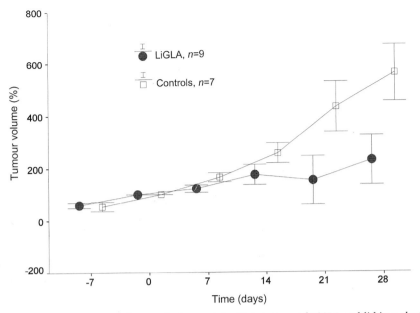

Figure 3. The mean tumour volumes of mice treated with intratumoral LiGLA and lithium oleate (control), presented as a percentage of the tumour volume at the beginning of therapy. A single injection of fatty acid was given at time = 0, followed by 4 weekly measurements. Vertical bars represent SEM.

239 μmol/l (mean, 95% CI: 213.4, 239–188). This was much higher than the LC90 values seen in the *in vitro* studies for MIA PaCa2 cell line, suggesting that the concentration of LiGLA necessary for growth inhibition *in vivo* may be much higher. Radiolabelled fatty acid uptake studies confirmed that following iv or ip administration the tumour uptake of GLA was poor compared with many other tissues in the body.

With intratumour administration, however, these factors can be overcome and a significant difference ($P < 0.05$, Mann–Whitney U-test) in tumour volumes was seen between the treatment and control groups at 3 and 4 weeks following the injection (Figure 3). Two tumours in the treatment group completely regressed following therapy and failed to reappear over a 4-week follow-up period. No tumour regressions were seen in the control group. Minor necrosis of skin overlying tumour occurred in three mice but healed spontaneously.

Clinical Trials of Fatty Acids in Pancreatic Cancer

An open phase I-II study in pancreatic cancer, using LiGLA, was reported recently (58). Forty-eight patients with irresectable pancreatic carcinoma were treated with LiGLA iv at doses ranging from 7–77 g/patient, followed by oral therapy. There were no significant side effects. Although overall median survival was not high (114 days), the survival was significantly prolonged compared with historical controls with demonstration of a dose-survival relationship (Table 1).

Table 1. Survival in phase I/II study of LiGLA in irresectable pancreatic carcinoma (Fearon et al. (58))

The dose of iv LiGLA received	Median survival from diagnosis (days)		Median survival from treatment (days)	
	All cases	Excluding possible misdiagnoses	All cases	Excluding possible misdiagnoses
(All patients)	228 ($n = 48$)	175 ($n = 43$)	126 ($n = 48$)	114 ($n = 43$)
0–40 g	105 ($n = 12$)	105 ($n = 11$)	58 ($n = 12$)	58 ($n = 11$)
41–60 g	228 ($n = 18$)	228 ($n = 17$)	121 ($n = 18$)	121 ($n = 17$)
61–80 g	431 ($n = 18$)	362 ($n = 15$)	327 ($n = 18$)	298 ($n = 15$)

LiGLA therapy was associated with an increase of DGLA, an immediate metabolite of GLA, in red cell phospholipids.

Subsequently a large phase III trial was conducted (data on file, Scotia Pharmaceuticals, Stirling, UK): 278 patients with irresectable pancreatic cancer were recruited from 17 centres in the UK and Europe for a randomised three-arm parallel study. Of these, 163 (59%) had histological confirmation. The treatment groups consisted of oral LiGLA ($n = 93$) (capsules containing LiGLA/GLA concentrate equivalent to 700 mg GLA daily for 15 days, administered on an out-patient basis), Low dose iv LiGLA ($n = 90$) (LiGLA 0.4 g/kg, equivalent 0.28 g/kg GLA) and high dose iv ($n = 95$) (1.2 g/kg LiGLA equivalent to 0.84 g/kg GLA), both administered as a continuous infusion dissolved in saline via a central venous catheter. The objectives were to determine the impact of LiGLA on survival and also to assess tumour response and effect on weight loss. As there is evidence that certain cytokines and acute phase response (APR) proteins implicated in the development of cancer cachexia can be influenced by EFAs, the effect on circulating cytokines and acute phase reactants, as well as that on serum Ca 19-9 were studied in a subset of 23 patients.

Table 2 lists the median survival times for the three treatment groups estimated using the Kaplan–Meier procedure; the survival curves are shown in Figure 4. While the median survival of both oral and low iv groups from the first day of treatment was similar at about 121–128 days, the survival of high-dose patients was, surprisingly in view of the phase II data, shorter. Three patients, one from each group, achieved a "complete response" and 10 patients achieved a partial response (oral: 4, low iv: 3, high iv: 3) giving an overall response rate of 4.7%. No side effects of conventional chemotherapy were seen. The commonest drug-related adverse event was asymptomatic and self-limiting haemoglobinuria,

Table 2. Median survival (days) in a phase III study of LiGLA in irresectable pancreatic carcinoma (data on file, Scotia Pharmaceuticals, Stirling, UK)

	Oral	Low iv	High iv
All patients from:			
Diagnosis	186 ($n = 92$)	160 ($n = 90$)	139 ($n = 94$)
Randomisation	129 ($n = 93$)	121 ($n = 90$)	94 ($n = 95$)
First day of treatment	128 ($n = 92$)	126 ($n = 84$)	90 ($n = 84$)
Histologically confirmed from:			
Diagnosis	179 ($n = 56$)	172 ($n = 52$)	132 ($n = 53$)
Randomisation	121 ($n = 57$)	120 ($n = 53$)	83 ($n = 53$)
First day of treatment	121 ($n = 57$)	126 ($n = 48$)	82 ($n = 49$)

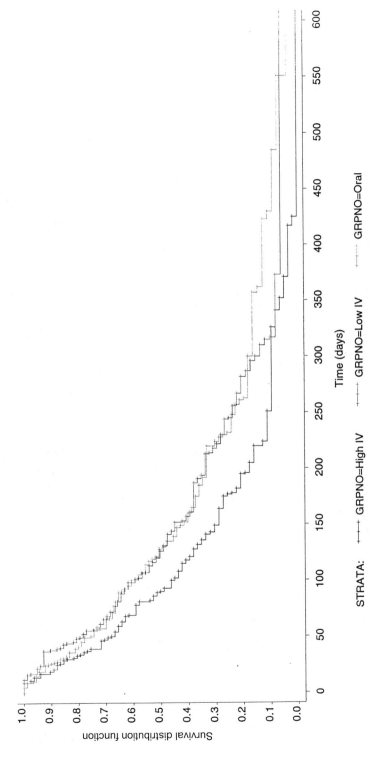

Figure 4. Phase III study of LiGLA in pancreatic carcinoma. The Kaplan-Meier survival curves from the first day of treatment. All patients by treatment group. (Data on file, Scotia Pharmaceuticals, Stirling, Scotland.)

mostly in the high-dose iv group. The commonest "drug-related" serious adverse events were deep vein thrombosis ($n = 3$) and anaemia ($n = 3$), especially in the high iv group, in line with the high incidence of haemoglobinuria. The maximum median serum lithium levels attained during the treatment period were oral: 0.2 mmol/l, low iv: 0.34, high iv: 0.74. Oral and low iv group patients lost weight at a similar rate while it was slightly more marked in the high dose iv group.

Serum Cytokines, CRP and Ca 19.9 in a Subgroup of Patients

Fifteen patients had an APR at the onset of therapy as demonstrated by a raised C-reactive protein (CRP) (> 10 mg/l). There was no significant change in the mean CRP level at the end of treatment although 10 of these patients had lower levels than previously. At 6 weeks follow-up the reduction just reached statistical significance ($P = 0.05$, paired t-test). This difference disappeared in those patients who survived up to 3 months. No IL-1β or IFγ was found in the serum of any patient. TNFα was detected only in three patients. However, 20 patients had abnormal IL-6 levels in plasma (> 1.6 pg/ml) and this included all patients with an APR. No significant difference was seen in IL-6 levels at any of the time points compared with the levels at the onset of therapy, although the levels decreased at the 6-weeks follow-up visit reflecting the pattern seen with CRP levels. Nineteen patients had abnormal levels of Ca 19.9 in the serum before therapy. No significant change in the levels were noted with therapy.

Summary

Fatty acids as antitumour therapy in pancreatic cancer is an interesting concept. They have none of the side effects of conventional chemotherapy, so quality of life is not impaired by treatment. However, preclinical studies have shown that although growth inhibition can be achieved *in vitro* at low micromolar range, modification of tumour fatty acid composition and growth inhibition are more difficult to achieve *in vivo*. In addition the concentration necessary for tumour growth inhibition appears to be higher *in vivo*. The results of the phase III study confirm these findings. Poor tumour response, measured both by tumour size and tumour markers, was associated with no improvement in survival. The success of intratumour therapy in nude mice, and promising results from animal and clinical studies with other tumours using this approach, however, confirms that an antitumour effect can be achieved *in vivo* by direct infusion of fatty acid into the tumour.

Further improvements are necessary in fatty acid delivery mechanisms that would ensure high fatty acid uptake by the tumour with conventional methods of administration. In the meantime locoregional administration of EFAs appears to offer the best chance of tumour growth inhibition *in vivo*. Locoregional chemotherapy such as intra-arterial or intratumoral therapy is feasible and effective in pancreatic carcinoma (59–61). Combination therapy with other anti-cancer agents is also worthwhile exploring. For example, a median survival of 200 days has been reported with a combination of LiGLA and 5-FU in advanced pancreatic cancer in a preliminary study (62). Further studies are in progress along all these avenues.

References

1. Guffy MM, North JA, Burns CP (1984) Effect of cellular fatty acid alteration on adriamycin sensitivity in cultured L1210 murine leukaemic cells. Cancer Res 44:1863–1866.
2. Kinsella JE, Black JM (1993) Effects of polyunsaturated fatty acids on the efficacy of anti-neoplastic agents toward L517Y lymphoma cells. Biochem Pharmacol 45:1881–1887.
3. Leary WP, Robinson KM, Booyens J, Dippenaar N (1982) Some effects of gamma linolenic acid on cultured human esophageal carcinoma cells. S Afr Med J 62:681–683.
4. Weber JM, Sircar S, Begin ME (1994) Greater sensitivity of human multidrug resistant (mdr) cancer cells to polyunsaturated fatty acids than their non-mdr counterparts. J Nat Cancer Inst 86:638–639.
5. Grammatikos SI, Subbaiah PV, Victor TA, Miller WM (1994) n-3 and n-6 fatty acid processing and growth effects in neoplastic and non-cancerous human mammary epithelial cell lines. Br J Cancer 70:219–227.
6. Anel A, Naval J, Desportes P, Gonzalez B, Uriel J, Pineiro A (1992) Increased cytotoxicity of polyunsaturated fatty acids on human tumoral B and T cell lines compared with normal lymphocytes. Leukaemia 6:680–688.
7. Begin ME, Das UN, Ells G, Horrobin DF (1985) Selective killing of human cancer cells by polyunsaturated fatty acids. Prostaglandins Leukot Med 19:177–186.
8. Begin ME, Sircar S, Weber JM (1989) Differential sensitivity of tumourogenic and genetically related non-tumourogenic cells to cytotoxic polyunsaturated fatty acids. Anticancer Res 9:1049–1052.
9. Sircar S, Cai F, Begin ME, Weber JM (1990) Transformation renders mdr cells more sensitive to polyunsaturated fatty acids. Anticancer Res 10:1783–1786.
10. Fugiwara F, Todo S, Imashuku S (1987) Fatty acid modification of cultured neuroblastoma cells by gamma linolenic acid relevant to its antitumour effect. Prostaglandins Leukot Med 30:37–49.
11. Begin ME, Ells G, Horrobin DF (1988) Selective killing of human cancer cells by polyunsaturated fatty acid induced cytotoxicity against tumour cells and its relationship to lipid peroxidation. J Natl Cancer Inst 80:188–194.
12. Chajes V, Sattler W, Stranzl A, Kostner GM (1995) Influence of n-3 fatty acids on the growth of human breast cancer cells in vitro: relationship to peroxides and vitamin-E. Breast Cancer Res Treatment 34:199–212.
13. Ghayur T, Horrobin DF (1981) Effects of essential fatty acids in the form of evening primrose oil on the growth of the rat R3230AC transplantable mammary tumour. ICRS Med Sci 9:582.
14. Karmali RA, Marsh J, Fuchs C, Hare W, Crawford M (1985) Effects of dietary enrichment with gamma linolenic acid upon growth of the R3230AC mammary adenocarcinoma. J Nutr Growth Cancer 2:41–51.
15. Pritchard GA, Jones DL, Mansel RE (1989) Lipids in breast carcinogenesis. Br J Surg 76: 1069–1073.
16. de Bravo MG, Schinella G, Tournier H, Quintans C (1994) Effects of dietary gamma and alpha linolenic acid on a human lung carcinoma grown in nude mice. Med Sci Res 22:667–668.
17. Siegel I, Liu TL, Yaghoubzadeh E, Keskey TS, Gleicher N (1987) Cytotoxic effects of free fatty acids on ascites tumor cells. J Natl Cancer Inst 78:271–277.
18. Ramesh G, Das UN, Koratkar R, Padma M, Sagar PS (1992) Effect of essential fatty acids on tumor cells. Nutrition 8:343–347.
19. Hayashi Y, Fukushima S, Kishimoto S et al. (1992) Anticancer effects of free polyunsaturated fatty acids in an oily lymphographic agent following intrahepatic arterial administration to a rabbit bearing VX-2 tumor. Cancer Res 52:400–405.
20. Botha JH, Robinson KM, Leary WP (1983) Parenteral gamma linolenic acid administration in nude mice bearing a range of human tumour xenografts. S Afr Med J 64:11–12.
21. Ramchurren N, Botha JH, Robinson KM, Leary WP (1985) Effects of gamma linolenic acid on murine cells in vitro and in vivo. S Afr Med J 68:795–798.

22. Gardiner NS, Duncan JR (1991) Possible involvement of delta-6-desaturase in control of melanoma growth by gamma-linolenic acid. Prostaglandins Leukot Essent Fatty Acids. 42:149–153.

23. Sakaguchi M, Imray C, Davis A et al. (1990) Effects of dietary n-3 and saturated fats on growth rates of the human colonic cancer cell lines SW-620 and LS 174T *in vivo* in relation to tissue and plasma lipids. Anticancer Res 10:1763–1768.

24. Sakaguchi M, Rowley S, Kane N et al. (1990) Reduced tumour growth of the human colonic cancer cell lines COLO-320 and HT-29 *in vivo* by dietary n-3 lipids. Br J Cancer 62:742–747.

25. Borgeson CE, Pardini L, Pardini RS, Reitz RC (1989) Effects of dietary fish oil on human mammary carcinoma and on lipid-metabolising enzymes. Lipids 24:290–295.

26. Gabor H, Blank EW, Ceriani RL (1996) Effect of dietary fat and monoclonal antibody therapy on the growth of human mammary adenocarcinoma MX-1 grafted in athymic mice. Cancer Lett 52:173–178.

27. Gonzalez MJ, Schemmel RA, Dugan L, Gray JI, Welsch CW (1993) Dietary fish oil inhibits human breast carcinoma growth: a function of increased lipid peroxidation. Lipids 28:827–832.

28. Welsch CW, Oakley CS, Chang CC, Welsch MA (1993) Suppression of growth by dietary fish oil of human breast carcinomas maintained in three different strains of immune-deficient mice. Nutr Cancer 20:119–127.

29. Istfan NW, Wan J, Chen ZY (1995) Fish oil and cell proliferation kinetics in a mammary carcinoma tumor model. Adv Exp Med Biol 375:149–156.

30. Rose DP, Connolly JM, Rayburn J, Coleman M (1995) Influence of diet containing eicosa-pentaenoic or docosahexaenoic acid on growth and metastasis of breast cancer cells in nude mice. J Natl Cancer Inst 87:587–592.

31. de Bravo MG, de Antueno RJ, Toledo J, De Tomas ME, Mercuri OF, Quintans C (1991) Effects of an eicosapentaenoic and docosahexaenoic acid concentrate on a human lung carcinoma grown in nude mice. Lipids 26:866–870.

32. Karmali RA, Reichel P, Cohen LA et al. (1987) The effects of dietary ω-3 fatty acids on the DU-145 transplantable human prostatic tumour. Anticancer Res 7:1173–1180.

33. Rose DP, Cohen LA (1988) Effects of dietary menhaden oil and retinyl acetate on the growth of DU-145 human prostatic adenocarcinoma cells transplanted into athymic nude mice. Carcinogenesis 9:603–605.

34. McIllmurray MB, Turkie W (1987) Controlled trial of gamma linolenic acid in Duke's C colorectal cancer. Br Med J 294:1260.

35. van der Merve CF, Booyens J (1987) Oral gamma linolenic acid in 21 patients with untreatable malignancy. An ongoing pilot open clinical trial. Br J Clin Pract 41:907–915.

36. van der Merwe CF, Booyens J, Joubert HF, van der Merwe CA (1990) The effect of gamma-linolenic acid, an *in vitro* cytostatic substance contained in evening primrose oil, on primary liver cancer. A double-blind placebo controlled trial. Prostaglandins Leukot Essent Fatty Acids 40:199–202.

37. Das UN, Prasad VVSK, Raia Reddy D (1995) Local application of gamma linolenic acid in the treatment of human gliomas. Cancer Lett 94:147–155.

38. Holoryde CP, Skutches CL, Reichard DG (1988) Effect of dietary enrichment with n-3 poly-unsaturated fatty acids (PUFA) in metastatic breast cancer. Proc ASCO 7:42 (abstract).

39. Reich R, Royce L, Martin GR (1989) Eicosapentaenoic acid reduces the invasive and metastatic activities of malignant tumour cells. Biochem Biophys Res Comm 160:559–564.

40. du Toit PJ, van Aswegen CH, du Plessis DJ (1994) The effect of gamma linolenic acid and eicosapentaenoic acid on urokinase activity. Prostaglandins Leukot Med 51:121–124.

41. DiBattista JA, Martel-Pelletier J, Fugimoto N, Obata K, Zafarullah M, Pelletier JP (1995) Prostaglandin E2 and E1 inhibit cytokine induced metalloprotease expression in human synovial fibroblasts. Mediation by cyclic AMP signalling pathway. Lab Invest 71:270–278.

42. Jiang WG, Hiscox S, Hallett MB et al. (1995) Regulation of the expression of E-cadherin on human cancer cells by gamma linolenic acid (GLA). Cancer Res 55:5043–5048.

43. Jiang WG, Hiscox S, Horrobin DF, Hallett MB, Mansel-RE, Puntis-MC (1995) Expression of catenins in human cancer cells and its regulation by n-6 polyunsaturated fatty acids. Anticancer Res 15:2569–2573.

44. Jiang WG, Hiscox S, Hallett MB, Scott C, Horrobin DF, Puntis MCA (1995) Inhibition of hepato-cyte growth factor-induced motility and *in vitro* invasion of human cancer cells by gamma linolenic acid. Br J Cancer 71:244–252.

45. Rose DP, Connolly JM, Liu X (1995) Effect of linolenic acid and gamma linolenic acid on the growth and metastasis of a human breast cancer cell line in nude mice and on its growth and invasive capacity *in vitro*. Nutr Cancer 24:33–45.

46. Honn KV, Nelson KK, Renaud C, Bazaz R, Diglio CA, Timar J (1992) Fatty acid modulation of tumour cell adhesion to microvessel endothelium and experimental metastasis. Prostaglandins 44:413–429.

47. Ziboh VA (1990) Biochemical basis for the anti-inflammatory action of gamma linolenic acid. In: Horrobin DF (ed) Omega-6 essential fatty acids. Pathophysiology and roles in clinical medicine. Liss, New York, pp 187–202.

48. McCarty MF (1996) Fish oil may impede tumour angiogenesis and invasiveness by down-regulating protein kinase C and modulating eicosanoid production. Med Hypotheses 46:107–115.

49. Karmali RA, Adams L, Trout JR (1993) Plant and marine n-3 fatty acids inhibit experimental metastasis of rat mammary adenocarcinoma cells. Prostaglandins Leukot Essent Fatty Acids 48:309–314.

50. Abbott WGH, Tezabwala B, Bennett M, Grundy SM (1994) Melanoma lung metastases and cytolytic effector cells in mice fed antioxidant-balanced corn oil or fish oil diets. Nat Immun 13:15–28.

51. Adams LH, Trout JR, Karmali RA (1990) Effect of n-3 fatty acids on spontaneous and experimental metastasis of rat mammary tumour 13762. Br J Cancer 61:290–291.

52. Hori T, Moriuchi A, Okuyama H, Sobajima T, Koizumi K, Kojima K (1987) Effect of dietary essential fatty acids on pulmonary metastasis of ascites tumour cells in rats. Chem Pharm Bull (Tokyo) 35:3925–3927.

53. Kort WJ, Weijma IM, Bijma AM, van Schalkwijk WP, Vergroesen AJ, Westbroek DL (1987) Omega-3 fatty acids inhibiting the growth of a transplantable rat mammary adenocarcinoma. J Natl Cancer Inst 79:593–599.

54. Lanson M, Bougnoux P, Besson P et al. (1990) n-6 polyunsaturated fatty acids in human breast carcinoma phosphatidylethanolamine and early relapse. Br J Cancer 61:776–778.

55. Falconer JS, Ross JA, Fearon KCH, Hawkins RA, O'Riordain MG, Carter DC (1994) Effect of eicosapentaenoic acid and other fatty acids on the growth in vitro of human pancreatic cancer cell lines. Br J Cancer 69:826–832.

56. Alley MC, Scudiero DA, Monks A et al. (1988) Feasibility of drug screening with panels of human tumour cell lines using a microculture tetrazolium assay. Cancer Res 48:589–601.

57. Bosanquet AG (1994) Short-term in vitro drug sensitivity tests for cancer chemotherapy. A summary of correlations of test result with both patient response and survival. Forum Trends Exp Clin Med 4:179–195.

58. Fearon KCH, Falconer JS, Ross JA et al. (1996) An open label phase I/II dose escalation study of the treatment of pancreatic cancer using lithium gammalinolenate. Anticancer Res 16:867–874.

59. Aigner KR, Muller H, Basserman R (1990) Intra-arterial chemotherapy with MMC, CCDP and 5-FU for non-resectable pancreatic cancer – a phase II study. Reg Cancer Treat 3:1–6.

60. Morai T, Makino TTI, Ishii K (1989) Intratumoural treatment of pancreatic cancer with mito-mycin C adsorbed to activated carbon particles. A clinical trial on 15 cases. Anticancer Res 9:1799–1804.

61. Link KH, Gansauge F, Pillasch J, Buchler M, Beger HG (1996) Regional treatment of advanced pancreatic carcinoma via coeliac axis infusion. In: Beger HG, Büchler MW, Schoenberg MH (eds) Cancer of the pancreas: molecular biology, recent progress in diagnostics and therapy. Universitatsverlag Ulm, Germany, pp459–465.

62. Bryce R, Lederman JA, Taylor I, Brennan C, Russell RCG, Hatfiedl A (1997) A phase II study of intravenous gamma linolenic acid (GLA) pre-treatment in patients with pancreatic or colorectal cancer treated with 5-fluorouracil (5-FU). Abstract submitted to the joint meeting of British Oncological Association, Association of Cancer Physicians and the Royal College of Radiologists, July 1997.

31 Imaging in Pancreatic Cancer: Spiral Computed Tomography (CT), CT Arterial Portography (CTAP) and Magnetic Resonance Imaging (MRI)

R.J. Heafield and C.N. Hacking

Imaging techniques for pancreatic cancer have evolved on a broad front over the past decade but the improving ability to reliably answer a variety of questions in a single procedure has made computed tomography (CT) the examination of choice for staging and preoperative planning. This chapter describes the recent advances in CT and the role of magnetic resonance imaging (MRI) in pancreatic cancer.

Computed Tomography

Since its invention in 1972, CT has gradually become the cornerstone of pre-operative staging for pancreatic cancer, superseding mesenteric angiography in the late 1980s by virtue of its ability to depict adequately the critical locoregional sites of spread in addition to vascular involvement (1). The proven ability of CT is in demonstrating irresectable disease and by the early 1990s many pancreatic radiologists and surgeons had produced CT data with surgical correlation achieving excellent sensitivities for irresectability of 85–95% (2).

Confidence in the CT technique has now greatly reduced the need for exploratory laparotomy as a staging procedure, notwithstanding the contribution of other staging methods and the impact of non-surgical palliation to this general trend. The factor underpinning such good results was the meticulous use of intra-venous contrast material, tumour conspicuity and spread being accentuated by maximising the enhancement difference of normal pancreas and vessels with low density tumour. From 1988, reports showed that dynamic incremental contrast-enhanced (DCT) imaging was able to demonstrate small lesions in the pancreas using rapid pump injections of contrast and narrow early phase CT sections even though the optimal timing requirements were not achievable on such CT scanners, which took 1–2 minutes to acquire images through the sagittal depth of the pancreas alone. Achieving pancreatic detail was possible only at the expense of the analysis of surrounding organs. Another concern particularly for small lesions was the problem of respiratory misregistration whereby variable respiratory movement would result in a small lesion being "missed out" of the acquired sections. Developments in MRI technique in the early 1990s were beginning to match the achievements of DCT, equalling CT sensitivities and positive predictive values for irresectability and it appeared that MRI would surpass CT as a staging investigation (3).

Ultrasonography

This chapter deals with the roles of CT and MRI but there is an extensive complementary and competing role for ultrasonography (US). This modality has different strengths and weaknesses from CT and MRI but is the initial imaging tool in the great majority of patients when it may provide all of the required diagnostic information. It is highly accurate in distinguishing obstructive from non-obstructive jaundice, which is a presenting feature in over 50% of patients. It may reveal liver metastases and peripancreatic spread and vascular changes can be seen with conventional and colour Doppler techniques (4). A recent report gives US equivalent accuracy to DCT for vascular involvement (5). Disadvantages of US are operator dependence, gaseous interference in the epigastrium and the restricted field of view affecting the satisfaction of search. Some of these limitations have been overcome with more invasive direct imaging of the gland using an endoscopic, intraoperative or laparoscopic approach. Endoscopic approaches have achieved high levels of specificity and sensitivity (6). These techniques are discussed in Chapter 33 and several papers show considerable improvement in positive predictive values for both resectability and irresectability when laparoscopic US is added to visual inspection. An element of bias due to the preselection is inevitable in these studies (7). Transabdominal US may give false-negative results and when a high clinical suspicion is present, CT should be performed after US.

Spiral CT

It was the evolution of X-ray tube engineering and detector hardware, accompanied by advances in computing which allowed the development of spiral (helical) CT. In short, the X-ray tube can now rotate continuously and move along the patient (and therefore "scan"). This has been achieved by "slip ring" high voltage electrode contacts which allow continuous data acquisition during table movement in the Z-axis covering up to 30 cm in 20–30 seconds. The consequence of continuous scanning is rapid tube heating but this problem has now been overcome with new tube construction methods and materials. For images to be immediately available (to determine the need for further acquisitions), advanced computer software for rapid image reconstruction is also required. The benefits of spiral CT apply in many parts of the body but in the upper abdomen the rapid speed of acquisition over a large field of view allows optimal contrast enhancement. Acquisition is completed within a single arrested respiration (breathhold) thus avoiding misregistration and reducing movement artefact. Success can be improved by scanning during the physiological "window of opportunity" (8,9) which is between 30 and 60 seconds after rapid injection for the pancreas (arterial phase) and 70–120 seconds for the liver (portal phase), an obligatory part of any examination for pancreatic cancer (10).

Theoretical Advantages of Spiral CT

Because the data are volumetric and are acquired continuously rather than separately in the Z-axis, spiral CT images can be more easily reconstructed in alternative planes and can be viewed at different slice intervals or locations, by reconstructing a different element of data. This reduces the effects of partial volume averaging (11). For example a series of 10-mm images may be reconstructed and viewed at 5-mm intervals to improve separation of anatomical structures. Multiplanar and three-dimensional (3D) reconstruction may be particularly valuable in vascular assessment prior to surgery (12,13). The patient room time is potentially reduced by spiral examinations, which is an important benefit for high capital cost equipment. Modern spiral capability equipment is also considerably faster in the conventional incremental or axial mode. Unlike MRI, with the evolution of spiral CT the basic image interpretation process is unchanged, indeed for a given section there is no appreciation of whether the acquisition is spiral or axial.

Improvements in Detection

The data on comparative quality of spiral CT remain incomplete at this time but the impression in our unit is that spiral CT produces dependable diagnostic images in almost all patients. Comparing the best images from a conventional CT pancreas examination may well provide equivalent data but consistency throughout the Z-axis cannot be matched. A recently published series with surgical correlation gives encouraging results with positive predictive values for irresectability of 92% and respectability of 87% (14), showing an improvement on initial experience (15).

Technique

We use dilute iodinated contrast for bowel opacification, 500 ml 20–30 minutes prior to examination. Plain unenhanced axial 10-mm contiguous sections are obtained through the upper abdomen and these are used to plan dual-phase intravenous (iv) enhancement with 100–150 ml Iohexol 300 injected at 2.5–4 ml/second via an 18-g iv cannula using a suitable pump. Images through the pancreas and duodenum are obtained at 30 seconds after starting the injection during suspended respiration with 5-mm beam collimation and a pitch of 1 to 1.3 depending on patient variables. These images are routinely reconstructed at 5-mm intervals. The scan direction is caudal. After a further delay of 20 seconds portal phase images are obtained during a second breathhold at approximately 70 seconds with 7-mm beam collimation and 7-mm reconstructions again varying the pitch accordingly, to include the liver and again to below the transverse duodenum in the caudal direction.

The CT Appearances of Pancreatic Cancer

Normal morphology of the pancreas includes a number of patterns, but arterial phase enhancement reveals well-marginated pancreatic tissue surrounded by fat and usually resolves the pancreatic duct, up to 3 mm diameter in body and tail and 5 mm in the head. Small tumours are best seen on arterial phase images as low density defects in the pancreas (Figure 1). The constant relationship to splenic, superior mesenteric and portal vein is readily appreciated (Figures 1, 2). Larger masses may also distort the outline of the surrounding pancreas or extend to or beyond the surface to involve adjacent fat. The size of a hypodense mass on CT correlates well with pathological measurements in a recent trial comparing spiral CT evidence with resection specimens (16).

Staging Classification

The 1981 American Joint Committee for Cancer (AJCC) Staging TNM system divides T staging into T1(a), < 2 cm; T1(b), > 2 cm; T2, limited direct extension into duodenum, bile duct or stomach; and T3, advanced direct extension not compatible with surgical resection (12). Table 1 defines Stages I to IV.

Hypodense masses on DCT are seen in 80% of cases; retrospective review of unenhanced examinations by comparison gives a detection rate of only 24% (18). Hyperdense lesions are seen in endocrine pancreatic tumours but are not described in ductal adenocarcinoma. Diffuse gland enlargement may occur in 4% of cases (19), and this should be considered in the investigation of pancreatitis. Approximately 70% of lesions are shown in the head and neck of the gland, secondary changes of duct dilatation here may assist CT diagnosis of small resectable lesions. However, the double duct sign on CT is often an indicator of poor prognosis. Biliary obstruction may also be due to nodal masses in the porta hepatis. The important differentials for the double duct sign are cholangio-carcinoma, ampullary tumour and chronic pancreatitis.

Many patients are referred for CT following ERCP and placement of biliary endoprosthesis. These can occasionally create artefact leading to diagnostic difficulty and our preference, particularly when ultrasonography has shown a mass, is to perform CT before ERCP. Changes in the peripancreatic fat after ERCP have been described and equally CT may give further diagnostic information to the endoscopist. Conversely, air or contrast introduced at ERCP may occasionally allow or improve the depiction of tumour. However small pancreatic ductal tumours may be only detected on ERCP or pancreatic duct endoscopy before they produce a mass or duct dilatation on CT.

Peripancreatic Changes

Contiguous tumour extending beyond the gland can be best appreciated when fat (of low attenuation) surrounds the pancreas and vessels. Alteration in fat volume and attenuation may indicate invasion or may be generalised due to increased fluid content resulting from a variety of mechanisms, e.g. cachexia, lymphatic obstruction. Ascites can have the same effect of reducing inherent tissue contrast. Where slight fat changes are reported with spiral CT, resection was still feasible in five of eight cases (14). Inevitably CT is unable to demonstrate microscopic involvement in this site, as shown in resected specimens.

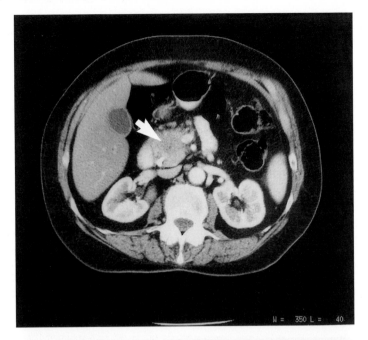

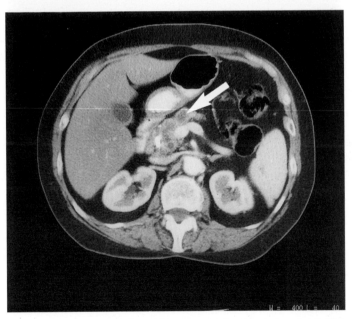

Figure 1. There is an area of low attenuation within pancreatic head (*top*). At a slightly higher level the dilated pancreatic duct is shown (*bottom*).

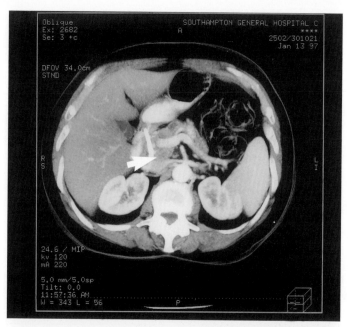

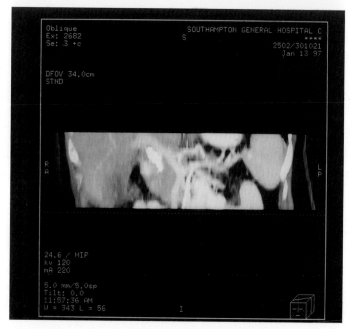

Figure 2. Axial image showing dense arterial opacification of the superior mesenteric artery and splenic vein (*top*). There is abnormal soft tissue around the vein which is better appreciated on a coronal reconstruction.

Table 1. AJCC staging classification for pancreatic cancer

Stage I	T1, T2, N0, M0: No (or unknown) direct extension, or limited direct extension, or limited direct extension of tumour to adjacent viscera, with no (or unknown) regional node extension and absence of distant metastases. Limited direct extension was defined as involvement of organs that could be removed *en bloc* with the pancreas if a curative resection was attempted.
Stage II	T3, N0, M0: Further direct extension of tumour into adjacent viscera with no (or unknown) lymph node involvement and no distant metastases, which precluded surgical resection.
Stage III	T1-3, N1, M0: Regional node metastases without clinical evidence of distant metastases.
Stage IV	T1-3, N0-1, M1: Distant metastatic disease in liver or other sites present.

Lymph Nodes

CT does not resolve the node groups draining directly from the gland but the second (porta hepatis, common hepatic, coeliac and proximal SMA) and third (periaortic, distal superior mesanteric artery (SMA)) echelons of nodes can be located. CT is sensitive to nodal enlargement, but malignant nodes may often be small giving a poor negative predictive value (20). This is clearly a limitation in providing full TNM staging data preoperatively, but spiral techniques do offer improved differentiation of nodes from vessels.

Vascular Spread

This characteristic feature of pancreatic cancer is rare in other GI malignancies and may be partly due to the vascular relations of the pancreas, but it is mostly attributed to rich interconnecting perivascular lymphatics and nerves which can transport a cuff of isolated perivascular involvement from a small remote tumour in the gland. This process explains the historical importance of angiography as a sensitive staging tool although it provided no direct imaging of the primary tumour. Spiral CT angiography is proving very accurate in the detection of arterial and venous encasement (Figure 3) and is replacing conventional angiography (21). A recent report suggests that recognisable changes in the small peripancreatic veins may be the most sensitive determinant of extrapancreatic spread as the veins lie on the anterior and posterior pancreatic surface (22). A comparison of angiography and DCT revealed no significant difference in 1988 (1) and we believe its role may now be limited to the facilitation of CT arterial portography (CTAP) (see below). Anomalous hepatic artery anatomy is often mentioned as a remaining reason for preoperative angiography when CT shows a resectable lesion (10), but these are usually recognisable particularly with 3D reformatting techniques (Figures 4, 5). A recent study confirms that spiral CT can be as sensitive as angiography for this finding (23).

Contiguous Organ Involvement

Gastric, hepatic and colonic invasion can all be appreciated by CT and may preclude resection. As the duodenum and distal CBD are part of the resected

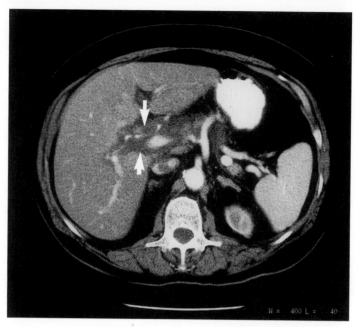

Figure 3. Arterial phase spiral CT image showing encasement of portal vein and hepatic artery in the porta hepatis.

Whipple's procedure specimen in these cases a technically complete removal may still be achieved.

Distant Spread

A focus on the primary pancreatic lesion must determine whether a curative resection is feasible technically, but the search for distant disease is also crucial, as revealing distant metastases confers a dismal prognosis making curative resection ineffectual. The peritoneum remains a blind spot on CT for solid surface nodules and some surgeons advocate laparoscopy and peritoneal lavage and cytology as a further staging procedure (24). CT has high sensitivity for small volumes of peritoneal fluid though ascites is usually accompanied by major signs of irresectable local disease. Liver metastases require a further dedicated examination which we perform with a dual-phase technique. Earlier spiral equipment was unable to achieve this prior to the equilibrium phase when tumour density approaches normal liver density. DCT has sensitivity for all metastases of 75–80% and there may be limited room for improvement in detection on spiral dual-phase examinations (25). The most sensitive technique for detection of liver metastases, however, is CTAP. Other sites of unusual distant spread shown on CT include the lower chest caudal to the dome of diaphragm and evaluation of this area on appropriate windows is necessary. These are hidden areas on the chest radiograph and it is important to review them in the preoperative patient.

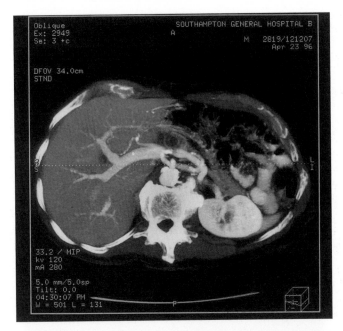

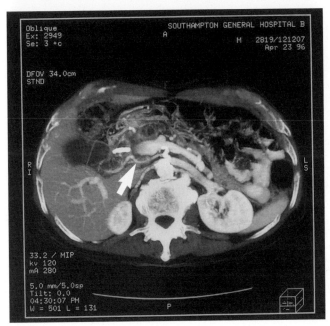

Figure 4. Multiplanar volume reformat (MPVR) images show arterial and portal venous opacification. The replaced right hepatic artery can be seen from its origin on the proximal superior mesenteric artery.

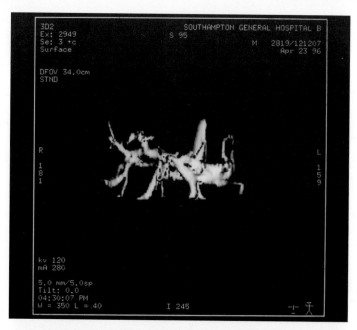

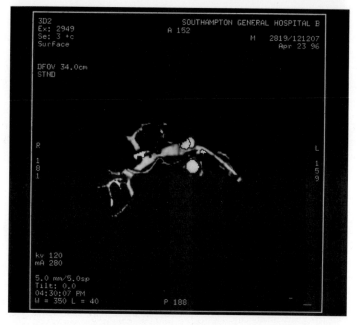

Figure 5. Three-dimensional reformatted images from the same examination allow assessment from anteriorly (*top*) and superiorly (*bottom*).

Oral contrast is essential to avoid difficulty with bowel related masses and occasionally further images are needed at selected levels to resolve the issue.

CT Arterial Portography (CTAP)

CTAP has been used increasingly to detect liver metastases from a number of primary sites but predominantly for colorectal secondaries where hepatic resection has a role. CTAP has produced the best sensitivity of any preoperative imaging technique with values from 85–96% (26). In pancreatic cancer the role is as yet unproven; however, our initial experiences would suggest a similarly high sensitivity in the detection of early liver metatases (Figure 6). An additional use for CTAP in assessing vascular involvement has been explored as this further information is "free" in the same field of view (27). Whilst useful in assessing portal vein involvement (Figure 7) arterial and peripancreatic vessel opacification is better seen on dual-phase spiral CT. Overall preoperative accuracy for vascular involvement in pancreatic resections has been reported at 96% in a group of 26 patients (28).

Comparison with angiography alone has shown superiority (27), but direct comparison with dual-phase intravenous spiral CT examination has not been performed.

Principle of CTAP

The underlying principle of CTAP is again to maximise liver/lesion contrast ratios, and introduce contrast preferentially into the portal vein alone rather than to the hepatic arterial and portal venous circulation together. This method exploits the dual blood supply of the liver and the absence of a portal supply to liver tumours to produce a bright liver vividly contrasting with hypodense tumour deposits. The theoretical direct portal injection is not feasible but the elegant alternative of selective superior mesenteric or splenic artery catheter contrast injection results in portal venous return and portal (only) liver enhancement after an interval of 20–30 seconds.

Technique

Under screening control, deep superior mesenteric artery catheter placement (or occasionally splenic artery) is performed and having established catheter stability and demonstrated any anomalous vascular anatomy, the patient is transferred to the CT suite. Iohexol 140, 200 ml, is injected at 4 ml/second and acquisition commences after a 25 second delay. Images are acquired with beam collimation of 5 mm, pitch 1–1.3 and reconstruction at 5-mm intervals. Further delayed images are obtained after 2 minutes. Both acquisitions are made during breathholding.

Specificity and False-Positive Findings

Dependence on vascular anatomy makes CTAP susceptible to a number of perfusion artefacts which must be recognised (Figures 8, 9). Straight line,

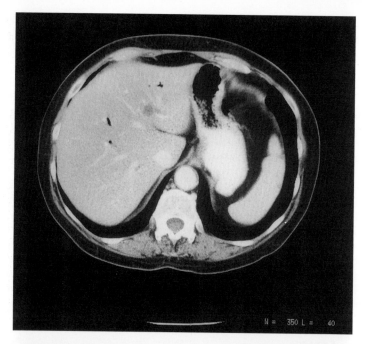

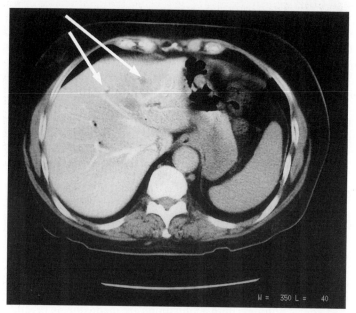

Figure 6. Arterial phase intravenous enhancement reveals a solitary lesion in segment 4 (*top*). A further two small lesions are revealed by CTAP. Note biliary duct air due to endoprosthesis.

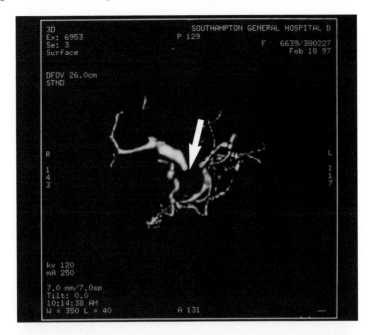

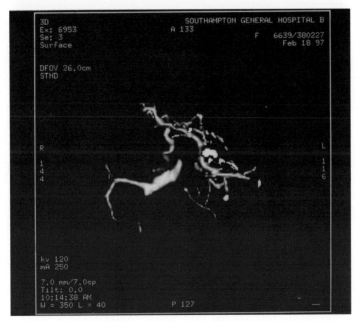

Figure 7. Three-dimensional reformatted images from CTAP examination showing a portal venous occlusion caudal to SMV and portal junction with large peripancreatic collaterals.

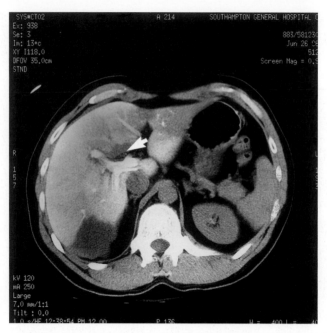

Figure 8. A large metastasis is seen in segment 6/7. Note the segment 4 non-tumorous perfusion defect due to venous supply from unopacified blood.

periligamentous and subcapsular perfusion abnormalities are common, particularly in segment 4 and must be treated with caution. The problems with perfusion artefacts and cysts can usually be resolved on the 2-minute images; however, small haemangiomata remain a problem and ultrasonography may be required to distinguish these from tumour. Clearly the technique is more complex and invasive but the high frequency of small liver metastases at presentation is a strong argument for its use in pancreatic cancer (29). Our belief is that CTAP should be reserved for detection of hepatic metastases where the tumour is otherwise resectable. Further evaluation of the superior mesenteric and portal veins is useful and can strengthen the impression of venous involvement suggested by the spiral CT examination. CTAP in the presence of biliary obstruction is difficult to interpret, because the dilated bile ducts show as filling defects in the liver. For this reason, we perform CTAP only if biliary decompression has been achieved.

Magnetic Resonance Imaging

Potential benefits of MRI are the high tissue contrast and a variety of pulse sequences which can evaluate different structures such as blood vessels, liver and the pancreas itself. MRI protocols for pancreas have been numerous. Conventional spin echo T1- and T2-weighted (T1W, T2W) sequences are being superseded by faster gradient echo (GRE) breathhold sequences (T1W) or fast spin echo (FSE T2W) or inversion recovery (STIR) sequences (30). The use of respiratory compensation, fat suppression (STIR) and enhancement with intravenous

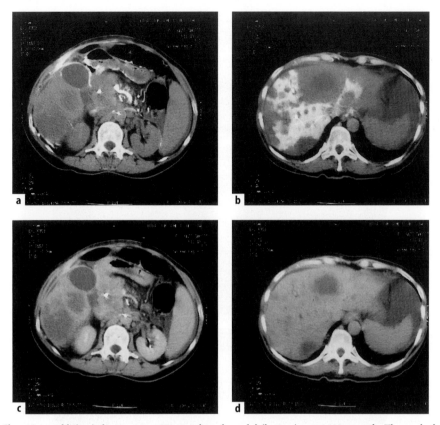

Figure 9. a and **b** (*top*) show scans at 30 seconds and **c** and **d** (*bottom*) are at 120 seconds. The marked perfusion defects in the right lobe overestimates true tumour size which is appreciated on later scans (**c** and **d**). Note that metastases down to 5 mm in diameter can be seen in the left lobe where perfusion defects are less marked.

gadolinium have been shown to improve resolution (31). Whether MRI can match CT in staging has been addressed in a large multicentre trial (3). Preference of sequences was given as T1W for tumour extent, GRE sequences, for vascular involvement T1W and T2W sequences for lymphadenopathy and for liver metastases T2W and STIR were preferred. This study showed comparable success with CT for respectability although both modalities had poor negative predictive value which was partly attributed to study design.

Appearances of Pancreatic Cancer on MRI

It is the biological nature of ductal adenocarcinoma as a scirrhous tumour with a desmoplastic response which results in hypointensity on T1W images. On T2 there is some variation as haemorrhage, necrosis and inflammation will all influence T2W. The gland is difficult to separate from surrounding fat and either fat suppression T1W or gadolinium-enhanced images improve conspicuity of the

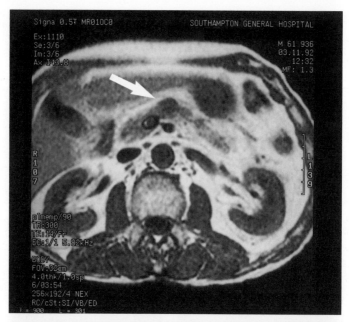

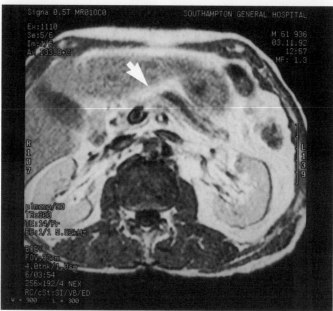

Figure 10. T1W (*top*) and T1W post-gadolinium images (*bottom*) show a low signal 2-cm nodule in the pancreatic body anterior to mesenteric vessels. Following enhancement the normal pancreas is bright and the hypointense tumour and dilated pancreatic duct are seen.

normal gland (Figure 10). The tumour is seen initially as a hypointense lesion after gadolinium with bright normal pancreas, but then reversal of this pattern occurs and bright tumour is seen after 3 minutes (32).

Neuroendocrine tumours represent a small proportion of pancreatic neoplasms but they may be characterised more reliably with MRI from their signal characteristics (33). They are hypervascular and show vivid enhancement after gadolinium and are typically hyperintense on T2W imaging. Recognition of these tumours is important as treatment options are different to those in ductal adenocarcinoma.

Recent Advances in MRI

MR versus Angiography

Comparison of dynamic MR portal venography with indirect portal venography by conventional angiography has shown some success for this limited role. A low false-positive rate was achieved thereby avoiding exclusion of an otherwise resectable lesion (34). However, this has not been compared with spiral CT angiography.

MR versus CT/CTAP

Improved dynamic sequences and the use of both oral, and liver-specific contrast improve the detection of metastases. Sensitivity equivalent to CT has been reported (35). As yet MR sensitivities are still lower than CTAP (36), but liver-specific contrast agents and newer subsecond sequences may change this in the near future.

MR versus ERCP

MR cholangiopancreatography (MRCP) offers a non-invasive alternative to diagnostic ERCP and early results are very promising (37,38,39).

Conclusion

Ultrasonography will continue to be useful in the many tumours presenting with jaundice. We confidently expect spiral CT to improve detection of the resectable T1(a) lesion but other non-imaging strategies for detecting early (treatable) disease are required. Late presentation remains an overwhelming problem and in this poor prognosis group spiral CT will provide adequate staging most of the time. Where the lesion appears resectable CTAP can probably improve on sensitivity for small liver metastases revealing further cases where surgery is not appropriate. Definitive evidence of increased sensitivity is not yet available however. MRI is valuable currently for neuroendocrine lesions, but in future as a non-invasive radiation-free method, MRI will challenge CTAP and spiral CT as an alternative staging technique and is presently useful when CT findings are uncertain.

References

1. Freeny PC, Marks WM, Ryan JA, Traverso LW (1988) Pancreatic ductal adenocarcinoma: diagnosis and staging with dynamic CT. Radiology 166:125–133.
2. Fuhrman GM, Charnsangavej C, Abbruzzese JL et al. (1994) Thin-section contrast-enhanced computed tomography accurately predicts the resectability of malignant pancreatic neoplasms. Am J Surg 167:104–111.
3. Megibow AJ, Zhou XH, Rotterdam H et al. (1995) Pancreatic adenocarcinoma: CT versus MR imaging in the evaluation of resectability: report of the Radiology Diagnostic Oncology Group. Radiology 195:327–332.
4. Garber S, Lees WR (1993) Pancreatic malignancy. In: Cosgrove D, Meire H, Dewbury K (eds), Abdominal and general ultrasound, vol 1. Churchill Livingstone, Edinburgh, pp 157–170.
5. Tomiyama T, Ueno N, Tano S, Wada S, Kimura K (1996) Assessment of arterial invasion in pancreatic cancer using color Doppler ultrasonography. Am J Gastroenterol 91:1410–1416.
6. Palazzo L, Roseau G, Gayet B et al. (1993) Endoscopic ultrasonography in the diagnosis and staging of pancreatic adenocarcinoma. Results of a prospective study with comparison to ultrasonography and CT scan. Endoscopy 25:143–150.
7. John TG, Greig JD, Carter DC, Garden OJ (1995) Carcinoma of the pancreatic head and periampullary region. Tumour staging with laparoscopy and laparoscopic ultrasonography. Ann Surg 221:156–164.
8. Bonaldi VM, Bret PM, Atri M, Garcia P, Reinhold C (1996) A comparison of two injection protocols using helical and dynamic acquisitions in CT examinations of the pancreas. AJR 167:49–55.
9. Lu DS, Vedantham S, Krasny RM, Kadell B, Berger WL, Reber HA (1996) Two-phase helical CT for pancreatic tumors pancreatic versus hepatic phase enhancement of tumour, pancreas, and vascular structures. Radiology 199:697–701.
10. Zeman RK, Silverman PM, Ascher SM, Patt RH, Cooper C, Al-Kawas F (1995) Helical (spiral) CT of the pancreas and biliary tract. Radiol Clin North Am 33:887–902.
11. Bluemke DA, Soyer P, Fishman EK (1995) Helical (spiral) CT of the liver. Radiol Clin North Am 33:863–886.
12. Johnson PT, Heath DG, Kuszyk BS, Fishman EK (1996) CT angiography with volume rendering: advantages and applications in splanchnic vascular imaging. Radiology 200:564–568.
13. Raptopoulos V, Steer ML, Sheiman RG, Vrachliotis TG, Gougoutas CA, Movson JS (1997) The use of helical CT angiography to predict vascular involvement from pancreatic cancer: correlation with findings at surgery. AJR 168:971–977.
14. Coley SC, Strickland NH, Walker JD, Williamson RCN (1997) Spiral CT and the preoperative assessment of pancreatic adenocarcinoma. Clin Radiol 52:24–30.
15. Bluemke DA, Cameron JL, Hruban RH et al. (1995) Potentially resectable pancreatic adenocarcinoma: spiral CT assessment with surgical and pathological correlation. Radiology 197:381–385.
16. Furukawa H, Takayasu K, Mukai K, Inoue K, Kosuge T, Ushio K (1996) Computed tomography of pancreatic adenocarcinoma: comparison of tumor size measured by dynamic computed tomography and histopathologic examination. Pancreas 13:231–235.
17. Cancer of the Pancreas Task Force (1981) Staging cancer of the pancreas. Cancer 47:1631–1642.
18. Megibow AJ (1992) Pancreatic adenocarcinoma: designing the examination to evaluate the clinical questions. Radiology 183:297–303.
19. Freeny PC, Traverso LW, Ryan JA (1993) Diagnosis and staging of pancreatic adenocarcinoma with dynamic computed tomography. Am J Surg 165:600–606.
20. Reznek RH, Stephens DH (1993) The staging of pancreatic adenocarcinoma. Clin Radiol 47:373–381.
21. Zeman RK, Davros WJ, Berman P et al. (1994) Three-dimensional models of the abdominal vasculature based on helical CT: usefulness in patients with pancreatic neoplasms. AJR 162:1425–1429.
22. Hommeyer SC, Freeny PC, Crabo LG (1995) Carcinoma of the head of the pancreas: evaluation of the pancreaticoduodenal veins with dynamic CT: potential for improved accuracy in staging. Radiology 96:233–238.
23. Chambers TP, Fishman EK, Bluemke DA, Urban B, Venbrux AC (1995) Identification of the aberrant hepatic artery with axial spiral CT. J Vasc Interv Radiol 6:959–964.
24. Leach SD, Rose JA, Lowy AM et al. (1995) Significance of peritoneal cytology in patients with potentially resectable adenocarcinoma of the pancreatic head. Surgery 118:472–478.

25. Hollett MD, Brooke Jeffrey R Jr, Nino-Murcia M, Jorgenson MJ, Harris DP (1995) Dual phase helical CT of the liver; value of arterial phase scans in the detection of small (< 1.5 cm) malignant hepatic neoplasms. AJR 164:879–884.
26. Redvanly RD, Chezmar JL (1997) CTAP; technique, indications and applications. Clin Radiol 52: 256–268.
27. Savader BL, Fishman EK, Savader SJ, Cameron JL (1994) CT arterial portography vs pancreatic arteriography in the assessment of vascular involvement in pancreatic and periampullary tumors. J Comput Assist Tomogr 18:916–920.
28. Soyer P, Lacheheb D, Belkacem A, Levesque M (1994) Involvement of superior mesenteric vessels and portal vein in pancreatic adenocarcinoma: detection with CT during arterial portography. Abdom Imaging 19:413–416.
29. National Cancer Institute (1991) Annual Cancer Statistics Review 1973–1988. Department of Health and Human Services, Bethesda (NIH publication No 91–2789).
30. Nghiem HV, Freeny PC (1994) Radiologic staging of pancreatic adenocarcinoma. Radiol Clin North Am 32:71–79.
31. Gabata T, Matsui O, Kadoya M et al. (1994) Small pancreatic adenocarcinomas: efficacy of MR imaging with fat suppression and gadolinium enhancement. Radiology 193:683–688.
32. Mergo PJ, Helmberger TK, Buetow PC, Helmberger RC, Ros PR (1997) Pancreatic neoplasms: MR imaging and pathologic correlation. Radiographics 17:281–301.
33. Pisegna JR, Doppman JL, Norton JA, Metz DC, Jensen RT (1993) Prospective comparative study of the ability of MR and other imaging modalities to localise tumours in patients with Zollinger–Ellison syndrome. Dig Dis Sci 38:1318–1328.
34. Rodgers PM, Ward J, Baudouin CJ, Ridgeway JP, Robinson PJ (1994) Dynamic contrast-enhanced MR imaging of the portal venous system: comparison with X-ray angiography. Radiology 191:741–745.
35. Ichikawa T, Haradome H, Hachiya J et al. (1997) Pancreatic ductal adenocarcinoma: assessment with helical CT versus dynamic MR imaging. Radiology 202:655–662.
36. Paulson EK, Baker ME, Paine SS, Spritzer CE, Meyers WC (1994) Detection of focal hepatic masses: STIR MR vs CT during arterial portography. J Comput Assist Tomogr 18:581–587.
37. Ishizaki Y, Wakayama T, Okada Y, Kobayashi T (1993) Magnetic resonance cholangiography for evaluation of obstructive jaundice. Am J Gastroenterol 88:2072–2077.
38. Low RN, Sigeti JS, Francis IR et al. (1994) Evaluation of malignant biliary obstruction: efficacy of fast multiplanar spoiled gradient-recalled MR imaging vs spin-echo MR imaging, CT, and cholangiography. AJR 162:315–323.
39. Schuster DM, Pedrosa MC, Robbins AH (1995) Magnetic resonance cholangiography. Abdom Imaging 20:353–356.

32 Laparoscopy and Laparoscopic Ultrasound in the Staging of Pancreatic and Periampullary Cancer

I.J. Martin, T.G. John and O.J. Garden

Given that malignant tumours of the pancreas are associated with a poor prognosis, the management of the majority of patients is focused on achieving optimal palliation of symptoms and maintaining quality of life. The diagnosis, staging and treatment of patients with malignancy of the pancreas and periampullary region remains a clinical challenge because of its retroperitoneal location, its complex relationship with blood vessels and viscera and the propensity for occult intraabdominal metastases at the time of presentation (1). The aim is therefore to select reliably patients for whom attempts at curative pancreatic resection are appropriate, while identifying those with factors which contraindicate surgery. Modern radiological imaging techniques may be misleading in the assessment of pancreatic malignancy; this is reflected by non-therapeutic laparotomy rates of 12 to 39% (2–5). The associated physical and psychological morbidity, and the cost-inefficiency of this strategy has led to increasing recognition that "laparotomy and biopsy" is an unacceptable primary method of assessing such patients (6).

Laparoscopy is the most sensitive investigation in detecting "occult" metastases to the liver and serosal surfaces without resorting to laparotomy. Laparoscopy with laparoscopic intraoperative ultrasonography (LapUS) provides a unique opportunity to evaluate pancreatic malignancy with respect to metastases and local invasion without resorting to dissection of peripancreatic tissue. These tools help provide an accurate diagnostic, staging and management algorithm for pancreatic cancer.

The utility of laparoscopy and LapUS in the evaluation of pancreatic cancer has emerged through direct comparison alongside other imaging modalities. The precise role of laparoscopy (and LapUS) may vary between individual institutions dependent upon the philosophy of the surgical team and also upon the available expertise of laparoscopy and other evolving modalities. This chapter illustrates the important role that staging laparoscopy with LapUS plays in the assessment of patients with pancreatic or periampullary cancer.

Laparoscopy Alone

Detection of Metastatic Disease

Laparoscopy has an important role in the preoperative assessment of patients with potentially resectable pancreatic cancers, largely due to its ability to detect

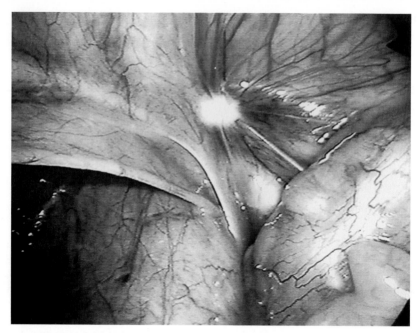

Figure 1. Malignant peritoneal seedlings discovered during laparoscopy over the parietal peritoneum of the left inguinal region. Radiological investigations had diagnosed a potentially resectable tumour of the periampullary region.

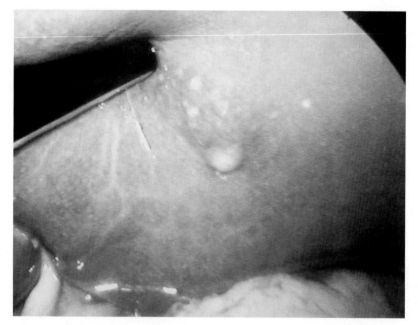

Figure 2. Small liver metastasis arising from the undersurface of hepatic segment III and discovered unexpectedly during staging laparoscopy for a potentially resectable pancreatic carcinoma.

Table 1. Staging laparoscopy and laparoscopic ultrasonography in the evaluation of pancreatic and periampullary cancer

Reference	Study details	Incidence of dissemination at laparoscopy (%)	Sensitivity for metastases (%)	Laparotomy avoided (%)
Cuschieri et al. 1978–1988 (7,9)	$n = 73$ Lap only	75	98	30
Ishida 1983 (8)	$n = 71$ Lap only	43	–	–
Warshaw et al. 1988–1993 (10,12)	$n = 86$ Lap only	41	96	41
John et al. 1995 (15)	$n = 40$ Lap / LapUS vs USS / CT	35	83	45[a]
Bemelman et al. 1995 (13)	$n = 73$ Lap vs USS	23	76	17[a]
Fernández-del Castillo et al. 1995 (14)	$n = 114$ Lap vs CT / SVA	24	93	24
Conlon et al. 1996 (16)	$n = 115$ Lap vs USS / CT	29	75[b]	36
John et al. 1998 (29)	$n = 50$ Lap / LapUS vs USS / CT / SVA	30	94	38[a]

Lap, laparoscopy; LapUS, laparoscopic ultrasonography; USS, ultrasonography; CT, abdominal computed tomography; SVA, selective visceral angiography.
[a] Includes LapUS findings; [b] liver metastases only.

intraabdominal metastases (7–16) (Figures 1 and 2, Table 1). The clinical information yielded by modern laparoscopy surpasses radiological imaging techniques of ultrasonography, CT, MRI and angiography in the detection of disseminated "minimal volume disease" within the abdominal cavity (7–11, 15–17). Warshaw and colleagues (10,11) found that unsuspected metastases are apparent during laparoscopy in up to 41% of patients considered candidates for pancreatic resection on the basis of prior USS and/or CT. Stepwise discriminant analysis confirmed the unique role played by staging laparoscopy in this context (11). More recent experience with staging laparoscopy in Edinburgh (15,17) and New York (16) has supported these findings in 29–35% of patients who were otherwise clinically and radiologically shown to have "curable" lesions.

Evaluation of Locoregional Disease

Whilst laparoscopy alone is excellent for detecting metastases, the retroperitoneal location of the pancreas, and in particular, the pancreatic head, restricts assessment of locoregional invasion. Nevertheless, various techniques of direct laparoscopic inspection to diagnose pancreatic malignancy have been reported (18–22). Indeed, using the supragastric approach, Ishida (8) successfully visualised tumours of the pancreatic body in 85% of cases, and achieved a laparoscopic-guided biopsy and/or cytological diagnosis of pancreatic malignancy in 74% of pancreatic head tumours and 87.5% of body and tail tumours (8).

However, several studies have revealed that laparoscopy alone fails to achieve a primary tumour diagnosis, and cannot assess accurately local tumour invasion of structures such as the portal and superior mesenteric veins (7,9–12,15,17). The role of laparoscopy alone to determine resectability of localised tumours in the head of the pancreas therefore appears limited.

Nevertheless, a laparoscopic approach to the locoregional staging of potentially resectable peripancreatic malignancy, aiming to mimic open surgical exploration and trial dissection of tumour has been adopted by Conlon and colleagues (16). In addition to demonstrating extrapancreatic tumour spread in 29% of patients (Table 1), laparoscopic evidence of vascular invasion was obtained in 16 patients (15%). Ultimately, pancreatic resection was performed in 61 of the 67 patients considered potentially resectable following laparoscopic staging (i.e. negative predictive value of 91%) (16). However, it remains to be seen whether such an invasive and time-consuming approach will be adopted widely as a prelude to exploratory laparotomy. In the Sloan–Kettering series, the laparoscopic dissection was undertaken under the same anaesthetic as the intended laparotomy. Such a laparoscopic staging approach may not be of great value to a specialist unit being referred patients with potentially resectable tumours which have been staged prior to referral. The development of relatively less intrusive techniques such as LapUS may be a more attractive means of staging pancreatic cancer in hospitals considering referral of cases to a specialist centre.

Laparoscopic Peritoneal Cytology

Positive laparoscopic peritoneal cytology occurs in 15–30% of radiologically "resectable" patients. The finding of malignant cells in the peritoneal cavity carries a grave prognosis and indicates advanced disease, early metastasis and short duration of survival (14,23–28). Our own experience in Edinburgh (28) with laparoscopic peritoneal cytology in the staging of patients with pancreatic and periampullary cancer is similar to that reported elsewhere (25,27). Laparoscopic peritoneal cytology was insensitive in identifying patients with irresectable tumours (18–22%). Furthermore, this technique provided little information over that obtained by laparoscopic inspection of the peritoneal cavity, as all patients with positive cytology in this study also exhibited obvious signs of extrapancreatic tumour dissemination. An overview of 49 patients with malignant peritoneal cytology reported in seven studies revealed that none have undergone curative pancreatic resection (14,23–28) and such patients were found to have a significantly shortened duration of survival.

Laparoscopic Ultrasonography

Laparoscopic intraoperative ultrasonography (LapUS) utilises the same principles as transabdominal ultrasonography during the laparoscopic examination.

The advantage of LapUS is that direct apposition with the intra-abdominal tissues allows the use of relatively high-frequency transducers (7.5–10 MHz) which achieve excellent image resolution, while minimising image degradation (or "acoustic attenuation") experienced when scanning from outside the body wall. LapUS helps overcome the tactile deficit present at laparoscopy and is particularly useful for detection of deep-seated intrahepatic metastases and regional lymph nodes. The relationships of pancreatic lesions with the peripancreatic vascular and ductal structures can be assessed without resorting to additional laparoscopic dissection (Figures 3 and 4). This is illustrated in a study of 38 patients considered to have potentially resectable tumours on the basis of ultrasonography and/or CT (15). Additional staging information such as the presence of vascular invasion, and regional lymphadenopathy, was obtained by LapUS in 20 patients (53%) and the clinical decision regarding tumour resectability was altered (i.e. up-staged) in 10 patients (25%). Laparoscopy combined with LapUS was more sensitive and accurate than laparoscopy alone in identifying tumour irresectability (88% and 89% versus 50% and 65%, respectively) (15).

Bemelman and colleagues (13) similarly reported the efficacy of staging laparoscopy with LapUS in 70 patients with pancreatic cancer considered to have potentially curable stage I disease following preoperative endoscopic retrograde cholangiopanreatography (ERCP) and Doppler ultrasonography. Laparotomy was avoided in 19% of patients due to the detection of liver, peritoneal and lymph node metastases, with 6 of 16 proven liver metastases detected solely by LapUS. Vascular invasion was identified accurately by LapUS, with one false-positive result demonstrated following portal vein resection in a patient with local fibrosis

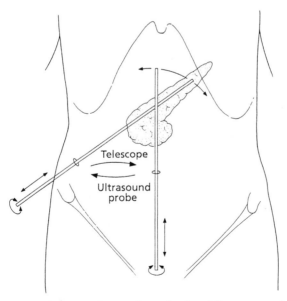

Figure 3. Position of the laparoscopic ports for evaluation of the pancreas. Sagittal/oblique cuts obtained with the probe inserted through the umbilical port provide cross-sectional scans of the pancreas, whereas scanning from the right lateral port in a transverse/oblique direction provides images orientated about the long axis of the gland.

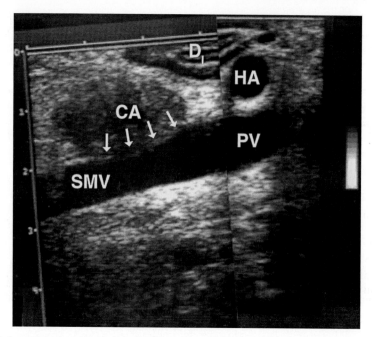

Figure 4. Laparoscopic sonogram obtained in a parasagittal plane with the probe inserted via the umbilical port and transducer placed upon the pancreatic head. A hypoechoic carcinoma (CA) is shown extending into the pancreatic neck anterior to the superior mesenteric vein (SMV) and portal vein (PV). Loss of the hyperechoic interface between tumour and vein indicate local tumour infiltration (*arrows*). The tumour is clear of the common hepatic artery (HA) and first part of duodenum (D$_1$) at the superior pancreatic border.

due to previous irradiation (96% specificity; 93% positive predictive value) (13). The TNM stage was altered in 41% of patients, and the therapeutic strategy changed in 18 patients (25%) when the LapUS findings of local tumour in-growth were confirmed by surgical exploration. However, histopathological validation of resection margins revealed that underestimation of local tumour stage still occurred despite the adoption of staging LapUS and was reflected by a 59% sensitivity and 74% negative predictive value.

Similarly, stringent surgical and histopathological validation of the TNM staging of pancreatic and periampullary cancer by laparoscopy with LapUS was performed in 50 patients in a recent study in Edinburgh, and comparison with ultrasonography, dynamic CT and angiography was undertaken (29). Laparoscopic staging was significantly superior to the other three investigations in detecting intra-abdominal metastases (94% versus 29%, 33% and 0%, respectively). However, unlike the experience of Bemelman and colleagues (13) the contribution of LapUS in detecting liver metastases not seen during laparoscopy was marginal. LapUS was most sensitive (96%) in detecting focal mass lesions (82% ultrasonography; 93% CT; 66% angiography).

In the Edinburgh study, laparoscopic ultrasonography was at least as sensitive as Doppler ultrasonography, CT and angiography in identifying locoregional invasion, although underestimation of T stage was encountered with all modalities (sensitivities of 68% versus 60%, 71% and 67% respectively). Importantly, however, LapUS did not overstage local tumour invasion in any patients reflecting a significantly better specificity (100%) than CT (47%) and ultra-sonography (64%) in defining irresectability by T stage. All investigations were unreliable in detection of malignant regional lymphadenopathy. The specificity and predictive value of LapUS (93% and 97%) were significantly superior to CT (54% and 79%) in defining overall tumour resectability. Angiography was an inaccurate method of tumour staging and provided no supplementary information over the other investigations.

Technical Considerations

It is the authors' preference to perform diagnostic laparoscopy with LapUS under general anaesthesia using a direct cutdown technique at the umbilicus for inser-tion of a 10-mm diameter port. A second 10/11-mm diameter port is inserted usually in the right flank (Figure 3). It is perhaps easier for the inexperienced ultrasonographer to employ a linear array I-shaped 5 or 7.5 MHz rather than a sectoral ultrasound probe, although the latter type of transducer enables exam-ination in all planes without the need to change ports. Other workers have pre-ferred to employ curvilinear array probes with small convex transducer footprints which require only a small cross-sectional area of contact (30,31). A

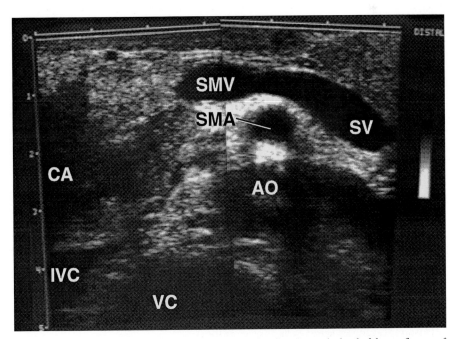

Figure 5. Laparoscopic sonograms obtained in the transverse direction at the level of the confluence of the superior mesenteric (SMV) and splenic veins (SV) with the probe inserted via the right flank port. An irregular, hypoechoic carcinoma of the pancreatic head (CA) is demonstrated. There is no evid-ence of tumour involvement of the peripancreatic blood vessels in this section. SMA, superior mesenteric artery; AO, abdominal aorta; VC, vertebral column; IVC, inferior vena cava.

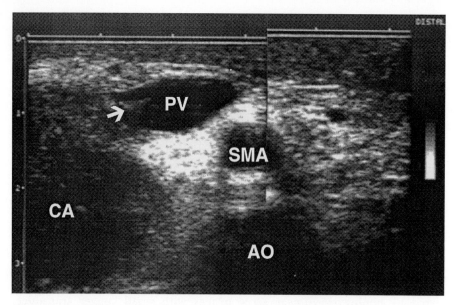

Figure 6. Laparoscopic sonograms during the same examination and at a slightly superior level to that shown in Figure 5. Hypoechoic carcinoma (CA) extends to invade the right lateral wall of the portal vein (PV) with loss of the normal hyperechoic parenchyma–vessel interface and irregularity of the vein wall (*arrow*). The superior mesenteric artery (SMA) and aorta (AO) appear to be clear of tumour.

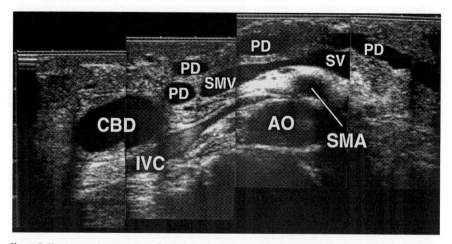

Figure 7. Transverse LapUS scans showing pancreatic duct (PD) and common duct (CBD) dilatation due to an isoechoic periampullary cancer invading the pancreatic head (left of picture). The inferior vena cava (IVC), aorta (AO), splenic vein (SV) and superior mesenteric vein (SMV) and artery (SMA) are seen.

systematic inspection of the peritoneal cavity is performed using a 30° telescope. Alteration of the telescope and LapUS probe between ports allows for LapUS scanning of the liver, biliary tree and pancreas in multiple planes. The portal vein and the common bile duct serve as the principal anatomical landmarks for examination of the pancreas when scanning through the umbilical port (Figure 4). The splenoportal venous confluence, superior mesenteric artery and inferior vena cava can be readily identified when the transducer is passed via the lateral port (Figures 5–7). In this way, detail regarding focal abnormalities of the pancreas and surrounding vessels may be observed (32–34).

Targeted biopsy may be performed freehand through a separate needle puncture (35). However, versatile LapUS probes equipped with guided needle biopsy channels are now available. The incorporation of a long Trucut biopsy needle in a sleeve which is secured to a sectoral transducer (SHARPLAN U Sight 9010, SHARPLAN Laser Industries, Tel Aviv, Israel) facilitates biopsy and avoids inadvertent puncture of vital structures before the needle is visualised on the scan.

Conclusion

The unparalleled sensitivity of laparoscopy in detecting and enabling biopsy of intra-abdominal metastases supports its routine use in patients with suspected resectable peripancreatic malignancy. Furthermore, laparoscopic contact sonography has comparable sensitivity and superior specificity compared with USS, CT and angiography in local evaluation of primary tumour invasion, thereby justifying its role in the staging algorithm of patients with potentially resectable pancreatic tumours. It could even be argued that laparoscopic ultrasonography should replace these conventional staging investigations.

Surgeons enthusiastic in acquiring the appropriate skills will note the very low patient morbidity and the opportunity to perform palliative laparoscopic biliary and/or duodenal bypass surgery. Anecdotal reports of malignant port site seeding have aroused concern although the two cases we have witnessed have been in the context of advanced peritoneal carcinomatosis (36–39).

References

1. Weiss SM, Skibber JM, Mohiuddin M, Rosato FE (1985) Rapid intra-abdominal spread of pancreatic cancer. Arch Surg 120:415–416.
2. Gudjonsson B (1987) Cancer of the pancreas. Cancer 60:2284–2303.
3. de Rooij PD, Rogatko A, Brennan MF (1991) Evaluation of palliative surgical procedures in unresectable pancreatic cancer. Br J Surg 78:1053–1058.
4. Watanapa P, Williamson RCN (1992) Surgical palliation for pancreatic cancer: developments during the past two decades. Br J Surg 79:8–20.
5. Bramhall SR, Allum WH, Jones AG, Allwood A, Cummins C, Neoptolemos JP (1995) Treatment and survival in 13 560 patients with pancreatic cancer, and incidence of the disease, in the West Midlands: an epidemiological study. Br J Surg 82:111–115.
6. Cuesta MA, Meijer S, Borgstein PJ (1992) Laparoscopy and the assessment of digestive tract cancer. Br J Surg 79:486–487.
7. Cuschieri A, Hall AW, Clark J (1978) Value of laparoscopy in the diagnosis and management of pancreatic carcinoma. Gut 19:672–677.
8. Ishida H (1983) Peritoneoscopy and pancreas biopsy in the diagnosis of pancreatic diseases. Gastrointest Endosc 29:211–218.
9. Cuschieri A (1988) Laparoscopy for pancreatic cancer: does it benefit the patient? Eur J Surg Oncol 14:41–44.
10. Warshaw AL, Tepper JE, Shipley WU (1986) Laparoscopy in the staging and planning of therapy for pancreatic cancer. Am J Surg 151:76–80.

11. Warshaw AL, Gu ZY, Wittenberg J, Waltman AC (1990) Preoperative staging and assessment of resectability of pancreatic cancer. Arch Surg 125:230–233.

12. Fernández-del Castillo C, Warshaw AL (1993) Laparoscopy for staging in pancreatic carcinoma. Surg Oncol 2:25–29.

13. Bemelman WA, de Wit LT, van Delden OM et al. (1995) Diagnostic laparoscopy combined with laparoscopic ultrasonography in staging cancer of the pancreatic head region. Br J Surg 82:820–824.

14. Fernández-del Castillo C, Rattner DW, Warshaw AL (1995) Further experience with laparoscopy and peritoneal cytology in the staging of pancreatic cancer. Br J Surg 82:1127–1129.

15. John TG, Greig JD, Carter DC, Garden OJ (1995) Carcinoma of the pancreatic head and periampullary region: tumor staging with laparoscopy and laparoscopic ultrasonography. Ann Surg 221:156–164.

16. Conlon KC, Dougherty E, Klimstra DS, Coit DG, Turnbull ADM, Brennan MF (1996) The value of minimal access surgery in the staging of patients with potentially resectable peripancreatic malignancy. Ann Surg 223:134–140.

17. Murugiah M, Paterson-Brown S, Windsor JA, Miles WFA, Garden OJ (1993) Early experience of laparoscopic ultrasonography in the management of pancreatic carcinoma. Surg Endosc 7:177–181.

18. Meyer-Berg J (1972) The inspection, palpation and biopsy of the pancreas. Endoscopy 4:99.

19. Ishida H, Furukawa Y, Kuroda H, Kobayashi M, Tsuneoka K (1981) Laparoscopic observation and biopsy of the pancreas. Endoscopy 13:68–73.

20. Ishida H, Dohzono T, Furukawa Y, Kobayashi M, Tsuneoka K (1984) Laparoscopy and biopsy in the diagnosis of malignant intra-abdominal tumors. Endoscopy 16:140–142.

21. Watanabe M, Takatori Y, Ueki K et al. (1989) Pancreatic biopsy under visual control in conjunction with laparoscopy for diagnosis of pancreatic cancer. Endoscopy 21:105–107.

22. Strauch M, Lux G, Ottenjann R (1973) Infragastric pancreoscopy. Endoscopy 5:30–32.

23. Martin JK, Goellner JR (1986) Abdominal fluid cytology in patients with gastrointestinal malignant lesions. Mayo Clin Proc 61:467–471.

24. Warshaw AL (1991) Implications of peritoneal cytology for staging of early pancreatic cancer. Am J Surg 161:26–30.

25. Lei S, Kini J, Kim K, Howard JM (1994) Pancreatic cancer. Cytologic study of peritoneal washings. Arch Surg 129:639–642.

26. Zerbi A, Balzano G, Bottura R, Di Carlo V (1994) Reliability of pancreatic cancer staging classifications. Int J Pancreatol 15:13–18.

27. Leach SD, Rose JA, Lowy AM et al. (1995) Significance of peritoneal cytology in patients with potentially resectable adenocarcinoma of the pancreatic head. Surgery 118:472–478.

28. John TG, McGoogan E, Wigmore SJ, Paterson-Brown S, Carter DC, Garden OJ (1995) Laparoscopic peritoneal cytology in the staging of pancreatic cancer. Gut 37:A3.

29. John TG, Paterson-Brown S, Wright A, Allan PL, Redhead DN, Carter DC, Garden OJ (1998) Laparoscopic ultrasonography in the TNM staging of pancreatic and periampullary cancer. World J Surg 1998: (in press).

30. Serio G, Fugazzola C, Iacono C et al. (1992) Intraoperative ultrasonography in pancreatic cancer. Int J Pancreatol 11:31–41.

31. Sigel B, Coelho JCU, Spigos D, Donahue PE, Wood DK, Nyhus L (1981) Ultrasonic imaging during biliary and pancreatic surgery. Am J Surg 141:84–89.

32. Garden OJ (1995) Intraoperative and laparoscopic ultrasonography. Blackwell Science, Oxford.

33. John TG, Garden OJ (1995) Ultrasonography in laparoscopy. In: Brooks D (edn) Current review of laparoscopy, 2nd edn. Current Medicine, Philadelphia, pp. 77–95.

34. John TG, Garden OJ (1994) Laparoscopic ultrasound: extending the scope of diagnostic laparoscopy. Br J Surg 81:5–6.

35. John TG, Garden OJ (1995) Laparoscopic targeted liver biopsies. In: Toouli J, Gossot D, Hunter JG (eds) Endosurgery. Churchill Livingstone, Edinburgh.

36. Jorgensen JO, McCall JL, Morris DL (1995) Port site seeding after laparoscopic ultrasonographic staging of pancreatic carcinoma. Surgery 117:118–119.

37. Siriwardena A, Samarji WN (1993) Cutaneous tumour seeding from a previously undiagnosed pancreatic carcinoma after laparoscopic cholecystectomy. Ann R Coll Surg Eng 75:199–200.

38. Nduka CC, Monson JRT, Menzies-Gow N, Darzi A (1994) Abdominal wall metastasis following laparoscopy. Br J Surg 81:648–652.

39. van Dijkum EJMN, de Wit LT, Obertop H, Gouma DJ (1996) Port-site metastases following diagnostic laparoscopy. Br J Surg 83:1793–1794.

33 The Role of Endoscopic Ultrasonography in the Assessment of Pancreatic Tumours

S.A. Norton and D. Alderson

Until recently, ultrasonography played a limited role in the investigation of pancreatic disease as transcutaneous scanning is limited by poor visualisation of deep structures, especially in the obese patient. This is due to the inverse relationship between the resolution of the image produced and the depth of penetration of the sound waves. In addition, the image is impaired by intervening bowel and other structures which cause further attenuation of the beam.

In recent years, technology has evolved to enable the incorporation of small ultrasound transducers into endoscopes allowing scanning of the pancreas to be performed via the stomach and duodenum. Because only a small depth of penetration is required, high frequency ultrasound can be used to improve image resolution.

This combination of endoscopy and ultrasonography was first introduced in 1980 but early echoendoscopes were difficult to manoeuvre due to the length of the rigid tip housing the transducer. The linear images produced made orientation difficult and it was not until Olympus developed smaller endoscopes incorporating mechanical rotating transducers that echoendoscopy became more feasible. Endoscopic ultrasonography (EUS) has been established for over 10 years in many countries including France, Japan and the USA, but has been slow to gain acceptance in the UK.

Equipment

Two basic scanning methods exist. Mechanically rotating or radial transducers produce a 360° image perpendicular to the long axis of the endoscope. Convex phased array scanners produce a sector image (100–120°) parallel to the axis of the scope. Although orientation is more difficult with the latter, fine-needle aspiration for cytology is easier. Both types of echoendoscope have forward-oblique viewing systems. A balloon at the tip of the echoendoscope is inflated with water to provide a sonic window, producing clearer images. They operate at frequencies of 7.5 and 12 MHz, compared with 2–5 MHz in conventional ultrasonography, with marked increases in image resolution. The effective image range is up to 12 cm.

An ultrasound miniprobe is also available which can be passed down the biopsy channel of a conventional endoscope and has been used to examine the pancreaticobiliary ductal systems (1,2).

Examination Technique

EUS of the upper gastrointestinal tract is performed in a similar way to standard endoscopy, as an outpatient procedure using intravenous sedation and anaesthetic throat spray. The patient lies in the left lateral position although the supine or prone position is occasionally useful to improve visualisation of certain structures. Care must be taken in the introduction of the scope as the long inflexible tip can potentially cause trauma, e.g. in the presence of a pharyngeal diverticulum. Care is also required in negotiating the duodenum when partial insufflation of the balloon after passing through the pylorus minimises the risk of trauma.

Unlike endosonography of the oesophagus which produces familiar cross-sectional images of the mediastinum, scanning of the pancreas is performed at a number of different angles resulting in anatomical sections that may be very difficult to interpret. As long as certain steps are followed, however, the whole of the pancreas can be reliably visualised with EUS.

The scanning frequency is usually set at 7.5 MHz with a range of 9 cm. The neck, body, tail and occasionally the upper, anterior part of the head of the pancreas are imaged through the posterior wall of the stomach. The splenic vein and

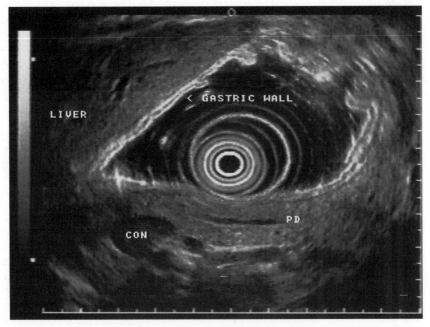

Figure 1. Pancreatic neck, body and duct visualised between posterior wall of stomach and portal/splenic vein confluence (CON, confluence; PD, pancreatic duct traversing body of gland).

its convergence with the superior mesenteric vein produces a tadpole like image which is usually easy to identify, above which will be found the neck of the gland. Following the splenic vein by gentle withdrawal of the scope with fine movements of the controls will reveal the entire body and tail. It is important to scan along the tail until the spleen is identified to be sure that the distal extremity of the pancreas is not missed. The pancreatic duct can usually be seen, even when not dilated, as a fine hypoechoic structure running through the gland (Figure 1).

To image the head it is necessary to scan through the duodenum. Initial placement of the scope in the second part of the duodenum, in the long position, will reveal the aorta and inferior vena cava in cross-section. Withdrawal of the scope into the short scope position will produce an image of the lower part of the head. The ventral pancreas (uncinate process) will be seen as a triangular structure which is less echogenic than the dorsal pancreas. It can be misinterpreted as pathological unless this feature is appreciated. The superior mesenteric and portal veins will be apparent in longitudinal section. The ampulla will be visible as a small hypoechoic nodule and small adjustments of the controls will reveal the terminal common bile duct and the pancreatic duct traversing the head to the ampulla. Positioning of the transducer in the bulb will enable the upper part of the head to be visualised. Lymph nodes may be apparent in the peripancreatic region, at the origin of the superior mesenteric artery (SMA) or at the coeliac axis, all of which are within the scanning range of EUS (Figure 2).

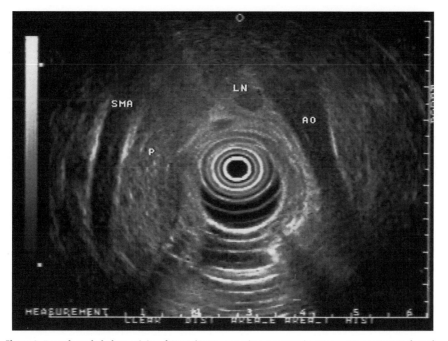

Figure 2. Lymph node below origin of SMA (SMA, superior mesenteric artery; AO, aorta; LN, lymph node; P, uncinate lobe of pancreas).

Role of EUS in the Management of Pancreatic Neoplasms

Diagnosis of Suspected Pancreatic Tumours

EUS is the most sensitive modality for the identification of small pancreatic tumours. It can reliably detect tumours of < 2 cm (accuracy 90%) when curative resection is more likely, compared with computed tomography (CT) and magnetic resonance imaging (MRI) which have an accuracy of 40% and 33%, respectively (3–5). It may therefore be useful in patients suspected of having pancreatic cancer on clinical grounds but with negative CT (Figure 3).

Tumour Staging

Endoscopic ultrasonography is of no value in large (> 4 cm) pancreatic tumours due to the limited range of the high-frequency ultrasound used. In addition, duodenal compression may make introduction of the scope difficult, resulting in incomplete views. Deviation of important structures, such as the portal vein, by the tumour displaces them to the edge of the scanning range. At this distance it is difficult to identify clearly tumour invasion as opposed to compression. Such tumours, however, are usually inoperable and are easily evaluated with other imaging modalities.

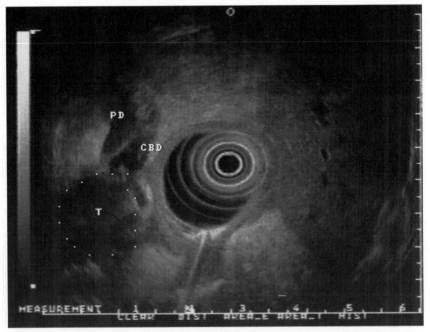

Figure 3. Small (1.7-cm) tumour of pancreatic head, not visible on CT scan, obstructing bile duct and pancreatic duct (CBD, common bile duct; PD, pancreatic duct).

Table 1. Accuracy rates for tumour and nodal staging of pancreatic cancer: results of meta-analysis (6). EUS, endoscopic ultrasonography; US, ultrasonography; CT, computed tomography; MRI, magnetic resonance imaging

	EUS	US	CT	MRI
Tumour staging	86%	35%	42%	57%
Nodal staging	71%	42%	53%	59%

EUS is useful in the T staging of potentially operable pancreatic tumours. A recent meta-analysis (6) involving 357 patients in 14 studies gave EUS an overall accuracy of 83%. The nodal staging in the same analysis was less accurate at 74% overall (ranging from 48% to 94%). A further meta-analysis (6) comparing EUS with conventional US, CT and MRI is shown in Table 1.

Anterior peripancreatic and gastric invasion can be reliably identified, aided by the clear definition of the gut wall seen with EUS, which is able to demonstrate five or more individual layers. CT appears to be particularly poor in this respect (7). Duodenal invasion or submucosal spread is similarly detected with an accuracy of around 83% (7). Early invasion of the three-layered bile duct wall is readily appreciated (5).

The presence of vascular invasion is probably the most important factor when considering the resectability of a pancreatic tumour (Figure 4). EUS can

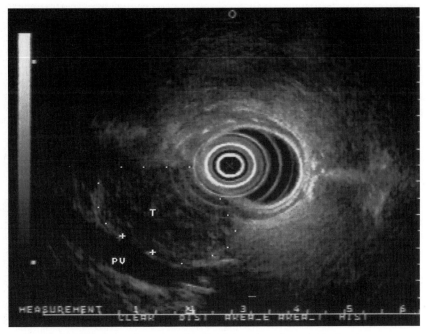

Figure 4. Large (3-cm) tumour of pancreatic head with invasion of portal vein seen between crosses (T, tumour; PV, portal vein).

determine such invasion with accuracy ranging from 66% to 100% of cases (6) compared with 63% for MRI (5), 20–80% for CT and 60–100% for angiography (6). It is particularly accurate in the detection of splenoportal venous invasion (sensitivity 88%, specificity 78%) (7,8) and may show involvement even when angiography reveals no abnormality (9). It may be less accurate in demonstrating arterial invasion but this is probably of little significance as arterial involvement without venous involvement is extremely rare (7,10).

The diagnosis of lymph node metastases relies on the identification of certain features including increase in size, homogeneity, hypoechogenicity, and a round well-demarcated appearance (11,12). Using these characteristics EUS identifies malignant nodes with greater accuracy than the other imaging modalities, described above. It does not, however, provide a histological diagnosis and cannot detect micrometastases in otherwise benign-looking nodes. EUS does not reliably differentiate malignant nodes from those seen in inflammatory disorders which have similar appearances.

Localisation of Neuroendocrine Tumours

Although rare, pancreatic endocrine tumours are notoriously difficult to localise when suspected on clinical and biochemical grounds. Conventional US and CT have a failure rate of 50–80% and angiography 30–50%. EUS, however, has been shown to detect 85% of tumours not visible with conventional imaging including MRI and scintigraphy (13–15). As EUS can visualise the gut wall with high definition, small tumours may be seen in extrapancreatic sites such as the stomach and duodenum although some lesions may be missed (13,15). EUS staging, including vascular invasion, of these tumours also appears to be accurate in many cases although numbers of reported cases are small (15). There could be advantages over intraoperative ultrasonography by facilitating subsequent surgery. Minimal access approaches can be used for anterior lesions in the body and tail of the gland whereas posterior head and uncinate lesions may require open surgery or major resections.

Limitations

In addition to the previous problems alluded to with respect to large tumours, a number of other factors can influence the accuracy of EUS. Previous operation especially total or partial gastrectomy, or duodenal stenosis, can make visual-isation of the full pancreatic region impossible. Large duodenal diverticula or biliary stents interfere with pancreatic imaging due to artefact produced by air. This problem may be overcome by the instillation of saline into the duodenum.

The differentiation between focal chronic pancreatitis and tumour may be difficult to make on ultrasonography (3,16,17) and will require further advances in the technique of fine-needle aspiration cytology using these scopes (18,19).

Summary

EUS has little to offer in the evaluation of large pancreatic tumours. In the case of small tumours EUS may provide useful staging information although it is operator-dependent and is no substitute for histology in lymph node assessment.

EUS is most useful when CT is equivocal or shows no lesion despite a clinical suspicion of pancreatic cancer. EUS is invaluable in the location of endocrine tumours.

EUS of the pancreatic region is a difficult technique to perfect and, like all ultrasound images, can easily be misinterpreted by the inexperienced. Experience with oesophageal and gastric EUS is advisable before progressing to the examination of this region.

Large studies are essential to determine accurately the precise role of EUS in the evaluation of pancreatic pathology and particularly to see if patient outcome is improved as a result of more accurate assessment. For these reasons, EUS should be confined to centres with a sufficient throughput of pancreatic disease. Advances in the technique of EUS guided fine-needle aspiration cytology will aid considerably in the accurate staging of nodal disease and in the differentiation of focal chronic pancreatitis from tumour.

References

1. Yasuda K, Mukai H, Nakajima M, Kawai K (1992) Clinical application of ultrasonic probes in the biliary and pancreatic duct. Endoscopy 24:370–375.
2. Furukawa T, Tsukamoto Y, Naitoh Y, Hirooka Y, Katoh T (1993) Evaluation of intraductal ultrasonography in the diagnosis of pancreatic cancer. Endoscopy 25:577–581.
3. Palazzo L, Roseau G et al. (1993) Endoscopic ultrasonography in diagnosis and staging of pancreatic adenocarcinoma. Endoscopy 25:143–150.
4. Snady H (1993) Clinical utility of endoscopic ultrasonography for pancreatic tumours. Endoscopy 25:182–184.
5. Mueller MF, Meyenberger C, Bertschinger P, Schaer R, Marincek B (1994) Pancreatic tumours: evaluation with endoscopic US, CT and MR imaging. Radiology 190:745–751.
6. Rosch T (1995) Staging of pancreatic cancer. Analysis of literature results. Gastrointest Endosc Clin North Am 5:735–739.
7. Yasuda K, Mukai H, Nakajima M, Kawai K (1993) Staging of pancreatic carcinoma by endoscopic ultrasonography. Endoscopy 25:151–155.
8. Rosch T, Lorenz R, Braig C, Classen M (1992) Endoscopic ultrasonography in diagnosis and staging of pancreatic and biliary tumours. Endoscopy 24:304–308.
9. Rosch T, Braig C, Gain T et al. (1992) Staging of pancreatic and ampullary carcinoma by endoscopic ultrasonography. Comparison with conventional sonography, computed tomography and angiography. Gastroenterology 102:188–199.
10. Snady H, Bruckner H, Siegel J et al. (1993) Endoscopic ultrasonographic criteria of vascular invasion by potentially resectable pancreatic tumours Endoscopy 25:182–184.
11. Grimm H, Hamper K, Binmoeller KF, Soehendra N (1992) Enlarged lymph nodes: malignant or not? Endoscopy 24:320–323.
12. Catalano MF, Sivak MV Jr, Rice T, Gragg LA, Van Dam J (1994) Endosonographic features predictive of lymph node metastasis Gastrointest Endosc 40:442–446.
13. Palazzo L, Roseau G, Salermon M (1992) Endoscopic ultrasonography in the preoperative localisation of pancreatic endocrine tumours. Endoscopy 24:350–353.
14. Rosch T, Lightdale CJ, Botet JF et al (1992) Localisation of pancreatic endocrine tumours by endoscopic ultrasonography. N Engl J Med 326:1721–1726.
15. Zimmer T, Zeigler K, Bader M, Hamm B, Riecken EO, Wiedenmann B 1994. Localisation of neuroendocrine tumours of the upper gastrointestinal tract. Gut 35:471–475.

16. Zuccaro G Jr, Sivak MV Jr (1992) Endoscopic ultrasonography in the diagnosis of chronic pancreatitis. Endoscopy 24:347–349.
17. Hayashi Y, Nakazawa S, Kimoto E, Naito Y, Morita K (1989) Clinicopathologic analysis of endoscopic ultrasonograms in pancreatic mass lesions. Endoscopy 21:121–125.
18. Wiersema MJ, Kochman ML, Cramer HM, Tao LC, Wiersema LM (1994) Endosonography-guided real-time fine-needle aspiration biopsy. Gastrointest Endosc 40:700–707.
19. Chang KJ, Albers G, Erickson RA et al. (1994) Endoscopic ultrasound-guided fine needle aspiration of pancreatic adenocarcinoma. Am J Gastroenterol 89:263–266.

34 Is Histological Diagnosis Essential Before Resection of Suspected Pancreatic Carcinoma?

C.R. Carter and C.W. Imrie

Carcinoma of the pancreas remains a major therapeutic challenge, its incidence is increasing on a global basis (1,2) and over 6000 patients die each year in Britain from the disease (3). Only 15–20% of patients are resectable at the time of diagnosis (4,5). Trede(6) has reported the best actual 5-year survival of 24%. However this was achieved only in those patients with R_0 resections. Most authors report a 2-year survival for resected patients in the region of 20% (7,8). In at least 90–95% of patients therefore, palliation of symptoms and optimising quality of life is the realistic aim of treatment.

In a review, Thomas (9) stated that histological confirmation should be obtained prior to instituting therapy. There is no doubt that, if easily achievable, preoperative histological confirmation of the diagnosis of malignancy is advantageous. The question lies in to what extent the surgeon strives when diagnostic studies are equivocal. Due to the variability of clinical presentation it is extremely difficult to suggest treatment algorithms that are universally applicable to patients. This is particularly true in the management of pancreatic carcinoma, where tumours may or may not have symptoms directly attributable to the mass effect of the tumour.

The need for surgical intervention is often determined by the presence or absence of jaundice, bleeding, or duodenal obstruction. In a patient with obstructive symptoms secondary to a mass lesion in the pancreatic head, resection may be a reasonable option for symptom relief regardless of the underlying diagnosis. By contrast, the subsequent management of a relatively asymptomatic tumour of the body or tail, or the non-operative management of a patient with advanced disease, and their potential inclusion in clinical trials, is dependent on accurate diagnosis. The need for histological confirmation is to a certain extent therefore, inversely proportional to the site and resectability of the lesion.

Differential Diagnosis of a Pancreatic Mass

Although the histological classification of pancreatic lesions is varied (Table 1), in practical terms the diagnosis of a focal pancreatic mass lies between a tumour and chronic pancreatitis. Cystic tumours are easily identified on ultrasound computed tomography (CT) on magnetic resonance imaging (MRI), whereas rapid

Table 1. Differential diagnosis of a pancreatic mass

Chronic pancreatitis		
Tumours	Benign	Microcystic serous adenoma
		Mature cystic teratoma
	Uncertain behaviour	Intraductal papillary tumour
		Intraductal mucin-secreting tumour
		Mucinous cystic tumour
		Solid and papillary (solid/cystic) tumour
	Malignant	Ductal adenocarcinoma
		Mucinous cystadenocarcinoma
		Acinar cell carcinoma (non-cystic)
		Microcystic serous cystadenocarcinoma
		Small cell carcinoma
		Combined exocrine/endocrine tumours
Lymphoma		
Metastases		
Endocrine tumours		Insulinoma
		Gastrinoma
		Other secreting tumours
		Non-functional tumours
Pancreatic pseudocyst		

tumour enhancement and specific clinical or biochemical features may suggest an endocrine tumour. Large, well-circumscribed tumours may suggest the presence of a non-functioning endocrine tumour; however, between 80% and 90% (10,11), are ductal carcinomas. Lymphoma and metastases are rare but their ident-ification has important consequences regarding subsequent treatment. Reports of late renal carcinoma metastases in the pancreas show this lesion may be amenable to effective surgical resection.

Staging Protocol

The evaluation of a patient with pancreatic carcinoma aims firstly to establish the diagnosis, and thereafter to assess the stage of disease and the fitness of the patient. The accuracy of various diagnostic techniques is summarised in Table 2. Imaging techniques may suggest the diagnosis or the potential for resection but histological or cytological techniques are required for confirmation. A core biopsy is the only definitive technique, but there are many reports suggesting that this may lead to tract contamination, potentiate dissemination (24) in addition to increasing the likelihood of subsequent peritoneal cytology being positive (25). The clinical significance of this last finding remains uncertain. Most clinicians will no longer perform a core biopsy whilst resection for potential cure remains a possibility. Our own investigative algorithm for the most common lesions in the head of pancreas is shown in Figure 1.

Positive pancreatic cytology has a specificity of 99% and is usually taken as sufficient confirmation to allow the patient to proceed to surgery, radiotherapy, chemotherapy or to be included in clinical trials. Most patients with a suspected pancreatic tumour will undergo an endoscopic retrograde cholangio pancreato-

Table 2. Accuracy of imaging techniques in pancreatic adenocarcinoma

Author	CT			US			MRI			EUS		
	Sens	Spec	Accuracy	Sens	Spec	Accuracy	Sens	Spec	Accuracy	Sens	Spec	Accuracy
Moskowitz (1984) (17)				84	92							
Neiderau (1985) (13)				81	90							
Rosch (1994) (14)			74			69						94
Palazzo (1993) (15)	69	53		65	60						96	73
Seroni (1995) (16)									79			
Muller (1994) (17)	69	64					83	100			94	100
Megibow (1995) (18)			73						70			
Forsmark (1993) (19)	56	71		44	80		67	86			77	88
Bakkevold (1992) (20)	81	79		73	68							
Yasuda (1993) (21)		38			46							81
Barthet (1996) (22)											100	58
Tio (1996) (23)												84

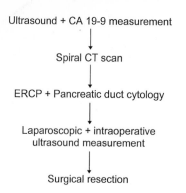

Ultrasound + CA 19-9 measurement

Spiral CT scan

ERCP + Pancreatic duct cytology

Laparoscopic + intraoperative
ultrasound measurement

Surgical resection

Figure 1. Investigative algorithm for suspected CA head of pancreas.

Table 3. False-negative percutaneous fine-needle aspiration patients with pancreatic adenocarcinoma

Author	Year	Patients (n)	False-negative
Alpern (26)	1992	52	42%
Hall Craggs (27)	1986	240	22.5%
Celle (28)	1986	82	23.5%
Athlin (29)	1990	79	24%
Bognel (30)	1988	27	15%
Geng (31)	1987	30	12%
Bakkevold (20)	1992	472	20%
Nakamura (32)	1994	67	28%

gram (ERCP) as part of the staging protocol, allowing brush cytology which has a sensitivity of 70%, which may be improved using duct-specific, over-the-wire techniques. Unfortunately percutaneous fine needle aspirate (FNA) has a sensitivity of only 80% (Table 3) and requires an additional percutaneous procedure. Such sensitivity means that in practice in one in five patients with a suspected pancreatic carcinoma may have no confirmed diagnosis having completed a standard staging protocol.

Pancreatic Cancer and Chronic Pancreatitis

The association between pancreatic cancer and chronic pancreatitis has been known for over 60 years (33). Most studies have been retrospective, postulating an incidence of up to 25% (34), although the median figure in published series is closer to 3%. Epidemiological studies indicate that patients with chronic pancreatitis have a 3–15 times risk of developing pancreatic carcinoma compared with a control population (35). Although these figures relate to cumulative risk, the development of obstructive symptoms in a patient with chronic pancreatitis raises the possibility of a concomitant pancreatic neoplasm. The recent work of Lowenfels coordinating an international prospective study of 2015 patients with chronic pancreatitis identified 56 patients who developed pancreatic carcinoma

Table 4. Mortality resectability and survival from pancreatic resection

Author	Year	Patients (n)	Resectability (%)	Mortality (%)	su
Trede (6)	1990	133	22	2.2%	24
Cameron (38)	1991	52	–	9%	19
Pelligrini (39)	1989	35	–	2%	8
Tsuchiya (40)	1986	106	–	4.2%	–
Baumel (41)	1994	555	21	8%	15
Van Heerden (42)	1984	146	10	4.1%	4 (3 years)
Funovics (43)	1989	100	17	13	5
Mosca (44)	1994	76	42	8	12
Bodner (45)	1988	274	28	6	11
Bradbeer Johnson (8)	1990				

over a mean follow up of 7.4 years (36). The standard incidence ratio was 26.3 (ratio of observed to expected cases). This represented a 1.8% and 4.0% risk of cancer of the pancreas for chronic pancreatitis patients at 10 and 20 years, respectively. They also reckoned this risk was independent of sex, country of origin or type of chronic pancreatitis.

The 1980s were associated with a nihilistic attitude to patients with pancreatic carcinoma because of the associated morbidity and mortality, and many potentially resectable patients were subjected to surgical, endoscopic or radiological palliation rather than risk resection. Bramhall et al. (37) reported representative results of pancreatic resection within the West Midlands with a mortality exceeding 20%. Many studies (Table 4) have shown that pancreatic resection for carcinoma can now be performed in specialist centres with a mortality of less than 5% making resection a viable alternative for the relief of obstructive symptoms.

Resection remains a valuable form of management for painful or complicated chronic pancreatitis. Only two randomised studies (46,47) have compared the efficacy of a standard Whipple resection with the currently more favoured duodenal-preserving procedures. These prospective studies, involving around 40 patients in each, highlighted that both procedures were effective in the alleviation of symptoms, and differences identified were mainly subjective. Although there may well exist a small benefit from duodenal preservation, the difference is small and as such standard or pylorus-preserving Whipple resection remains a reasonable option where neoplasia is a possibility.

Carcinoma of the Pancreatic Body and Tail

The resectability and consequently the prognosis of ductal adenocarcinoma of the body and tail is much lower than that of head, periampullary and ampullary tumours. The symptoms arising from body and tail lesions are later in presentation and potentially less responsive to surgical resection. Moossa's review (48) of the results of resection of body tumours over four decades found only one patient surviving more than 12 months following resection. Recent results from specialist centres (49,50), however, have suggested that improved results may be a possibility due to the earlier diagnosis associated with the widespread adoption of CT scanning for abdominal pain.

Histology at All Costs?

The assessment of patients with suspected pancreatic carcinoma described above will provide histological or cytological confirmation of the diagnosis in up to 90% of patients. In the 10% without such confirmation, subsequent management will be determined by the clinical presentation and the results of the staging investigations. Patients may therefore be divided into three subgroups:

1. Those unfit for resection or with a non-resectable lesion
2. Those without obstructive symptoms and a potentially resectable lesion
3. Those with obstructive symptoms and a mass lesion.

In patients unfit for resection or those with advanced disease, the ability to include these patients in trials of therapy, referral for non-surgical palliative treatments and the identification of unusual tumours that may respond well to alternative treatments (e.g. lymphoma) are dependent on obtaining a tissue diagnosis. Continuing uncertainty surrounding the diagnosis also raises specific difficulties in counselling patients or relatives. The initial results regarding percutaneous FNA reported no morbidity but cutaneous seeding, pancreatic ascites, bruising/bleeding, and peritonitis have all been documented. The risks associated with percutaneous puncture are in practice very small, and where pathological confirmation of diagnosis will alter the treatment algorithm, there is little debate that reasonable efforts should be made to establish the diagnosis, including percutaneous core biopsy if necessary.

Those patients with a descrete mass lesion without obstructive symptoms raise a further dilemma. Asymptomatic tumours are often outwith the pancreatic head, and all resections therefore must in practice be primarily considered palliative. Those lesions considered resectable commonly present as a chance finding, or with minimal symptoms. An asymptomatic focal mass secondary to chronic pancreatitis may require little direct treatment and there is therefore limited prospect of symptom relief. Percutaneous confirmation of the diagnosis is then a reasonable precaution before considering resection.

Most pancreatic surgeons agree that, where appropriate, resection provides the best option for symptomatic pancreatic adenocarcinoma. The aim of therapy is to relieve pain, biliary obstruction or occasionally gastric outflow obstruction. Having positive or negative cytology does not alter the need for surgical decompression, and a Whipple type of resection is a reasonable treatment option. *The majority of patients with pancreatic carcinoma will have the diagnosis confirmed preoperatively by brush cytology.* Subjecting the remainder to further percutaneous aspiration will not alter the treatment algorithm, will not exclude a carcinoma, and exposes the patients to an admittedly small risk of complications. We would therefore suggest that for this group of patients the next rational step in management is to go forward to surgical resection after confirmation of the lack of small surface metastases on the liver or local evidence of non-resectability by laparoscopic ultrasonography, which also provides a more accurate assessment than spiral CT alone. The only drawback to this policy is the occasional unnecessary resection in a patient with chronic pancreatitis and no carcinoma.

References

1. Muir C, Waterhouse J, Mack T, Powell J, Whelan S. Cancer incidence in five continents, vol V. IARC Lyon, (No. 88).
2. Fontham ETH, Correa P. Epidemiology of pancreatic cancer. Surg Clin North Am.
3. Williamson RCN (1988) Pancreatic cancer: the greatest oncological challenge. Br Med J 296:445–446.
4. Trede M (1985) The surgical treatment of pancreatic carcinoma. Surgery 97:28–35.
5. Connelly MM, Dawson PJ, Michaelassi F, Moossa AR, Lowenstein F (1987) Survival in 1001 patients with carcinoma of the pancreas. Ann Surg 122:827–829.
6. Trede M, Schwall G, Saeger HD (1990) Survival after pancreaticoduodenectomy: 118 consecutive patients without operative mortality. Ann Surg 211:447–458.
7. Braasch JW, Rossi RL, Watkin E (1986) Pyloric and gastric preserving pancreatic resection. Ann Surg 204:411–418.
8. Bradbeer J, Johnson CD (1990) Pancreaticogastrostomy after panceaticoduodenectomy. Ann R Coll Surg Eng 72:266–269.
9. Thomas CR, Ngheim HV, Pelligrini CA (1996) Pancreatic cancer: diagnosis and therapy 1995. In Beger HG et al. (eds) Cancer of the pancreas. Universitätsverlag, pp 419–434
10. Baumel H, Deixonne B (1986) Exocrine pancreatic cancer. Springer, Berlin Heidelberg New York.
11. Eelkema EA, Stevens DH, Ward EM (1984) CT Features of non-functioning islet cell carcinoma. AJR 143:943–944.
12. Moskowitz G (1984) Analysis of abdominal imaging procedures. Gastroenterology 87:1408–1413.
13. Neiderau C, Grendell JH (1985) Diagnosis of chronic pancreatitis Gastroenterology 88:1973–1995.
14. Rosch T (1994) Endoscopic ultrasonography. Endoscopy 26:806–807.
15. Palazzo L, Roseau G, Gayet B (1993) Endoscopic ultrasound in the diagnosis and staging of pancreatic adenocarcinoma. Results of a prospective study with comparison to ultrasonography and CT scan. Endoscopy 25:143–150.
16. Sironi S, De Cobelli F, Zerbi A et al. (1995) Pancreatic carcinoma: MR assessment of tumor invasion of the peripancreatic vessels. J Comput Assist Tomogr 19:739–744.
17. Muller MF, Meyenberger C, Bertschinger P et al. Pancreatic tumors: evaluation with endoscopic US, CT, and MR imaging. Radiology 190:745–751.
18. Megibow AJ, Zhou XH, Rotterdam H et al. (1995) Pancreatic adenocarcinoma: CT versus MR imaging in the evaluation of resectability: report of the radiology diagnostic oncology group. Radiology 195:327–332.
19. Forsmark CE, Albert CA, Lambiasc L (1993) Diagnostic test for pancreatic carcinoma. Gastrointestinal Endosc 39:A336.
20. Bakkevold KE, Arnesjo B, Kambestad B (1992) Carcinoma of the pancreas and papilla of Vater: assessment of resectability and factors influencing resectability in stage I carcinomas. A prospective multicentre trial in 472 patients. Eur J Surg Oncol 18:494–507.
21. Yasuda K, Mukai H, Nakajima M, Kawai K (1993) Staging of pancreatic carcinoma by endoscopic ultrasonography. Endoscopy 25:151–155.
22. Barthet M, Portal I, Boujaoude J et al. (1996) Endoscopic ultrasonographic diagnosis of pancreatic cancer complicating chronic pancreatitis. Endoscopy 28:487–491.
23. Tio TL Sie LH, Kallimanis G et al. (1996) Staging of ampullary and pancreatic carcinoma: comparison between endosonography and surgery. Gastroint Endosc 44:706–713.
24. Weiss SM, Skibber JM, Mohiuddin M, Rosato FE (1985) Rapid intra-abdominal spread of pancreatic cancer. Influence of multiple operative biopsy procedures. Arch Surg 120:415–416.
25. Warshaw AL (1991) Implications of peritoneal cytology for staging of early pancreatic cancer. Am J Surg 161:26–30.
26. Alpern GA, Dekker A (1985) Fine needle aspiration cytology of the pancreas. An analysis of its use in 52 patients. Acta Cytol 2:873–878.
27. Hall Craggs MA, Lees WR (1986) Fine-needle aspiration biopsy: Pancreatic and biliary tumors. Am J Roent 1986:147;2,399–403.

28. Celle G, Savarino V, Biggi E (1986) Fine-needle aspiration cytodiagnosis: A simple and safe procedure for cancer of the pancreas. Gast Clin Biol 10:545–548.

29. Athlin L, Blind PJ, Angstrom T (1990) Fine-needle aspiration biopsy of pancreatic masses. Acta Chir Scand 156:91–94.

30. Bognel C, Rougier P, Leclere J et al. (1988) Fine needle aspiration of the liver and pancreas with ultrasound guidance. Acta Cytol 32:22–26.

31. Geng JZ, Qin PR, Hui LD Po PD (1987) CT guided fine needle aspiration biopsy of biliopancreatic lesions: Report of 30 cases. Jpn J Surg 17:461–464.

32. Nakamura R, Machado R, Amikura K et al. (1994) Role of fine needle aspiration cytology and endoscopic biopsy in the preoperative assessment of pancreatic and peripancreatic malignancies. Int J Pancreatol 16:17–21.

33. Walton AJ, Willcox W, Dods EC (1933) Chronic pancreatitis. Trans Med Soc Lond 56:220.

34. Pauline-Netto A, Dreiling DA, Baronofsky ID (1960) The relationship between pancreatic calcification and pancreatic cancer Ann Surg 151:530–537.

35. Neiderau C, Neiderau MC, Heintges T, Luthen R (1996) Relationship between chronic pancreatitis and pancreatic carcinoma. In: Begert HG et al. (eds) Cancer of the pancreas. Universitätsverlag, pp 9–15.

36. Lowenfels AB Maisonneuve P Cavallini G et al. (1993) Pancreatitis and the risk of pancreatic cancer. N Engl J Med 328:1433–1437.

37. Bramhall SR, Allum WH, Jones et al. (1995) Treatment and survival in 13 560 patients with pancreatic cancer, and incidence of the disease, in the West Midlands: an epidemiological study Br J Surg 82:111–115.

38. Cameron JL, Crist DW, Sitzmann JV et al. (1991) Factors influencing survival after pancreatico-duodenectomy for pancreatic adenocarcinoma. Am J Surg 161:120–125.

39. Pellegrini CA, Heck CF, Raper S, Way LW (1989) An analysis of the reduced morbidity and mortality rates after pancreaticoduodenectomy. Arch Surg. 124:778–781.

40. Tsuchiya R, Noda T, Harada N (1986) Collective review of small carcinomas of the pancreas. Ann Surg 203:77–81.

41. Baumel H, Huguer M, Manderscheid JC, Fabre JM, Houry S, Fagot H (1994) Results of resection of cancer of the exocrine pancreas: a study from the French Association of Surgery. Br J Surg 81:102–107.

42. Van Heerden JA (1984) Pancreatic resection for carcinoma of the pancreas Whipple vs total pancreatectomy: an institutional perspective. World J Surg 8:880–888.

43. Funovics JM, Karner J, Pratschner T, Fritsch A (1989) Current trends in the management of carcinoma of the pancreatic head. Hepatogastroenterology 36:450–455.

44. Mosca F, Guilianomi PC, Balestracci T et al. (1994) Preservation of the pylorus in duodeno-cephalo-pancreatectomy in pancreatic and periampullary tumours. Chir Ital 46:59–67.

45. Bodner E (1988) Achievements in tumour surgery in tumours of the pancreas. Langenbecks Arch Chir 2:133–8.

46. Buchler MW, Friess H, Muller MW, Wheatley AM, Beger HG (1995) Randomised trial of duodenum-preserving pancreatic head resection versus pylorus-preserving Whipple in chronic pancreatitis. Am J Surg 169:65–69.

47. Izbicki JR, Bloechle C, Knoefel WT, Kuechler T, Binmoeller KF, Broelsch CE (1995) Duodenum-preserving resection of the head of the pancreas in chronic pancreatitis. A prospective randomised trial. Ann Surg 4:350–358.

48. Moossa AR (1982) Pancreatic cancer. Approach to diagnosis, selection for surgery and choice of operation. Cancer 50:2689–2698.

49. Johnson CD (1991) Why resect pancreatic cancer? In: Johnson CD, Imrie CW (eds) Pancreatic disease. Springer, London, pp 97–102.

35 Pancreatic Resection for Pancreatic Cancer: Outcome in Specialist Units

M.D. Finch and J.P. Neoptolemos

Amongst the earliest published experience of partial pancreaticoduodenectomy was that by Kausch from Germany in 1912 (1) and Whipple from the USA in 1935 (2). Despite technical improvements over the ensuing 40 years many clinicians remained sceptical of resection for pancreatic ductal adenocarcinoma because of previously high postoperative mortality rates and early cancer-related deaths (3,4). However, it is now evident that acceptable morbidity and mortality rates are achievable and that surgical intervention can improve survival. These improved results have come from specialist units (5–14), while the recent results of non-specialist general surgeons demonstrate a high, albeit improved, mortality of 28% in the 1980s compared with earlier years and only a small improvement in survival (15). Continued reluctance to refer patients for consideration of resection is therefore not surprising. The relationship between specialist surgical experience and outcome which has been shown to be important in breast and colon cancer surgery (16,17) has recently been examined with respect to resection for pancreatic cancer.

Postoperative Deaths in General Surgical Units

A recent survey of experience in the West Midlands region of England used Cancer Registry data to identify virtually every case of resected and non-resected pancreatic cancer between 1957 and 1986 inclusive, comprising 13 560 patients in total (15). The data were divided into two time periods comprising an earlier 20-year period and a recent 10-year period. In the recent period from 1977 to 1986 postoperative mortality was 28%; it was 45% in the earlier period. The 5-year survival was also improved to 9.7% from 2.6%. These results relate to the experience of general surgeons in 28 district general hospitals situated within a region of 5.5 million population.

A comparable study to this was carried out by the New York State Department of Public Health using data on 1972 patients who underwent pancreatic resection for malignancy between 1984 and 1991 (11) (Table 1). The difference in the latter study was that both specialist and non-specialist centres were included. The mortality rate was 16% in patients operated on by surgeons performing fewer than nine cases per year but the mortality rate was less than 5% for those performing

Table 1. Hospital mortality rates following resection for ductal adenocarcinoma of the pancreas reported in multi-institutional surveys since 1990

Authors	Population base	Number of institutions (number of surgeons)	Period	Number of resections	Mean number of resections per institution per year	Hospital deaths	% Mortality
Bakkevold & Kambestad 1993 (26)	Norwegian multicentre study	38 (NA)	1984–87	84	0.22	9	10.7[a]
Edge et al. 1993 (23)	University Hospital Consortium, USA	26 (91)	1989–90	128[b]	2.46	10	7.8
Baumel et al. 1994 (25)	French Association of Surgeons	148[d] (NA)	1982–88	787	0.89	77	9.8[c]
Bramhall et al. 1995 (15)	West Midlands region, UK	28 (NA)	1977–87	145	0.52	40	27.6[a]
Wade et al. 1995 (24)	Department of Veterans Affairs Hospitals, USA	98[a] (NA)	1987–91	252	0.43	21	8.3[a]
Lieberman et al. 1995 (11)	State of New York, USA	184 (748)	1984–91	1972	1.53 1.4 (124 units) 1.4–10 (57 units) 10.1–11.4 (1 unit) >11.5 (2 units)	254	12.9 18.9 11.8 12.9 5.5
Gordon et al. 1995 (13)	State of Maryland, USA	39 (NA)	1988–93	502	2.86 <1 (20 units) 1.1–2.2 (9 units) 2.2–3.3 (6 units) 3.3–4.4 (3 units) >4.4 (1 unit)	37	7.7 19.1 14.3 13.0 8.9 2.2
Glasgow et al. 1996 (18)	State of California, USA	298	1990–94	1705	1.43 <1.25 (210 units) 1.35–2.5 (53 units) 2.6–5.0 (20 units) 5.1–7.5 (9 units) 7.6–12.5 (4 units) >12.5 (2 units)	168	9.9 14.1 9.6 8.7 6.9 8.3 3.5
UKPACA 1997 (12)	Pancreatic surgeons (UKPACA), UK	21 (33)	1976–96	421	3.41	25	5.9

NA, not available
[a] 30-Day mortality
[b] Kausch–Whipple resections only
[c] Mortality at 1 month
[d] 3% Response from private units and 19% response from academic units.

more than 41 cases per year. In addition, mortality and hospital caseloads were negatively correlated. In a logistic regression analysis of factors contributing to mortality, individual surgeon caseload was significant but became insignificant when hospital caseload was controlled. The logistic regression curve demonstrating the relationship between caseload and mortality (11) (Figure 1) is virtually superimposable on that of a more recent UK study which analysed non-specialist, specialist and multicentre studies together (12) (Figure 2).

A study in Maryland, USA also showed a significantly improved mortality of 2.2% in the main specialist centre, the Johns Hopkins Hospital, Baltimore, compared with 14% in the remaining centres in Maryland State (13,14) (Table 1). The patients treated outside the main specialist centre, however, were older and had more renal dysfunction, while a much larger percentage of patients at the specialist unit may have had benign disease (14). These data were not standardised for risk factors in contrast to the New York study and another similar study

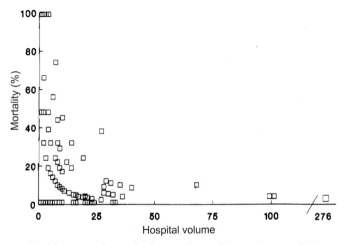

Figure 1. Relationship between hospital volume and mortality in the New York State study (11).

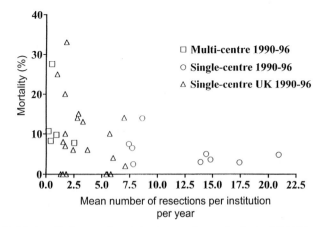

Figure 2. Relationship between hospital volume and mortality in the UKPACA study (12).

from California (18) (Table 1). The California study, comprising 1705 patients, also showed a correlation between hospital caseload and survival (Table 1).

Individual Specialist Experience

The large published series of pancreatic resection from single units have been associated with the lowest mortality rates. In single unit series published between 1990 and 1996 reporting more than 50 cases, mortality rates ranged from 2.2% to 15% (Table 2) (5–10,19–22). Morbidity rates have not been reported consistently enough in most of these studies to permit proper comment. Several of the reports indicated a decrease in operative mortality over time, further supporting the concept that experience is related to outcome.

Collective Specialist Experience

Recent studies which fall into this category are those which focus on surgeons from university hospitals or referral units, the results of which are summarised in Table 1. The study by Edge et al. in 1993 (22) audited 26 US university hospitals. The overall postoperative mortality was 7.8% with a major morbidity rate of 21%. Morbidity but not mortality rate was correlated with a surgeon caseload of less than four per year, but there were too few events (deaths versus total cases per surgeon) to be able to show with any confidence a relationship between mortality rate and individual surgeon caseload (Type II statistical error).

Reports from the US Veterans' Administration hospitals (23) and from the French Association of Surgeons (24) largely reflect specialist practice. In the former case (23), although the number of cases per hospital was low, the surgeons performing these operations often had simultaneous appointments at university hospitals where their caseload was probably higher. Such an affiliation accounted for the majority of surgeons in the study. The study found no significant correlation of hospital outcome with specific university affiliation but the data were not analysed according to individual surgeon caseload. There was no significant correlation between mortality and hospital caseload but the events for each hospital were again too few to be able to demonstrate a significant relationship (Type II statistical error). The French study (24) was performed using a voluntary questionnaire and the response rate was only 3% for private units and 19% for academic units. With this type of data collection, those units with good results and with large patient numbers kept in active databases are most likely to participate. The mortality rate of 10% therefore must be considered reflective largely of specialist practice in France. No attempt was made in this study to correlate mortality with surgeon or hospital caseload.

In a multicentre trial of adjuvant chemotherapy in Norway (25,26) morbidity and mortality data were collected prospectively on 84 patients undergoing Whipple's resection for pancreatic ductal adenocarcinoma. Operative mortality among 20 institutions was 10.7%. Although the mean number of cases recorded per hospital was low, this number did not include patients undergoing resection who were not in the trial, and the authors indicated that accrual was slow. No correlation with surgeon or hospital caseload was attempted. Because resections

Table 2. Hospital mortality rates following resection for ductal adenocarcinoma of the pancreas from single institutions with 50 or more cases published since 1990

Authors	Institution	Period	Number of resections	Mean number of resections per year	Hospital deaths	% Mortality
Trede et al. 1990 (6)	Mannheim, Germany	1972–89	133	7.8	3	2.2
Gall et al. 1991 (19)	Erlangen, Germany	1969–87	138	7.7	9	6.5
Geer & Brennan 1993 (8)	Memorial Sloan-Kettering Cancer Center, New York, USA	1983–90	146	20.9	7	4.8
Hanyu et al. 1993 (22)	Women's Medical College, Tokyo, Japan	1978–90	167	13.9	5	3.0
Takahashi et al. 1994 (21)	Keio University, Tokyo, Japan	1976–92	137	8.6	19	13.9
Allema et al. 1995 (9)	Amsterdam Medical Centre, Holland	1983–92	67	7.4	5	7.5
Nitecki et al. 1995 (10)	Mayo Clinic, Rochester, USA	1981–91	174	17.4	5	2.9
Yeo et al. 1995 (20)	Johns Hopkins, Baltimore, USA	1970–94	201	14.4	10	5.0
Beger et al. 1996 (7)	Ulm, Germany	1982–95	193	14.8	7	3.6

Table 3. Summary of logistic regression analyses on the sets of data from the UKPACA (12) series, published multi-institutional series, and published specialist units, using the caseload to model the mortality statistics

Series	Improvement χ^2 for using caseload	Goodness of fit χ^2	Logit slope (standard error)	Constant (standard error)
UKPACA series (12)	$\chi^2_1 = 7.17$ $P = 0.007$	$\chi^2_{15} = 14$ $P = 0.53$ (NS)	0.3 (0.12)	1.68 (0.43)
Multi-institutional series (11,12,15,23,26)	$\chi^2_1 = 14.18$ $P < 0.001$	$\chi^2_4 = 29.6$ $P < 0.001$	0.29 (0.08)	1.82 (0.12)
Specialist units (6–10,19,21,22)	$\chi^2_1 = 5.38$ $P = 0.02$	$\chi^2_7 = 18.6$ $P = 0.009$	0.07 (0.03)	2.1 (0.37)

NS, not significant.

were only performed in 20 of 38 hospitals eligible for the trial it is reasonable to infer that specialist experience was concentrated in these 20 units.

Recently a comprehensive survey of morbidity and mortality in UK specialist units was undertaken by the UK Pancreatic Cancer Group (UKPACA) (12). The study was specifically designed to answer questions related to caseload. In contrast to the USA, surgeons in the UK largely perform this type of surgery in a single institution, so such an analysis is more straightforward in the UK. Only recognised units with relatively high caseloads were included. Logistic regression analysis of the UKPACA data, of large single institution studies and five other multi-institutional studies published since 1990 showed that institutional caseload was a significant predictor of mortality for all three groups (Table 3, Figure 1). The goodness of fit χ^2 statistic of the logit model for the UKPACA data was not significant, indicating that caseload was the single most important variable related to mortality. The logit models for the UKPACA and for the other multi-institutional studies, including the UK West Midlands study were not significantly different from each other. Thus the 5.9% versus 27.6% difference in outcome in the two UK studies appears to be directly related to hospital caseload.

Complications

Postoperative morbidity is much more difficult to quantify as definitions of specific complications and consistency of reporting vary from unit to unit. In both of the recent UK multicentre studies (12,15) these data were too incomplete for analysis. Multicentre studies that have reported complications include the Norwegian study (25,26), the US veterans study (23) and the US university hospitals study (22). Bakkevold et al. (25) reported haemorrhage in 15%, intra-abdominal abscess in 8%, pancreatitis and septicaemia in 4% and general complications not specifically related to pancreas surgery in 15% in a series of 84 cases. The US university hospitals study reported an overall major complication rate of 22% and a correlation between complication rate and the experience of the surgeon (22). In the US veterans study, septic complications were recorded in 15% and pancreatic leak in 5% (23). The other most common complications were pneumonia, gastrointestinal bleeding, wound dehiscence, wound infection, and postoperative bleeding (23). Preoperative biliary drainage was associated with a non-significant decrease in mortality from 9% to 3%, but the morbidity rate was significantly increased in the drained group from 33% to 56% due to increased rates of sepsis, wound dehiscence and postoperative bleeding.

In the Johns Hopkins experience, delayed gastric emptying was the most frequent complication at 36%, followed by pancreatic fistula in 19%, intra-abdominal abscess in 9%, wound infection in 8%, pancreatitis and bile leak in 6% and cholangitis in 5%; there was no mention of postoperative bleeding (20). There was no significant difference for any of these complications in relation to the indication for operation or to the age of the patient.

Sperti et al. (27) reported an overall morbidity rate of 10% including pancreatic leak in 3% and intra-abdominal abscess in 2% and no intraoperative bleeding after a standard Kausch–Whipple's resection.

The literature needs to be interpreted cautiously over the issue of whether the morbidity rate is increased in older patients undergoing resection. Whilst some studies have cited age as a risk factor for morbidity and mortality, others have shown that it is possible to achieve respectable results in the over 70 years age group. Declore et al. (28) reported an overall morbidity of 14% and a mortality of 5% in this group while Spencer et al. (29) reported figures of 28% and 12% respectively. Clearly good results can be achieved in older patients but this must involve a degree of patient selection based on sound clinical judgement.

Survival

The trend toward improving 5-year survival for patients who have undergone resection for pancreatic cancer is more apparent than real. Five-year survival rates following pancreaticoduodenectomy for pancreatic ductal adenocarcinoma

Table 4. Five-year survival rates from single institutions

Institution	Year published	Overall 5-year survival rate %
Memorial Sloan Kettering (8)	1993	24
Mannheim (6)	1990	24
Johns Hopkins (20)	1995	21
Keio University, Tokyo (21)	1994	14
Kyoto, Japan (48)	1990	14
Erlangen (33)	1996	13
Boston (49)	1993	13
Copenhagen (50)	1994	13
Padua (28)	1996	12
Erlangen (19)	1991	11
Rotterdam (51)	1993	11
Mayo Clinic (10)	1995	6.8
Munich (35)	1992	6
Amsterdam (9)	1995	0

(excluding other periampullary tumours) from specialist units reported over the past 5 years ranged from 0 to 24% (Table 4).

The reasons for this degree of range are not entirely clear but include variations in disease stage, tumour size, resection margin involvement and the inclusion of cases other than ductal adenocarcinoma of the pancreas, all of which have been shown to affect survival (22,30,31). The absence of lymph node metastases for example is associated with an improvement in 5-year survival of between 19% and 45% (10,20,23,25,32–34).

The survival rates from the West Midlands Region seem to indicate that survival was not related to specialist experience or to operative mortality (15). Surprisingly, in a significant proportion of the multi-institutional series, resections were carried out in the face of advanced disease. This perhaps accounts for the somewhat lesser survival in some of these series than has been seen in non-specialist reports, where such patients are rarely resected. Nevertheless, factors which would seem to be related to specialist experience have also been related to longer survival. Cameron et al. (34) found a significant correlation between operative blood loss and survival in a multivariate analysis. Trede et al. (6) and Bakkevold et al. (25,26) have confirmed that a clear microscopic as well as macroscopic resection using a standard Kausch–Whipple resection is associated with an appreciably increased 5-year survival rate.

Beyond Conventional Surgery

In many centres with a large experience surgical technique has been extended beyond the classical Kausch–Whipple procedure, either in an attempt to preserve normal gastric function in the case of the pylorus-preserving procedure, or for the purpose of radically removing otherwise unresectable tumours by the use of extended resection. In the recent UKPACA series, 32% of all pancreatic cancers and 41% of all ampullary cancers resected in specialist units were by pylorus-preserving methods (12). Although there is no completed randomised study all but one of the published comparisons of pylorus-preserving versus standard resection of the head of the pancreas have indicated a similar survival (31,35–39).

Nagakawa et al. (40) reported a 5-year survival of 27% for macroscopically resected tumours and 40% after microscopic clearance. Care is needed in interpreting the results of such reports because of the problem of stage migration in retrospectively allocating patients to more or less favourable survival groups (already knowing the survival of patients allocated). The technique used involved radical clearance of the lymph nodes and nerve plexus from the coeliac axis down to the aortic bifurcation, and when necessary portal vein resection, with a post-operative mortality of 9.4%. Takahashi et al. (41), using a similar technique, reported a similar mortality rate but with a 5-year survival of 15% after curative resection. Klempnauer et al. (42) reported using a radical lymphadenectomy and as needed resection of the hepatic portal vein, various branches of the coeliac axis, superior mesenteric artery or adjacent involved organs with an overall 5-year survival of 13.3%. The 5-year survival ranged from 13% to 21% depending on which vessels were resected. But when other organs were resected in addition to the hepatic portal vein, including the colon, liver, adrenal gland, kidney or other organ, the 5-year survival rate was nil with a median survival of only 3 to 7 months. The mortality rate was high except in the case of simultaneous hepatic

Table 5. Five-year survival rates from multi-institution reports

	Overall 5-year survival rate (%)	5-year survival for stages I & II (%)	5-year survival for stages III & IV (%)
Norwegian study (26)	< 1	< 2	0
French Association of Surgeons (24)	12	20	4
US Veterans study (23)	9		
US Commission on Cancer (30)	3–4	17	
West Midlands (15)	9.7		

portal vein resection or hepatectomy. Furhman et al. (43) have reported that *en bloc* resection of the superior mesenteric–portal vein confluence had no significant impact on morbidity or mortality. Perhaps for some patients the operative risk was worthwhile considering that prolonged survival would have been impossible otherwise.

Resection involving excision of the portal–superior mesenteric vein or other adjacent organs such as the transverse mesocolon may help to convert a locally advanced tumour into a resection. There is no convincing evidence that extended pancreatic resections and extended lymphadenectomy improve long-term survival, whilst the latter is associated with severe side effects including protracted hospital stay, refractory diarrhoea and sustained weight loss. Apparently good results are related to the phenomenon of stage migration especially when the results using the Japanese staging classification are compared with the UICC or the American Cancer Society Staging Systems (44,45). Critical comparisons show an improvement for each stage yet the overall survival of the resected group remains directly comparable to that obtained using non-radical procedures. Pedrazzoli et al. (46) have carried out a randomised trial comparing traditional pancreaticoduodenectomy with or without the addition of a more extensive lymph node dissection. The results of this study are discussed in Chapter 36.

Conclusion

Several recent studies have indicated that morbidity and mortality rates following resection for pancreatic adenocarcinoma are optimal in specialist centres and that resection can be undertaken with equally good results in older patients in such centres. The West Midlands study (15) showed that the mortality rate in general surgical units improved in the 1980s compared with earlier years but was still unacceptably high. While the survival in that study was reasonable considering the stage of disease, one cannot ignore the fact that many of these patients were not given this chance for survival. Even so, in specialist centres long-term survival was still very poor. Several small studies have demonstrated promising improvements using adjuvant therapies (26,47). As these and other modalities are developed and placed into larger clinical trials only patients who have recovered from resection will have the opportunity to participate. In addition to the negative impact on quality of life, postoperative complication can delay and sometimes preclude trial entry, and hence can slow progress toward finding effective adjuvant treatments. Concentration therefore of major pancreatic resection into specialist centres should not only optimise immediate outcome, it is also the most appropriate means of improving the present dismal results in survival.

References

1. Kausch W (1912) Das Carcinom der Papilla duodeni und seine radikale Entfemung. Beitr Klin Chir 78:439–486.
2. Whipple AO, Parsons WB, Mullins CR (1935) Treatment of cancer of the ampulla of Vater. Am Surg 102:763–779.
3. Crile GC (1970) The advantages of bypass operations over radical pancreaticoduodenectomy in the treatment of pancreatic carcinoma. Surg Gynecol Obstet 130:1049–1053.
4. Carter DC (1980) Surgery for pancreatic cancer. Br Med J I:744–746
4a. Gall FP, Kessler H, Hermanek P (1991) Surgical treatment of ductal pancreatic carcinoma. Eur J Surg Oncol 17: 173–181.
5. Hanyu F, Suzuki M, Imaizumi T (1993) Whipple operation for pancreatic carcinoma: Japanese experience. In: Beger HG, Bnchler M, Malfertheiner P (eds). Standards in pancreatic surgery. Springer, Berlin Heidelberg New York, pp 646–653.
6. Trede M, Schwall G, Saeger H-D (1990) Survival after pancreatoduodenectomy: 118 resections without an operative mortality. Ann Surg 211:447–458.
7. Beger HG, Link KH, Poch B, Gansauge F (1996) Pancreatic cancer: recent progress in diagnosis and treatment. In: Neoptolemos JP, Lemoine NR (eds). Pancreatic cancer: molecular and clinical Advances. Blackwell Science, Oxford, pp. 227–235.
8. Geer RJ, Brennan MF (1993) Prognostic indicators for survival after resection of pancreatic adenocarcinoma. Am J Surg 165:68–73.
9. Allema JH, Reinders ME, van Gulik TM et al. (1995) Prognostic factors for survival after pancreaticoduodenectomy for patients with carcinoma of the pancreatic head region. Cancer 75:2069–2076.
10. Nitecki SS, Sarr MG, Colby TV, van Heerden JA (1995) Long-term survival after resection for ductal adenocarcinoma of the pancreas. Is it really improving? Ann Surg 221:59–66.
11. Lieberman MD, Kilburn H, Lindsay M, Brennan MF (1995) Relation of perioperative deaths to hospital volume among patients undergoing pancreatic resection for malignancy. Ann Surg 222:638–645.
12. The UK Pancreatic Cancer Group (UKPACA) (1997) Low mortality following resection for pancreatic and periampullary tumours in 1026 patients: UK survey of pancreatic specialist units. Br J Surg (in press).
13. Gordon TA Burleyson GP, Tieslch JM, Cameron JL (1995) The effects of regionalization on cost and outcome for one general high-risk surgical procedure. Ann Surg 221:43–49.
14. Cameron JL, Pitt HA, Yeo CJ, Lillemoe KD, Kaufman KS (1993) One hundred and forty-five pancreaticoduodenectomies without mortality. Ann Surg 217: 430–438.
15. Bramhall SR, Allum WH, Jones AG, Allwood A, Cummins C, Neoptolemos JP (1995) Treatment and survival in 13 560 patients with pancreatic cancer, and incidence of the disease in the West Midlands: an epidemiological study. Br J Surg 82: 111–115.
16. McCardle CS, Hole D (1991) Impact of variability among surgeons on post-operative morbidity and mortality and ultimate survival. Br Med J 301: 1501–1505.
17. Gillis CR, Hole DJ (1996) Survival outcome of care by specialist surgeons in breast cancer: a study of 3786 patients in the west of Scotland. Br Med J 312:145–148.
18. Glasgow RE, Mulvihill SJ (1996) Hospital volume influences outcome in patients undergoing pancreatic resection for cancer. West Med J 165:254–300.
19. Gall FP, Kessler H, Hermanek P (1991) Surgical treatment of ductal pancreatic carcinoma. Eur J Surg Oncol 17:173–181.
20. Yeo CJ, Cameron JL, Lillemoe KD et al. (1995) Pancreaticoduodenectomy for cancer of the head of the pancreas: 201 patients. Ann Surg 221:721–723.
21. Takahashi S, Ogata Y, Tsuzuki T (1994) Combined resection of the pancreas and portal vein for pancreatic cancer. Br J Surg 81:1190–1193.
22. Edge SE, Schmieg RE, Rosenlof LK, Wilhelm MC (1993) Pancreas cancer resection outcome in American university centres in 1989–1990. Cancer 71:3502–3508.

23. Wade TP, El-Ghazzaway AG, Virgo KS, Johnson FE (1995) The Whipple resection for cancer in US Department of Veterans' Affairs Hospitals. Ann Surg 221: 2141-2148.
24. Baumel H, Hugyuier M, Manderscheid JC, Fabre JM, Houry S, Fagot H. (1994) Results of resection in cancer of the exocrine pancreas. A study from the French Association of Surgeons. Br J Surg 81:102-107.
25. Bakkevold KE, Kambestad B (1993) Long-term survival following radical and palliative treatment of patients with carcinoma of the pancreas and papilla of Vater: the prognostic factors influencing the long-term results. A prospective multicentre trial. Eur J Surg Oncol 19:147-161.
26. Bakkevold KE, Amesjo Bo, Dahl O, Kambestad B (1993) Adjuvant combination chemotherapy (AMF) following radical resection of carcinoma of the pancreas and papilla of vater: results of a controlled, prospective, randomised multicentre study. Eur J Cancer 29A: 698-703.
27. Sperti C, Pasquali A, Piccoli A, Pedrazzoli S (1996) Survival after resection for ductal adenocarcinoma of the pancreas. Br J Surg 83:625-631.
28. Declore R, Thomas JH, Hermreck A (1991) Pancreaticoduodenectomy for malignant pancreatic neoplasms in elderly patients. Am J Surg 162:532-535.
29. Spencer MP, Sarr MG, Nagorney DM (1989) Radical pancreatectomy for pancreatic cancer in the elderly: is it safe and justified? Ann Surg 212:140-143.
30. Janes RH, Niederhuber JE, Chmeil JS et al. (1996) National patterns of care for pancreatic cancer. Ann Surg 223:261-272.
31. Grace PA, Pitt HA, Tomkins RK, DenBesten L, Longmire W (1986) Decreased morbidity and mortality after pancreatoduodenectomy. Am J Surg 151:141-149.
32. Tannapfel A, Wittekind C, Hunefeld G (1992) Ductal adenocarcinoma of the pancreas. Histopathological features and prognosis. Int J Pancreatol 12:145-152.
33. Declore R, Rodriguez FJ, Forster J, Hermaneck AS, Thomas JH (1996) Significance of lymph node metastases in patients with pancreatic cancer undergoing curative resection. Am J Surg 172:463-469.
34. Cameron JL, Crist DL, Sitzman JV et al. (1991) Factors influencing survival after pancreatico-duodenectomy for pancreatic cancer. Am J Surg 161:120-125.
35. Roder JD, Stein HJ, Huttl W, Siewert JR (1992) Pylorus-preserving versus standard pancreatico-duodenectomy: an analysis of 110 pancreatic and periampullary carcinomas. Br J Surg 79:152-155.
36. Klinkenbijl JHG, van der Schelling GP, Hop WCJ, van Pel R, Bruining HA, Jeekel J (1992) The advantages of pylorus-preserving pancreatoduodenectomy in malignant disease of the pancreas and periampullary region. Ann Surg 216:142-145.
37. Braasch JW, Deziel DJ, Rossi RL, Watkins E, Jr, Winter PF (1986) Pyloric and gastric preserving pancreatic resection. Experience with 87 patients. Ann Surg 204:411-418.
38. Grace PA, Pitt HA, Longmire WP (1990) Pylorus-preserving pancreatoduodenectomy: an overview. Br J Surg 77:968-974.
39. Zerbi A, Balzano G, Patuzzo R, Calori G, Braga M, Di Carlo V (1995) Comparison between pylorus-preserving and Whipple pancreatoduodenectomy. Br J Surg 82:975-979.
40. Nagakawa T, Masanori N, Futakami F et al. (1996) Results of extensive surgery for pancreatic carcinoma. Cancer 77:640-645.
41. Takahashi S, Ogata Y, Miyazaki H (1995) Aggressive surgery for pancreatic duct cell cancer: feasibility, validity, limitations. World J Surg 19:653-660.
42. Klempnauer J, Ridder GJ, Bektas H, Pichlmayr R (1996) Extended resections of ductal pancreatic cancer: impact on operative risk and prognosis. Oncology 53:47-53.
43. Fuhrman GM, Leach SD, Staley CA et al. (1996) Rationale for en bloc vein resection in the treatment of pancreatic adenocarcinoma adherent to the superior mesenteric-portal vein confluence. Ann Surg 223:154-162.
44. Ishikawa O, Ohigashi H, Sasaki Y (1988) Practical usefulness of lymphatic and connective tissue clearance for the carcinoma of the pancreas head. Ann Surg 208:215-220.
45. Kobari M, Sunamura M, Ohashi O, Saitoh Y, Yusa T, Matsuno S (1996) Usefulness of Japanese staging in the prognosis of patients treated operatively for adenocarcinoma of the head of the pancreas. J Am Coll Surg 182:24-32.
46. Pedrazzoli S, Di Carlo V, Dionigi R, Michelassi F, Mosca F, Pederzoli P (1993) Preliminary results of traditional and extended lymphadenectomy in resection of pancreatic head cancer. Digestion 54:299 (abstract).
47. The Gastrointestinal Tumor Study Group (1987) Further evidence of effective adjuvant combined radiation and chemotherapy following urative resection of pancreatic cancer. Cancer 59:2006-2010.

48. Manabe T, Ohshio G, Bab N, Tobe T (1990) Factors influencing prognosis and indications for curative pancreatectomy for ductal adenocarcinoma of the head of the pancreas. Int J Pancreatol 7:137–143.

49. Willet CG, Lewandrowski K, Warshaw AL, Efird J, Compton CC (1993) Resection margins in carcinoma of the head of the pancreas. Implications for radiation therapy. Ann Surg 217:144–148.

50. Anderson HB, Baden H, Brabe NE, Bucharth F (1994) Pancreaticoduodenectomy for periampullary adenocarcinoma. J Am Coll Surg 179:545–552.

51. Klinkenbijl JHG, Jeekel J, Schmitz PIM et al. (1993) Carcinoma of the pancreas and periampullary region: palliation versus cure. Br J Surg 80: 1575–1578.

36 Resection in Cancer: Lymph Node Dissection

C. Bassi, M. Falconi, S. Pedrazzoli, C. Pasquali and P. Pederzoli

Radical resection of ductal carcinoma of the pancreas affords the only realistic chance of a cure. Though the disappointing results achieved to date in terms of overall long-term survival of resected patients still prompt many surgeons to refrain from surgical intervention (1), over the years there has been a progressive increase in resection rates, which have steadily risen from around 20% some 15 to 20 years ago to an average of 35% of cases observed today and which now even exceed 50% in some centres (2).

We believe it to be ethically mandatory to regard "taking it out" as the primary aim of curative treatment of carcinoma of the pancreas in those centres where the morbidity (around 30%) and mortality rates (< 5%) make this a feasible proposition. Clearly, this can only apply in those cases in which the preoperative staging has ruled out both remote metastases and locoregional irresectability.

Unfortunately, however, even when carried out by expert investigators with all the benefits of advanced technology, clinical staging tells us little or nothing about the presence and extent of lymph node involvement (3). In other words, the N factor can be clarified only after surgical resection, and the reliability of lymph node negativity is directly related to the size of the specimen sent to the pathologist and thus to the extent of the lymphadenectomy performed.

The risk of false-negatives, particularly in Western surgical practice with its comparative reluctance to perform extended lymphadenectomies (though, as we shall see later, the classic Whipple procedure removes most of the commonly involved lymph nodes), is a result of the lack of anatomical contiguity in the lymphatic invasion pattern of the pancreatic carcinoma, with positivity in remote lymph node stations and negative peripancreatic lymph nodes. In addition, there is frequently a lack of any correlation between tumour diameter and lymph node positivity, which, in some case series, may be present in half of cases with a small tumour (T < 2 cm) (4).

The result of this bizarre behaviour of the N factor, of its as yet unclear specific prognostic significance as distinct from other cofactors, and of the lack of any correlation between lymph node positivity and adjuvant therapeutic options, and unlike the situation in other digestive and non-digestive tract cancers (e.g. of the colon and breast), is that the effective need for a more or less extended lymphadenectomy accompanying the resection in carcinoma of the pancreas remains a hotly debated issue.

In this chapter we shall attempt to tackle the problems associated with the pattern of lymph node involvement in pancreatic carcinoma and its prognostic significance. This type of analysis is the necessary forerunner to any attempt to interpret the usefulness of extended lymphadenectomy compared with basic traditional resection.

Frequency and Pattern of Lymph Node Involvement in Pancreatic Cancer

In pancreatic ductal carcinoma, the percentage of resected patients with lymph node involvement is around 70% in the patient samples described in the literature (5–22).

The different, more aggressive surgical approach adopted in Japan might be thought to lead to a generally higher incidence of lymph node positivity in case series in the Far East. In fact, the percentage distribution in the various studies shows no significant difference. The figure reported by the Japan Pancreas Society (74.6% positivity) (15) is comparable to the rates reported in European (10) and USA (18) studies (67.5 and 71.6%, respectively). In our own more recent series of 54 patients undergoing pancreaticoduodenectomy of the head of the pancreas for ductal carcinoma, 32 (60%) were lymph node-positive.

Particularly interesting, in this connection, are the studies conducted by Cubilla and Fitzgerald (7), which show that the classic Whipple pancreaticoduodenectomy successfully removes 80% of the lymph node sites most commonly involved in the carcinoma. We shall discuss later whether or not the remaining 20% of sites potentially at risk of presenting malignant residues justify a more extended resection.

Apart from the above-mentioned study, the literature contains very few reports of pathological analyses of surgical specimens aimed at establishing the topographical distribution of the lymph node areas affected by metastatic spread (4,8,23). In this sector, the Japanese literature is by far the most informative, thanks above all to Nagakawa's study (4), where the patterns of lymph node metastases are analysed in 42 specimens from resections of the pancreatic head with particular reference to the correlation between the frequency of para-aortic lymph node involvement and the extent of the primary tumour. The intention is clearly to assess, on the basis of quantitative evidence, whether lymphadenectomy should be also extended to the remote lymph nodes and whether this is a rational step.

Thirty-three of 42 patients (79%) had lymph-node metastases, and threequarters of these lymph node-positive subjects showed simultaneous positivity of the resection margin of the posterior surface of the pancreas. The lymph node areas most affected, according to the Japanese general rules for the study of pancreatic cancer (15) (Table 1), were areas 13 (posterior to the head of the pancreas; 29/33), 17 (anterior to the head of the pancreas; 17/33) and 14 (root of the mesentery; 16/33), followed by areas 12 (hepatoduodenal ligament; 9/33) and 16 (along the abdominal aorta; 7/33). All other sites were only sporadically affected. In particular, in area 16 (along the aorta) 16% of patients had nodal involvement. The highest incidence (70% of affected nodes) in this group was in the interaortocaval region.

The extent of lymphatic metastasis tends to increase with tumour diameter, though the finding of two cases of small tumours (diameter < 2 cm) which had already metastasised to area 16 provided evidence of a poor correlation, with unpredictable involvement and distribution of the N factor as compared with the T factor.

Table 1. Regional lymph node of the pancreas

Area number	Location
1	Right cardiac region
2	Left cardiac region
3	Along the lesser curvature of the stomach
4	Along the greater curvature
5	Suprapyloric region
6	Infrapyloric region
7	Along the left gastric artery
8a	Anterior-posterior region of the common hepatic artery
8p	Posterior region of the common hepatic duct
9	Coeliac axis
10	Hilum of the spleen
11	Along the splenic artery
12h	Hepatoduodenal ligament
12a1	Upper portion of the proper hepatic artery
12a2	Lower portion of the proper hepatic artery
12p1	Upper portion of the portal vein
12p2	Lower portion of the portal vein
12b1	Along the proximal bile duct
12b2	Along the distal bile duct
12c	Along the cystic duct
13	Posterior to the head of the pancreas
13a	Superior and posterior to the head of the pancreas
13b	Inferior and posterior to the head of the pancreas
14	Mesenteric root
14A	Along the superior mesenteric artery
14a	Root of the superior mesenteric artery
14b	Root of the inferior pancreaticoduodenal artery
14c	Root of the middle colic artery
14d	Root of the jejunal artery
14V	Along the superior mesenteric vein
15	Along the middle coelic artery
16	Along the abdominal aorta
17	Anterior to the head of the pancreas
17a	Superior and anterior of the head of the pancreas
17b	Inferior and anterior of the head of the pancreas
18	Along the inferior border of pancreatic body–tail

According to the General Rules for Cancer of the Pancreas (15).

This unpredictability is further confirmed by our own experience: in a study aimed at detecting small tumours of the pancreatic head (14), none of the four cases prospectively identified out of 72 consecutive observations were node-positive. By contrast, three of seven small tumours identified retrospectively in 56 historical patients were node-positive; even one of the more recent lymph node-positive cases (in a total of 32 node-positive cases) had a diameter of 1.5 cm.

These data, along with those of other studies in both animals (24) and human subjects (25), would appear to suggest that the pathway of para-aortic metastases passes via a retroperitoneal lymphatic route from area 13 to area 14 before reaching area 16. On the basis of this analysis, Nagakawa et al. (4) conclude that "an extensive dissection including areas 14 and 16 is necessary for radical resection".

Can this pattern of lymph-node involvement also be regarded as valid for Western case series? To answer this question we analysed 54 consecutive resections of the head of the pancreas performed recently in the University of Verona Surgical Department in patients with pancreatic ductal carcinoma.

Thirty-two cases were node-positive. The lymph-node sites mainly affected were the pancreatic-paraduodenal areas 13 and 17 (30/32) followed by the hepatoduodenal ligament area 12 (positive nodes in 7/27 radical lymphadenectomies performed in that site) and the mesenteric area 14 (positive in 3/16 radical lymphadenectomies performed in that site). A similar pattern to the Japanese one is thus confirmed in a Western patient sample.

Failure to perform a standard lymphadenectomy in all patients in our series might be interpreted as the result of a variable surgical approach by the surgeons performing the resections (P.P., C.B. and M.F.). In fact, Western surgeons often find themselves having to operate on patients who, despite the disease, have major intra-abdominal obesity of a type which, for anthropomorphic and dietetic reasons, is comparatively rare in Eastern populations. This technical obstacle often proves insurmountable except by prolonging the operative times and increasing the risks of the procedure.

For this reason, our series included only 15 node-positive cases (47%) potentially capable of providing data on the ill-famed area 16. Two patients (13%) had positive nodes in this area, both in lymph nodes of interaortocaval origin. The similarities to Nagakawa's findings (4), in terms of both frequency and site, are striking.

In one of our two cases, sequential involvement of areas 13 → 14 → 16 was observed, whereas, in the other, the area 16 positivity coincided with positivity only of area 13, all the other areas yielding negative findings. The erratic pattern of lymph node involvement is also confirmed by two cases which were lymph node negative in area 13, but positive at the level of the hepatoduodenal ligament (area 12): one of these tumours had a diameter of 1.5 cm (the above-mentioned small node-positive tumour) and the other a diameter of 4 cm.

Despite these incongruities, which make any correlation between N and T factors unreliable, in our case series the mean diameter of the node-negative tumours was less than that of the node-positive malignancies (26.3 mm, range 10 to 40; and 30.5 mm, range 15 to 40, respectively).

Lymph Node Involvement and Prognosis

Despite the generally widespread conviction that the presence of lymph node metastases is a highly prejudicial factor for the prognosis of pancreatic carcinoma, this is by no means an established fact in the literature. While a number of recent reports (1993–1996) support this view (5,18,26,27), others regard the N stage as being of secondary prognostic importance, as compared, particularly, with tumour diameter and the T stage (28–31). All these discordant opinions are supported by statistical analyses conducted, with a sole exception (31), in sizeable patient samples.

A number of the studies, including very recent ones (5,9,10), failed to tackle the issue on the basis of multivariate analysis, leaving the reader with the suspicion that some other cofactor potentially capable of affecting the prognosis (such as, for instance, patient age, type of surgery, tumour diameter, invasion of retroperitoneal vascular and nerve structures, tumour grading, units of blood transfused, invasion or otherwise of the resection margin, aneuploidy and adjuvant therapy, if any) may to some extent blur the real significance of lymph node involvement.

In 1991, an elegant study by Cameron et al. (22) showed, however, that, in multivariate analysis, the strongest predictive factor is lymph node status with a median survival of 55.8 months in node negative patients as against 11 months in node-positive subjects. The relative risk (3.31) was even greater than that of vascular invasion (2.19).

In 1995, the same group (18) substantially confirmed the findings for lymph node status, associating it, additionally, with tumour diameter (> 3 cm) and the state of the resection margin, with relative risks of 1.6, 1.7 and 1.4, respectively. In a subpopulation of patients who were also studied in terms of tumour DNA status, however, aneuploidy was the element with the highest relative risk (2.7), followed by tumour diameter (2.2), lymph node status (1.7) and resection margin involvement (1.6).

We can therefore reasonably conclude that lymph node status is an independent factor capable of affecting survival times in patients undergoing resection for pancreatic ductal carcinoma. In our own series, too, node-positive patients have a mean survival of 9 months (range: 3 to 20.5 months) as opposed to a 15.1 month mean survival in the node-negative patients (range: 3 to 35.4 months).

The N stage also appears to be decisive with regard to long-term survival (beyond 5 years): in a recent study aimed at identifying the characteristics of patients destined to survive for longer periods (28), all the patients surviving for more than 10 years were node-negative. On the other hand, it is by no means rare to find node-positive patients surviving for 5 years, with death occurring as a result of the disease after 5 years or more (5,27,32).

Finally, it is important to make sure, in the more recent studies, that the use of adjuvant radio- or chemotherapy has not affected the relationship between the N stage and patient survival (5,26,27). The results of these studies, however, which are neither controlled nor well matched as regards treatment and which refer to a limited patient sample (mainly node-positive), should be viewed with extreme caution.

Results of Extended versus Traditional Lymph Node Dissection

As a consequence of the uncertain relationship between lymph node involvement and survival in carcinoma of the pancreas, the value of systematic lymph node dissection in the oncologically radical surgical treatment of ductal tumours is still a much debated issue. This refers, of course, to the need, if any, for extending lymph node removal after pancreatic resection, which, in itself, involves a lymphadenectomy adjacent to the gland.

In fact, it is not only problems of pattern and prognostic significance that create differences of opinion and attitude: lymphadenectomy, which is taken for granted in other tumours such as those of the breast, stomach and colon, yields no information that will influence adjuvant therapy for the pancreas on the basis of positivity or otherwise.

The advocates of this "extended" approach can do no more than base their rationale on the intrinsic therapeutic efficacy of lymphadenectomy as such (removal of potential malignant foci and interruption of lymphatic tumour spread).

This theoretical benefit can only be demonstrated by a significantly enhanced survival in patients treated radically as compared with those undergoing standard surgery. Isikawa et al. (11), in 1988, showed a significant increase in survival after extended lymphadenectomy albeit in a limited number of cases. Since then, other reports – predominantly Japanese – have described the benefits obtainable with the use of extended lymphadenectomy (2,6,9).

Nagakawa (33), however, stresses that, if we want to offer the individual patient the maximum chance of survival, we cannot confine ourselves to extended lymphadenectomy alone, but must also remove the retroperitoneal laminar tissue including the coeliac nerve plexus. The resulting benefit in terms of survival is, however, questioned by the Japanese authors themselves, inasmuch as these patients are liable to experience devastating diarrhoea syndromes requiring very lengthy periods of hospitalisation (34).

Western surgeons have always tended to have misgivings with regard to the radical approach. Gall et al. (13) reported results which are distinctly at variance with the Japanese findings: in their study, the mean survival was no more than 9 months in node positive patients as against 60 months in the node-negative group. Henne-Bruns and co-workers (35) claimed, on the strength of preliminary data, that only patients with early-stage tumours are likely to benefit from this approach.

Why this discrepancy between East and West? Bearing in mind, in the first place, the basic importance of interpreting survival curves properly, after first establishing whether the survival is real or actuarial, we can say that, from the strictly morphological and biological standpoints, cancer of the pancreas is the same the world over, despite the fact that well-differentiated forms appear to predominate in Japan as compared with the USA and Europe (34). This finding, however, is dependent upon the pathologist's subjective judgement, although it may reflect either less aggressive biological processes or, perhaps, an earlier diagnosis with a more careful selection of cases to be submitted to radical resection.

As we see it, however, the factor which more than any other may account for the East–West discrepancy is the very different way in which pancreatic malignancies are staged. The UICC classification system used in Western countries tends to underestimate locoregional invasion and to place greater emphasis on lymph node invasion. The system used in Japan is undoubtedly more accurate in its analysis of local invasion factors (pancreatic capsule, vessels and retroperitoneum), thus proving much more predictive of the individual patient's prognosis (3).

The discrepancies between the two systems emerge clearly when they are applied simultaneously to the same patient population, as demonstrated by Tsunoda et al. (36) in a Japanese patient sample and by Zerbi et al. (37) in a European sample. The Japanese system is unquestionably more reliable in prognostic terms, but, unlike the UICC system, it is by no means simple to apply. We clearly need to come up with new classification parameters in future which combine the simplicity of the UICC system and the reliability of the Japanese classification (3,38). The fact remains, as stressed by Osaki (34), that the 5-year survival rate in Japan is 40% after extirpative surgery alone in patients with UICC stage I cancer and 5% in those with UICC stage III tumours – which is exactly the same as in Western countries.

All things considered, then, the discrepancies between East and West are only apparent: different classification systems and selection of patients for treatment are probably responsible for what are now no more than "historical" mis-understandings. On the other hand, analysis of the cumulative data from studies in the literature favouring an extension of lymphadenectomy has failed to demonstrate any advantage in terms of survival (39). By way of confirmation of this, in 185 cases of small tumours resected and analysed in the context of a Japanese multicentre study (40), no differences in survival were observed in patients treated with the standard or extended methods (27% in both groups). These findings have been confirmed in an American study (27).

In effect Nagakawa's claim (4) for the need to extend lymph node dissection also to sites remote from the tumour on the basis of the haphazard pattern of lymphatic invasion, though perfectly convincing from the anatomico-topographical standpoint, gives rise to a certain amount of perplexity, when we see that four of seven patients with metastases in area 16 died within 1 year and that the longest period of survival was little more than 2 years. Our own two patients with positive lymph nodes in area 16 also died of their cancer within one year. In conclusion, the suspicion arises that surgery, even when it is as extensive as possible, cannot be acceptable as the only treatment for these patients, in view of the fact, amongst other things, that the subjects in our case series who underwent classic Whipple resections presented a mean survival of 14.8 months with a range of 2.1 to 35.4 months.

No definitive judgement, however, can be expressed without prospective controlled clinical trials. We report below on our experience with an Italian multicentre study conducted by the Lymphadenectomy Study Group.

Lymphadenectomy Study Group Multicentre Prospective Randomised Study

Over the period from March 1991 to March 1994, a total of 83 patients with adenocarcinoma of the head of the pancreas were recruited into a prospective randomised stratified study by six contributing centres (41).

Patients undergoing laparotomy were eligible to enter the trial if the entire macroscopic tumour could be excised. In the course of thorough surgical exploration, the tumour diameter was evaluated and frozen sections of peri-pancreatic nodes suspected of being metastatic were obtained. Randomisation was carried out during laparotomy. If the study inclusion criteria were met, patients were stratified as follows: (1) lymph node-negative pancreatic tumours measuring less than 4 cm in diameter (2) lymph node-positive pancreatic tumours and node-negative tumours measuring more than 4 cm in diameter.

Patients were then allocated to traditional or extended lymphadenectomy by means of random numbers generated on a personal computer. Classic Whipple or pylorus-preserving pancreaticoduodenectomy was performed on the basis of the operating surgeon's preference.

Traditional lymphadenectomy included resection of the following groups of lymph nodes: anterior and posterior pancreaticoduodenal, inferior head, pyloric, common bile duct, superior head, superior mesenteric and superior and inferior pancreatic body nodes. In addition to the latter, extended lymphadenectomy also entailed removal of the following: hepatic duct, mid-coelic, coeliac axis and para-aortic region (from the diaphragmatic crura to the inferior mesenteric artery and between the right and left renal hila). Reconstruction was allowed according to the surgeon's preference.

Forty-two patients were randomised to traditional and 41 to extended lymphadenectomy. Histological specimens from 76 of the 83 patients (all 3-year survivors included) were reviewed by two independent pathologists (G. Kloppel and K. Dhaene, from Kiel). Two patients in the traditional lymphadenectomy group were subsequently excluded, one because of a suspected endocrine pancreatic tumour, confirmed by the histological reviewers, and the other because of postoperative histological demonstration of hepatic metastasis. The survival analysis was conducted in the remaining 81 patients.

The characteristics of the two patient groups were comparable for age, sex, length of follow-up, tumour stage, tumour diameter and grading.

The number of lymph nodes removed with the extended procedure was significantly greater than with the traditional one. There were no significant differences between the two groups as regards the number of patients undergoing intraoperative radiotherapy (IORT) or a pylorus-preserving procedure. No adjuvant treatment was given to either group postoperatively.

The overall survival was the same in the two groups ($P < 0.05$). Neither age, sex, surgical department, pylorus-preserving procedures nor IORT influenced survival. Worse survival was observed in patients with high-grade tumours ($P = 0.001$), tumour diameters > 2 cm ($P = 0.002$) and lymph node metastases ($P = 0.006$). Lymph node-positive patients had significantly better survival after extended than after traditional lymphadenectomy ($P = 0.026$); moreover, survival was the same in node-negative patients (whatever the type of lymphadenectomy) and in node-positive patients treated with an extensive approach (41).

Operation Times and Safety of Extended Lymphadenectomy

The experience outlined above also appears to confirm that, as reported by other authors (11,13,35,40), there are no significant differences in postoperative morbidity and mortality in the patient groups undergoing classic lymphadenectomy as compared with those undergoing the extended procedure: of a total of four deaths, two occurred in each group, and there were complications up in 22 and 27 patients in the traditional and extended lymphadenectomy groups, respectively.

At the same time, both the numbers of transfusion recipients and of blood units used showed no significant difference between the two treatment groups. Post-operative hospitalisation was also comparable. On the basis of these considerations we may reasonably conclude that the radical procedure is as safe as traditional lymphadenectomy, at least in centres where pancreatic surgery is common practice.

Finally, as regards operation times, extended lymphadenectomy took on average only about 30 min longer to perform than the classic operation. This does not contradict what we said earlier regarding the difficulties often encountered by Western surgeons when operating in the context of abdominal cavities presenting particularly large amounts of fat. In day-to-day practice, unlike what may happen in the setting of a controlled clinical trial, extension of the lymphadenectomy may still meet with substantial resistance in conceptual terms owing to the contradictory results reported in the literature.

Conclusions

Ductal carcinoma of the pancreas remains one of the main causes of cancer mortality in industrialised countries; in Italy it comes sixth on the list (42). Despite the fact that flattering reports have suggested an improvement in long-term prognosis, this is true only in specifically selected subgroups. Tumour size, lymph node positivity and DNA status would appear to be the decisive factors (5,9,10,13,14,18,22,26,42).

One interesting point emerging from a recent review (42) is that four of nine patients surviving beyond year 5 were submitted to surgery with a preoperative diagnosis of pancreatitis. This means that early identification of such cancers still belongs largely to the realm of wishful thinking. In fact, the overall long-term survival of resected patients is still below 10% (26,42).

How meaningful, then, today is a lymphadenectomy procedure involving a greater measure of radicality? The only controlled data provided by a prospective, randomised study are those reported in this chapter, and these would appear to suggest strongly that extended lymphadenectomy is capable of favourably affecting prognosis, in the subgroup of node-positive patients, who, however, constitute the majority of those resected.

As extensive a lymphadenectomy as possible now appears to be the most effective means of enhancing survival in these patients, whose lymph node involvement in most cases cannot be detected except by pathological analysis of the entire surgical specimen.

Our scanty knowledge of the biology of pancreatic cancer prevents us today from being able to identify any form of effective postoperative adjuvant therapy either in the resected population as a whole or, even less so, specifically in lymph node positive patients, unlike the situation obtaining in other types of malignancy. Extended lymphadenectomy as proposed here therefore also falls within the domain of the fairly unsophisticated "take-it-out" concept mentioned at the beginning of this chapter, inasmuch as it proves useful only in node-positive cases. As a therapeutic approach, this is fairly uninspiring on the threshold of the year 2000.

References

1. Gudjonson B (1995) Carcinoma of the pancreas: critical analysis of costs, results of resections and the need of standardized reporting. J Am Coll Surg 181:483–503.
2. Büchler MW, Wagner M, Friess H (1996) Surgery for pancreatic cancer. In: Dervensis CG (ed) Advances in pancreatic disease. Georg Thieme Verlag, Stuttgart, pp. 309–323.
3. Bassi C, Falconi M, Zamboni G, Iacono C, Talamini G, Pederzoli P (1996) How should we go about staging cancer in the future? In: Beger HG et al. (eds), Cancer of the pancreas. Universitatsverlag Ulm, Germany, pp 125–131.
4. Nagakawa T, Kobayashi H, Ueno K et al. (1993) The pattern of lymph node involvement in carcinoma of the head of the pancreas. Int J Pancreatol 13:15–22.
5. Delcore R, Rodriguez FJ, Forster J, Hermreck AS, Thomas JH (1996) Significance of lymph node metastases in patients with pancreatic cancer undergoing curative resection. Am J Surg 172:463–469.
6. Ishikawa O (1993) What constitutes curative pancreatectomy for adenocarcinoma of the pancreas? Hepatogastroenterology 40:414–417.
7. Cubilla AL, Fitzgerald PJ (1980) Surgical pathology of tumors of exocrine pancreas. In: Moossa AR (ed) Tumors of the pancreas. Williams & Wilkins, Baltimore pp 159–193.

8. Nagakawa T, Kobayashi H, Ueno K, Ohta T, Kayahara, Miyazaki I (1994) Clinical study on lymphatic flow to the paraaortic lymph nodes in carcinoma of the head of the pancreas. Cancer 73:1155–1162.

9. Yamamoto M, Saitoh Y (1996) Does lymph node dissection prolong survival? In: Beger HG et al. (eds) Cancer of the pancreas. Universitatsverlag Ulm, Germany, pp 409–418.

10. Kockerling F, Kessler H, Hermanek P, Gall FP (1996) The role of lymph node dissection in the treatment of ductal carcinoma of the pancreas. In: Beger HG et al. (eds) Cancer of the pancreas. Universitatsverlag Ulm, Germany, pp 403–408.

11. Isikawa O, Ohhigashi K, Sasaky J et al. (1988) Pratical usefulness of lymphatic and connective tissue clearance for the carcinoma of the pancreas head. Ann Surg 208:215–220.

12. Nagai H, Kuroda A, Morioka Y (1986) Lymphatic and local spread of T1 and T2 pancreatic cancer. Ann Surg 80:65–71.

13. Gall FP, Kessler H, Hermanek P (1991) Surgical treatment of ductal pancreatic carcinoma. Eur J Surg Oncol 17:173–181.

14. Bassi C, Falconi M, Talamini G et al. (1995) Prospective study of the detection and treatment of small tumours of the head of the pancreas. J Hepat Bil Pancr Surg 2:347–351.

15. Japan Pancreas Society (1996) Classification of pancreatic carcinoma (English edn). Kanehara, Tokyo.

16. Yamamoto M, Ohashi O, Ishida H, Kamigaki T, Onoyama H, Saitoh Y (1994) Relationship between survival and cancer extension. Int J Pancreatol 16:118–120.

17. Lillemoe KD (1995) Current management of pancreatic carcinoma. Ann Surg 221:133–148.

18. Yeo CJ, Cameron JL, Lillemoe KD et al. (1995) Pancreaticoduodenectomy for cancer of the head of the pancreas. Ann Surg 221:721–733.

19. Ceuterick M, Gelin M, Rickaert F et al. (1989) Pancreaticoduodenal resection for pancreatic or periampullary tumours: a ten-year experience. Hepatogastroenterology 36:467–473.

20. Cameron JL, Pitt HA, Yeo CJ, Lillemoe KD, Kaufmann HS, Coleman J (1993) One hundred and forty five consecutive pancreaticoduodenectomies without mortality. Ann Surg 217:430–438.

21. Tsuchiya R, Harada N, Tsunoda T, Miyamoto T, Ura K (1988) Long-term survivors after operation on carcinoma of the pancreas. Int J Pancreatol 3:491–496.

22. Camenron JL, Crist DW, Sitzmann JV et al. (1991) Factors influencing survival after pancreaticoduodenectomy for pancreatic cancer. Am J Surg 161:120–125.

23. Kawarada Y, Yanagisawa K, Isaji S, Mizumoto R (1994) The prevalence of pancreatic cancer lymph node metastasis in Japan and pancreatic cancer categories. Int J Pancreatol 16:101–104.

24. Hagiwara K (1990) Experimental and clinicopathological studies on lymphatic flow of the pancreas. Igaku Kenkiu 52:61–85.

25. Nagai H (1987) Involvement of paraaortic lymph nodes by pancreatic cancer and its lymphatic flow. Jpn J Surg 88:308–317.

26. Nitecki SS, Sarr MG, Colby TV, van Heerden JA (1995) Long-term survival after resection for ductal adenocarcinoma of the pancreas. Is it really improving? Ann Surg 221:59–66.

27. Geer RJ, Brennam MF. Prognostic indicators for survival after resection of pancreatic adenocarcinoma. Am J Surg 165:68–73.

28. Klempnauer J, Ridder GJ, Bektas H, Pichlmayr R (1995) Surgery for exocrine pancreatic cancer: who are the five and ten year survivors? Oncology 52:353–359.

29. Allema JH, Reinders ME, van Gulik TM et al. (1995) Prognostic factor for survival after pancreaticoduodenectomy for patients with carcinoma of the pancreatic head region. Cancer 75:2069–2076.

30. Staley CA, Lee JE, Cleary KR et al. (1996) Preoperative chemoradiation, pancreaticoduodenectomy and intraoperative radiation therapy for adenocarcinoma of the pancreatic head. Am J Surg 171:118–125.

31. Fortner JG, Klimstra DS, Senie RT, Maclean BJ (1996) Tumor size is the primary prognosticator for pancreatic cancer after regional pancreatectomy. Ann Surg 223:147–143.

32. Trede M, Chir B, Schwall G, Saeger HD (1990) Survival after pancreatoduodenectomy. Ann Surg 211:447–458.

33. Nagakawa T, Konishi I, Ohta T et al. (1991) The results and problems of extensive radical surgery for carcinoma of the head of the pancreas. Jpn J Surg 21:262–267.

34. Osaki H (1994) Modern surgical treatment of pancreatic cancer. Int J Pancreatol 16:121–129.

35. Henne-Bruns D, Kremer B, Meyer-Pannwitt U, Schroder VS (1993) Partial duodenopancreatectomy with radical lymphoadenectomy in patients with pancreatic and periampullary carcinomas: initial results. HepatoGastroenterology 40:145–149.

36. Tsunoda T, Ura K, Eto T, Matsumoto T, Tsuchiya R (1991) UICC and Japanese stage classification for carcinoma of the pancreas. Int J Pancreatol 8:205–214.

37. Zerbi A, Balzano GP, Bottura R, Di Carlo V (1994) Reliability of pancreatic cancer classifications. Int J Pancreatol 15:13–18.
38. Bassi C, Butturini G, Falconi M et al. (1996) Prognosis of pancreatic carcinoma: why are differences to be found between European and Japanese patients? In: Dervenis CG (ed) Advances in pancreatic diseases. Georg Thieme Verlag, Stuttgart, pp 303–308.
39. Yeo CJ, Cameron JL (1994) Arguments against radical (extended) resection for adenocarcinoma of the pancreas. Adv Surg 27:273–284.
40. Satake K, Nishimaki H, Yokomatsu H et al. (1992) Surgical curability and prognosis for standard versus extended resections for T1 carcinoma of the pancreas. Surg Gynecol Obstet 175:259–265.
41. Pedrazzoli S, Di Carlo V, Dionigi R and the Lymphadenectomy Study Group (1998). Traditional versus extended lymphadenectomy associated with pancreatoduodenectomy in surgical treatment of pancreatic head cancer. Multicenter prospective randomized trial. Ann Surg (in press).
42. Sperti C, Pasquali C, Piccoli A, Pedrazzoli S (1996) Survival after resection for ductal adenocarcinoma of the pancreas. Br J Surg 83:625–631.

37 Results of Radical Lymphadenectomy in Pancreatic Carcinoma

H. Zirngibl, J. Schmidt, E. Heinmöller, S. Mann, U. Mann, A. Agha and J. Rüschoff

Radical lymphadenectomy has been performed since the late 1970s, especially in the surgical departments of Japanese universities. Excellent results were reported for extended lymphadenectomy in gastric and oesophageal cancer when wide local excision was combined with systematic extended lymph node dissection. Overall 5-year survival of over 50% for the large number of patients undergoing gastric resection for cancer seems to demonstrate convincingly the value of the extended lymphadenectomy. All Oriental studies published to now are uncontrolled as are most reports from Western countries. The role of extended lymphadenectomy is therefore far from certain. On the other hand there is evidence that extended lymph node dissection in the treatment of pancreatic cancer might be of benefit to patients with small stage I and II tumours (1). All available data from published studies suggest that lymph node involvement is an important prognostic factor in patients with carcinoma of the head of the pancreas. Lymph node metastases occur in as many as 50% of the cases of even the smallest pancreatic cancers now being diagnosed and resected, especially those less than 2 cm in diameter (2). Classification of the critical areas of lymph node dissection in patients with carcinoma of pancreatic head show that perigastric lymph node involvement is found at about 14%. Para-aortic lymph node involvement in these patients is about 26% (3). Studies with radioactive colloids to determine lymphatic spread from the head of the pancreas to the para-aortic lymph nodes (area 16) showed that the main lymphatic route was found to pass through the nodes of the posterior region of the head of the pancreas (area 13) and around the superior mesenteric artery (area 14). Lymphatic metastases in area 16 are mainly seen in the lower segment of the middle region from the coeliac artery to the inferior mesenteric artery. Nagakawa et al. (4) concluded that lymph node dissection in area 16 should be extended toward the dorsal side of the renal artery rather than be performed widely along the abdominal aorta to make the radical operation for pancreatic cancer more effective.

Patients with stage I or II disease experience recurrence significantly less often than patients with stage III or IV disease. Local retroperitoneal recurrence is discovered in about 80% of post-mortem examinations. Hepatic metastases are found in about 65%, peritoneal dissemination at 55% and recurrent lymph node metastases in about 5%. Almost all patients with liver metastases also have local retroperitoneal recurrence. This frequency of retroperitoneal recurrence, especially in carcinoma of the head of pancreas, suggests that retroperitoneal dissection including nerve plexus and lymph nodes should be included in curative resection for patients with stage I or II of pancreatic cancer (5).

Published Data

In the past 20 years, especially in the early 1980s, many studies originating from Japan elucidated the prognostic relevance of radical lymphatic dissection in pancreatic carcinoma and carcinoma of the periampullary region (6). In the late 1980s and the early 1990s there was little information regarding this technique. In Western countries the promising results from Japanese centres could not be achieved until now. Taking into consideration prospective studies of the past 10 years (Table 1) we find that together with an overall operative mortality rate of 7.6%, the overall 5-year survival for patients with pancreatic carcinoma who underwent radical lymphadenectomy is 21.5%.

Periampullary carcinoma was falsely integrated within the studies of radical lymphadenectomy of pancreatic carcinoma in the early 1980s. As this tumour shows a different biology and long-term prognosis all those studies have to be looked at separately. We found three studies of periampullary cancer published in the past 3 years gathering about 200 patients where, together with an operative mortality rate of 6.6%, the overall 5-year survival rate reached 28.4% (13,14,15).

In a study published in 1996 (16) including 129 resected patients with pancreatic carcinoma, intrapancreatic neural infiltration was demonstrated in 90%. There was a statistically relevant correlation between intrapancreatic neural infiltration and extrapancreatic infiltration of the neural plexus. These patients showed a significantly lower survival rate. In this group 68 patients had a portal infiltration of the tumour and presented a 100% mortality rate by the thirteenth postoperative month. Thus the relevance of vascular resections in order to gain oncological radicality remains uncertain.

Personal Results

Since 1992 150 patients were admitted to our institution. All patients had standard diagnostic procedures done including laboratory investigations, tumour

Table 1. Radical lymphadenectomy in pancreatic carcinoma (7–12)

Study	Year	Patients (n)	Operative mortality (%)	5-Year survival (%)
Ozaki (7)	1996	15	0	29
Nagakawa (8)	1996	53	9, 4	27, 4
Takahashi (9)	1995	149	10	15
Manabe (10)	1989	32	0	33, 4
Miyazaki (11)	1989	31	3, 2	22, 6
Ishikawa (12)	1988	22	9, 6	27
Total		302	7, 6	21, 5

markers (CEA, CA19–9), chest X-ray, abdominal sonography, endoscopic sonography, ERCP and spiral computed tomography with intravenous contrast enhancement. If biliary stenosis was present an endoscopic prosthesis was placed or drainage via PTC was achieved. There were 115 patients with pancreatic ductal adenocarcinoma in the head region, 14 patients had the tumour location in the body and seven within the pancreatic tail. Additionally there were 14 cases with periampullary carcinoma. Within the group of carcinoma of the pancreatic head ($n = 115$) the mean age was 62.2 ± 11.2 years, and there were 52 women. Postoperative hospitalisation was for 16.9 ± 11.9 days after resection and 13.1 ± 6.7 days after palliative procedures.

After prediction of operability, patients underwent exploratory laparotomy. The greater omentum was dissected free from the transverse colon. Then the Kocher manoeuvre was performed. If the lymph nodes posterior to the bile duct in the hepatoduodenal ligament were not suspicious a needle biopsy of the pancreatic tumour was done. In case of primary pancreatic carcinoma or periampullary carcinoma the operation was completed as a partial or subtotal duodenopancreatectomy (DPE). Reconstruction was performed with a retrocolic jejunal Roux-Y-loop building a terminolateral hepaticojejunostomy and a laterolateral isoperistaltic gastrojejunostomy (technique of Hofmeister–Finsterer). The pancreatic remnant was sealed by ethibloc (Ethicon, Germany) instillation into the pancreatic duct, which was secured with a purse string suture. If a pancreatogastrostomy was done, the reconstruction was performed with the same technique locating the pancreatic anastomosis behind the gastrojejunostomy at a distance of at least 3 cm. Pancreatojejunostomy was sewed in two suture lines for both anterior and posterior wall using a Roux-Y jejunal loop.

In all cases of either portal or mesenteric venous and arterial resections the anastomosis was completed directly without interposition of prostheses or peripheral veins. This is possible after mobilisation of the ascending colon which reduces the tension on the mesenteric trunk significantly. Total mortality rate for duodenopancreatectomy was 3.8% (2/52). In 10 cases we had to perform a resection of portal vein and in one case together with the resection of the superior mesenteric artery. In this group there were no deaths (Table 2). The overall mortality rate of operative and non-operative palliation procedures was 9.2% (6/65).

In pancreatic carcinoma 24 of 38 R0 patients without vascular resection had clinical stage III, four patients were at clinical stage I and six at clinical stage II. In the vascular resection group (R0, $n = 6$) one of six patients was at clinical stage II and one at clinical stage I, three at clinical stage III and one at stage IV.

The overall complication rate was 28% (15/52), but only three patients had to be reoperated (5.8%). In the palliation group overall complication rate was 57% (37/65). Within these complications in the resection group there were only

Table 2. Operation-related deaths in carcinoma of pancreatic head ($n = 52$, R0 + R1, December 1992–June 1996)

Operation	Patients	Deaths
DPE	42	2 (4.8%)
DPE + vascular resection	10	0
DPE total	52	2 (3.8%)

DPE, duodenopancreatectomy.

Table 3. Complications after DPE and palliative procedures in pancreatic and periampullary carcinoma

	Resection (n = 31)	Palliation (operative/non-operative)
Intra-abdominal haemorrhage	1	–
Intraintestinal haemorrhage	1	4
Mesenteric thrombosis	–	2
Pancreatic fistula	3	1
Biliary fistula	1	4
Pleural effusion	2	10
Pneumonia	3	5
Wound infection	1	4
Total	12 (42%)	30 (47%)
Major complications	6 (19%)	11 (17%)
Reoperation	1 (3%)	4 (6%)

nine major complications (17.3%), all the other complications were of minor importance (Table 3).

The resection rate for carcinoma of the pancreatic head was 45.2% (Table 4). There was a total of 66 lymph nodes (mean) removed with every specimen of ductal adenocarcinoma (Table 5). The lymph node ratio was 0.1 ± 0.06 (infiltrated lymph nodes/total of removed lymph nodes). The sites of nodal metastases are shown in Figure 1. In the vascular resection group there was macroscopic vascular invasion determined intraoperatively in all 10 patients, histological vascular invasion was confirmed in only four. In this group the postoperative survival was 6.5 months (mean). In ductal adenocarcinoma without vascular resection and R0 situation (UICC) the overall 4-year survival rate is actually 28% (Figure 2).

Table 4. Operative and non-operative procedures in pancreatic carcinoma

	n	R0 (UICC)	R1 (UICC)	Palliative surgery
Ductal adenocarcinoma	105	38	4	40
Ductal adenocarcinoma + vascular resection	10	6	4	–

R0 resection (UICC) (44/115) 38.3%; R1 resection (UICC) (8/115) 6.9%.

Table 5. Lymph node ratio (involved nodes/removed nodes) in carcinoma of pancreatic head (n = 32, R0 + R1, N1, December 1992–June 1996)

	Dissected lymph nodes (mean)	Lymph node ratio
Ductal adenocarcinoma	67	$0.1 \pm 0.07^*$
Ductal adenocarcinoma + vascular resection	66	$0.1 \pm 0.02^*$
Ductal adenocarcinoma (total)	66	0.1 ± 0.06

* No statistical difference ($P < 0.01$).

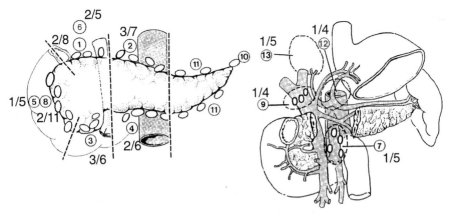

Figure 1. Localisation of lymph node metastases (UICC) in pancreatic carcinoma ($n = 32$, R0 + R1, N1, December 1992–June 1996).

Summary and Conclusion

The outcome of patients with pancreatic carcinoma remains poor as the tumour has often trespassed the margins of the organ at an early stage. In a prospective study conducted at our institution radical lymphadenectomy for pancreatic and periampullary carcinoma has been performed since 1992. We have demonstrated feasibility and low operation-associated complication rates, including mortality. Patients with low-risk clinical stages (I/II, UICC) may gain higher survival rates than without radical lymphatic dissection. In Figure 2 the overall survival includes all patients with R0 resection ($n = 44$). As our patient number is very small, statistical differentiation between clinical stages is not possible at this point.

If major regional vessels are invaded by the tumour, neither dissection nor vascular resection brings benefit to these patients as more than 90% die within 7 months after the operation. These results have been demonstrated already by several institutions in Europe. The rather good results coming from Japan may not be reproducible in Europe (17). On the other hand the operated population at our institution is too small and the observation time is still too short to produce statistically valid results. But the results show a trend towards higher survival rates after radical lymphatic dissection.

Our future aim is to achieve studies where adjuvant therapies should be integrated. Lygidakis presented a prospective randomised study in 1996 where 80 patients with pancreatic carcinoma of the head were treated in one arm with partial duodenopancreatectomy and regional lymphadenectomy and in the second arm two arterial catheters were implanted into the splenic and middle colic arteries. Immunostimulation with interleukin-2 and interferon-γ together with chemotherapy (including mitomycin C, cisplatin, 5-fluorouracil and leucovorin) were given. Chemotherapy was performed after immunostimulation over 10 days in the postoperative period. This therapy was repeated every 3 months during the first year and every 4 months during the second and third postoperative year. The survival rate according to Kaplan–Meier showed a

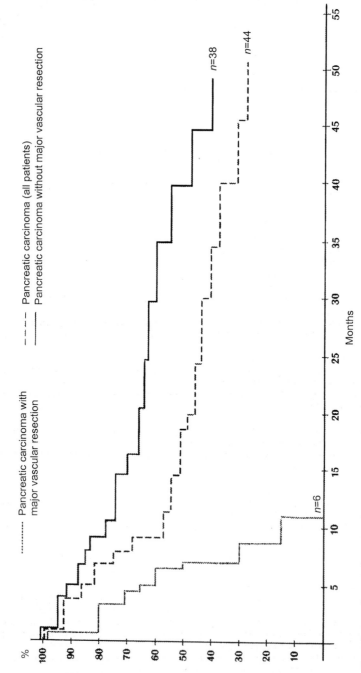

Figure 2. Overall survival rate (Kaplan–Meier) for patients with and without vascular resection in pancreatic carcinoma (*n* = 44, R0, December 1992–June 1996).

significant difference in favour of the immunochemotherapy group (18). Also Gansauge et al. (19) were able to demonstrate a protective effect of postoperative adjuvant regional chemotherapy in patients with advanced stage of pancreatic carcinoma where resection was not curative (R1, UICC). Chemotherapy was performed with mitoxantrone, 5 FU and folinic acid together with cisplatin and patients developed significantly fewer hepatic metastases.

Ohigashi et al. (20) used methotrexate via the splenic or gastroduodenal artery (through two catheters) in irresectable pancreatic carcinoma. Together with this treatment intravenous infusion with 5 FU was given. In this patient group, where expected survival rate is 6 months, median survival was 14 months.

The combination of adjuvant trials with radical lymphadenectomy should be tested in future in low-stage pancreatic malignancy (clinical stages I and II) to demonstrate any effect on postoperative outcome.

References

1. Taat CW, van Laschot JJ, Gouma DJ, Obertop H (1995) Role of extended lymph node dissection in the treatment of gastrointestinal tumours: a review of the literature. Scand J Gastroenterol 212(Suppl):109–116.
2. Reber HA, Ashley SW, McFadden D (1995) Curative treatment for pancreatic neoplasms. Radical resection. Surg Clin North Am 75:905–912.
3. Nakao A, Harada A, Nonami T et al. (1995) Lymph node metastases in carcinoma of the head of the pancreas region. Br J Surg 82:399–402.
4. Nagakawa T, Kobayashi H, Ueno K, Ohta T, Kayahara M, Miyazaki I (1994) Clinical study of lymphatic flow to the paraaortic lymph nodes in carcinoma of the head of the pancreas. Cancer 73:1155–1162.
5. Kayahara M, Nagakawa T, Ueno K, Ohta T, Takeda T, Miyazaki I (1993) An evaluation of radical resection for pancreatic cancer based on the mode of recurrence as determined by autopsy and diagnostic imaging. Cancer 72:2118–2123.
6. Ishikawa O, Ohigashi H, Imaoka S et al. (1992) Preoperative indications for extended pancreatectomy for locally advanced pancreas cancer involving the portal vein. Ann Surg 215:231–216.
7. Ozaki H, Kinoshita T, Kosuge T et al. (1996) An aggressive therapeutic approach to carcinoma of body and tail of the pancreas. Pancreas 77:2240–2245.
8. Nagakawa T, Nagamori M, Futakami F et al. (1996) Results of extensive surgery for pancreatic carcinoma. Cancer 77:640–645.
9. Takahashi S, Ogata Y, Miyazaki H et al. (1995) Aggressive surgery for pancreatic duct cell cancer: feasibility, validity, limitations. World J Surg 19:653–659.
10. Manabe T, Ohshio G, Baba N et al. (1989) Radical pancreatectomy for ductal cell carcinoma of the head of the pancreas. Cancer 64:1132–1137.
11. Miyazaki I (1989) Significance of extensive surgery for pancreatic cancer. Gan To Kagaku Ryoho 16:1064–1069.
12. Ishikawa O, Ohhigashi H, Sasaki Y et al. (1988) Practical usefulness of lymphatic and connective tissue clearance for the carcinoma of the pancreas head. Ann Surg 208:215–220.
13. Burcharth F, Andersen HB, Brahe NE, Baden H (1995) Pancreaticoduodenectomy for periampullary cancer. Ugeskr Laeger 157:5544–5548.
14. Shirai Y, Tsukada K, Ohtani T, Hatakeyama K Carcinoma of the ampulla of Vater: is radical lymphadenectomy beneficial to patients with nodal disease? J Surg Oncol 61:190–194.
15. Roder JD, Schneider PM, Stein HJ, Siewert JR (1995) Number of lymph node metastases is significantly associated with survival in patients with radically resected carcinoma of the ampulla of Vater. Br J Surg 82:1693–1696.
16. Nakao A, Harada A, Nonami T, Kaneko T, Takagi H (1996) Clinical significance of carcinoma invasion of the extrapancreatic nerve plexus in pancreatic cancer. Pancreas 12:357–361.
17. Matsuda M, Nimura Y (1983) Perineural invasion of pancreas head carcinoma. Nippon Geka Gakkai Zasshi 84:719–728.

18. Lygidakis NJ, Stringaris K (1996) Adjuvant therapy following pancreatic resection for pancreatic duct carcinoma: a prospective randomized study. Hepatogastroenterology 43:671–680.
19. Gansauge F, Link KH, Rilinger N, Kunz R, Beger HG (1996) Adjuvant regional chemotherapy in advanced pancreatic cancer. Chirurgie 67:362–365.
20. Ohigashi H, Ishikawa O, Imaoka S et al. (1996) A new method of intraarterial regional chemotherapy with more selective drug delivery for locally advanced pancreatic cancer. Hepatogastroenterology 43:338–345.

38 Multimodal Therapies for Pancreatic Ductal Adenocarcinoma

M.H. Schoenberg, K.H. Link, F. Gansauge and H.G. Beger

Patients with pancreatic cancer expect an extremely low 5-year survival rate of 1%. Resection of the primary tumour at an early stage may offer the only chance for cure, although this treatment result is rare, since only 5% of resected patients live beyond 5 years after surgery with curative intent. The overall fatal outcome of this disease is due to the fact that frequently the tumour has either already metastasised at the time of diagnosis or is locally advanced, so that resection without residual tumour is not possible. In spite of the large surgical experience of our own institution, resection could be performed in only 36% of 471 patients between 1982 and 1993; the 5-year survival rate was 8% and median survival time 11.3–12.1 months (1).

In our opinion, the treatment outcome may be improved by increasing the resectability rate and influencing the biology of the tumour which rapidly leads to local relapses, hepatic progression or development of peritoneal carcinomatosis.

Recent data from studies treating irresectable patients with radiochemotherapy (2,3) have brought substantial evidence that primarily irresectable cases could be down-staged and resected with the result of 33 months median survival time (4). The aim of down-staging pancreatic cancer may also be reached with intra-arterial infusion chemotherapy (5). The regional chemotherapeutic approach in our experience may also prolong survival by preventing hepatic progression (6,7).

Since local relapses/progression and hepatic metastases are the most frequent causes of death (8–10), these predicted sites of disease progression should be treated prophylactically. We reviewed the literature and came to the conclusion that locally advanced pancreatic cancer should be treated with radiotherapy and intra-arterial infusion for better local and hepatic disease control.

If this combination of two locoregional treatment modalities can down-stage and improve palliation and survival in locally advanced irresectable cases, regional chemotherapy and radiotherapy, combined with postoperative intra-arterial infusion chemotherapy via the coeliac axis could be a useful additional option for neoadjuvant/adjuvant treatment of all patients with pancreatic adenocarcinoma stages I–III UICC.

Biology of Ductal Pancreatic Cancer

Weiss et al. (8) performed a detailed analysis of the metastatic patterns revealed at autopsy of patients with pancreatic cancer. They found sufficient evidence, that

..ctastasis of pancreatic cancer takes place in a stepwise manner via venous routes, first to the liver, next to the lungs and finally, via arterial routes, to other organs. The presence of lymph node metastases was often associated with increased risk of extralymphatic metastases, but this association was not invariable in individual cases. No evidence was found for a causal relationship between lymph node involvement and haematogenous metastases. Peritoneal involvement occurred in early disease, and progressively increased in more advanced disease in association with pulmonary metastases, but did not correlate with either nodal involvement or primary tumour size. At death, cancer was confined to the pancreatic primary site in 17% of cases, and in an additional 29% there were distant, overt metastases limited to the liver.

Another important site of disease progression is the retroperitoneum; pancreatic cancer cell growth obviously has a high affinity to nerves in the retroperitoneum. Uncontrolled and frequent biopsy procedures, including transabdominal or endoscopically controlled needle biopsies, might lead to early and rapid intra-abdominal spread of pancreatic cancer (11–13). The spontaneous course of the disease, including retroperitoneal infiltration, and early presence of microscopic disease in the peritoneum (12–15) and the liver (16,17) and the critical topographic anatomy leading to tumour infiltration into life-important structures, such as the superior mesenteric vein, artery, and the portal venous system (12,18) clearly limit the curability by surgery.

Two studies have analysed the recurrence patterns after pancreatectomy for pancreatic cancer (9,10). They found local relapses with or without other locations of progressive disease in 86–92%, liver metastases with or without other manifestations of progression in 62–92%, while local relapses without liver metastases were present in 8% and isolated liver metastases without local relapses were observed in 14%. Peritoneal (42%) and hepatic failures (62%) were common. Extra-abdominal metastases were documented in only 27% of cases, but never as sole site (10). Patients who received postoperative adjuvant radiochemotherapy with a radiation treatment of 55 Gy had improved local control and cure when compared with patients treated with lower doses of radiation (10). From these analyses it is clear that local recurrence, hepatic metastases, and peritoneal seeding are the major problems after pancreatic cancer surgery with curative intent.

Although better surgical techniques or better patient selection might contribute to improvement of the results from pancreatic cancer surgery (12), the outcome for the pancreatic cancer patients, resectable or not resectable, and with or without metastases, can only be improved by the development of more efficient palliative treatment that eventually can be used as effective treatment modalities for preoperative, intraoperative and postoperative neoadjuvant/ adjuvant treatment.

Palliative Treatment

Irresectable pancreatic cancers may be treated with either chemo- or radio-chemotherapy. The systemic standard treatment, in spite of numerous efforts to improve on its results, remains 5-FU alone (19). Trials testing 5-FU modulations with folinic acid or interferon-alpha have produced contradictory results. While

Table 1. Systemic chemotherapy of advanced pancreatic cancer with 5-FU modulations

Author	Year	Patients	UICC stage	Treatment	Response (%)				Median survival (months)
					CR	PR	NC	PD	
Cascini (20)	1993	22	III, IV	5-FU, FA, IFNa	CR + PR = 9			5.0	
Bernhard (23)	1995	54	II–IV	5-FU, FA IFNa	0	14	63	23	10.0
Moore (21)	1993	22	III, IV	5-FU, FA, IFNa	0	14	19	67	6.0
Derderian (62)	1991	46	III, IV	5-FU, FA, IFNa	2	7	?	?	n.d.
Schneider (63)	1995	14	IV	5-FU, FA IFNa	0	0	14	86	n.d.
Isacoff (24)	1995	41[a]	III	5-FU, FA c.i. MMC, DP	10	31	0	59	15.0
Louvet (22)	1995	20	III, IV	5-FU, FA	0	11	32	57	6.0
De Caprio (64)	1989	27	III, IV	5-FU, FA	0	8	?	?	8.0

[a] For patients resected after CT.
5FU, 5 fluorouracil; FA, folinic acid; IFNa, interferon alpha; MMC, mitomycin C; DP, dipyridanole; ci, continuous infusion; CR, complete response; PR, partial response; NC, no change; PD, progressive disease.

several protocols did not achieve response rates and survival times better than 5-FU (20–22), the combinations of 5-FU, folinic acid, and interferon-alpha (23) and 5-FU, folinic acid, mitomycin-C and dipyridamol (24) were associated with median survival times in UICC II–IV patients of 10 and 15 months, respectively (Table 1). The median survival in irresectable cancer patients treated with 5-FU + CDDP was 7 months (25) and with 5-FU, mitomycin-C, and adriamycin 8.3 months (26). This last study was a randomised comparison of FAM-chemotherapy versus no chemotherapy and demonstrated a significant survival benefit for the patients receiving FAM-treatment. The other protocols need confirmation in controlled trials to confirm their impact on prolongation of survival compared with no- or 5-FU chemotherapy. One study, which has generated great interest due to a significant survival benefit, is the comparison of gemcitabine versus 5-FU in advanced stage pancreatic cancer patients, reported in abstract form by Moore et al. (27). The median survival time in the patient group receiving gemcitabine was 5.7 months. This was significantly superior to 5-FU with 4.4 months median survival time, and the quality of life was better in the gemcitabine group. Although the improvement in quality of life is an important parameter of chemotherapeutic treatment, it must be noted that merely symptomatic treatment can also improve quality of life significantly, and the gain of survival due to gemcitabine therapy was only 1.3 months (Table 2).

Obviously, chemotherapeutic concepts that are more effective in disease control are required. The rationale to deliver drugs via intra-arterial infusion is promising, since drugs exert clear concentration response behaviour (28–30). The method has improved response rates, survival and quality of life in colorectal liver metastases (31,32), is anatomically practicable for treatment of pancreatic cancer (33) and justified by what we know of tumour biology (8). The results of

Table 2. Systemic chemotherapy of advanced pancreatic cancer with combination protocols

Author	Year	Patients	UICC stage	Treatment	Response (%)				Median survival (months)
					CR	PR	NC	PD	
Wils (65)	1993	33	(III), IV	CDDP	6	15	0	79	4.0
Rougier (25)	1993	38	III, IV	5-FU c.i., CDDP	3	24	24	45	7.0
Berthault (66)	1993	14	III, IV	5-FU c.i. chronomodulated	0	21	36	43	
Bukowski (67)	1993	71	III, IV	5-FU, ADM MMC, STP	CR + PR = 11				4.8
		32		MGBG	CR + PR = 6				
		29		DHAD	CR + PR = 0				3–4
		21		AZQ	CR + PR = 0				
Palmer (26)	1994	23	III, IV	5-FU, MMC, ADM					8.3[a]
		20	III, IV	no chemotherapy					3.8
Moore (27)	1995	123	III, IV	5-FU			n.d.		4.4
				GEM			n.d.		5.7[a]
Rougier (68)	1995	27	IV	Doxetaxel	0	22	30	48	n.d.
		12	III	Doxetaxel	0	25	25	50	n.d.
Wils (69)	1993	21	IV	IFO	0	0	?	?	n.d.
Asbury (70)	1994	26	III, IV	DHAD	CR + PR = 0				2.3
		22		ACLA	CR + PR = 0				2.8
		26		SPIRO	CR + PR = 0				2.8
		23		VP16	CR + PR = 0				3.0
Bartolomeo (71)	1993	10	III, IV	EPI VP16, CDDP	CR + PR = 0				n.d.
Orita (72)	1995	22	III, IV	OHF-1	5	8	55	22	9.0

[a] Randomised study, $P < 0.05$

CDDP, cisplatinum; ADM, adriamycin; STP, streptozotocin; MGBG, methyl-glyoxal-bis-guanylhydrazone; EPI, epirubicin; OHF-1, interferon-α + TNFα; DHAD, dihydroxyanthracinedone; AZQ, aziridinylbenzoquinone; GEM, gemcitabine; IFO, ifosfamide; ACLA, aclacinomycin-A; SPIRO, spirogermanium; VP16, vepesid. For other abbreviations see Table 1.

Table 3. Regional chemotherapy of advanced pancreatic cancer

Author	Year	Patients	UICC Stage	Treatment	Response (%)				Median survival (months)
					CR	PR	NC	PD	
Aigner (73)	1990	26	IV	5-FU MMC, CDDP	4	65	12	19[a]	9–14
Aigner (5)	1993	99	IV	various		n.d.			10–12
Link (6)	1995	36	III, IV	NOV 5-FU, FA, CDDP	0	21	38	41	7.5
Ohigashi (35)	1994	20	III, IV	ADM MTX, ATII		n.d.			12.0
Miura (74)	1994	48	?	5-FU MMC, +RT/ HT/etc.		n.d.			7.0
Ohigashi (55)	1993	19	III	ADM MTX, 5-FU		n.d.			11.0

[a] Tumour marker response.

MTX, methotrexate; RT, radiotherapy; HT, hyperthermia; ATII, angiotensin II; NOV, Novantrone (mitoxantrone). Other abbreviations as in Tables 1 and 2.

the first trials applying regional chemotherapy for treatment of advanced pancreatic cancer may be regarded as positive. Regional chemotherapy delivered via the coeliac axis induced longer survival times ranging from 7 to 14 months in stage III–IV, UICC patients, compared with the 3 to 6.5 months achieved with systemic chemotherapy of combination regimens or 5-FU monotherapy (19) (Table 3). Although intra-arterial infusion via the coeliac axis requires greater technical efforts, down-staging of the tumour size, facilitating resection in previously irresectable cases, is possible (5) and pain can be controlled (6). We have treated 32 patients (17 UICC III, 15 UICC IV) with advanced irresectable pancreatic cancer using a combination chemotherapeutic protocol of mitoxantrone, 5-FU + folinic acid, and cisplatinum, delivered cyclically via the coeliac trunk (6). The median survival times compared with untreated historical controls were 12 versus 4.8 months ($P < 0.006$) in UICC III patients, and 4 versus 2.7 months (n.s.) in UICC IV patients (34). Surprisingly, the patients rarely developed liver metastases but died either of peritoneal carcinomatosis, local progression or lung metastases. Two patients underwent resection after local response. Better control of hepatic progression with intra-arterial chemotherapy was also reported by Ohigashi et al. (35). The feasibility and toxicity of our palliative regional chemotherapeutic protocol was acceptable (6).

Similar response rates (Table 4) and survival times (Table 5) in irresectable pancreatic cancer may be achieved with radiochemotherapy. Radiochemotherapy was superior to radiation or chemotherapy alone in randomised controlled trials (36,37) and the results are consistent in the non-randomised studies. The advantage of the combination treatment with radio- and chemotherapy may be attributed to effective local control, while extraregional progression into the liver and development of peritoneal carcinosis cannot be prevented. After radiochemotherapy Bruckner et al. (2,3) reported local control in all treated patients; however, progression occurred in the peritoneum (60%), liver (35%) and other locations (20%). Radiochemotherapy may also convert irresectable to resectable tumours (4). The treatment is time consuming and may be associated with high toxicity (2,3,38).

Table 4. Response rates after multimodal palliative therapy in irresectable pancreatic cancer

Author	Year	Patients	Radiotherapy dose (Gy)	Treatment	Response (%)			
					CR	PR	NC	PD
Whittington (75)	1984	20	^{125}I + 55–60	5-FU, MMC, CCNU	CR + PR = 81			19
Mohiuddin (76)	1992	81	^{125}I + 55–60	SFU, MMC, CCNU	CR + PR = 71			29
Wagener (77)	1989	19	40	FAP pre/5-FU	16	32	52	0
Kamthan (78)	1992	35	40–54	+FSP/5-FU, FA[a]	17	26	29	29
Bruckner (2)	1993	20	54	+5-FU c.i. STP, CDDP/ 5-FU+FA	44	31	19	6
Jessup (79)	1993	16	45	+5-FU c.i.				31
Bronn (80)	1995	9	60	+5-FU, CDDP c.i./ +5-FU, CDDP c.i.	44	44	12	0

[a] Chemotherapy during RT/Chemotherapy after RT.
FSP, 5-fluorouracil, streptozotocin, cisplatinum.

Table 5. Survival after multimodal palliative therapy in irresectable pancreatic cancer

Author	Year	Patients	Radiotherapy dose (Gy)	CT treatment	Median survival (months)
Moertel[a]	1981	25	60	–	5.5
(GITSG) (36)		83	40	+5-FU/5-FU[b]	10.5[c]
GITSG[a] (37)	1988	86	60	+5-FU/5-FU	10
		21	–	SMF	8
		22	54	+5-FU/SMF	10.5[b]
Schein (MAOP) (81)	1983	21	45	FAM pre/post RT	12
Whittington (75)	1984	20	I^{125} + 55–60	5-FU, MMC, CCNU	12.5
Mohiuddin (76)	1992	81	I^{125} + 55–60	5FU, MMC, CCNU	12
Komaki (82)	1988	16	61 + 23 hep.	+5-FU/5-FU	14
Komaki (83)	1992	79	61 + 23 hep.	+5FU/5FU	8.4
Wagener (77)	1989	19	40	FAP pre RT/5-FU	14
Wagener (EORTC) (84)	1992	50	40	EP pre RT, +5-FU/5-FU	12
Kamthan (78)	1992	35	40–54	+FSP/5-FU, FA	12
Bruckner (3)	1993	20	54	+5-FU c.i., STP, CDDP/ 5-FU + FA	12
Earle (85)	1993	44	40–50	+5-FU	8.5
		43	40–50	+Hycanthone	8.5
Jeekel (86)	1991	20	50	+5-FU	10
Jessup (79)	1993	16	45	+5-FU c.i.	8
Moertel (38)	1994	22	45–54	+5-FU, FA/5-FU, FA	13, 5

[a] Randomised study.
[b] Chemotherapy during RT/chemotherapy after RT.
[c] $P < 0.05$.
SMF, streptozotocin, 5-FU, mitomycin-C; hep, hepatic irradiation; EP, epidoxorubicin, cisplatinum. Other abbreviations as in earlier tables.

No effective alternative treatments inducing some response or proving prolongation of survival in patients with advanced irresectable pancreatic cancer have been reported in the literature (12). Intraoperative radiotherapy may achieve local disease control without impact on survival (39).

Adjuvant Therapy

Since resection alone results in inadequate disease control, adjuvant chemotherapy and radiochemotherapy have been used to improve outcome. Bakkevold et al. (40) were able to extend median survival from 11 to 23 months after resection in patients with ductal and periampullary pancreatic cancers in a controlled study comparing postoperative FAM-chemotherapy versus surgery only. This extension of the median survival time did not translate into improved 5-year survival rates (4% versus 8%, n.s.).

Adjuvant postoperative radiochemotherapy added to surgical treatment in a GITSG study improved the short- and long-term prognosis in patients with R0-resected ductal pancreatic cancer. The median survival times and 5-year survival rates with 20 versus 11 months and 20% versus 5% were significantly higher in the patient group receiving postoperative radiochemotherapy. This survival benefit persisted, so that after 10 years 19% of the patients treated with radiochemotherapy and no patient of the surgical control group were living (41–43). Foo et al. (44) confirmed the median survival time achievable by postoperative adjuvant radiochemotherapy and found that a higher dose of radiotherapy increases local disease control. The better local disease control by higher doses of radiation therapy, associated with longer survival, was also described by Griffin et al. (10). While the local relapse rates (33% versus 47–55%) in the GITSG patient groups receiving 40 Gy radiotherapy were not improved (41), other patients treated with 54 Gy had only 9% local relapses (44); disease progression in the liver (52%) and peritoneum (52%) limited the prognosis of those patients in spite of improved local disease control (44).

Regional adjuvant chemotherapy improved the survival time in two studies, comparing intra-arterial chemotherapy versus historical controls. Our group was the first to treat resected pancreatic cancer patients with cyclic postoperative coeliac axis infusions using the same protocol as in an irresectable patient group (6). The median survival time of 20 patients (1 UICC I, 3 UICC II, 16 UICC III; 16 R0/R1-resected, 4 R2-resected) with ductal adenocarcinoma (18 patients) or cystadenocarcinoma (2 patients) was 17.8 months versus 9.3 months in historical controls ($P < 0.05$). Again, disease progression was rarely noted in the liver, since tumour regrowth or metastases occurred either locally or in the peritoneum (7). Coeliac artery infusion delivers the drugs not only to the rest of the pancreas and upper abdominal organs but also intraportally via the splenic vein. The combination of hepatic arterial and portal vein infusion, as practised in resected pancreatic cancer patients by Ishikawa et al. (17) reduced the hepatic progression and improved survival significantly in comparison with historical controls, mainly due to suppression of hepatic disease progression. Other forms of successful adjuvant therapy have not yet been reported. Postoperative immunotherapy with a murine monoclonal antibody did not improve survival (46).

Neoadjuvant Therapy

The rationales of neoadjuvant preoperative therapy have been outlined by Goldie and Coltman (47) from a tumour biology point of view. The need to down-stage tumours effectively results from the low resectability rates which range from 5% to 22% in large collective reviews or series (12). The approach to treat all tumours before resection has been successfully applied in childhood (hepatoblastoma, Wilm's tumour), sarcomas, and breast cancer, either to achieve better survival rates or to allow more conservative and less mutilating surgery. Bruckner et al. (4) found that previously irresectable cases treated with radiochemotherapy, down-staged and resected, had a median survival time of 33 months that compares well with the median survival times reported in the literature. A Fox Chase Cancer Center group treated all stage I–III UICC resectable pancreatic cancer patients with preoperative radiochemotherapy using 50.4 Gy external beam radiotherapy and 5-FU continuous infusion plus mitomycin-C bolus infusion as radiation enhancers. Surgical resection was scheduled 4–6 weeks after the completion of radiotherapy. Subsequently this programme was extended to other institutions of the Eastern Cooperative Oncology Group (ECOG). Eighteen percent of the patients developed extrapancreatic disease progression during neoadjuvant treatment, and in 5/39 (13%) the primary tumour increased in size (48). In the multicentre FCCC/ECOG study involving 53 patients, 41 were explored via laparotomy, and 23 could be resected, a resection rate of 56% in the explored and 43% in all patients (49). There were two treatment-related deaths and grade IV ECOG toxicity was 34% (49). A treatment break (1–14 days) was necessary in 31% of the patients. The operative morbidity and mortality (5.3%) was not higher than in patients who had pancreatic resection without prior chemoradiation, although total pancreatectomy was the preferred surgical method at the beginning of the study to avoid radiotherapy-induced anastomotic troubles. With increasing experience Whipple's procedure was also performed if indicated (50). Interestingly, in the patients who had total pancreatectomy, in addition to brittle diabetes, six of nine patients also developed severe ascites that was eventually reversible (48). There was no complete response of the resected primary tumour, and a reduction of the tumour area was seen in only one patient. Pathologically the tumours showed abundant fibrosis, necrosis, and hyalinisation with scattered islands of malignant cells. Surgical margins were negative for malignancy in all resected cases, in spite of frequent intraoperative portal vein or SMV adherence. Lymph node metastases were present in only 17% of the resected specimens (50). Recurrence sites were the liver, peritoneum, pleura or multiple, and local recurrence occurred in only 10% (48,50). The median survival time in the 23 resected patients of the cooperative group study was 16.6 months (49) and actuarial 5-year survival was 58% (50). As a conclusion from this study, the authors stated that lymph nodes and margins seemed to be down-staged, complete resection was facilitated and local recurrences were prevented with a procedure that could be performed safely even in a cooperative study group setting. These hypotheses and the question whether neoadjuvant chemoradiation according to the FCCC/ECOG protocol prolongs survival must be examined in a randomized controlled phase III trial. The method seems to be effective as well in duodenal cancer (50). Preoperative radiation alone also seems to devitalise the tumour and facilitate resection, improving the short-term, but not the long-term survival (16).

Conclusions and Future Directions

Up to now, only 22% or less of operated patients have received some form of chemotherapy, radiotherapy or the combination of both (51). In resected patients multimodal treatment is even less often used. This may be because many physicians believe that the disease has an uncontrollable early fatal outcome, that cannot be influenced by currently available standard methods. The literature and our own experiences with adjuvant therapy in resected pancreatic cancer patients have shown that life can be significantly prolonged by multimodal therapy. Adjuvant systemic chemotherapy, postoperative radiochemotherapy or postoperative intra-arterial infusion chemotherapy seem to extend the median survival time by $\geq$ 9 months (7,17,40–44) and increase 5-year survival rates by > 10% (41–44) with tolerable side effects. Preoperative radiotherapy/ radiochemotherapy may down-stage the primary tumour, increase resectability and reduce local recurrences (16,48–50) and improve survival (4), and this neoadjuvant treatment seems to be superior to postoperative radiochemotherapy or surgery concerning cost-effectiveness (54).

There is therefore an intriguing rationale to combine preoperative radiotherapy with pre- and postoperative intra-arterial coeliac axis infusion chemotherapy. Preoperative radiotherapy tumours can down-stage the tumour and sterilise margins. High-concentration local chemotherapy in addition may contribute to destruction of chemosensitive micrometastatic foci in the distribution area of the coeliac axis including the liver. In our palliative trial, the primary tumours showed a partial remission according to WHO criteria (56) in 29% and did not resume growth in another 35% of the patients. Preoperative radiochemotherapy induced a partial response in only one patient (50), so that the substitution of systemic by regional chemotherapy might result in a better response and a lower progression rate, not only locoregionally but also in the liver. It can be assumed that the drugs used in our combination protocol appear – at reduced plasma levels – also in the systemic circulation, as has been demonstrated for 5-FU and folinic acid during hepatic arterial infusion (57). Our protocol, based on *in vitro* studies with human pancreatic cancer cell lines (30), contains mitoxantrone, 5-FU + folinic acid and cisplatinum which are active even in systemic chemotherapy. Preoperative radiochemotherapy can be safely applied, even in a multicentre setting (48,49). Intra-arterial drug delivery in our hospital is standardised from the medical and nursing care points of view, and is safely practised in other hospitals. Toxicity does not include the toxic side effects of "conventional" systemic chemotherapy or radiochemotherapy (6). Postoperative regional chemotherapy, perfusing the non-irradiated upper abdominal organs including the pancreatic remnant, most probably prolongs survival with the major effect on hepatic progression (7,17). For the irradiated area it must be assumed that 8–12 weeks after radiation the peripheral arterial blood flow is substantially decreased. The "adjuvant" intra-arterial treatment should therefore be continued for at least four cycles, making a total of six cycles of regional chemotherapy.

The problem of peritoneal progression most probably will not be resolved with this multimodality approach. Peritoneal carcinomaosis might be generated by direct tumour infiltration of the peritoneum and tumour cell shedding, by contamination due to surgical or diagnostic manipulations or by tumour cells outflowing from disrupted lymphatic vessels (12,14,15). Intraperitoneal hyperthermic intraoperative chemotherapy might be an additional approach to be added to a multimodality concept to treat pancreatic cancer (14). Intraperitoneal chemotherapy takes advantage of the concentration response behaviour of drugs (28,29), is effective in malignant ascites (29), in small nodule or superficial peritoneal carcinomatosis, especially if applied under hyperthermic conditions (58) and as adjuvant treatment of locally advanced gastrointestinal cancers (59–61).

An alternative option for neoadjuvant/adjuvant therapy of pancreatic cancer would be systemic chemotherapy, if sufficiently active protocols were available. The 5-FU modulation protocols induce response rates from 0 to 41%, and are associated with median survival times of 5–15 months (20–24, 62–64). Although with the combination of 5-FU continuous infusion, folinic acid, mitomycin-C and dipyridamol, which induces extremely good responses (10% CR, 31% PR, 59% PD), down-staging and resection is possible (H. Reber, UCLA, personal communication, (24)), the responses of the other protocols, including the combination of 5-FU with other drugs or of other drugs without 5-FU, are low, so that these therapies, especially if not yet proven to be more active than 5-FU monotherapy, currently do not qualify for neoadjuvant treatment protocols involving only chemotherapy.

We have started a protocol treating non-resectable pancreatic cancer patients with radiotherapy and intra-arterial chemotherapy in an interdisciplinary approach ("Ulmer Forschungsgruppe Onkologie Gastrointestinaler Tumoren, protocol UFOGT-1"). If this protocol proves to be tolerable and successful and can lead to a down-staging and a higher resectability rate in primarily non-resectable cases, it will be used in a controlled study for neoadjuvant/adjuvant therapy of all pancreatic cancer patients. If peritoneal carcinomatosis remains a major problem within this treatment concept, the next step would be to add intraperitoneal intraoperative hyperthermic chemotherapy as the fourth treatment modality to this multimodality neoadjuvant/adjuvant treatment approach.

References

1. Beger HG, Büchler MW, Friess H (1994) Chirurgische Ergebnisse und Indikation zu adjuvanten Mabnahmen beim Pankreascarcinom. Chirurg 65:246–252.
2. Bruckner HW, Kalnicki S, Dalton J et al. (1993) Combined modality therapy increasing local control of pancreatic cancer. Cancer Invest 11:241–246.
3. Bruckner HW, Kalnicki S, Dalton J et al. (1993) Survival after combined modality therapy for pancreatic cancer. J Clin Gastroenterol 16:199–203.
4. Bruckner HW, Snady H, Cooperman A et al. (1995) Combined modality therapy for effective local control in stage II and III unresectable pancreatic carcinoma. Proc ASCO 14:216 (abstract).
5. Aigner KR, Gailhofer S (1993) Regional chemotherapy for nonresectable, locally metastasized pancreatic cancer: four studies including 164 cases. Reg. Cancer Treat. Suppl. 1:2 (abstract).
6. Link KH, Gansauge F, Pillasch J et al. (1994) Regional treatment of advanced nonresectable and of resected pancreatic cancer via celiac axis infusion. First results of a single institution study. Dig Surg 11:414–419.
7. Gansauge F, Link KH, Rilinger N et al. (1996) Adjuvante regionale Chemotherapie beim resezierten fortgeschrittenen Pankreascarcinom. Chirurg 67:362–365.
8. Weiss L, Harlos JP, Hartveit F et al. (1992) Metastatic pattern from cancers of the pancreas: an analysis of 558 autopsies. Reg. Cancer Treat 4:265–271.
9. Andrén-Sandberg A, Westerdahl J, Ihse I (1992) Recurrence after pancreatectomy for pancreatic cancer. Digestion 52:67–137 (abstract).
10. Griffin JF, Smalley SR, Jewell W (1990) Patterns of failure after curative resection of pancreatic carcinoma. Cancer 66:56–61.
11. Weiss SM, Skibber JM, Mohiuddin M, Rosato FE (1985) Rapid intra-abdominal spread of pancreatic cancer. Arch Surg 120:415–416.
12. Warshaw AL, Fernández-Del Castillo C (1992) Pancreatic carcinoma. N Engl J Med 326:455–465.
13. Warshaw AL (1991) Implications of peritoneal cytology for staging of early pancreatic cancer. Am J Surg 161:26–30.
14. Ettinghausen SE (1995) Rationale for intraperitoneal chemotherapy in the treatment of adenocarcinoma of the pancreas. Reg Cancer Treat 8:20–24.
15. Heeckt P, Safi F, Binder T, Büchler M (1992) Freie intraperitoneale Tumorzellen beim Pankreascarcinom-Bedeutung für den klinischen Verlauf und die Therapie. Chirurg 63:563–567.
16. Ishikawa O, Ohigashi H, Imaoka S et al. (1994) Is the long-term survival rate improved by preoperative irradiation prior to Whipple's procedure for adenocarcinoma of the pancreatic head? Arch Surg 129:1075–1080.
17. Ishikawa O, Ohigashi H, Sasaki Y et al. (1994) Liver perfusion chemotherapy via both the hepatic artery and portal vein to prevent hepatic metastasis after extended pancreatectomy for adenocarcinoma of the pancreas. Am J Surg 168:361–364.

18. Warshaw AL, Swanson RS (1988) Pancreatic cancer in 1988. Possibilities and probabilities. Ann Surg 208:541–553.
19. Arbuck SG (1990) Overview of chemotherapy for pancreatic cancer. Int J Pancreatol 7:209–222.
20. Cascinu S, Fedeli A, Fedeli SL, Catalano G (1993) 5-Fluorouracil, leucovorin and interferon alpha 2b in advanced pancreatic cancer: a pilot study. Ann Oncol 4:83–84.
21. Moore MJ, Erlichman C, Kaizer L, Fine S (1993) A phase II study of 5-fluorouracil, leucovorin and interferon-alpha in advanced pancreatic cancer. Anticancer Drugs 4:555–557.
22. Louvet C, Beerblock K, De Gramont A et al. (1993) High-dose folinic acid, 5-fluorouracil bolus and infusion in advanced pancreatic adenocarcinoma: a pilot study. Eur J Cancer 29A:1217–1218.
23. Bernhard H, Jager AE, Bernhard G et al. (1995) Treatment of advanced pancreatic cancer with 5-fluorouracil, folinic acid and interferon alpha-2A: results of a phase II trial. Br J Cancer 71:102–105.
24. Isacoff WH, Reber H, Tompkins R et al. (1995) Continuous infusion (CI) 5-fluorouracil (5-FU), calcium leucovorin (LV), mitomycin-c (Mito C), and dipyridamole (D); treatment for patients with locally advanced pancreatic cancer. Proc ASCO 14:198 (abstract).
25. Rougier P, Zarva JJ, Ducreux M et al. (1993) Phase II study of cisplatin and 120-hour continuous infusion of 5-fluorouracil in patients with advanced pancreatic adenocarcinoma. Ann Oncol 4:333–336.
26. Palmer KR, Kerr M, Knowles G et al. (1994) Chemotherapy prolongs survival in inoperable pancreatic carcinoma. Br J Surg 81:882–885.
27. Moore M, Andersen J, Burris H et al. (1995) A randomized trial of gemcitabine (GEM) versus 5-FU as first-line therapy in advanced pancreatic cancer. Proc ASCO 14:199 (abstract).
28. Link KH, Staib L, Beger HG (1989) Influence of exposure concentration and exposure time cxt on toxicity of cytostatic drugs to HT29 human colorectal carcinoma cells. Reg Cancer Treat 2:189–197.
29. Link KH, Hepp G, Butzer Z et al. (1995) Rationales for intraperitoneal chemotherapy: chemo-sensitivity testing and pharmacokinetic considerations. Clinical experience with intraperitoneal chemotherapy. Acta Chir Austr 27:95–100.
30. Link KH, Kindler D, Hummel M, Büchler M (1992) Dose response treatment studies with two pancreatic carcinoma cell lines in vitro. Digestion 52:102 (abstract).
31. Rougier P, Laplanche A, Huguier M et al. (1992) Hepatic arterial infusion of floxuridine in patients with liver metastases from colorectal carcinoma: long-term results of a prospective randomized trial. J Clin Oncol 10:1112–1118.
32. Allen-Mersh TG, Earlam S, Fordy C et al. (1994) Quality of life and survival with continuous hepatic-artery floxuridine infusion for colorectal liver metastases. Lancet 344:1255–1260.
33. Donatini B, Rougier P (1992) Anatomical basis for pancreatic locoregional chemotherapy. Reg Cancer Treat 4:272–276.
34. Gansauge F, Link KH, Rilinger N (1995) Regionale Chemotherapie beim fortgeschrittenen Pankreaskarzinom. Med Klin 90:501–505.
35. Ohigashi H et al. (1994) Pancreatic cancer: arterial infusion chemotherapy for advanced pancreatic cancer. In: Tagachi T, Nakamura H (eds) Arterial infusion chemotherapy. pp 416–426.
36. Moertel CG, Frytak S, Hahn RG et al. (Gastrointestinal Tumor Study Group) (1981) Therapy of locally unresectable pancreatic carcinoma: a randomized comparison of high dose (6000 rads) radiation alone, moderate dose radiation (4000 rads + 5-fluorouracil) and high-dose radiation and 5-fluorouracil. Cancer 48:1705–1710.
37. Gastrointestinal Tumour Study Group (1988) Treatment of locally resectable carcinoma of the pancreas: comparison of combined-modality therapy (chemotherapy plus radiotherapy) to chemotherapy alone. J Natl Cancer Inst 80:751–755.
38. Moertel CG, Gunderson LL, Mailliard JA et al. (1994) Early evaluation of combined fluorouracil and leucovorin as a radiation enhancer for locally unresectable, residual, or recurrent gastrointestinal carcinoma. J Clin Oncol 12:21–27.
39. Bodner E (1994) Intraoperative Bestrahlung beim Pankreascarcinom. Chirurg 65:241–245.
45. Riethmüller G, Schneider-Gädicke E, Schlimok G et al. (1994) Randomised trial of monoclonal antibody for adjuvant therapy of resected Dukes' C colorectal carcinoma. Lancet 34:1177–1183.
46. Büchler M, Friess H, Schultheis KH et al. (1991) A randomized controlled trial of passive immunotherapy (murine monoclonal antibody 494/32) in resectable pancreatic cancer. Cancer 68:1507–1512.
47. Goldie JH, Coldman AJ (1986) Application of theoretical models to chemotherapy protocol design. Cancer Treat. Rep 70:127–131.

48. Hoffman JP, Weese JL, Solin LJ et al. (1993) A single institutional experience with preoperative chemoradiotherapy for stage I–III pancreatic adenocarcinoma. Am Surg 59:772–780.
49. Hoffman JP, Weese JL, Lipsitz S et al. (1995) Preoperative chemoradiation for patients with resectable pancreatic adenocarcinoma: an eastern cooperative oncology group (ECOG) phase II study. Proc ASCO 14:201(abstract).
50. Yeung RS, Weese JL, Hoffman JP et al. (1993) Neoadjuvant chemoradiation in pancreatic and duodenal carcinoma – A phase II study. Cancer 72:2124–2133.
51. Baumel H, Huguier M, Manderscheid JC et al. (1994) Results of resection for cancer of the exocrine pancreas: a study from the French Association of Surgery. Br J Surg 81: 102–107.
52. Gall FP, Zirngibl H (1986) Maligne Tumoren des Pankreas und der periampullären Region. In: gall FP et al. (eds) Chirurgische Onkologie: Histologie- und stadiengerechte Therapie maligner Tumoren. Springer, Berlin Heidelberg New York, pp 416–460.
53. Gudjonsson B (1987) Cancer of the pancreas: 50 years of surgery. Cancer 60:2284–2303.
54. Farber LA, Fier CM, Mandeli J, Bruckner HW (1996) Efficacy, cost and quality of life considerations applicable to periadjuvant therapy for pancreatic cancer (Sixth International Congress on Anti-Cancer Treatment). SOMPS 118(abstract).
55. Ohigashi H, Ishikawa O, Nakamori S et al. (1993) Evaluation of intra-arterial infusion chemotherapy and radical pancreatectomy in patients with locally advanced pancreatic cancer. Gan To Kagaku Ryoho 20:1672–1675.
56. Miller AB, Hoogstraten B, Staquet M, Winkler A (1981) Reporting results of cancer treatment. Cancer 47:207–214.
57. Link KH, Kreuser ED, Safi F et al. (1993) Die intraarterielle Chemotherapie mit 5-FU und Folinsäure (FA, Rescuvolin) im Therapiekonzept bei nicht resektablen kolorektalen Lebermetastasen. Tumordiagn u Ther 14:224–231.
58. Fujimoto S, Shrestha RD, Kokubun M et al. (1990) Positive results of combined therapy of surgery and intraperitoneal hyperthermic perfusion for far-advanced gastric cancer. Ann Surg 212:592–596.
59. Hagiwara A, Takahashi T, Kojima O et al. (1992) Prophylaxis with carbon-absorbed mitomycin against peritoneal recurrence of gastric cancer. Lancet 339:629–631.
60. Sugarbaker PH, Gianola FJ, Speyer JL et al. (1985) Prospective randomized trial of intravenous v. intraperitoneal 5-FU in patients with advanced primary colon or rectal cancer. Semin Oncol XII:101–111.
61. Fujimoto S, Shrestha RD, Kokubun M et al. (1988) Intraperitoneal hyperthermic perfusion combined with surgery effective for gastric cancer patients with peritoneal seeding. Ann Surg 208:36–41.
62. Derderian P, Pazdur R, Adjani J et al. (1991) Phase II study of 5-fluorouracil (5FU) and recombinant alpha-2a interferon (rIFN) in the treatment of advanced pancreatic carcinoma. Proc Am Soc Clin Oncol 10:147(Abstract).
63. Schneider CJ, Vaughn DJ, Holroyde C et al. (1995) Phase II trial of 5-FU, leucovorin and interferon alpha 2A in metastatic pancreatic carcinoma: A Penn Cancer Clinical Trials Group (PCCTG) trial. Proc ASCO 14:189(Abstract).
64. DeCaprio JA, Arbuck SG, Mayer RJ (1989) Phase II study of weekly 5-fluorouracil (5FU) and folinic acid (FA) in previously untreated patients with unresectable measurable pancreatic adenocarcinoma. Proc Am Soc Clin Oncol 8:100(Abstract).
65. Wils JA, Kok T, Wagener DJT et al. (1993) Activity of cisplatin in adenocarcinoma of the pancreas. Eur J Cancer 29A:203–204.
66. Bertheault-Cvitkovic F, Lévi F, Soussan S et al. (1993) Circadian rhythm-modulated chemotherapy with high-dose 5-fluorouracil: a pilot study in patients with pancreatic adenocarcinoma. Eur J Cancer 29A:1851–1854.
67. Bukowski RM, Fleming TR, MacDonald JS et al. (1993) Evaluation of combination chemotherapy and phase II agents in pancreatic adenocarcinoma. Cancer 71:322–325.
68. Rougier P, Adenis A, Ducreux M et al. (1995) Phase II study of docetaxel in pancreatic adenocarcinoma (PAC): final results after extra-mural review. Acta Chir Scand
69. Wils JA, Kok T Wagener DJT et al. (1993) Phase II trial with ifosfamide in pancreatic cancer. Eur J Cancer 29A:290.
70. Asbury RF, Cnaan A Johnson L et al. (1994) An eastern cooperative onocology group phase II study of single agent DHAD, VP-16, aclacinomycin, or spirogermanium in metastatic pancreatic cancer. Am J Clin Oncol 17:166–169.
71. Di Bartolomeo M, Zampino MG, DiLeo A, Bajetta E (1993) Epirubicin, etoposide and cisplatin in advanced pancreatic carcinoma. Eur J Cancer 29:1215–1216.

72. Orita K, Tanaka N, Gochi A et al. (1995) Clinical trial of immunochemotherapy with OH-1 preparation (IFN-α and TNF-α) and UFT (uraciltegafur) in unresectable pancreatic cancer. Proc ASCO 14:162(abstract).
73. Aigner KR, Müller H, Bassermann R (1990) Intra-arterial chemotherapy with MMC, CDDP and 5-FU for nonresectable pancreatic cancer: a phase II study. Reg Cancer Treat 3:1-6.
74. Miura T (1994) Arterial infusion chemotherapy for pancreatic cancer. In: Taguchi T, Nakamura H (ed) Arterial infusion chemotherapy. pp 427-436.
75. Whittington R, Solin L, Mohiuddin ME (1984) Multimodality therapy of localized unresectable pancreatic adenocarcinoma. Cancer 54:1991-1998.
76. Mohiuddin M, Rosato F, Barbot D et al. (1992) Long-term results of combined modality treatment with J125 implantation for carcinoma of the pancreas. Int J Radiat Oncol Biol Phys 23:305-311.
77. Wagener DJT, v. Hoesel WGCM Yap SHE (1989) Phase II trial of 5-fluorouracil, adriamycin and cisplatin (FAP) followed by radiation and 5-fluorouracil in locally advanced pancreatic cancer. Cancer Chemother Pharmacol 25:131-134.
78. Kamthan A, Morris JC, Chesser MR et al. (1992) Combined modality therapy for effective local control in stage II and III pancreatic carcinoma. Proc Am Soc Clin Oncol 11:160.
79. Jessup JM, Jr Steele G, Mayer RJ et al. (1993) Neoadjuvant therapy for unresectable pancreatic adenocarcinoma. Arch Surg 128:559-564.
80. Bronn D, Franklin R, Krishnan R et al. (1995) Rapid radiographic response in pancreatic cancer with concurrent continuous infusion (DI) 5-fluorouracil and cisplatin and hyperfractionated radiotherapy. Proc ASCO 14:193(abstract).
81. Schein PS, Smith FP, Dritschillo A et al. (1983) Phase I-II trial of combined modality FAM (5-fluorouracil, adriamycin, mitomycin-C) plus splitcourse radiation (FAM-RT-FAM) for locally advanced gastric cancer and pancreatic cancer: a mid-atlantic oncology program study. Proc ASCO 2:126(abstract)
82. Komaki R, Hansen R, Cox JD et al. (1988). Phase I-II study of prophylactic hepatic irradiation with local irradiation and systemic chemotherapy for adenocarcinoma of the pancreas. Int J Radiation Oncol Biol Phys 15:1447-1452.
83. Komaki R, Wadler S, Peters T et al. (1992) High-dose local irradiation plus prophylactic hepatic irradiation and chemotherapy for inoperable adenocarcinoma of the pancreas. Cancer 69:2807-2812.
84. Wagener DJT, Rougier P, Wils JA (1992) Combined chemoradiotherapy for locally advanced pancreatic cancer. Proc ASCO 11:166(abstract).
85. Earle JD, Foley JF, Wieand HS et al. 1993. Evaluation of external-beam radiation therapy plus 5-fluorouracil (5-FU) versus external-beam radiation therapy plus hycanthone (HYC) in confined, unresectable pancreatic cancer. Int J Radiat Oncol Biol Phys 28:207-211.
86. Jeekel J, Treurniet-Donker AD (1991) Treatment perspectives in locally advanced unresectable pancreatic cancer. Br J Surg 78:1332-1334.

39 Adjuvant Therapy in Pancreatic Cancer

Paula Ghaneh, Anthony Kawesha, J.D. Evans and J.P. Neoptolemos

Pancreatic cancer continues to present a difficult clinical problem with an overall 5-year survival rate of only 0.4% (1,2). Nevertheless, improvements in surgical techniques, supportive care and referrals to specialised centres (3) have resulted in resection rates of 7–14% (4,5) and decreasing operative mortality rates of less than 10%. Yet the median survival time after surgery is only 10–18 months, with overall 5-year survival rates of 10–24% (6–13). In reality this means that very few patients are actually cured in spite of the advances that have been made in conventional treatment (10).

The main purpose of adjuvant therapy is to improve survival following curative resection, which should be accompanied by a reasonable quality of life. The extent of toxicity is therefore an important factor when considering the particular choice of regimen. The rationale for the range and combination of agents currently being tested in the adjuvant setting is based on the result of treatments in patients with advanced disease.

Neoadjuvant Therapy

For patients with locally advanced disease preoperative chemoradiotherapy may offer a better chance for curative surgery and improved survival. The main benefits of preoperative therapy are a reduction in the high frequency of positive resection margins; that radiation is more effective on oxygenated tumour cells which have not been traumatised by previous surgery; that treatment is not delayed by a protracted postoperative recovery; possible peritoneal tumour cell spread may be prevented; and the proportion of patients suitable for resection may be increased. The concept of preoperative radiotherapy was first published by Tepper et al. in 1975 (14). Early studies of preoperative radiotherapy resulted in a 30% 5-year survival in those patients who subsequently underwent resection (15,16). A more recent study of patients receiving preoperative external beam radiation therapy (EBRT) alone demonstrated a high resection rate but similar survival to that of surgery alone (17). A limiting factor affecting the resection rate may be the size of the tumour. Two studies found that tumours greater than 4–5 cm or which obstructed the portal vein/SMV or encased the SMA were unlikely to be resected (18–19) following neoadjuvant therapy.

In some studies of resection only, a high proportion of positive resection margins has been reported (20), but neoadjuvant treatment seems to demonstrate a much lower rate. One study found just one of 11 patients had a positive resection margin (19). Another demonstrated a resection rate of 60% with a negative resection margin rate of 82% (21). A recent study using 30–50 Gy with continuous infusion 5-FU and IORT in 39 patients showed a high negative margin rate (82%) and median survival time of 19 months (22). The high rates of negative resection margins seen may be due to a number of other factors such as more detailed preoperative imaging of the tumour using spiral/contrast enhanced CT and angiography to identify arterial involvement/anatomy and a standardised resection technique.

Median survival for preoperative chemoradiation has been reported as high as 19–27 months from tissue diagnosis (17,19,22,23). Results of preoperative regimens seem encouraging, especially for locally advanced tumours (Table 1). Toxicity can be considerable: increased hospitalisation can be required in a high proportion of cases and treatment-related deaths may be higher than without preoperative chemotherapy (19). The use of neoadjuvant therapy will need to be endorsed by randomised clinical trials before it can be considered as part of a standard treatment for pancreatic cancer.

Intraoperative and Postoperative Radiotherapy

A number of studies have demonstrated advantages of radiotherapy in terms of local control and pain relief with some increase in survival times (Table 2). In a comparative study of IORT and EBRT in patients who have undergone pancreatic resection, the median survival for the IORT group was 18 months versus 12 months for the EBRT group (25). In a non-randomised trial comparing IORT with no radiotherapy in patients with resected pancreatic cancer, the local recurrence rate was 50% less in the IORT group but survival was not significantly different (31). Two reports combining radical and extended radical excision in combination with IORT reported a 3-year survival of 53% and 5-year survival of 29% (27,32). Overall however the long-term survival figures for adjuvant EBRT or IORT seem to be similar to those for surgery alone.

High doses of IORT have been associated with visceral and vascular damage and septic complications (33), although operative blood loss was reported not to be high in one study (31). Both IORT and EBRT appear to decrease local recurrence rates but there is no reduction in the rate of distant metastases (Table 3) and long-term survival rates are not apparently increased. Overall current data suggest that radiation therapy is probably inadequate as a single modality treatment in the adjuvant setting but can provide good local control with alleviation of pain in most patients. There appears to be no significant difference between EBRT and IORT in terms of their activity and survival; moreover IORT requires specialised equipment and dedicated operating space.

The liver has been suggested as a specific target for irradiation due to the high rate of hepatic recurrence. The toxicity of this approach can be considerable, as shown in one study of hepatic irradiation and chemotherapy in patients due to have pancreatic resection, in which the excessive toxicity resulted in early termination (37).

Table 1. The results of neoadjuvant therapy in pancreatic cancer

Series	Number	EBRT(Gy)	Chemotherapy	Resection rate		Operative mortality		Resection margin +ve		Survival
				n	(%)	n	(%)	n	(%)	
Pilepich & Miller 1980 (15)	17	40–50	–	6/17	35	0	0	2/6	33	2 × 5 year survivors
Kopelson et al. 1983 (16)	4	40–45	–	4/4	100	0	0	0/4	0	1 > 7 years
Weese et al. 1990 (24)	16	40–60	5FU + mitomycin C	10/16	62	2/10	20	0/10	0	MST 11 months
Evans et al. 1992 (21)	28	50.4	5FU	17/28	61	1/17	6	3/17	18	–
Ishikawa et al. 1994 (17)	23	50	–	17/23	74	0/17	0	–	–	22% 5-year survival
Coia et al. 1994 (18)	27	50.4	5FU + mitomycin C	13/27	48	–	–	0/13	0	MST 16 months 43% 3-year survival
Hoffman et al. 1995 (19)	34	50	5FU + mitomycin C	11/34	32	1/11	9	1/11	9	40% 5-year survival
Staley et al. 1996 (22)	39	30–50	5FU + IORT	39/39	100	1/39	2	7/39	18	MST 19 months 19% 4-year survival

5FU, fluorouracil; MST, median survival time; IORT, intraoperative radiation therapy; EBRT, external beam radiation therapy.

Table 2. The results of adjuvant radiotherapy in pancreatic cancer.

Series	Period	Number	Pancreatic resection	IORT (Gy)	EBRT (Gy)	Actuarial survival			
						MST	1 year (%)	3 years (%)	5 years (%)
Sindelar (1989) (25)	–	11	tp	20	–	12 months	–	–	–
		6	tp	–	45–50	10 months	–	–	–
Shibamoto et al. 1990 (26)	1983–89	17	c	–	50–55	14 months	82	25	25
	1983–89	11	n-c	–	55–60	12 months	61	0	0
Hiraoka 1990 (27)	1966–75	19	c	–	–	8 months	27	0	0
	1976–81	15	c	30	–	8 months	38	0	0
	1982–83	9	r/c	–	–	8 months	44	12	0
	1984–89	16	r/c	–	–	26 months	65	50	29
Bosset et al. 1992 (28)	1985–90	14	c	–	54	23 months	100	50	18
Brachet et al. 1993 (29)	1985–92	18	kw	18	36–44	–	57	23	–
			tp	–	13	–			
Johnstone et al. 1993 (30)	1980–84	26	kw	20	45–55	18 months	–	–	–
Zerbi et al. 1994 (31)	1985–93	43	c	12.5–20	–	13 months	71	24	–
		47	c	–	–	8 months	49	16	–

tp, total pancreatectomy; kw, Kausch–Whipple resection; c, curative; r, radical; n-c, noncurative; MST, median survival time; IORT, intraoperative radiation therapy; EBRT, external beam radiation therapy.

Table 3. The incidence of tumour local recurrences and metastases following adjuvant therapy for pancreatic cancer.

Series	Number	EBRT/IORT	Chemotherapy	Recurrence overall		local		hepatic		peritoneal		distant	
				n	%	n	%	n	%	n	%	n	%
GITSG 1987 (34)	30	EBRT	5FU	–	–	11	37	9	30	–	–	–	–
Whittington et al. 1991 (35)	37	EBRT	5FU	29	78	14	38	13	35	13	35	5	14
Bosset et al. 1992 (28)	14	EBRT	–	12	86	7	50	5	36	2	14	–	–
Foo et al. 1993 (36)	29	EBRT	5FU	24	83	3	10	12	41	12	41	–	–
Johnstone et al. 1993 (30)	15	EBRT/IORT	–	11	73	14	93	8	53	5	33	5	33
Willet et al. 1993 (20)	72	EBRT	5FU	–	–	48	67	–	–	–	–	–	–
Zerbi et al. 1994 (31)	37	IORT	–	22	59	10	27	12	32	–	–	4	10

Adjuvant Chemotherapy

Regimens of chemotherapy alone allow for cytotoxic doses which can be commenced soon after surgery. The use of chemotherapy alone would perhaps have the drawback of inadequate local control but one study demonstrated similar rates of recurrence (33% locoregional) to that observed after EBRT alone (38). In a non-randomised study using the FAM regimen 16 patients had adjuvant treatment and 36 did not, with 3-year survival rates which were 24% and 28%, respectively (38). The FAM regimen has also been used in a randomised trial in which 30 patients were given chemotherapy following surgery and 31 patients had resection alone (Table 4). The median survival was significantly greater for the adjuvant group (23 months versus 11 months for the resection only group) but the 5-year survival figures were not significantly different (39).

The toxic affects of combination chemotherapy can be significant. In the study by Bakkevold et al. (39) only 13 of 24 patients managed to complete all the courses of adjuvant treatment. Gastrointestinal toxicity was the major problem and approximately half the patients needed hospitalisation. One patient died of septic complications. The role of chemotherapy alone as an adjuvant treatment still needs confirmation from other randomised clinical trials.

Adjuvant Regional Therapy

The main aim of hepatic infusional chemotherapy is to control hepatic metastases and improve the results seen with systemic chemotherapy alone. Simultaneous infusion of 5FU via both portal vein and hepatic artery in 20 patients for 28–35 days (compared with a group of historical controls with and without adjuvant therapy) was used in one study (41). The treatment was well tolerated by the patients and 3-year survival was 54%. Death from hepatic metastases alone was 8% compared with 34% in the control groups and death from locoregional recurrence was similar for all groups.

Regional intra-arterial chemotherapy is limited by the lack of a single definable vascular source for the blood supply of the pancreas and many of the adjacent organs are sensitive to the chemotherapeutic agents. To increase the selectivity of this approach the splenic and or the gastroduodenal artery have been used with simultaneous infusion of angiotensin II to increase blood flow in tumour tissue (42). Link et al. (43) used a regimen consisting of mitoxantrone, folinic acid, 5-FU and cisplatin for coeliac artery infusion in 20 patients following resection. Median survival was an impressive 21 months with a 2-year survival rate of 40%. Regional therapy seems to reduce the rate of liver metastases but has no effect on local recurrence. There is a substantial dropout rate associated with these approaches but the results are encouraging and should be assessed further.

Combined Adjuvant Therapy

The first prospectively randomised trial of postoperative adjuvant therapy was instituted by the GITSG in 1973. Patients were randomised to receive a split course of 40 Gy combined with 5FU (500 mg/m^2 bolus), or no adjuvant treatment.

Table 4. Results of adjuvant chemotherapy in pancreatic cancer

Series	Period	Number	Regime	Actuarial survival			
				MST	1 year (%)	3 years (%)	5 years (%)
Splinter et al. 1989 (38)	1980–84	16	5FU DOX MITC	–	–	24	–
Bakkevold et al. 1993[a] (39)	1984–87	30	5FU DOX MITC	23 months	70	70	4
		31	–	11 months	45	30	8
Baumel et al. 1994 (40)	1982–88	43	not specified	12 months	–	–	–

[a] Randomised controlled study.
DOX, doxorubicin; MITC, mitomycin C.

After 43 patients had been accrued, median survival in the control group was 11 months and in the treatment group 20 months, with a 2-year survival of 15% in those who did not receive adjuvant treatment and 42% for those that did (44). A further 30 patients received treatment and in this confirmatory group the median survival was 18 months and 2-year survival was 46% (34).

In a study from Whittington et al. (35), between 1981 and 1984 a total of 33 patients underwent pancreatectomy and did not receive adjuvant therapy. Local recurrence was 85% and there was a 41% 2-year survival in patients with negative resection margins. Then 19 patients received 45–48.6 Gy and eight also received bolus 5FU; the local recurrence was reduced to 55% but the 2-year survival was 33%. In about half of these patients the resection margin was grossly involved with tumour, again confirming that positive resection margins have a major effect on survival. A third group of patients received 5FU infusion concurrently with radiotherapy and a single dose of mitomycin C. Local recurrences were 25% and 2-year survival in patients with no residual disease was 59% (Table 5).

In the UK a study of combined treatment was devised by the UK Pancreatic Cancer Trials Group (UKPACA). Forty patients were recruited between 1987 and 1993. Following resection, patients received 40 Gy (with 5FU) then received weekly follow-on chemotherapy with 5FU. There was moderate toxicity with treatment discontinued in four patients. The median survival was 23 months and the 5-year survival was 15%. Significant prognostic factors were negative lymph node status and positive resection margins (46). Thus an improved long-term survival of more than 20% remains to be confirmed by much larger randomised trials to justify the routine use of adjuvant therapy in the treatment of pancreatic cancer.

The European Organisation for Research and Treatment of Cancer (EORTC) organised a randomised trial comparing adjuvant EBRT and concurrent 5FU with no adjuvant treatment (J. Jeekel, personal communication). One of the objectives was to demonstrate an improved 2-year survival from 30% to 50%. A total of 218 patients were randomised to receive EBRT + 5FU or observation only. There were 60 patients with ampullary tumours, 22 with bile duct tumours, two with duodenal tumours and the remainder had pancreatic ductal adenocarcinoma. The treatment was well tolerated with no major toxicity. The early results indicated no difference in median and 2-year survival between the two groups (and no difference between ampullary and ductal carcinomas). Analysis of the pattern of recurrence revealed it to be the same for both groups. The regimen in this study consisted of EBRT and concomitant 5FU without follow-on systemic chemotherapy, which may prove to be an important factor.

The European Study Group for Pancreatic cancer (ESPAC) is currently undertaking a large trial (ESPAC 1) to compare adjuvant radiotherapy (40 Gy course) and concurrent bolus of 5FU (500 mg/m^2), with systemic chemotherapy (folinic acid 20 mg/m^2 followed by 425 mg/m^2 5FU at weekly intervals for 6 months) and a combination of both of these treatments with a control arm (47). The patients are stratified by the presence of negative or positive resection margins. At the present time over 350 patients have been randomised through randomisation centres in the UK, Switzerland and Germany with further major centres in Spain, France, Italy and Greece. The target number is 450 patients in total. This is the largest pancreatic cancer trial so far and will provide invaluable information for the standardisation of pancreatic cancer adjuvant treatment.

Table 5. The results of adjuvant combined treatment in pancreatic cancer

Series	Period	Number	Radiotherapy (Gy)	Chemotherapy	Actuarial survival				
					MST	1 year (%)	2 years (%)	3 years (%)	5 years (%)
Kalser and Ellenberg 1985[a] (44)	1974–82	21	EBRT 40	5FU	20 months	67	43	24	18
		22	–	–	11 months	50	18	7	8
GITSG 1987 (34)	1982–85	30	EBRT 40	5FU	18 months	77	43	–	17
Whittington et al. 1991 (35)	1984–89	19	EBRT 45–49	5FU	–	–	55	–	–
		20	EBRT 54–63	5FU + Mit C	25	–	–	–	–
Willett et al. 1993 (20)	1978–91	16 (nm)	EBRT 40–50	5FU	21 months	–	–	–	29
		23 (pm)	EBRT 40–50	5FU	11 months	0	–	–	–
Yeo et al. 1995 (12)	1991–94	56	EBRT 45	5FU	20 months	–	35	–	–
1997 (45)	1991–95	99	EBRT 45	5FU	21 months	80	44	–	–
UKPACA 1997 (46)	1987–93	35	EBRT 40	5FU	13 months	56	38	29	15

[a] Randomised controlled trial.
Mit C, mitomycin C; nm, negative margins; pm, positive margins.

Towards the Millenium

Several classes of novel agents are now under early clinical investigation in advanced disease. Immunotherapeutic approaches using cytokines such as IL-2, IFNα, IFNγ and cytotoxic monoclonal antibodies have yet to show significant activity (48–50). IFNα has also been used as a modulator of 5-FU along with folinic acid with promising results (51). Early clinical trials of topoisomerase I inhibitors and thymydilate synthase inhibitors also are ongoing (52,53). The theory that tumour growth is angiogenesis dependent (54) has resulted in the use of various inhibitors of angiogenesis such as TNP-470 and IL-12 in early clinical studies (55). New drugs such as gemcitabine (a nucleoside analogue structurally similar to cytosine arabinoside) are currently being assessed. In a phase III study of 126 patients comparing gemcitabine to 5FU, median survival time was 5.6 months for gemcitabine and 4.4 months for 5FU (56). The orally bioactive matrix metalloproteinase inhibitor marimastat (BB 2516), which can also act as an inhibitor of angiogenesis, has shown encouraging early results, with a median survival time of over 6 months in patients with advanced pancreatic cancer (57). Tumour cytotoxicity can also be enhanced using gene therapy approaches (58–60) which are likely to lead to clinical trials in the near future. The studies in patients with advanced cancer have been and continue to be invaluable in ruling out toxic and ineffective drugs as well as indicating promising agents for use in the adjuvant setting.

Already major adjuvant trials using novel biological agents are under way including a study of marimastat versus placebo aiming to recruit 200 patients in the USA and Europe. An intergroup study in the USA is being planned to compare EBRT with radiosensitising 5FU against systemic gemcitabine. As the millenium approaches, these large trials will come to fruition and point the way for a standardised scientific approach to the adjuvant therapy of pancreatic cancer.

References

1. Gudjonsson B (1987) Cancer of the pancreas: 50 years of surgery. Cancer 60:2284–2303.
2. Bramhall SR, Allum WH, Jones AG, Allwood A, Cummins C, Neoptolemos JP (1995) Incidence, treatment and survival in 13,560 patients with pancreatic cancer: an epidemiological study in the West Midlands. Br J Surg 82:111–115.
3. Lieberman MD, Kilburn H, Lindsey M, Brennan MF (1995) Relation of perioperative deaths to hospital volume among patients undergoing pancreatic resection for malignancy. Ann Surg 222:638–645.
4. Neiderhuber JE, Brennan MF, Menck HR (1995) The national cancer data base report on pancreatic cancer. Cancer 76:1671–1677.
5. Wade TP, Halaby IA, Stapleton DR, Virgo KS, Johnson FE (1996) Population-based analysis of treatment of pancreatic cancer and Whipple resection: Department of Defense hospitals 1989–1994. Surgery 120:680–687.
6. Grace PA, Pitt HA, Tompkins RK, DenBesten L, Longmire Jr WP (1986) Decreased morbidity and mortality after pancreatectomy. Am J Surg 151:141–149.
7. Trede M, Schwall G, Saeger H-D (1990) Survival after pancreatoduodenectomy: 118 consecutive resections without an operative mortality. Ann Surg 211:447–458.
8. Russell RCG (1990) Surgical resection for cancer of the pancreas. Baillière's Clin Gastroenterol 4:889–916.
9. Cameron JL, Pitt HA, Yeo CJ, Lillimoe KD, Kaufman HS, Coleman J (1993). One hundred and forty five consecutive pancreaticoduodenectomies without mortality. Ann Surg 217:430–438.

10. Edge SB, Schmieg Jr R, Rosenlof LK, Willhelm MC (1993) Pancreas cancer resection outcome in American university centers in 1989–1990. Cancer 71:3502–3508.

11. Nitecki SS, Sarr MG, Colby TV, Van Heerden JA (1995) Long-term survival after resection for ductal adenocarcinoma of the pancreas. It is really improving? Ann Surg 221:59–66.

12. Yeo CJ, Cameron JL, Lillimoe KD et al. (1995) Pancreatoduodenectomy for cancer of the head of the pancreas in 201 patients. Ann Surg 221:721–733.

13. Conlon KC, Klimstra DS, Brennan MF (1996) Long-term survival after curative resection for pancreatic ductal adenocarcinoma. Clinicopathologic analysis of 5 year survivors. Ann Surg 223:273–279.

14. Tepper J, Nardi G, Suit H (1976) Carcinoma of the pancreas: review of MGH experience from 1963 to 1973: analysis of surgical failure and implications for radiation therapy. Cancer 37:1519–1524.

15. Pilepich MV, Miller HH (1980) Preoperative irradiation in carcinoma of the pancreas. Cancer 46:1945–1949.

16. Kopelson G (1983) Curative surgery for adenocarcinoma of the pancreas/ampulla of Vater: the role of adjuvant pre- or post-operative radiation therapy. Int J Radiat Oncol Biol Phys 9:911–915.

17. Ishikawa O, Ohigashi H, Imaoka S et al. (1994) Is the long-term survival rate improved by pre-operative irradiation prior to Whipple's procedure for adenocarcinoma of the pancreatic head? Arch Surg 129:1075–1080.

18. Coia L, Hoffman J, Schier R et al. (1994) Preoperative chemoradiation for adenocarcinoma of the pancreas and duodenum. Int J Radiat Oncol Biol Phys 30:161–167.

19. Hoffman JP, Weese JL, Solin LJ et al. (1995) A pilot study of preoperative chemoradiation for patients with localised adenocarcinoma of the pancreas. Am J Surg 169:71–78.

20. Willett CG, Lewandrowski K, Warshaw AL, Efird J, Compton CC (1993) Resection margins in carcinoma of the head of the pancreas. Implications for radiation therapy. Ann Surg 217:144–148.

21. Evans DB, Rich TA, Byrd DR et al. (1992) Preoperative chemoradiation and pancreatico-duodenectomy for adenocarcinoma of the pancreas. Arch Surg 127:1335–1339.

22. Staley CA, Lee JE, Clearly KR et al. (1996) Preoperative chemoradiation pancreatico-duodenectomy and intraoperative radiation therapy for adenocarcinoma of the pancreatic head. Am J Surg 171:118–124.

23. Tyler DS, Evans DB (1994) Reoperative pancreaticoduodenectomy. Ann Surg 219:211–221.

24. Weese JL, Nussbaum ML, Paul AR et al. (1991) Increased resectability of locally advanced pancreatic and periampullary carcinoma with neoadjuvant chemoradiotherapy. Int J Pancreatol 7:177–185.

25. Sindelar WF (1989) Clinical experience with regional pancreatectomy for adenocarcinoma of the pancreas. Arch Surg 124:127–132.

26. Shibamoto Y, Manabe T, Baba M (1990) High dose external beam and intraoperative radio-therapy in the treatment of resectable and unresectable pancreatic cancer. Int J Radiat Oncol Biol Phys 19:605–611.

27. Hiraoka T (1990) Extended radical resection of cancer of the pancreas with intraoperative radiotherapy. Baillière's Clin Gastroenterol 4:985–993.

28. Bosset JF, Pavy JJ, Gillet M, Mantion G, Pelissier E, Schraub S (1992) Conventional external irradiation alone as adjuvant treatment in resectable pancreatic cancer: results of a prospective study. Radiother Oncol 24:191–194.

29. Brachet A, Gilly FN, Braillon G (1993) IORT and surgery for pancreatic adenocarcinoma: a series of 56 patients treated according to the Lyon intraoperative system. Digestion 54:266–267 (abstract).

30. Johnstone PA, Sindelar WF (1993) Patterns of disease recurrence following definitive therapy of adenocarcinoma of the pancreas using surgery and adjuvant radiotherapy correlations of a clinical trial. Int J Radiat Oncol Biol Phys 27:831–834.

31. Zerbi A, Fossati V, Parolini D et al. (1994) Intraoperative radiation therapy adjuvant to resection in the treatment of pancreatic cancer. Cancer 73:2930–2935.

32. Ozaki H, Kinoshita T, Kosuge T, Egawa S, Kishi K (1990) Effectiveness of multimodality treatment for resectable pancreatic cancer. Int J Pancreatol 7:195–200.

33. Abe M, Takahashi M (1981) Intraoperative radiotherapy: the Japanese experience. Int J Radiat Oncol Biol Phys 7:863–868.

34. GITSG (1987) Further evidence of effective adjuvant combined radiation and chemotherapy following curative resection of pancreatic cancer. Cancer 59:2006–2010.

35. Whittington R, Bryer MP, Haller DG, Solin LJ, Rosato EF (1991) Adjuvant therapy of resected adenocarcinoma of the pancreas. Int J Radiat Oncol Biol Phys 21:1137–1143.

36. Foo ML, Gunderson LL, Nagorney DM et al. (1993) Patterns of failure in grossly resected pancreatic ductal adenocarcinoma treated with adjuvant irradiation ± 5 fluorouracil. Int J Radiat Oncol Biol Phys 26:483–489.

37. Evans DB, Abbruzzese JL, Cleary KR (1995) Preoperative chemoradiation for adenocarcinoma of the pancreas: excessive toxicity of prophylactic hepatic irradiation. Int J Radiat Oncol Biol Phys 33:913–918.

38. Splinter TA, Obertop H, Kok TC, Jeekel J (1989) Adjuvant chemotherapy after resection of adenocarcinoma of the periampullary region and the head of the pancreas. A non-randomised pilot study. J Cancer Res Clin Oncol 115:200–202.

39. Bakkevold KE, Arnesjo B, Dahl O, Kambestad B (1993) Adjuvant combination chemotherapy (AMF) following radical resection of carcinoma of the pancreas and papilla of Vater: results of a controlled, prospective, randomised multicentre study. Eur J Cancer 5:698–703.

40. Baumel H, Huguier M, Manderscheid JC, Fabre JM, Houry S, Fagot H (1994) Results of resection for cancer of the exocrine pancreas: a study from the French Association of Surgery. Br J Surg 81:102–107.

41. Ishikawa O, Ohigashi H, Sasaki Y et al. (1994) Liver perfusion chemotherapy via both the hepatic artery and portal vein to prevent hepatic metastasis after extended pancreatectomy for adenocarcinoma of the pancreas. Am J Surg 168:361–364.

42. Ohigashi H, Ishikawa O, Imaoka S et al. (1996) A new method of intraarterial regional chemotherapy with more selective drug delivery for locally advanced pancreatic cancer. Hepatogastroenterology 43:338–345.

43. Link KH, Gansuage F, Rilinger N, Beger HG (1997) Celiac artery adjuvant chemotherapy: results of a prospective trial. Int J Pancreatology 21:65–69.

44. Kalser MH, Ellenberg SS (1985) Pancreatic cancer: adjuvant combined radiation and chemotherapy following curative resection. Arch Surg 120:899–903.

45. Yeo CJ, Abrams RA, Grochow LB et al. (1997) Pancreaticoduodenectomy for pancreatic adenocarcinoma: postoperative adjuvant chemoradiation improves survival. A prospective single-institution experience. Ann Surg 225:621–636.

46. UKPACA (1993) Adjuvant radiotherapy following resection of pancreatic cancer. Gut:34:1296 (abstract).

47. Neoptolemos JP, Baker P, Beger H et al. (1997) Progress report: A randomised multicentre European study comparing adjuvant radiotherapy, six months chemotherapy and combination therapy versus no adjuvant treatment in resectable pancreatic cancer. Int J Pancreatol (in press).

48. Tempero MA, Sivinski C, Steplewski Z, Harvey E, Klassen L, Kay HD (1990) Phase II trial of interferon gamma and monoclonal antibody 17-1A in pancreatic cancer. Biologic and clinical effects. J Clin Oncol 8:2019–2026.

49. Büchler M, Friess H, Schultheiss HK (1991) A randomised controlled trial of adjuvant immunotherapy (murine monoclonal antibody 494/32) in resectable pancreatic cancer. Cancer 68:1507–1517.

50. Weiner LM, Harvey E, Padavic-Shaller K, Willson JK, Walsh C, Lacreta F (1993) Phase II multicenter evaluation of prolonged murine monoclonal antibody 17-1A therapy in pancreatic carcinoma. J Immunother 13:110–116.

51. Bernhard H, Jagerarand E, Bernhard G et al. (1995) Treatment of advanced pancreatic cancer with 5-fluorouracil, folinic acid and interferon alpha 2A: results of a phase II trial. Br J Cancer 71:102–105.

52. Wagener DJ, Verdonk HE, Dirix LY, Catimel G, Siegenthaler P, Buitenhuis M (1995) Phase II trial of CPT-11 in patients with advanced pancreatic cancer, an EORTC early clinical trials group study. Ann Oncol 6:129–132.

53. Rinaldi HA, Dorr FA, Woodworth JG, Kuhn JR, Eckhardt JR (1995) Initial phase I evaluation of the novel thymidilate synthetase inhibitor, LY231514, using the modified continual reassessment method for dose escalation. J Clin Oncol 13:2842–2850.

54. Folkman J (1995) Angiogenesis in cancer, vascular, rheumatoid and other disease. Nat Med 1:27–31.

55. Voest EE, Kenyon BM, Truitt G et al. (1995) Inhibition of angiogenesis in vivo by interleukin 12. J Nat Cancer Inst 87:581–586.

56. Moore MJ, Andersen J, Burris H, Tarassoff P, Green M, Casper E (1997) A randomised trial of gemcitabine versus 5-FU as first line therapy in advanced pancreatic cancer. J Clin Oncol (in press).

57. Evans JD, Bramhall SR, Stark A et al. (1996) A phase II trial of marimastat (BB-2516) in advanced pancreatic cancer. Int J Pancreatology 19:218 (abstract).

58. Dimaio JM, Clary BM, Via DF, Coveney E, Pappas TN, Lyerly HK (1994) Directed enzyme prodrug gene therapy for pancreatic cancer *in vivo*. Surgery 116:205–213.
59. Yang L, Hwang R, Pandit L, Gordon EM, Anderson F, Parekh D (1996) Gene therapy of metastatic pancreas cancer with intraperitoneal injections of concentrated retroviral herpes thymidine kinase vector supernatant and gancyclovir. Ann Surg 224:405–417.
60. Green NK, Youngs DJ, Neoptolemos JP (1997) Sensitization of colorectal and pancreatic cancer cell lines to the prodrug 5-(aziridin-1-yl)-2, 4-dinitrobenzamide (CB1954) by retroviral transduction and expression of the E. coli nitroreductase gene. Cancer Gene Therapy (in press).

40 Quality of Life Assessment in Pancreatic Cancer

D. Fitzsimmons and C.D. Johnson

Pancreatic cancer is well known to have a short duration of survival after diagnosis, and despite advances in treatment and therapies, little progress has been made regarding the outcome of prolonging quantity of life. Indeed, the majority of patients (80%) will receive palliative medical or surgical interventions aimed at control of symptoms only. Within this context of limited survival, quality of life assumes great importance. Clinicians should be concerned not only with advancing knowledge regarding the biophysical disease process but also with the consequences of illness on the well-being of their patients and how the patients cope with their illness, treatment and care. Such knowledge can only help to advance our understanding of pancreatic cancer.

Quality of Life

The term "quality of life" is a key catchphrase in cancer medicine today (1,31,52). However, a precise definition remains vague and no gold standard exists. Indeed some aspects of what influences a person's evaluation of the quality of life (for example, level of education, housing, income) are outside the remit of what can be influenced by the clinician (24). Such aspects of health-related quality of life (or subjective health status) include the impact of symptoms, physical functioning, occupational (role) functioning, cognitive, and psychological and social well-being (11,18). Clinicians need to take a well informed decision with colleagues, patient and family as to whether the benefit of treatment in terms of increased survival and relief of symptoms outweighs the potential risk of toxicity and side effects which may severely compromise the patient's well-being.

There are a number of specially designed quality of life instruments available to the clinician. These may be loosely grouped into three categories: generic, disease-specific and dimension-specific (11). Each one comprises various constructs of quality of life. A comprehensive evaluation of the most commonly used measures is given by Bowling (10) and Newman and McDowell (42).

Some of the issues covered in these instruments are applicable to all cancer patients. However, some issues are specific to pancreatic cancer, and their assessment, which is necessary for a full picture of each patient's quality of life, requires construction of a pancreatic cancer-specific instrument. Before an appropriate pancreatic cancer-specific questionnaire can be developed, the clinical and psychosocial features of the disease must be considered.

Symptoms of Pancreatic Cancer

The number and magnitude of symptoms depends on the stage, site and treatment of the disease. Presenting symptoms may be non-specific such as pain, weight loss and dyspepsia, whilst in the advanced patient there may be a multiplicity of distressing symptoms (30).

One of the main challenges is to relieve the symptoms caused by malignant *bile duct obstruction*. This not only brings about the clinical symptoms of jaundice but also the distress of pruritus and skin changes. Jaundice may affect the patient's psychological and social well-being. Changes in perceived body image may be of great concern for the patient as the jaundice emphasises their illness. Social activities may be curtailed as the patient is aware of the change in physical appearance. Recurrent jaundice after palliative treatment is an ominous sign for many patients, with significant psychological impact.

Nausea and vomiting has been reported in 30–40% of pancreatic cancer patients although true mechanical obstruction occurs in only 5% of cases (51,58). Because of the effect of the disease, patients may suffer *indigestion* and *early satiety*. Dietary changes are usually inevitable as the patient is no longer able to consume the same volume or types of food. For example, some patients are unable to tolerate a high fat/protein diet and diabetes mellitus may occur (39). This can have repercussions on the patient and family as they try to find an adequate diet which is both palatable and tolerated by the patient and ensures an adequate level of nutrition. *Other symptoms* include gastric stasis, steatorrhoea, altered bowel habit, flatulence and indigestion (30).

Weight loss and *cachexia* occur in over 90% of patients with pancreatic cancer (15). As in other advanced cancer patient populations, this can have a significant effect on patient well-being. With such pronounced energy depletion, the pancreatic cancer patient may have muscle wasting resulting in weakness and fatigue (44). This can result in changes in body image and also is used by many patients as a marker to assess the stage of their illness. Weight loss is seen as a crucial indication that there is disease progression.

Pain is a well-reported problem in pancreatic cancer (13,29,30). Frequently the patient presents with dull epigastric pain, and as the disease progresses, pain can radiate to the back (13,32) and can become severe. Pain may also result from metastases in the cervical or thoracic spine. The patient may find mobility and sleeping are affected as it may be difficult to lie supine (13) and pain may have a profound impact on psychological well-being, with anxiety and depression being associated with pain (29). Such pain is difficult for the clinician to manage.

The Psychosocial Impact of Advanced Cancer

Few studies have examined the impact of pancreatic cancer on the well-being of the patient. One study has investigated the observation of increased depression in these patients (29). Explorations of this link have postulated an association between pain and anxiety and depression, or that the patient has to face the demands that a diagnosis of advanced cancer brings (4,46).

Pancreatic cancer is less common than colon, breast, lung and gynaecological cancers, therefore patients may have not heard of the disease before.

Alternatively, they may associate it with other cancers such as colorectal cancer, where the clinical picture is different and treatment options and prognosis are more favourable. Before we review quality of life assessment it will be helpful to consider what is known about quality of life in other advanced cancers.

The diagnosis of cancer can have an overwhelming impact on the patient and his or her family (18). With advanced cancer, not only do they have to face the dilemmas of being labelled as a cancer patient, but also it is usually clear that treatment is limited and survival will be short. Despite changes in public education and in the media, cancer is still associated with thoughts of a painful, long and undignified death (18). There may well be repercussions of stigma associated with a label of advanced cancer resulting in isolation of patient and family. They have to enter the health care arena which for many is a new and frightening experience as they cope with the demands of treatment and hospitalisation and with the realisation that their advanced cancer may be incurable. There is a potential conflict in the need for truth-telling and optimism. Clinicians are faced with the task of breaking bad news yet may often have very little preparation for this. A common response of the clinician is distancing from the patient yet this has the potential to further isolate the patient and to ensure that psychological morbidity goes unrecognised (19).

Coping with Advanced Cancer

Several studies have investigated how patients and their families cope with the "cancer experience" and the consequent uncertainty about the future (16,21,37). One commonly identified coping mechanism is denial or avoidance. Despite attempts to provide the patient with accurate and truthful information he or she either disregards the news that they have cancer or selectively assimilates only the most optimistic news, giving them an unrealistic expectation of their illness. Although frustrating for those caring for such patients, it may be a necessary defence mechanism for the patient.

In the face of adversity some patients cope by finding an acceptable explanation for their illness. This may involve rationalising their illness through past behaviour or life events, such as smoking or blaming the illness on the actions of others (19). Patients commonly ask the question 'Why me?', and in the case of pancreatic cancer, the disease often cannot be attributed to any definite cause. Some patients may be frustrated by this lack of knowledge regarding their illness.

Control

One factor which influences the way that patients cope successfully or otherwise with their illness is their perceived control over their illness and treatment. Patients adapt more easily if they feel that they can contribute to the outcome of their illness. This may be manifest in strategies such as the need for information regarding their illness and treatment or by direct action to fight against the cancer. Such patients may want surgery or other treatment at any cost and are willing volunteers for clinical trials. The concept of maintaining hope is crucial for many when faced with such adversity. Helplessness is associated with a strong risk of later depressive illness (37).

Psychosocial support it a crucial element of coping with cancer. This includes not only support from family and friends and the ability to talk honestly about the illness and future plans, but also support and feedback from the health care team.

Quality of Life Assessment in Pancreatic Cancer

Little research has been published examining quality of life in pancreatic cancer. An extensive literature search of the Embase, Medline and CINAHL information databases revealed only 78 articles, pertaining to quality of life in pancreatic neoplasm. A number of these papers are reviews only mentioning "quality of life" with no formal assessment. Of the remainder, the majority has been published in the past 5 years and are cross-sectional or retrospective studies (Figure 1). Many are subject to methodological flaws in the design and assessment of quality of life and most are primarily concerned with assessing the outcome of a particular treatment or intervention. Quality of life assessment is used to this end, but is not reported as an end to itself. We will review the published work in detail before describing our own work on the development of a specific assessment tool.

Published Work

A few studies purporting to measure quality of life as an outcome of intervention did not use any formal assessment tool but applied their own criteria to assess quality of life with the conclusion drawn that quality of life was satisfactory or good (12,25,55). Such observations are open to methodological criticism in light of small sample sizes and selection bias of patients. An evaluation of pancreatic resection in 158 patients with either stage III or IV disease used hospital-free survival as an indication of quality of life (60). This crude indicator takes no account

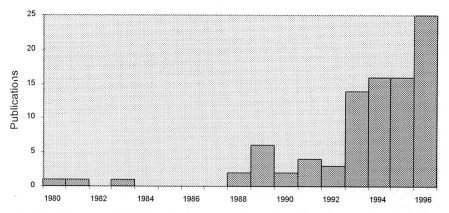

Figure 1. Numbers of publications by year from 1980 to 1996 quoting quality of life in pancreatic cancer.

of the multidimensional construct of quality of life. Although the authors of the study consider that survival and hospital-free survival are the best general means to measure quality of life, there is no evidence from a professional or patient viewpoint to support such as assumption.

Other studies have taken a similar approach to measuring aspects of health status from retrospectively defined criteria. In a phase II clinical trial of gemcitabine in advanced pancreatic cancer, an attempt has been made to quantify symptomatic improvement in the calculation of a "clinical benefit response" using measures including pain intensity, analgesic consumption, weight loss and performance status (41). Although the authors state that this is a valid and reliable method (5), caution should be given to the interpretation of such "response" in regards to patient improvement, when the defined criteria are "objective expert" viewpoint.

Similarly, other studies have used unidimensional indicators as measures to ascertain quality of life. A widely used measure in this context is the Karnofsky Index (27) which only allows a crude observer indicator of a patient's physical performance. Such approaches have been used in a comparison of low/high dose regimens of octreotide (17), comparison of radical resection versus palliative bypass (6) and a retrospective study of outcome of patients with pancreatic and periampullary carcinomas, which assessed complaints of symptoms with the Swiss Group for Clinical Cancer Research (SAKK) score and disease duration. These studies indicated that symptoms impairing quality of life were loss of physical performance, pain, jaundice and vomiting. These studies attempt to consider a range of important symptoms and a basic measure of function but do not take a standardised and comprehensive approach to measuring quality of life. A limitation of these approaches is that they fail to consider the impact of psychological and social well-being on quality of life.

Other approaches to quality of life assessment include the cost of treatment in terms of impact on quality of life and survival. Glimelius et al. (23) measured the cost of pancreatic cancer on quality of life adjusted years (QUALYs) in a study of primary chemotherapy versus best supportive care in 61 inoperable

Table 1. Quality of life assessment tools used in pancreatic cancer studies

Measures of quality of life	Reference
Rotterdam Symptom Checklist	Palmer et al. 1994 (45)
EORTC QLQ-C30	Bloche et al. 1995 (9)
	Luman et al. 1996 (36)
	Glimelius et al. 1996 (23a)
Hospital Anxiety and Depression	Taylor et al. 1993 (56)
Score (HADS)	Palmer et al. 1994 (45)
	Ballinger et al. 1994 (7)
Functional Assessment of Cancer	Sherman et al. 1996 (50)
Therapy (FACT) questionnaire	
Functional Living Index – Cancer	Kelsen et al. 1995 (29)
Beck Depression Inventory (BDI)	
Hopelessness Scale	
Memorial Pain Assessment Card	
Sickness Impact Profile	McLeod et al. 1995 (40)
GI Quality of Life Index	
Visick Scale	
Utility Measures	McLeod et al. 1995 (40)
	Glimelius et al. 1995 (23)

gastrointestinal tumours, 22 of which were pancreatic. This small study indicated a 50% increase in the QALY cost of treatment compared with other disease sites, but acknowledged that such results need to be interpreted cautiously with the limited knowledge of quality of life assessment in pancreatic cancer. McLeod et al. (40) showed that mean utility measures as assessed by the time trade-off technique were between 0.98 and 1, suggesting a near normal well-being. However, this apparent stability is suspect as the pancreatic cancer patients are biased in terms of best outcome, had no recurrence at time of follow-up and had good functional scores. However, with the increasing proliferation of interest in quality of life research, the use of utility measures is recognised as increasingly important in the allocation of the most appropriate cost effective resources.

Other studies have used a variety of subjective health measures in their studies (Table 1). In a randomised placebo-controlled trial of tamoxifen in 44 patients with irresectable tumours, the Karnofsky Index and Hospital Anxiety and Depression Scale failed to indicate any difference in quality of life (56). In an investigation of the effect of pain and depression on quality of life in 130 newly diagnosed cancer patients, only those with moderate or increased pain showed significantly poorer quality of life scores and impaired functional ability, with chemotherapy patients using significantly more analgesics and having higher depression scores (29). Problems were acknowledged regarding the poor compliance at the beginning of the study as patients were unable to complete the large array of instruments and that in the advanced stages of disease problems affecting quality of life may be more prevalent. Similarly, in a study examining the quality of life in 25 patients after Whipple resection compared with age/sex matched patients after cholecystectomy, a variety of quality of life assessment tools was used, including a clinical assessment of nutritional status. The results indicated that quality of life was excellent in the Whipple's group and not significantly different from the control group. In regards to the nutritional status, there was no significant difference in gastrointestinal symptoms although five of the Whipple's patients complained of greasy bowel movements, six required a diabetic diet and one had difficulty maintaining weight. A limitation in interpreting such promising results is that the Whipple's group included patients with both malignant and benign neoplasm, therefore the data can only be used to address the benefits of operation and not the disease. Also, the use of so many different instruments can be cumbersome. However, such approaches are in the right direction towards patient-centred, standardised quality of life assessment.

A limited number of recent studies have compared the outcome of medical and surgical interventions for pancreatic cancer in terms of quality of life in specially designed cancer quality of life measures. In the follow-up of 19 patients who had undergone endoscopic insertion of a stent, Ballinger et al. (8) assessed quality of life prior to ERCP and then at 1, 4, 8 and 12 weeks. After stenting there was complete relief of jaundice and pruritus, and anorexia was significantly better at 1 week and there was complete relief at 8 weeks. Fifteen patients felt that their mood was good or very good before stent insertion and this was unchanged at 12 weeks. In a recent study, Luman et al. (36) used the EORTC QLQ-C30 in 31 patients with malignant biliary obstruction with two additional questions on jaundice and pruritus. Patients reported significant improvement in emotional, cognitive and global health scores. In addition to the expected improvement in pruritus and jaundice, anorexia, diarrhoea and sleep patterns were also reported to be improved. Recently the EORTC QLQ-C30 has been used in a randomised controlled trial comparing 90 patients randomised to receive a chemotherapy regime of 5FU, leucovorin with/without etoposide plus best supportive care against best supportive care only (23a). The results indicated that patients in the chemotherapy group had significantly better emotional functioning, with increases in role functioning, pain and appetite. Overall quality of life-adjusted survival was 4 months in the chemotherapy group versus 1 month in the best supportive care group. Although this study highlighted some methodological problems of assessment tools at present, including the apparent stability of quality of life scores and that the sickest patients whose quality of life would be impaired were lost to follow up, the move towards using a standardised, valid and reliable assessment tool ensures that we can now begin to address the outcome of treatment and new therapies in pancreatic cancer in terms of quality of life.

In summary then, although the question of quality of life in pancreatic cancer is beginning to be addressed in research studies, there is still little standardised and comprehensive approach to its assessment. Little consideration has been given to the patient's viewpoint of what affects their quality of life, while no studies exist that allow patients to rate the relevance of each issue with regard to their own experience of pancreatic cancer. Some studies, although using well-described quality of life assessment tools, have to supplement the chosen tool with additional items which may have influenced the validity and reliability of the results obtained (26). What appears obvious is the lack of significant results between disparate groups which suggests that the various approaches used have not been sensitive or specific enough to assess quality of life in pancreatic cancer. The studies that did obtain significant differences tended to use a number of instruments in their studies. Psychometrically, triangulation of measurement approaches increases content and construct validity as a greater proportion of the conceptual domains of quality of life will be tapped (11,26). However, this should be carefully balanced with the realities of clinical practice, where there is a need for a quick, easy to measure assessment tool, whose findings can be easily interpreted. This will improve compliance, as the patient may find it difficult to complete lengthy questionnaires. This is particularly pertinent to the pancreatic cancer patient as these patients may be simply too unwell to complete such lengthy questionnaires. Follow-up of such patients at particularly vulnerable times when their quality of life is compromised could be difficult. Consensus of specialist opinion has suggested that there is a need for a pancreatic cancer-specific quality of life questionnaire (3,34,57).

Development of a Pancreatic Cancer Quality of Life Questionnaire

In developing a valid and reliable questionnaire for use in the evaluation of clinical trials, attention should focus on the developmental process itself and the methodology employed. In 1980, the EORTC established the Quality of Life Study Group to address such issues. In 1986 the study group began to develop a generic cancer-specific quality of life assessment tool. A core cancer module, the QLQ-C30 has been developed and refined. It has demonstrated validity and reliability across a range of cancer patient populations and cultures (2,43,48).

Attention has now focused on the development of add-on specific modules to supplement the QLQ-C30. A lung cancer module has been developed and breast, colorectal, head and neck, oesophageal modules are now completing the final stages of development. In March 1996 we established the European Quality of Life in Pancreatic Cancer (EQoLiPA) study group, involving 12 clinicians across 10 countries. This group is committed to the multilingual development of a pancreatic cancer-specific module using published guidelines for module development (2) which consist of four phases. From our phase 1 and 2 work, which has been completed, we can highlight some important issues for patients with pancreatic cancer.

Phase 1: Generation of Quality of Life Issues

There are three key steps in generating a list of relevant disease-specific issues: extensive literature review, interviews with specialists and interviews with patients. The literature review was largely unproductive (59). In order to ensure the most important and relevant issues were generated from the patient's perspective, a qualitative study was undertaken to gain an insight into pancreatic cancer patient's perception of their illness, treatment and care.

A convenience sample of 21 patients was interviewed to identify important concepts. Interviews with a further five patients were conducted to validate the concepts raised. This sample encompassed a broad spectrum of the disease and treatment.

Five multidisciplinary health professionals were interviewed using a semi-structured approach to ask which issues they perceived to be important and also to check for significant omissions or irrelevant issues. These results were then analysed in parallel to the patient's responses.

A social sciences methodology known as Grounded Theory was used to guide the data collection and analysis (20,22,53). This produced a conceptual framework of how quality of life is perceived by professionals and patients with pancreatic cancer. This was validated by interview of further groups of patients and professionals.

The interviews with health professionals and patients generated a range of similar issues. Both groups included specific symptoms and side effects of pancreatic cancer and also additional health-related quality of life issues. After comparison with issues already covered by the QLQ-C30, 42 issues were identified as specific and relevant for potential inclusion in a pancreatic cancer module.

Differences Between Patients and Professionals

The main differences in perception between the groups arose when the responses to why each particular issue were compared. Health professionals took a mechanistic approach to quality of life perception, with the presence of each symptom encountered having a direct impact on a patient's quality of life. This approach assumes that with increasing severity of symptom, there will be a reciprocal impact on quality of life.

However, unlike the professionals, patients did not attribute the changes in quality of life directly to the impact of symptoms. Instead, these issues were placed in context, with the process of coping acting as a mediating process. Two key factors were involved: perceived threat and maintenance of control. Figure 2 provides an explanatory framework to illustrate the patient's evaluation of a

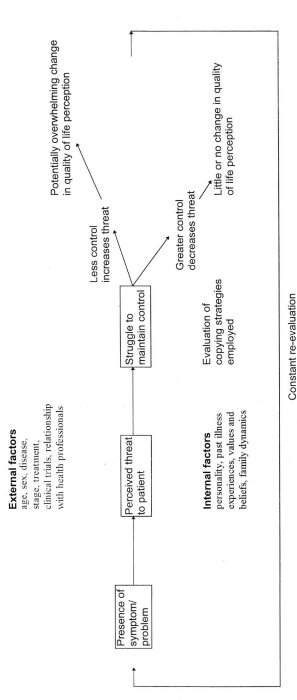

Figure 2. Interaction of perceived threat of symptom, maintaining control and influence on quality of life perception.

Table 2. Main coping strategies

Strategy	Example
Defending/avoidance	Symptom or problem ignored for as long as possible, e.g. selective assimilation of information
Blaming	Symptom is blamed on external event, e.g. initial onset of pain is blamed on a recent fall, other disease, or blamed on past behaviour
Rationalising	Symptom is rationalised as a "normal part of the illness", e.g. pain seen in the postoperative patient as expected consequence of surgery, or as ageing
Turning to others	Patient turns to family and/or health professionals to explain symptoms and provide support in tackling symptom
Taking direct action	Patient takes affirmative action against symptom, e.g. takes analgesia or volunteers for participation in clinical trials

symptom in relation to overall quality of life perception. First, the patient saw the impact of symptoms in terms of a perceived threat. This was placed within the context of their illness and was dependent on both internal and external variables. To maintain control was seen by patients as paramount to minimise the impact of these threats on quality of life. This was undertaken using coping strategies (Table 2). If the threat was mild to the patient coping strategies would allow successful control and consequently there would be little or no impact on quality of life. However, if the threat was severe and coping strategies were unable to control the threats, the effect on quality of life could be overwhelming. Throughout the disease process such evaluation of each threat in relation to quality of life was re-evaluated.

In addition to enabling the developing of a pancreaitic cancer-specific module, our study has provided an important insight into how the pancreatic cancer patient copes with their illness and care. It supports the assumptions that quality of life perception is multidimensional and subjective and can only be described accurately by patients themselves. It also demonstrates some limitations of quality of life questionnaires. This has been described by Portenoy (47) in a theoretical model (Figure 3). Most questionnaires do not allow symptom severity to be taken into account, i.e. they assume that the impact of a symptom on quality of life is constant, regardless of severity. Although specialists regarded symptom severity as having a direct impact on quality of life, the patient's perspective was mediated through coping strategies. As Cella (14) suggests "A limitation of quality of life measures is that they neglect the underlying cognitive processes that mediate patient's perception of quality of life". In short, we may be overoptimistic in such measurements. What we really are measuring is aspects of subjective health status. Only when such information is placed in context, can we really be confident in measuring health-related quality of life.

Phase 2: Operation of a Pancreatic Cancer Quality of Life Module

A pancreatic cancer module has now been developed to supplement the EORTC QLQ-C30. It has undergone reviews by patients and a panel of international specialists to check for appropriate face and content validity. Following review and refinement from the EORTC QoL modular development committee, a

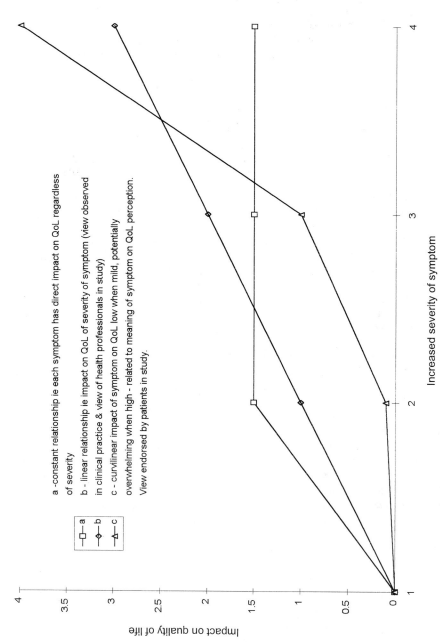

a -constant relationship ie each symptom has direct impact on QoL regardless of severity

b - linear relationship ie impact on QoL of severity of symptom (view observed in clinical practice & view of health professionals in study)

c - curvilinear impact of symptom on QoL low when mild, potentially overwhelming when high - related to meaning of symptom on QoL perception. View endorsed by patients in study.

Figure 3. Symptom intensity and quality of life: three hypothesised relationships (47).

26-item module has been constructed and approved. The issues covered are broadly shown in Table 3. It has been translated into eight European languages and is currently undergoing parallel multilingual pretesting by EQoLiPA. This will ensure internal reliability, cross-cultural appropriateness and ensure no significant omissions of items. At present it is intended for assessment in all treatments of pancreatic adenocarcinoma, ductal cell carcinomas and periampullary tumours.

Interventions to Improve Quality of Life

Over the past two decades there has been considerable advance in medical and surgical interventions for pancreatic cancer; however, these have failed to have a significant impact on the long-term survival of patients. There is still much debate on what constitutes "appropriate treatment" for pancreatic cancer. Using quality of life as an outcome measure may help us address the risks and benefits of such interventions.

Surgical resection is the only form of intervention that can provide patients with a chance of long-term survival. Although we have seen a decrease in mortality and morbidity associated with the procedure, patients are still faced with threats to their quality of life. The postoperative period and recovery may be long and characterised by postoperative complications. The patient may be faced with the onset of diabetes or exocrine insufficiency resulting in medication and dietary modification for the remainder of life. Surgery also has been reported to have a negative effect on patient's perceived body image (18). The impact on the family may be significant as they cope with the demands of care giving. However, a positive effect on quality of life may be observed, with the hope that there may be change in the fight against disease. Such attitude has influenced quality of life perception in other radical surgical procedures for cancer (38,54). Surgical palliation may benefit the patient by giving one-off relief of symptoms for the remainder of life. However, against this must be placed the associated risks such as postoperative complications and longer hospitalisation. Similarly, interventions such as coeliac plexus blocks may improve symptoms and quality of life (28). As demonstrated earlier little research has been conducted to support or disprove such assumptions. What is urgently required is the assessment of such interventions in terms of their effect on quality of life.

For a significant number of patients, who present at an advanced stage, the benefits of endoscopic palliation on quality of life appear significant (7,36,50). These factors in combination with the overall general health and age of the patient and projected survival should all be considered when deciding on the management of care in the inoperable patient.

The potential benefit of adjuvant therapies continues to be a source of debate, with the majority still undergoing clinical trials. The assessment of quality of life should be paramount. Some therapies, for example chemotherapy and radiotherapy, are associated with known side effects and toxicity. Yet these risks must be assessed in relation to any benefits to quality of life. Symptoms and physical functioning may be improved. As in other cancer studies, there may be a psychological benefit to receiving adjuvant therapy or clinical trial participation as patients perceive that having a degree of control over their disease assumes greater importance than mild or moderate side effects (52). Yet, again we must be cautious of such assumptions with such limited evidence. As Lionetto (35) concluded from a review of 21 adjuvant trials, future studies should focus on screening of new drugs or combinations supported by a strong biological rationale and the development of a valid and acceptable tool for evaluation of quality of life in such patients. Such recommendations should be followed in the evaluation of novel approaches, for example fatty acids and matrix metalloproteinase inhibitors where the intended therapeutic benefit is control of disease rather than cure.

Future Directions

Quality of life assessment in pancreatic cancer is still in its infancy and provides an exciting opportunity for future research and development. This should focus on the standardisation of quality of life assessment and the application of such measurement in research studies particularly in randomised controlled trials. A key issue rests on greater understanding of the clinical application of quality of life assessment and appreciation of the contribution of other research methodologies which can enhance our knowledge of all aspects of disease and illness.

In regards to the individual management of care of the pancreatic cancer patient, quality of life should be a prime concern when deciding on the best course of action for each patient, especially for the patient whose survival is limited. Supportive care interventions have an important role. Not only should these be concerned with strategies to relieve symptoms associated with the disease but also to facilitate the patient and family to adjust to their illness and treatment and to optimise their quality of life.

As clinicians are increasingly aware that the illness is much more than a biological disease process but represents the impact on all aspects of a person's life, management of pancreatic cancer should not be conducted in isolation but should be a process of decision making between patient, family, surgeon, physician, oncologist, radiologist, general practitioner, nurse and other health care professionals to ensure that all research and clinical endeavours are aimed at maximising the quality of life for patient.

References

1. Aaronson NK, Meyerowitz BE, Bard M et al. (1991) Quality of life research in oncology: past achievements and future priorities. Cancer 67:839–843.
2. Aaronson NK, Cull A, Kaasa S, Sprangers MA (1994) The European Organisation for Research and Treatment of Cancer (EORTC) modular approach to quality of life assessment in oncology: an update. In: Spilker B (ed) Quality of life and pharmacoeconomics in clinical trials, 2nd edn. Raven Press, New York.
3. Ahlgren JD (1996) Chemotherapy for pancreatic carcinoma. Cancer 78:654–663.
4. Alter CL (1996) Palliative and supportive care of patients with pancreatic cancer. Semin Oncol 23:229–240.
5. Andersen JS, Burris HA, Casper E et al. (1994) Development of a new system for assessing clinical benefit for patients with advanced pancreatic cancer. Proc Am Soc Clin Oncol 13:461 (abstract).
6. Bakkevold KE, Kambestad B (1995) Palliation of pancreatic cancer. A prospective multicentre study. Eur J Surg Oncol 21:176–182.

7. Ballinger AB, McHugh M, Catnach SM, Alstead EM, Clark ML (1994) Symptom relief and quality of life after stenting for malignant bile duct obstruction. Gut 35:467–470.

8. Ballinger AB, McHugh M, Catnach SM et al. (1994) Symptom relief and quality of life after stenting for malignant bile duct obstruction. Gut 35:476–470.

9. Bloechle C, Izbicki JR, Knoefel WT et al. (1995) Quality-of-life in chronic-pancreatitis — results after duodenum-preserving resection of the head of the pancreas. Pancreas 11:77–85.

10. Bowling A (1991) Measuring health: a review of quality of life measurement scales. Open University Press, Buckingham.

11. Bowling A (1991) Measuring disease. Open University Press, Buckingham.

12. Carter JP, Saxe GP, Newbold V, Peres CE, Campeau RJ, Bernal Green L (1993) Hypothesis: dietary management may improve survival from nutritionally linked cancers based on analysis of representative cases. J Am Coll Nutr 12:209–226.

13. Carter DC (1995) Clinical features and management of carcinoma of the pancreas. Br J Hosp Med 54:459–464.

14. Cella DF (1994) Quality of life: concepts and definitions. J Pain Symptom Management 9:186–192.

15. De Wys WD (1986) Weightloss and nutritional abnormalities in cancer patients: incidence, severity and significance. In: Calman KC, Fearon KCH (eds) Nutritional support for the cancer patient. Baillière Tindall, London.

16. Dunkel-Schatter C, Feinstein LG, Taylor SE, Falke RL (1991) Patterns of coping with cancer. Health Psychol 11:79–87.

17. Ebert M, Friess H, Beger HG, Büchler M (1994) Role of octreotide in the treatment of pancreatic cancer. Digestion 55 (Suppl 1):48–51.

18. Fallowfield L (1990) Quality of life: the missing measurement in health care. Souvenir Press, London.

19. Faulkner A, Maguire P (1994) Talking to cancer patients and their families. Oxford Medical Publications, Oxford.

20. Fitzsimmons D (1998) Differences in perception of quality of life issues between health professionals and patients with pancreatic cancer. Psycho-Oncology (in press).

21. Gammon J (1991) Which way out of the crisis? Professional Nurse May:488–493.

22. Glaser BG and Strauss AL (1986) The discovery of grounded theory: strategies for qualitative research. Aldine, Chicago.

23. Glimelius B, Hoffman K, Graf W et al. (1995) Cost-effectiveness of palliative chemotherapy in advanced gastrointestinal cancer. Ann Oncol 6:267–274.

23a. Glimelius B, Hoffman K, Sjoden PO et al. (1996) Chemotherapy improves survival and quality-of-life in advanced pancreatic and biliary cancer. Ann Oncol 7:593–600.

24. Hopkins A (1992) Measures of quality of life and the uses to which such measures may be put. Royal College of Physicians, London.

25. Ishikawa O, Ohigashi H, Nakaizumi A et al. (1993) Surgical resection of potentially curable pancreatic cancer with improved preservation of endocrine function: further evaluation of intraoperative cytodiagnosis. Hepatogastroenterology 40:443–447.

26. Jaloweic A (1990) Issues in using multiple measures of quality of life. Semin Oncol Nursing 6:271–277.

27. Karnofsky DA, Abelman WH, Craver LF et al. (1948) The use of nitrogen mustards in the palliative treatment of carcinoma. Cancer I:634–656.

28. Kawamata M, Ishitani K, Ishikawa K et al. (1996) Comparison between celiac plexus block and morphine treatment on quality of life in patients with pancreatic cancer pain. Pain 64:597–602.

29. Kelsen DP, Portenoy RK, Thaler HT (1995) Pain and depression in patients with newly diagnosed pancreas cancer. J Clin Oncol 13:748–755.

30. Krech RL, Walsh D (1991) Symptoms of pancreatic cancer. J Pain Symptom Management 6:360–367.

31. Lancet Editorial (1995) Quality of life and clinical trials. Lancet 346:1–2.

32. Lebovits AH and Lefkowitz M (1989) Pain management of pancreatic carcinoma: a review. Pain 36:1–11.

33. Lebovits AH, Lefkowitz M (1988) Pain management of pancreatic carcinoma: a review. Pain: 36,1–11.

34. Lionetto R, Pugliese V, Bruzzi P and Rosso R (1995) No standard treatment is available for advanced pancreatic cancer. Eur J Cancer 31A:882–887.

35. Lionetto R, Pugliese V, Bruzzi P, Rosso R (1995) No standard treatment is available for advanced pancreatic cancer. Eur J Cancer 31A:882–887.

36. Luman W, Cull A, Palmer KR (1996) Quality of life following endoscopic stenting for malignant biliary obstruction. Abstract Presented at the British Society of Gastroenterology, Brighton, March, 1996.
37. Maguire (1992) Improving the recognition and treatment of affective disorders in cancer patients. In: Granville-Grasson K (ed) Recent advances in psychiatry 7. Churchill Livingstone, Edinburgh.
38. Maguire P (1985) Barriers to psychological care of the dying. BMJ 291:1711–1713.
39. McLaughlin S. (1994) Pancreatic cancer and diabetes. Diabetes Educ. 20, 20, 24, 26.
40. McLeod RS. Taylor BR. O'Connor BI et al. (1995) Quality of life, nutritional status, and gastrointestinal hormone profile following the Whipple procedure. Am J Surg 169:179–85.
41. Moore H (1996) Activity of gemcitibine in patients with advanced pancreatic carcinoma. Cancer 78:633–638.
42. Newman, I, McDowell C (1992) A guide to rating scales and questionnaires. Oxford University Press, Oxford.
43. Niezgoda HE, Pater JL (1993) A validation study of the domains of the core EORTC quality of life questionnaire. Qual Life Res 2:129–148.
44. Ottery F (1996) Supportive nutritional management of the patient with pancreatic cancer. Oncology 10:26–32.
45. Palmer KR, Kerr M, Knowles G, Cull A et al. (1994) Chemotherapy prolongs survival in inoperable pancreatic carcinoma. Br J Surg 81:882–885.
46. Passik SD and Breitbart WS (1996) Depression in patients with pancreatic carcinoma. Diagnostic and treatment issues. Cancer 78:615–626.
47. Portenoy RK (1991) Pain and quality of life: clinical issues and implications for research. In: Tchelmedigion NS and Cella DF (eds) Quality of life in oncology: practice and research. New York.
48. Ringdal GI, Ringdal K (1993) Testing the EORTC quality of life questionnaire on cancer patients with heterogeneous diagnoses. Qual Life Res 2:129–140.
49. Schumate CR, Baron TH (1996) Palliative procedures for pancreatic cancer: when and which one? South Med J 89:27–32.
50. Schoeman MN, Huibregtse K (1995) Pancreatic and ampullary carcinoma. [Review.] Gastrointest Endosc Clin North Am 5(1):217–236.
51. Singh SM, Reber HA (1989) Surgical palliation for pancreatic cancer. Surg Clin North Am 69:599–611.
52. Slevin ML (1992) Quality of life: philosophical question or clinical reality? Br Med J 305:466–469.
53. Strauss A, Corbin J (1990) Basics of qualitative research: grounded theory procedures and techniques. Sage, New York.
54. Sugarbaker PH, Barosky I, Rosenberg SA, Gianola FJ (1982) Quality of life assessment of patients in extremity sarcoma clinical trials. Surgery 91:17–23.
55. Tamura K, Kin S, Nagami H et al. (1992) Heterotopic autotransplantation of the distal pancreas segment after total pancreatectomy for cancer of the head of the pancreas. Pancreas 7:664–671.
56. Taylor OM, Benson EA, McMahon MJ. 1993. Clinical trial of tamoxifen in patients with irresectable pancreatic adenocarcinoma. The Yorkshire Gastrointestinal Tumour Group. Br J Surg 80:384–386.
57. Trede M, Carter DC (1987) Surgery of the pancreas. Churchill Livingstone, Edinburgh.
58. Watanapa P, Williamson RCN (1992) Surgical palliation for pancreatic cancer: developments during the past two decades. Br J Surg 79:8–20.
59. Webster S, Johnson CD (1994) Quality of life in pancreatic cancer. Fourth-year medical student study-in-depth project. University of Southampton (unpublished).
60. Yasue M, Sakamoto J, Morimoto T et al. (1995) Evaluation of the effect of pancreatic resection in advanced pancreatic cancer with special reference using hospital-free survival as a measure of quality of life. Jpn J Clin Oncol 25:37–45.

Subject Index

461